# The Multifactorial Etiology of Congenital Heart Disease:

## Insights from Teratology, Genetics, and Exposomics

Ramya Raghavan
https://orcid.org/0000-0002-9953-543X
*Sri Sathya Sai University for Human Excellence, India*

IGI Global
Scientific Publishing
Publishing Tomorrow's Research Today

| | |
|---|---|
| Vice President of Editorial | Melissa Wagner |
| Director of Acquisitions | Mikaela Felty |
| Director of Book Development | Jocelynn Hessler |
| Production Manager | Mike Brehm |
| Cover Design | Jose Rosado |

Published in the United States of America by
IGI Global Scientific Publishing
701 East Chocolate Avenue
Hershey, PA, 17033, USA
Tel: 717-533-8845 | Fax: 717-533-7115
Website: https://www.igi-global.com E-mail: cust@igi-global.com



Library of Congress Cataloging-in-Publication Data

LCCN: 2025944126 (CIP Data Pending)
ISBN13: 979-8-3373-3735-7
Isbn13Softcover: 979-8-3373-3736-4
EISBN13: 979-8-3373-3737-1

British Cataloguing in Publication Data
A Cataloguing in Publication record for this book is available from the British Library.

# Table of Contents

# Detailed Table of Contents



Congenital heart disease (CHD) affects approximately 9 per 1,000 live births globally and is a leading cause of infant mortality. The integration of Developmental Origins of Health and Disease (DOHaD) theory with Social Determinants of Health (SDOH) frameworks provides a comprehensive understanding of how early-life programming and social inequities interact to influence CHD development, progression, and outcomes. Multiple studies identified risk factors for congenital heart disease including demographic characteristics (maternal age, consanguinity, birth order, socioeconomic status), environmental exposures (pollution, occupational hazards, urban residence), and maternal health indicators (diabetes, obesity, stress, nutritional factors), showing regional variations. Current evidence demonstrate that CHD outcomes are significantly shaped by parental environmental exposures, genetic susceptibility, epigenetic modifications, and multilevel social determinants. The DOHaD-SDOH framework provides a roadmap for developing equitable, and sustainable prevention approaches. Ongoing research advocates for longitudinal and case-control studies to assess environmental exposures and their implications of on cardiovascular health.



Gene polymorphisms involved in cardiac development are increasingly recognized as key contributors to congenital heart disease (CHD), often co-occurring with neonatal anomalies and malignancy risk. Disruptions in developmental pathways such as RAS/MAPK, Notch, and Wnt not only affect cardiac morphogenesis but also exert pleiotropic effects across multiple organ systems. Syndromic CHDs, including Noonan, Alagille, and 22q11.2 deletion syndromes, demonstrate well-established links between specific genetic variants, structural anomalies, and elevated cancer susceptibility. Non-syndromic CHD genes, such as NKX2-5, GATA4, and TBX20, typically lead to isolated cardiac defects, though emerging evidence suggests subtle associations with oncogenic processes. Polygenic risk, copy number variations, and gene–environment interactions further complicate the genetic landscape. Understanding these interrelated mechanisms supports the integration of genomic data into early diagnosis, clinical management, and personalized surveillance strategies for both cardiac and oncologic outcomes.



Congenital heart disease (CHD) is the most common congenital anomaly worldwide, affecting 8–12 per 1,000 live births and contributing significantly to infant morbidity and mortality. Concurrently, assisted reproductive technologies (ART), including in vitro fertilization (IVF) and intracytoplasmic sperm injection (ICSI), have become increasingly prevalent, resulting in over 8 million births globally. Evidence indicates a modest but consistent elevation in CHD risk among ART-conceived offspring, particularly non-syndromic ventricular septal defects, atrial septal defects, and conotruncal anomalies such as tetralogy of Fallot. Population-based registries report a 1.3–2.0-fold increased relative risk, with ICSI and multiple gestations conferring higher susceptibility. Mechanistic studies suggest multifactorial pathways involving ART-related interventions, maternal factors (advanced age, metabolic disorders), pregnancy complications (multiple gestations, preterm birth), and epigenetic dysregulation during critical windows of cardiac development.



Endocrine disrupting chemicals (EDCs) such as Dibutyl Phthalate exposure affects the expression of male germ cell genes expression associated with cardiac development pathways. Phthalates exposure, in males affects spermatogenesis, increasing offspring's susceptibility to congenital heart disease (CHD). In silico analysis confirmed that phthalates induce gene changes in cardiomyopathy, aortic aneurysms, and septal hypertrophy pathways, suggesting the intergenerational transmission of congenital heart disease risk. The Gene Ontology of MYBPC3,

Congenital Heart Disease (CHD) is a multifactorial disorder, which is caused and predisposed by a set of interrelating genetic factors along with epigenetic, environmental, and developmental risk factors. This rich heterogeneity is frequently not reflected in more traditional approaches to risk assessment, diagnosis, and prediction of outcomes. The chapter will look at how artificial intelligence and machine learning will transform the way we know more about the CHD etiology and improve clinical care. We provide an extensive survey of the role of AI and ML methods in key areas that are pertinent to CHD, such as genomic and epigenomic data integration, exposomic and teratogenic risk modeling, advanced cardiac imaging interpretation and dynamic risk stratification. The chapter describes the technical underpinnings of these methods, their contemporary use in prenatal and postnatal care, and how they may benefit precision cardiology through integration of disparate data sources into personalized prediction. Concurrently, we discuss the issues that arise in the potential application of AI in pediatric and perinatal settings, including limited data volumes, model levels of generalizability, interpretability, and ethical concerns as critically. We end by summarising a vision of AI-enabled precision congenital cardiology: where transdisciplinary research, information infrastructures with strong data governance, and transparent algorithmic governance are combined to redefine knowledge about CHD, its diagnosis and management along the lifespan.



Congenital heart disease (CHD) affects around 1% of live births globally, with environmental teratogens contributing significantly to its complex causes. This chapter introduces an engineering framework combining signal processing, machine learning, and embedded systems for real-time detection of cardiac teratogens during fetal development. The system fuses maternal physiological signals, environmental data, and fetal metrics using adaptive Kalman filtering and wavelet transforms. A custom CNN with temporal attention enables teratogen classification and uncertainty quantification. Edge computing ensures real-time performance through model compression and power-aware strategies. To address data scarcity, GAN-based synthetic data generation preserves physiological realism. Results show over 92% sensitivity in detecting teratogens across exposure scenarios. This interdisciplinary solution links electrical engineering and prenatal care, enabling proactive CHD prevention via early intervention.



Congenital heart disease (CHD) affects nearly 8 in 1,000 live births and remains a major contributor to infant mortality worldwide. Traditional CHD risk assessments often rely on retrospective data and limited environmental tracking, leaving critical gaps in early detection. This chapter proposes a system engineering framework for intelligent biosensor networks that integrate artificial intelligence with multi-modal sensing for real-time prenatal CHD risk evaluation. The system merges environmental sensors for detecting teratogens, maternal-fetal physiological monitors, and advanced AI models for predictive analytics. Using convolutional neural networks, LSTMs, and ensemble methods, it enables personalized, real-time risk assessment based on exposomic and physiological data streams. Clinical validation highlights the system's promise in identifying high-risk pregnancies early, facilitating proactive care and potentially lowering CHD incidence while improving outcomes for mothers and infants.



Congenital heart diseases (CHD) are a major cause of morbidity and mortality in children and involve abnormal development of heart chambers and valves, along with the origin, course, or structure of the vessels (aorta, pulmonary and coronary artery anomalies, anomalous pulmonary veins, vascular rings, etc.). This chapter presents an algorithm for 3D reconstruction from two uncalibrated fluoroscopic angiography views, addressing the resulting inaccuracies by using an optimization algorithm to minimize the reconstruction error. The study provides the vessels geometry (length, curvature, diameter) along with the generated quantitative coronary angiography (QCA). The 3D reconstruction errors were compensated by an optimization algorithm, and the results were validated by comparison with the vessels' absolute length acquired using dedicated angiographic software. The key contributions of the manuscript are a detailed phenotyping that can help the linking of structure to development of the disease, proving insights into genetic studies and hemodynamic analysis.

# Preface

Congenital Heart Disease (CHD) remains one of the most prevalent and challenging congenital anomalies, affecting approximately one in every 100 children born worldwide. By synthesizing contemporary research, this book elucidates how gene polymorphisms, parental factors, and environmental exposures shape cardiac morphogenesis and CHD susceptibility. The economic burden of complex congenital heart defects alone costs the United States $74 billion annually, with individual patients facing lifetime healthcare costs averaging $2.2 million. Public-private partnerships and non-governmental organizations address the financial burden of CHD in low- and middle-income countries (LMICs). This volume is inspired by and dedicated to the pioneering efforts of organizations committed to bridging this massive healthcare gap. At the forefront is the Sri Sathya Sai Sanjeevani Research Foundation in India. The economic challenges faced by children with congenital heart disease significantly contribute to morbidity and mortality. This book is a direct response to this challenge, highlighting the systemic barriers that underscore the urgent need for research on CHD prevention. The chapters are also designed to bring awareness of reproductive toxicities for adolescents and young adults, as well as future parents.

The study of CHD transcends traditional disciplinary boundaries, requiring integration across molecular biology, teratology, epidemiology, and clinical medicine. This book, The Multifactorial Etiology of Congenital Heart Disease: Insights from Teratology, Genetics, and Exposomics, was conceived as a collaborative platform to capture these intersections and bridge the gap between molecular research and translational outcomes. Understanding the causes of heart problems in babies can help doctors prevent them. Suppose we know that specific genes or environmental factors are linked to heart problems. In that case, we can take steps to reduce the risk for future babies. By analyzing environmental exposures, family histories, genomic or exome sequencing data, we aim to enhance prevention, diagnosis, and management. The book will present case studies and examples of how exposomic data can be integrated into clinical decision-making, offering practical guidance for pediatric cardiology healthcare professionals. Public health professionals will benefit from etiology and environmental factors. The technological solutions, AI-driven diagnostic tools, and remote monitoring systems offer pathways to democratize access to high-quality CHD care. Our comprehensive volume is an essential resource for everyone pursuing careers in environmental health sciences, toxicology, epidemiology, and embryology. The journey from the early days of CHD care to today's sophisticated, multidisciplinary approach represents one of medicine's greatest success stories. The survival rate for CHD patients has improved due to groundbreaking innovations, including the heart-lung machine, neonatal cardiac surgery, and transcatheter interventions. A new era of precision healthcare, where artificial intelligence, genomics, and advanced imaging technologies are revolutionizing how we understand, diagnose, and treat congenital heart disease.

The key selling points of our project lie in its ability to provide a comprehensive view of pollutants, endocrine disruptors, and toxic exposures. Overcrowding, poor sanitation, and a lack of green spaces can indirectly increase the risk of CHD by contributing to exposure to pollutants. Exposure to heavy metals, including lead and other toxins from paints, water, and industrial emissions, is a recognized risk factor for cardiovascular anomalies and CHD. Pesticides, industrial chemicals, and persistent organic pollutants contribute to CHD risk, going beyond traditional studies that focus on single environmental factors.

Gene therapy approaches and artificial intelligence systems that can predict and prevent complications before they occur are no longer distant possibilities but emerging realities. The table of contents reflects the book's comprehensive nature, addressing the complex interplay among teratogenic, genetic, and exposomic factors in both syndromic and non-syndromic CHD. The structure allows for a thorough exploration of each factor while also emphasizing the integrative approach required to understand CHD etiology. The book will be an accessible yet comprehensive resource for researchers, students, and healthcare professionals interested in the molecular aspects of CHD.

## SECTION 1: ENVIRONMENTAL, PARENTAL, AND SOCIAL DETERMINANTS

The exposomics framework provides conceptual and methodological tools for characterizing complex exposure mixtures and their biological consequences, enabling precision environmental health approaches. The book begins by exploring the historical perspective on CHD etiology, tracing the evolution of our understanding from embryology. It will then delve into the specific teratogenic factors associated with CHD, with a particular focus on parental contributions. The chapters will cover environmental factors linked to CHD, including parental health conditions, medications, infectious diseases, environmental pollutants, and nutritional factors. Maternal factors remain a significant global concern in LMICs. Environmental exposures, including maternal phenylketonuria, assisted reproductive technologies, paternal phthalate exposure, and air pollution, contribute substantially to CHD etiology. The social determinants of health add to teratogenic mechanisms, epigenetic alterations, and gene-environment interactions. Gene polymorphisms influence not only cardiac development but also associated neonatal anomalies and tumor risk. The book sections will explore the current state of preventive measures and screening programs for CHD risk factors. The lifestyle modifications, maternal health condition management, and vaccination strategies reduce CHD risk. The chapters will also present current screening methodologies, from risk assessment tools to non-invasive imaging techniques, and discuss their potential applications in CHD prevention.

## Chapter 1: Developmental Origins of Heart and Congenital Heart Diseases (CHD): Environmental Risk Factors and Genomic Correlations

Congenital Heart Disease (CHD) remains one of the most prevalent and challenging congenital anomalies worldwide. The developmental origins of health and disease (DOHaD) framework posits that in utero environmental conditions program cardiovascular structure and function. Heart development begins with cardiac progenitor specification in the gastrulating embryo, followed by migration to bilateral heart fields, where cells concomitantly assemble into tubular structures and differentiate into cardiomyocytes. Adverse intrauterine environments, including maternal metabolic disorders, malnutrition, hypoxia, and toxicant exposures, induce adaptive responses in the developing fetus. Chapter one aims to provide an embryology exploration of the teratogenic, genetic, and exposomic influences on the development of both syndromic and non-syndromic CHD.

## Chapter 2: Association of Gene Polymorphisms With Neonatal Anomalies and Tumor Risks in CHD Patients: Gene Polymorphisms in CHD-Linked Anomalies and Tumors

Epidemiological evidence reveals a substantially elevated cancer risk among children and young adults with CHD compared to the general population. The chapter explores the genetic architecture of CHD between chromosomal abnormalities, copy number variations (CNVs), and single-nucleotide polymorphisms (SNPs). Single-gene defects leading to syndromes associated with CHD have been extensively characterized through advances in genomic technologies following the

Human Genome Project. The role of gene polymorphisms in predisposing CHD patients to neonatal anomalies and tumor development is discussed. The advances in high-throughput sequencing, genome-wide association studies (GWAS), and the integration of genetic data with other omics to elucidate of risk mechanisms. Identification and functional validation of gene variants associated with both congenital heart defects and related tumor risks highlight clinical implications. The identification of specific genotype-phenotype correlations enables improved prognostic counseling. The anticipatory management of associated comorbidities might consider increased cancer risk among patients with syndromic CHD.

### Chapter 3: Risk of Congenital Heart Disease in Assisted Reproductive Pregnancies: Mechanisms, Evidence, and Clinical Implications

Emerging studies propose increased CHD risk with assistive reproductive technologies. The chapter contents explore proposed contributors as the relative risk increase appears statistically significant, the absolute risk increase is modest. The overall incidence showcases CHD risk due to underlying parental infertility factors, epigenetic changes induced by embryo culture conditions. Additionally, the general population risk can vary due to hormonal stimulation protocols that affect the endometrial environment and confounding factors such as maternal age and metabolic factors.

### Chapter 4: The Paternal Link to Congenital Heart Disease: Phthalate Exposure Alters Sperm Gene Expression and Increases Offspring Cardiac Risk.

Preconception environmental conditions have been shown to shape sperm epigenetics and, in turn, influence offspring health and development. Paternal preconception exposure to di(2-ethylhexyl) phthalate (DEHP), a widely used plasticizer, induces genome-wide DNA methylation changes in sperm with potential intergenerational effects. Paternal factors (advanced paternal age, occupational chemical exposures), and ambient environmental pollutants (air pollution, pesticides, heavy metals) have been identified. This chapter highlights the male preconception environment's sensitivity to chemical exposures. It underscores the need to consider paternal factors in risk assessment analyses.

## SECTION 2: GENETIC AND MOLECULAR MECHANISMS OF CONGENITAL HEART DISEASE

The chapters in the second section of the book focus on the genetic factors underlying CHD. Gene polymorphisms in cardiac developmental genes, chromatin modifiers, and metabolic pathways contribute to CHD. Multiple inheritance patterns, including autosomal dominant monogenic disorders (RASopathies), de novo variants, and oligogenic rare variants. Chromosomal abnormalities, copy-number variants (CNVs), and single-gene disorders are associated with syndromic CHD. The book contents will also delve into non-syndromic CHD, discussing monogenic models, genetic heterogeneity, and the emerging understanding of polygenic and oligogenic contributions to CHD risk. Single-cell and multi-omics technologies have revolutionized the understanding of cardiac development by revealing cellular heterogeneity, lineage trajectories, and gene regulatory networks with unprecedented resolution. Integration of transcriptomics, proteomics, metabolomics, and epigenomics provides comprehensive molecular landscapes of heart morphogenesis, identifying novel genes, regulatory interactions, and metabolic programs.

Single-cell omics technologies provide unprecedented insights into the cellular heterogeneity of developing hearts, revealing previously unknown pathways in cardiac morphogenesis. Epigenetic-mediated regulatory mechanisms have emerged as central governors of cardiac gene expression during development. The miRNA target sites within 3'-UTRs of critical cardiac transcription factors exemplify how non-coding genetic variation can disrupt regulatory networks. MicroRNA-mediated regulatory mechanisms are unveiled as critical controllers of heart morphogenesis, offering new therapeutic targets and diagnostic biomarkers.

### Chapter 5: Integrating Exposomics with Genomics and Epigenomics: A Holistic Approach to Unraveling the Etiology of Congenital Heart Disease

This chapter advocates integrating exposomics, environmental exposure assessment, with genomics and epigenomics to provide a systems-level understanding of CHD etiology. Advanced methodologies enable precise characterization of both external exposome (environmental chemicals, radiation, lifestyle factors) and internal exposome (metabolic products, oxidative stress, inflammation, gut microbiome). The epigenetic regulatory mechanisms account for approximately 10% of severe CHD cases overall. The extracardiac abnormalities and neurodevelopmental delays with CHD also highlight the need for multi-omics and systems biology approaches.

## Chapter 6: Polygenic and Oligogenic Risk in Congenital Heart Disease- A Systems View of Multifactorial Etiology

The chapter provides a summary of genomic studies showing that CHD exhibits oligogenic inheritance, in which multiple rare genetic variants combine to produce disease phenotypes. The coordinated expression patterns of cardiac transcription factors (NKX2.5, GATA4, TBX5, MEF2C, HAND1/2, TBX1, FOXH1, TBX20) during critical embryonic weeks 3-8 drive normal cardiac development, and disruption leads to CHD. The oligogenic inheritance test detects risk genes and their interactions. CHD probands harbor significantly more oligogenic gene sets than pseudo-sibling controls, which are enriched for known CHD risk genes. Diagnosis-specific oligogenic sets have been identified in phenotypically similar subgroups, including Ebstein's anomaly, pulmonary atresia with intact ventricular septum, truncus arteriosus, tetralogy of Fallot, and hypoplastic left heart syndrome (HLHS).

## Chapter 7: MicroRNA-Mediated Regulatory Mechanisms in the Etiopathogenesis of Congenital Heart Disease

Cardiac muscle is enriched with numerous miRNAs, including miR-1, miR-133, miR-499, and miR-208, which are abundantly expressed in cardiac tissue. The presence of SNPs in the 3'-untranslated regions (3'-UTRs) of miRNA target genes plays a vital role in CHD susceptibility by altering miRNA binding affinity. This chapter shows that high-throughput technologies combining bioinformatic and molecular analyses reveal that miRNAs modulate cardiac transcription factors. The iRNA biogenesis and its function as a post-transcriptional regulator are emerging as biomarkers and therapeutic targets in CHD. Therapeutic modulation of miRNA activity represents a promising avenue for the prevention and treatment of CHD. However, clinical translation requires substantial additional research.

# SECTION 3: TECHNOLOGICAL INNOVATIONS AND FUTURE DIRECTIONS

Despite advancements in medical science, children with CHD globally lack access to essential cardiac care. The core obstacles are low public awareness, delayed diagnosis and referral, and the severe issues of inaccessibility and unaffordability of life-saving medical interventions. Artificial intelligence and machine learning applications are transforming CHD diagnosis, risk stratification, and management across the lifespan. AI-enhanced fetal echocardiography improves prenatal detection. Deep learning models enable ECG-based screening and optimize surgical planning and perioperative care. From automated detection of cardiac anomalies in fetal ultrasounds to predictive algorithms for post-surgical outcomes, AI is transforming every aspect of CHD management. Advanced biosensor networks and edge computing systems promise real-time monitoring capabilities that could prevent complications before they become life-threatening emergencies. Three-dimensional reconstruction technologies and advanced imaging modalities are providing unprecedented visualization of cardiac anatomy, enabling precision surgical planning and personalized treatment approaches. These innovations, combined with an emerging understanding of genetic regulators and environmental exposures, are paving the way for truly personalized medicine in CHD care. Integration of AI with wearable biosensors and edge computing architectures promises real-time monitoring and early detection of complications. However, substantial validation and regulatory challenges must be addressed.

## Chapter 8: Artificial intelligence and Machine learning Applications

The technological revolution in CHD care is perhaps nowhere more evident than in the applications of artificial intelligence and machine learning. Artificial intelligence has demonstrated transformative potential in CHD diagnosis, risk stratification, and outcome prediction. Machine learning algorithms enhance diagnostic accuracy, reduce interobserver variability, and enable prediction of long-term outcomes in complex CHD. This chapter presents AI applications for improved anatomic diagnosis, cardiac function assessment, and risk stratification for mortality and morbidity. ML algorithms improve the identification of structural defects and procedural planning in interventional cardiology. AI with tele-echocardiography could enable effective CHD detection at the prenatal stage in low-resource settings, addressing healthcare access disparities.

## Chapter 9: Signal Processing and Machine Learning Architectures for Real-Time Fetal Cardiac Teratogen Detection: An ECE-Driven Approach to Exposomic Monitoring

Signal processing and machine learning architectures for real-time fetal cardiac monitoring leverage Doppler ultrasound (DUS) signals to assess fetal cardiac activity and detect potential teratogenic effects non-invasively. Integration of maternal stress level estimation from heart rate variability, body temperature, and physical activity provides contextual information for interpreting fetal cardiac parameters. Translational exposomics approaches combine exposome data with genomic variation to enhance causal inference and identify biomarkers, exposure-response relationships, and disease prediction mechanisms.

## Chapter 10: AI-Driven Biosensor Networks for Real-Time Prenatal Monitoring and CHD Risk Assessment: A Systems Engineering Approach

AI-driven biosensor networks for real-time prenatal monitoring are integrated systems that combine wearable sensors, wireless communication, edge computing, cloud analytics, and clinical decision-support interfaces. Systems engineering principles guide architectural design, ensuring reliability and scalability. The chapter compares wearable biosensors employed for CHD. Medical-grade devices for heart rhythm assessment and consumer-grade devices need interoperability and user-centered functionality. The FDA clearance of wireless wearable pulse oximeters and heart rate monitors depends on validation data from CHD populations.

## Chapter 11: 3D Reconstruction of Cardiovascular Anatomy for Investigating the Etiology of Congenital Heart Disease

3D-reconstructed models contribute to a mechanistic understanding of CHD etiology by enabling detailed morphometric analyses of malformed structures. Computational modeling using patient-specific 3D anatomy enables simulation of hemodynamic consequences of structural malformations, revealing relationships between anatomical defects and physiologic dysfunction. Finite element analyses of 3D-reconstructed hearts can test hypotheses about mechanical forces during cardiac development that may contribute to specific malformation patterns. Three-dimensional reconstruction technologies provide powerful tools for visualizing complex cardiac anatomy, improving surgical decision-making, and investigating relationships between structural malformations and hemodynamic consequences. A combination of 3D anatomical data with genomic, epigenomic, and exposomic information creates comprehensive datasets for elucidating multifactorial CHD etiologies.

## Chapter 12: Integrating AI and Edge Computing in Congenital Heart Disease Management

For CHD management, edge architectures enable real-time decision support at the point of care without delays inherent in cloud round-trip communications. Deep learning models optimized for deployment on resource-constrained edge processors achieve clinically relevant accuracy while meeting the power and computational constraints of wearable devices. Translational objectives encompass developing risk prediction models that integrate genetic, epigenetic, and environmental data for personalized counseling and creating targeted prevention interventions for high-risk populations.

In conclusion, the book offers a unique opportunity to address a critical knowledge gap in CHD research and to make a significant contribution to cardiovascular medicine. Advances in genomic technologies, single-cell biology, exposomics, and artificial intelligence provide unprecedented opportunities to improve prevention, diagnosis, and treatment.

Public health implications can inform prevention strategies, potentially reduce the incidence of these defects, and improve maternal and fetal health outcomes. Realizing this potential requires sustained commitment to basic and translational research and to interdisciplinary collaboration worldwide. Further meaningful public-private partnerships and societal investments are recommended to reduce environmental hazards and health inequities.

Progress in mitigating the burden of CHD will not emerge from a single discovery but from a concerted, interdisciplinary effort. Ultimately, The Multifactorial Etiology of Congenital Heart Disease aims to serve as a reference and catalyst for future investigation. By converging expertise from teratology, genetics, systems biology, and artificial intelligence, this volume advocates for a unified approach to congenital heart disease. The technological roadmap for the next generation of research aims for a future characterized by enhanced prediction, targeted prevention, and personalized intervention.

The edited volume advocates for empowering practitioners, policymakers, and researchers committed to ensuring that every child, regardless of their socioeconomic background, has access to a healthy heart.

Wishing Best Wishes for One World and One Family

**Ramya Raghavan**

*Sri Sathya Sai University for Human Excellence, India*

# Chapter 1
# Developmental Origins of Heart and Congenital Heart Diseases (CHD): Environmental Risk Factors and Genomic Correlations

**Shanthagoud P. Biradar**
https://orcid.org/0009-0001-9080-2300
*Sri Sathya Sai University for Human Excellence, India*

## ABSTRACT

*Congenital heart disease (CHD) affects approximately 9 per 1,000 live births globally and is a leading cause of infant mortality. The integration of Developmental Origins of Health and Disease (DOHaD) theory with Social Determinants of Health (SDOH) frameworks provides a comprehensive understanding of how early-life programming and social inequities interact to influence CHD development, progression, and outcomes. Multiple studies identified risk factors for congenital heart disease including demographic characteristics (maternal age, consanguinity, birth order, socioeconomic status), environmental exposures (pollution, occupational hazards, urban residence), and maternal health indicators (diabetes, obesity, stress, nutritional factors), showing regional variations. Current evidence demonstrate that CHD outcomes are significantly shaped by parental environmental exposures, genetic susceptibility, epigenetic modifications, and multilevel social determinants. The DOHaD-SDOH framework provides a roadmap for developing equitable, and sustainable prevention approaches. Ongoing research advocates for longitudinal and case-control studies to assess environmental exposures and their implications of on cardiovascular health.*

DOI: 10.4018/979-8-3373-3735-7.ch001

## INTRODUCTION

Congenital heart disease (CHD) demonstrates significant global variation in prevalence, mortality, and outcomes, with the greatest burden falling on low- and middle-income countries. In 2021, global CHD prevalence in children under five exceeded 4.18 million cases, representing a 3.4% increase since 1990. CHD outcomes reflect cumulative effects of disadvantage across the life course, from preconception through adulthood. Early programming during fetal development interacts with postnatal social environments to determine long-term cardiovascular health trajectories. In developed countries, over 90% of cases are now survivable due to advancements in early treatment options. A growing trend in CHD research was observed over the last decade, with the majority of publications originating from the United States, China, and the United Kingdom. The ECHSA-CCDB is the second largest congenital cardiac database in the world, documenting 377,606 procedures in 294,206 patients over 25 years, from 1999 to August 2024. The focus in congenital heart disease (CHD) care is increasingly shifting from just procedural success to longer-term patient survival and quality of life (Jonas, 2025). Significant advances in surgical techniques over the past few decades have dramatically improved short-term survival rates for children with CHD, with 1-year survival after surgery increasing from approximately 90.7% to 96.5% in recent years, and 5-year survival rates have also shown improvement. However, improving survival beyond the immediate postoperative period into adulthood remains a critical challenge. Especially for patients with complex heart defects. For example, a potential association between genetically predicted congenital anomalies of great vessels and an increased risk of atrial fibrillation, unspecified stroke, and ischemic stroke. The specific odds ratios and confidence intervals reported survival rates vary markedly by CHD complexity, associated with poorer long-term survival (Krishnan et al., 2025).

In Quito, Ecuador, from January 2019 to December 2022, a total of 1,000 pediatric medical records were reviewed, revealing that 56.0% of the patients were female and 65.2% lived at high altitudes (2,500-3,500 m), with acyanotic CHD being the most common type (71.4%). The most prevalent specific condition was patent ductus arteriosus (48.7%), while Tetralogy of Fallot was the most common among cyanotic CHD cases (28.1%). The study reported a mortality rate of 5.3% among patients, primarily affecting those with acyanotic CHD. It highlighted a significant burden of disability associated with CHD conditions despite the low mortality rate (Izquierdo-Condoy et al., 2025).

The Developmental Origins of Health and Disease (DOHaD) hypothesis, initially proposed by David Barker in the 1980s, postulates that environmental factors during critical periods of development can permanently program disease susceptibility in adulthood. Social determinants of health (SDOH) has evolved to encompass a broader understanding of developmental programming across multiple life phases, including preconceptional, periconceptional, fetal, neonatal, and early childhood periods (Raghavan & Ahamad, 2025). The periconceptional period (one month before conception through the first trimester) emerges as the most critical window for CHD development. During cardiac organogenesis occurs, making the developing heart vulnerable to environmental insults. Different CHD types may have distinct susceptibility windows, with complex lesions potentially requiring exposures during multiple critical periods (Safi-Stibler & Gabory, 2020).

Environmental factors, maternal diabetes mellitus, represent well-established risk factors through underlying mechanisms. Advanced maternal age, low education, and multiple pregnancies increase CHD risk (Dolk et al., 2020).

Recent large-scale studies have shown associations with air Pollution. A 2024 Korean study found strong correlations between prenatal exposure to sulfur dioxide ($SO_2$) and cadmium, and an increased risk of ventricular septal defects (VSD) (OR for $SO_2$: 6.843; for cadmium: 1.513) (Jin et al., 2024).

Social determinants (race, SES, education, insurance, geography) influence both exposure to risk factors and access to care, driving disparities in CHD prevalence and outcomes. Factors contributing to higher odds of GIC include being older than 10.5 years, having simple CHD, living farther from care facilities, receiving public insurance, and having a low Child Opportunity Index. Addressing social determinants of health, such as insurance status and neighborhood opportunities, is essential for reducing GIC in patients with CHD. (Zaidi et al., 2024). Social deprivation increased exposure to environmental pollutants, which is linked to higher CHD incidence (Safi-Stibler & Gabory, 2020). Mouse models with Tbx1 or Fgfr1/Fgfr2 mutations exhibit increased CHD severity when exposed to gestational hypoxia (Yasuhara et al., 2025).

## CRITICAL WINDOWS OF CARDIAC DEVELOPMENT

Cardiac development begins in the third week of gestation, with the formation of the First Heart Field (FHF) and Second Heart Field (SHF) from cardiogenic progenitor cells. The heart tube forms by day 21, followed by looping (days 23–28) and chamber formation. Genetic and molecular pathways tightly regulate processes and are highly sensitive to environmental insults (Zachariah et al., 2024). Early-life environmental exposures (teratogens, infections, nutritional deficiencies) during critical developmental windows can disrupt cardiac development, in genetically susceptible individuals.

Organogenesis involves the coordinated development of various cell lineages, exemplified by the transformation of the cardiac crescent into a four-chambered heart. Cardiomyocytes arise from the first and second heart fields, each contributing differently to the formation of the definitive heart. The development of the human heart is among the earliest and most intricate. The events of embryogenesis related to heart embryological process begins during the third week of gestation, alongside the establishment of the trilaminar germ layers during gastrulation. From the splanchnic layer of the lateral plate mesoderm, two bilateral populations of cardiogenic progenitor cells emerge to form the First Heart Field (FHF) and Second Heart Field (SHF). Two progenitor sources contribute distinctively to the forming heart: the FHF largely contributes to the left ventricle and parts of the atria, while the SHF contributes to the right ventricle, outflow tract, and remaining atrial regions.

First heart field cells originate from a juxtacardiac field near the extraembryonic mesoderm. The second heart field cells come from a multilineage-primed progenitor population through specific pathways. The FHF and SHF, derived from the lateral head mesoderm, lack a distinct anatomical boundary and function as a continuum influenced by morphogenetic movements and local environments (Wolton et al., 2025). Single-cell sequencing technology enables precise observation of gene expression and cell fate in first heart field (FHF) and second heart field (SHF) cells, revealing that primitive streak cells that contribute to the ventricles exhibit distinct molecular signatures compared to those that form the outflow tract and atrium. Technological advances, combined with systems biology frameworks, offer the potential to construct predictive models (S. et al., 2025). Machine learning and artificial intelligence can identify at-risk pregnancies and guide personalized interventions (Kelly, 2023) (GVS et al., 2025).

## Heart Tube Formation

Cardiac development is a complex process regulated by numerous molecular signals, including growth factors and signaling pathways such as WNT, retinoic acid, and Notch signaling. Cardiopulmonary progenitor cells (CPPs) during organogenesis highlight the coordinated development of the heart and lungs. The mesoderm surrounding the developing heart and anterior foregut endoderm is crucial for guiding cardiopulmonary development. It serves as a source of Wnt2-expressing CPPs. The lineage tracing of Wnt2 expressing CPPs and single-cell RNA sequencing to create a comprehensive cell atlas (Wen et al., 2025). In week 3, bilateral endocardial tubes form from the fusion of angiogenic clusters in the cardiogenic mesoderm. Heart tubes migrate medially and coalesce into a single linear heart tube by day 21. The heart tube in the pericardial cavity consists of endocardium, cardiac jelly (acellular matrix), and myocardium. The formation and fusion of the heart tube are tightly regulated by BMP2, FGF8, and WNT-inhibitory factors such as DKK1. Key developmental milestones include the establishment of the basic cardiac layout by

4.5 weeks, completion of septation at the venous pole by 6 weeks, incorporation of the outflow tract into the ventricles between 5.5 and 6.5 weeks, and completion of remodeling of the interventricular foramen by 7 weeks (Hikspoors et al., 2022). Factors such as cilia, the extracellular matrix, epigenetic modifications, hypoxia, autophagy, metabolic transition, and macrophages play significant roles. Disruptions in pathways due to hypoxia, retinoid imbalance, or toxic chemical exposures may result in cardia bifida or early embryonic lethality. The integration of spatial mapping, computational analysis of cell trajectories, and transcriptional profiling provides insights into the molecular and cellular mechanisms underlying cardiopulmonary development.

## Cardiac Looping

The role of epicardium-myocardium crosstalk in heart development, highlighting its influence on processes such as epithelial-to-mesenchymal transition, cell fate specification, myocardial growth, and coronary vasculature development. By day 23–28, the heart tube undergoes looping, transforming from a straight tube into a helical structure. The D-looping process correctly positions the atrial and ventricular chambers, creating spatial orientation critical for normal heart architecture. The looped configuration of vertebrate hearts, characterized by curved and twisted components, is phylogenetically conserved and significantly influences cardiac pumping function. Cardiac looping, which occurs during embryonic development, enhances the pumping efficiency of valveless embryonic hearts. Bilaterally asymmetric (chiral) looping is crucial for the proper alignment and separation of pulmonary and systemic flow paths in the multichambered hearts of tetrapods. Chiral looping is not necessary for the efficient pumping of the two-chambered hearts found in fish. In contrast, the sigmoidal curvature of the flow path improves pumping efficiency in both lower and higher vertebrates.

Abnormal looping may result in conditions such as dextrocardia, L-transposition, or heterotaxy. Inadequate remodeling of the heart tube's inner curvature and variability in the connection of the primary atrial segment led to incomplete formation of atrial and atrioventricular septal structures. Left-right patterning genes like NODAL, LEFTY, and PITX2 are central to this process. Environmental teratogens, such as valproic acid, maternal diabetes, or nicotine, can affect nodal cilia function, disrupt morphogen flow, and result in laterality defects. Hexafluoropropylene oxide trimer acid (HFPO-TA) in global water environments affects gene expression related to heart development and the vascular endothelial growth factor (VEGF) pathway, leading to disrupted embryonic vascular development and decreased erythrocyte numbers. Exposure to HFPO-TA induced oxidative stress and altered transcriptional levels of genes associated with cell cycle and apoptosis, suggesting potential harm to both cardiovascular and hematopoietic systems. Exposure to D-tetramethrin results in downregulation of transcription factors associated with cardiac looping (Myh6, Nkx2.5) and heart function (Gata4, Vmhc) (Ye et al., 2025). The accumulation of ROS due to pesticide exposure alters gene transcription related to cardiac development, cardiac looping failure in zebrafish embryos.

## Chamber Development and Septation

From weeks 4 to 8, the linear heart tube undergoes ballooning to form the primitive atria and ventricles. Chamber septation proceeds through the septum primum / secundum formation in the atria. The muscular ridge expansion in the ventricles and endocardial cushion fusion at the atrioventricular junctions are also observed. Atrioventricular septal defect with a common valvar orifice is prevalent in patients with Down syndrome. Two critical developmental factors contributing to atrioventricular septal defects were identified: (a) an alteration in the heart tube configuration leading to inadequate remodeling of the inner heart curvature, and (b) variability in the connection of the primary atrial cardiac segment to the dorsal mesocardium, affecting its relationship with the extracardiac mediastinal mesoderm. Hypoplasia and apical filling of the right ventricle were significantly more common in patients with Down syndrome ($p < 0.001$), indicating distinct anatomical differences (Belhadjer et al., 2025). There was little difference in the connection between normal and trisomic embryos at early stages (20-25 somites). Many significant changes occurred later, with trisomic embryos exhibiting a larger area of attachment to the mediastinal mesoderm. In trisomic embryos, the right pulmonary ridge did not accumulate the necessary extracardiac mesoderm. It failed to undergo the expected forward growth, resulting in incomplete formation of both atrial and atrioventricular septal structures.

The transcription factors and signaling molecules, such as TBX5, GATA4, NKX2-5, and CRELD1, are part of the genetic mechanisms underlying the embryological development. The cardiovascular system structures are influenced by transcription factors such as GATA4, TBX5, and NKX2.5, and their association with CHDs (Kukshal et al., 2023). The development of the atrioventricular mesenchymal complex is sensitive to teratogens such as alcohol, which alter retinoic acid gradients and transcriptional regulation. The gross anatomy of the fossa ovalis (FO) and anatomical variations due to incomplete fusion of the septum primum and septum secundum, including atrial septal pouches and left atrial septal ridges, are observed in CHDs.

## Neural Crest Cells(NCCs)

Neural crest cells are migratory and multipotent, originating from the neural folds and undergoing epithelial-mesenchymal transition (EMT) to migrate within vertebrate embryos. Splicing factors are crucial for mRNA maturation and play a significant role in neural crest development in the craniofacial region. The splicing factors in vagal neural crest cells are involved in the development of the outflow tract and the enteric nervous system (ENS). The cardiac neural crest is essential for normal heart development, and its surgical ablation in chicken model mimics common human congenital heart defects, including 'Common Arterial Trunk' and 'Double Outlet Right Ventricle' (DORV). The survival rate of embryos subjected to right cardiac neural crest ablation was lower than that of those subjected to left cardiac neural crest ablation, suggesting potential asymmetrical differences in the roles of left versus right cardiac neural crest in heart development (Solovieva & Bronner, 2025). The volatile organic compounds (VOCs) benzene, toluene, and xylene, as well as solvents, racquet, and pollution, are associated with outflow tract defects and neural crest defects (Nagashri et al., 2024). MVOCs interrupt WNT and NOTCH signaling and compromise SHF and NCC contributions. Disruption of CXCR4/SDF1 signaling results in disorganization of the neural tube basement membrane; it does not affect the epithelial-mesenchymal transition (EMT) of neural crest cells. Oxidative stress modifies the β-catenin signaling. PAHs, coal, and smoke downregulate traits in the BMP and WNT axes and epigenetic mechanisms.

Additionally, neural crest cells (NCCs) migrate into the outflow tract and pharyngeal arches, contributing to conotruncal septation. Ankrd11 knockout in neural crest cells disrupts the expression of transcription factors, chromatin remodelers, and key signaling pathways, including mTOR, BMP, and TGF-β, which are crucial for heart development and function. Impairment of NCC migration by agents such as retinoic acid, methotrexate, or diabetes-associated hyperglycemia can result in persistent truncus arteriosus, Tetralogy of Fallot, or double-outlet right ventricle. The effects of serotonin receptor modulation, specifically 5-HT2B and 5-HT2C receptors, on cNCC migration and the development of cardiac derivatives, emphasizing the relevance of serotonergic drug safety during pregnancy (Wells et al., 2025).

Developmental timing and teratogenic vulnerability during the developmental trajectories of various cardiac progenitor populations emphasize the importance of combining genome-wide association studies with single-cell and spatial atlases to identify non-coding risk variants. Innovative platforms such as cardiac organoids and engineered developmental models are being used to validate gene function and model lineage-specific defects, contributing to a mechanistic understanding of CHD and paving the way for precision diagnostics and targeted therapies (Byalahunasishetter et al., 2025).

Each morphogenetic event has a precise temporal window

- Heart tube formation: days 18–22
- Looping: days 23–28
- Septation and valve formation: weeks 4–8

Neural crest cells (NCCs), including cardiac neural crest (CNC) cells, play a crucial role in the embryogenesis of cardiac and vascular structures. Teratogenic exposures within critical windows have distinct outcomes. For example:

- Alcohol exposure at 3–4 weeks disrupts looping and FHF derivatives. Ethanol abolishes retinoic acid (RA) signaling and the transcription factors, GATA4 and TBX5. Apoptosis of the SHF develops as a result of oxidative stress.
- Rubella infection at 5–7 weeks affects endothelial and valvular development.
- BPA exposure during SHF proliferation impairs right ventricular development and NCC-derived septation. Cardiovascular neurocristopathy encompasses genetic disorders affecting NCC-derived structures, manifesting as cardiac septation disorders, great vessel and vascular disorders, myocardial dysfunction, or a combination of CHD phenotypes.

Common phenotypic characteristics of cardiovascular neurocristopathies, such as a bicuspid aortic valve and a thoracic aortic aneurysm. Toxic exposures may result in functional rather than structural impairments or go unnoticed (Soliman et al., 2024). The hyperglycemic intrauterine environment led to significant morphological alterations in conal ridges. It increased the risk of conotruncal heart defects, including double-outlet right ventricle and atrioventricular (AV) canal defects. Unlike early teratogenic exposures, which cause structural congenital heart defects, perinatal risk factors, anomalies, maternal illnesses, and exposure to drugs are more likely to affect functional maturation, vascular patterning, and cardiomyocyte proliferation. Techniques such as in vivo labeling, cell tracking, and models such as gastruloids and organoids enhance understanding of cardiac morphogenesis and its links to congenital heart diseases (Lakshmaiah et al., 2025).

## Cardiac Maturation

The fetal heart undergoes major transformations from a simple looping tube into a complex, multichambered, and functional organ. Neural crest cells (NCCs) and cardiac neural crest cells (cNCCs) are crucial for the development of ventricular outflow tracts (OFTs) and the embryonic conus. Key maturation processes include histodifferentiation and myocardial growth. From the beginning of the second trimester, cardiomyocytes proliferate and differentiate into specialized cell types, including contractile, pacemaker, and conduction cells. The fetal myocardium also matures in architecture, transitioning from striated muscle to a defined trabecular network and compact myocardial layer. Cardiomyocyte differentiation is regulated by transcription factors such as MEF2, GATA4, and HAND1/2, and modulated by local environmental cues, including oxygen tension, hormones, and extracellular matrix signals. Maternal hypoxia, placental insufficiency, or toxins can cause cardiomyocyte immaturity, contributing to cardiac remodeling and impaired function (Soliman et al., 2024). Specific associations between maternal health factors identify high-risk groups for CHD development. The metabolic disorders and pregnancy complications, placental dysfunction issues related to a hyperglycemic intrauterine environment, and prevention strategies are recommended (Ramírez-Fuentes et al., 2025).

## Vascular Development and Coronary Formation

The epicardium plays a crucial role in heart development by serving as a paracrine signaling hub and a source of progenitor cells, facilitating communication with the myocardium.

Bidirectional communication between the epicardium and myocardium is essential for proper cardiac morphogenesis and involves tightly regulated signaling networks. The fetal heart also requires the establishment of the coronary vasculature and systemic–pulmonary connections. The coronary arteries arise from epicardial-derived cells (EPDCs), which differentiate into vascular smooth muscle and endothelial cells. VEGF (Vascular Endothelial Growth Factor) and PDGF (Platelet-Derived Growth Factor) signaling are critical for epicardial epithelial-to-mesenchymal transition, cell fate specification, myocardial growth, and coronary vasculature development. Disruption of VEGF by anti-angiogenic drugs, hypoxia, or environmental pollutants (dioxins) can impair epicardium-myocardium crosstalk on various developmental processes, including epithelial-to-mesenchymal transition (EMT), fate specification of epicardium-derived cells (EPDCs), myocardial proliferation, and coronary vasculature development (Nusrat & Wu, 2025).

Congenital Rubella Syndrome (CRS) leads to downregulation of VEGF, NOTCH, and FGF signaling during teratogenic infection. Abnormalities of the fetus due to maternal rubella in the first trimester, before week 8, are reported as septal defects, Patent ductus arteriosus (PDA), and stenosis of the pulmonary artery. The Atrial (ASD) and ventricular (VSD) septal defects arise from fetal endothelial cells infected by the rubella virus and impede vascular remodeling. It disrupts neural crest cell (NCC) migration and destroys the mesenchyme of the endocardial cushion. Infants of diabetic mothers, for instance, may show abnormal coronary artery growth, altered capillary density, and impaired perfusion, all of which relate to later cardiovascular risks. Cardiotoxicity is defined as a chemically induced condition and is a significant cause of drug attrition. Furthermore, fetal vascular development is sensitive to maternal metabolic conditions. The cardiac anomalies that are comprised in fetal alcohol spectrum disorders cause myocardium and septal defects, conotruncal malformations.

The toxicity can arise from both functional effects, such as alterations in contractile and electrical regulation, and structural changes in cardiomyocytes and other cardiac cells, leading to conditions such as arrhythmias and reduced left ventricular ejection fraction (LVEF).

For example, anticancer drugs can impair the function of cardiomyocytes, cardiac fibroblasts, and cardiac endothelial cells, disrupting autocrine and paracrine signaling and altering cardiac cellular homeostasis. New lineage-tracing techniques for understanding cardiovascular development and physiology, highlighting their role in identifying cellular origins, fates, and plasticity across various cell populations (Ananthakumar et al., 2025).

## Conduction System Development

Endothelial cells and cardiomyocytes communicate via paracrine signaling to maintain cardiac homeostasis and influence both cardiac development and function. From the second trimester onward, the cardiac conduction system (sinoatrial node, atrioventricular node, bundle branches, and Purkinje fibers) undergoes specification and insulation from surrounding myocardium. The functional isolation is vital for synchronous contraction. RGS proteins regulate G protein signaling, which is essential for maintaining conduction physiological homeostasis. Both genetic and nongenetic factors affecting G protein signaling in cardiomyocytes contribute to the development of dilated cardiomyopathy (DCM). Dynamic changes in gene expression, cell-state determination, and cell-fate conversion across multiple cell lineages contribute to pathophysiological processes. Defects in G protein regulation by RGS proteins are believed to cause structural damage to cardiomyocytes and reduced contractile function (Garcia et al., 2025).

The paracrine signals released by endothelial cells affect cardiomyocyte growth, hypertrophy, and contractility. The signals from cardiomyocytes that impact angiogenesis and vascular tone. Disrupted communication between endothelial cells and cardiomyocytes can lead to cardiomyopathy, driven by inflammatory cytokines and viral infections (Coxsackie B virus). Fetal myocarditis and conduction defects, as well as structural heart disease, have been ascribed to Cytomegalovirus (CMV) and Coxsackie B high-density virus. Inflammatory cytokines, such as IL-6 and TNF-α, affect cardiomyocyte proliferation and matrix remodeling during the second trimester.

Exogenous toxins can cause arrhythmias and fetal bradycardia, underscoring the crucial role of mitochondrial quality control in regulating mitochondrial function in cardiomyocytes and influencing mitochondrial morphology and function. Other transcription mechanisms underlying inflammation, hypertrophy, and fibrosis are modulated by TBX3 (which represses the working myocardial gene program in nodal tissue) and NKX2.5 (which modulates conduction zone boundaries). SHOX2 and ISL1 (which specify pacemaker identity) emphasize the importance of mitophagy and mitochondrial dynamics in the disease's pathogenesis (Vey et al., 2025).

Understanding the role of endothelial-cardiomyocyte crosstalk is essential for insights into tissue homeostasis, regeneration, and disease mechanisms, potentially leading to new diagnostic and therapeutic targets. The lineage-tracing techniques and single-cell omics of cardiovascular biology can reveal new insights into cellular origins, fates, plasticity, and heterogeneity in cardiomyocyte, endothelial, and mesenchymal cell populations (Biradar et al., 2025). Epigenetics and mechanobiology are implicated in the pathogenesis of CHD, with aberrant regulation contributing to disease. Advancements in genome sequencing are enhancing our knowledge of CHD genetics, including the roles of oligogenic inheritance, epigenetic modifications, genetic mosaicism, and noncoding variants in gene expression (P. et al., 2025). Novel epigenetic biomarkers and environmental risk factors are highlighted for improved diagnosis and understanding of CHD etiology (Choudhury et al., 2025).

*Table 1. Examples for Genetic Basis of Congenital Heart Diseases*

| Inheritance Pattern | Genetic Basis | Common Cardiac Anomalies |
|---|---|---|
| Noonan Syndrome | PTPN11, SOS1 | Pulmonary stenosis, hypertrophic cardiomyopathy |
| Alagille Syndrome | JAG1, NOTCH2 | Pulmonary branch stenosis, bile duct paucity |
| Holt-Oram Syndrome | TBX5 | Atrioventricular septal defects, conduction defects |
| Down Syndrome | Trisomy 21 | Atrioventricular septal defects |
| DiGeorge Syndrome | 22q11.2 Deletion | Conotruncal defects |
| Turner Syndrome | Turner Syndrome | Coarctation of the aorta |
| Autosomal Dominant | NKX2-5 | Atrial septal defects, ventricular septal defects |
| Autosomal Dominant | GATA4 | Atrioventricular septal defects |
| Autosomal Dominant | TBX20 | Tetralogy of Fallot |

## SOCIOECONOMIC ENVIRONMENTAL RISK FACTORS

Socioeconomic status influences CHD risk through multiple pathways, including access to healthcare, nutritional adequacy, environmental exposures, and health-seeking behaviors. Lower socioeconomic groups demonstrate 1.8-2.9-fold increased CHD risk, with educational attainment emerging as the strongest predictor within socioeconomic indicators. Social determinants of health were found to explain as much, or more, variability in both operative and longitudinal mortality than clinical comorbidities or prior cardiac surgeries, indicating their significant impact on patient outcomes (Zaidi et al., 2024).

The inclusion of social determinants in risk models improved model discrimination, enabling better classification of survivors and deaths. Socio-demographic factors such as age at marriage, education, residence, and economic status significantly influence the prevalence of consanguinity. Consanguinity is associated with various social benefits, including family stability and increased social security. However, it also poses risks to reproductive health, leading to higher rates of congenital and medical disorders. Although it only minimally enhanced predictive performance, emphasizing the need for careful integration in clinical risk assessments (Crook et al., 2024). The CREATE registry demonstrates transparent inverse gradients between socioeconomic position and CHD-related mortality. However, disparities diminish when adjusted for treatment differences, highlighting healthcare access as a critical mediating factor (Gupta et al., 2008).

*Table 2. Key Gene-Environment Interactions in CHD (Kalisch-Smith et al., 2020)*

| Genetic Factor | Environmental Exposure | Outcome/Mechanism |
|---|---|---|
| NKX2-5 mutation | Gestational hypoxia | Embryo lethality, increased CHD severity |
| TBX1, FGF8 mutations | Hypoxia, retinoid imbalance | Increased incidence/severity of heart defects |
| SHF/FHF gene variants | BPA, alcohol, and maternal diabetes | Disrupted chamber formation, septal/conotruncal defects |

## MATERNAL HEALTH AND REPRODUCTIVE FACTORS

Maternal underweight status (BMI <18.5 kg/m$^2$) demonstrates significant associations with CHD (OR: 1.28-2.1), reflecting chronic nutritional insufficiency that affects fetal cardiac development. The median weight-for-age Z-score of Indian children undergoing cardiac surgery is -3.2, compared to -0.59 for healthy

Indian children. Folic acid deficiency during pregnancy was linked to a significant increase in CHD risk (OR = 2.02, 95% CI: 1.51–2.70). The evidence supports the role of folate supplementation in preventing CHD. Women with low folate levels or inadequate supplementation during pregnancy had a significantly higher risk of delivering infants with CHD (Tyagi et al., 2022). The nutritional burden creates a vicious cycle where CHD children face additional risks due to pre-existing malnutrition, complicating surgical outcomes and recovery (Dolk et al., 2020). Maternal infections (rubella, syphilis), drug use, nutrition (folate deficiency), air pollution, and other environmental toxins. Maternal education emerges as the strongest predictor of racial and ethnic disparities in CHD outcomes (Safi-Stibler & Gabory, 2020).

Maternal infections were strongly associated with a higher risk of CHD (OR = 2.48, 95% CI: 1.88–3.28). An association indicates that children born to mothers who experienced rubella or other viral infections during pregnancy had more than twice the risk of developing congenital heart defects compared to children of uninfected mothers.

## Maternal Malnutrition And Micronutrient Deficiencies

Maternal malnutrition and micronutrient deficiencies constitute major modifiable risk factors with substantial public health implications. Black patients with CHD have significantly higher mortality than White patients (OR 1.62 for non-critical CHD in infants). Structural racism and systemic inequities affect access to care and outcomes (Tran et al., 2022). Periconceptional folic acid deficiency is consistently associated with an increased risk of CHD (OR: 1.4-2.3), with only 30.9% of mothers in Indian studies reporting adequate folic acid supplementation during the periconceptional period (Zaqout et al., 2021). Maternal food diversity emerges as a protective factor, with diets of medium and high diversity reducing CHD risk by 6% compared with low-diversity diets. Women smoking ≥25 cigarettes per day during the periconceptional period show increased risk for septal defects (OR: 2.1) and right-sided obstructive defects. The association demonstrates a dose-response relationship, with heavier smoking conferring greater risk (Dolk et al., 2020).

Advanced maternal age emerges as a consistent risk factor across multiple studies, with women aged 30 years and above demonstrating 2.5-3.9-fold increased odds of CHD offspring compared to younger mothers. Advanced maternal age (≥35 years) was associated with a slightly increased risk of CHD (OR = 1.26, 95% CI: 1.03–1.54). While maternal age has a negligible effect compared to other risk factors, it still increases the likelihood of CHD (Choudhury et al., 2025). The heterogeneity in maternal age and CHD association was relatively low ($I^2 = 27\%$). CHD association increases with maternal age, reflecting age-related chromosomal abnormalities and cumulative environmental exposures that affect cardiac embryogenesis (Zachariah et al., 2024).

## Maternal Diabetes

Maternal diabetes emerges as the strongest modifiable risk factor, encompasses both pre-gestational diabetes and gestational diabetes mellitus. The diabetic mothers show significantly higher rates of cardiac malformations, septal defects and outflow tract anomalies. Hyperglycemia is identified as the primary teratogen in diabetic pregnancies, affecting fetal cardiac development (Xu et al., 2025). Maternal diabetes increased the odds of CHD by 1.8 times (OR = 1.81, 95% CI: 1.24–2.65). Diabetes in pregnancy was found to be a significant risk factor for CHD, with mothers who had pre-existing diabetes or gestational diabetes showing a higher likelihood of having children with heart defects. The plot showed moderate heterogeneity ($I^2 = 39\%$). ROS-mediated effects and alterations in signaling pathways, such as the Wnt, Notch, and TGFβ pathways, are key mechanisms by which hyperglycemia impacts heart development. The underlying mechanism is complex and multifactorial, involving oxidative stress and changes in gene expression. Children born to mothers under 18 or with less than 12 years of education have higher CHD mortality. Multiple pregnancies and prematurity, influenced by SDOH, increase risk (Tran et al., 2022). The pathophysiological mechanisms involve maternal hyperglycemia disrupting cardiac neural crest cell migration and altering expression of cardiac transcription factors during critical developmental windows.

## Pollution

Exposure to air pollution during pregnancy represents an emerging risk factor with particular relevance to Indian populations, given that 21 of the world's 30 most polluted cities are located in India. Ambient particulate matter (PM2.5) concentrations in major Indian cities range from 150 to 300 $\mu g/m^3$ during the winter season, exceeding the WHO guidelines by a significant margin. Population-weighted mean annual PM2.5 exposure in India was 89.9 $\mu g/m^3$ in 2017, with 76.8% of the population exposed to levels exceeding 40 $\mu g/m^3$. Exposure to high levels of air pollution was associated with a moderate increase in the risk of CHD (OR = 1.35, 95% CI: 1.02–1.80). The association with air pollution exposure, in urban areas with high vehicular emissions, supports the growing body of evidence linking environmental pollutants to developmental defects, including CHD (Jin et al., 2024). Heterogeneity in the studies was high ($I^2 = 56\%$), likely due to varying pollution levels across regions. The biological mechanisms linking air pollution to CHD include maternal and fetal inflammation, oxidative stress, and epigenetic modifications that affect cardiac developmental pathways (Zachariah et al., 2024). Household air pollution from solid fuel combustion compounds risks, in rural areas where 42% of children are underweight. The combination of ambient and household air pollution creates sustained exposures throughout pregnancy that may disrupt normal cardiac morphogenesis.

## FUTURE DIRECTIONS

Comprehensive pre-conceptional care need to address modifiable risk factors, including smoking cessation, diabetes management, nutritional optimization, and environmental exposure reduction. Interventions should be integrated with broader social determinants approaches addressing education, economic opportunity, and environmental justice (Raghavan et al., 2025). Prenatal Screening amniocentesis, chorionic villus sampling (CVS), Non-Invasive Prenatal Testing (NIPT) are vital. Nuchal translucency measurement with serum markers (PAPP-A, β-hCG) to assess chromosomal abnormality risk detects ~90% of trisomies linked to CHD. Second-trimester ultrasound, 4-chamber view (4CV) identifies 63% of major CHD. Outflow tract views (OFTVs) increases sensitivity to 91% for critical CHD. Fetal echocardiography is the gold standard for structural CHD diagnosis has 90% sensitivity for major defects in high-risk pregnancies. Echocardiography detects ductal-dependent lesions (hypoplastic left heart syndrome). Cell-free DNA (cfDNA) screening allows non-invasive detection of trisomies and microdeletions (22q11.2) with >99% specificity.

Regulation of environmental toxins, including pesticides, heavy metals, and air pollutants, can protect reproductive-age women during critical windows of fetal development. Deep learning algorithms are being developed to automate and improve the accuracy of fetal echocardiography. Automated image acquisition guide sonographers to obtain optimal cardiac views. Identifying cardiac structures and anomalies more quickly and accurately than human interpretation alone. Automated chd detection and classification flag suspicious findings and even suggesting specific CHD diagnoses. Quantification of cardiac function by measuring ventricular volumes, ejection fraction, and other functional parameters to standardize image interpretation and reduce variability (Lakshmaiah et al., 2025).

## 3D/4D Ultrasound With Spatiotemporal Image Correlation (STIC)

STIC captures a 3D volume of the fetal heart over a complete cardiac cycle, allowing for offline analysis and multiplanar reconstruction.

Virtual Planes and "En Face" septa, valves Views: Enabling visualization of cardiac structures that are difficult to obtain with standard 2D ultrasound.

Non-Invasive Prenatal Testing (NIPT) Functional Assessment: Measuring myocardial mass, contractility, and developing 4D-based myocardial performance indices.

Fetal cardiac magnetic resonance imaging and advanced motion correction algorithms measure fetal movement and rapid heartbeats. Research is focused on developing more robust motion correction techniques and cardiac gating strategies. It is often using external Doppler ultrasound devices synchronized with the MRI scanner to obtain clearer images. 4D Flow MRI technique allows for 3D, time-resolved visualization and quantification of blood flow throughout the fetal cardiovascular system. It holds significant promise for detailed Assessment of intricate vasculature, shunts, and connections. 4D Flow MRI characterize Flow patterns like coarctation of the aorta or pulmonary atresia with aortopulmonary collaterals, which can be challenging with echocardiography alone (GVS et al., 2025).

- Assessing Oxygenation and Hemodynamics: Investigating the relationship between the heart, brain, and placenta with regard to blood flow and oxygenation.
- Higher Resolution Imaging: Continuous efforts to improve spatial and temporal resolution for better visualization of small fetal cardiac structures.

Fetal MRI is increasingly seen as a valuable adjunct to echocardiography, especially in late gestation or when echocardiography views are limited. Genomic and Genetic Screening Advancements and Next-Generation Sequencing (NGS) for Monogenic CHD rely on expanded gene panels beyond common aneuploidies. Research is expanding to include broader panels for detecting single-gene defects associated with syndromic and some asyndromic CHDs (genes related to Noonan syndrome, DiGeorge syndrome). Whole Exome Sequencing (WES) and Whole Genome Sequencing (WGS) comprehensive genomic approaches are increasingly used in cases of suspected genetic etiology, especially when targeted gene panels are inconclusive or in fetuses with multiple anomalies. Prenatal Microarray Analysis for smaller chromosomal deletions or duplications (copy number variants) supplement traditional karyotyping. Polygenic Risk Scores (PRS) research is ongoing to develop and validate PRS for CHD. These scores combine information from multiple common genetic variants, each with a small effect, to estimate an individual's overall genetic predisposition to CHD. PRS could potentially be integrated into preconception risk assessment. Liquid Biopsy (Cell-Free Fetal DNA beyond Aneuploidy) detect single-gene disorders. Efforts are underway to expand to detect specific single-gene mutations associated with CHD from cell-free fetal DNA in maternal blood, reducing the need for invasive procedures. Investigating epigenetic modifications (DNA methylation) in cell-free fetal DNA, for viral bacterial or fungi infections for CHD risk will allow early diagnosis (Nanjundeshwara et al., 2025). Novel biomarkers metabolomics and proteomics profiles or protein biomarkers in maternal blood or amniotic fluid could indicate an increased risk of CHD, even before structural anomalies are apparent on imaging.

## Clinical Trials and Research Initiatives

Key areas of focus in these trials include validation of Artificial intelligence (AI) algorithms in fetal echocardiography.

### Clinical Artificial Intelligence Fetal Echocardiography (CAIFE) Study

To develop machine-learning models for real-time detection of abnormalities in fetal hearts, collecting large datasets of ultrasound images and videos for training. Trials compare AI-assisted screening to traditional methods to assess diagnostic accuracy, efficiency, and impact on workflow. Implementation of Advanced Fetal Cardiac MRI trials establish normative data for fetal heart dimensions and function using advanced MRI sequences (4D Flow MRI) to improve the reliability of detecting subtle abnormalities. Studies evaluate the clinical utility of fetal cardiac MRI as a complementary tool to echocardiography, particularly in complex or difficult cases (coarctation of the aorta, pulmonary atresia).

### Expanded Genomic Screening

Clinical trials assessing the effectiveness and cost-effectiveness of integrating broader prenatal genetic sequencing (WES/WGS) into high-risk pregnancies for CHD. The impact of genetic counseling alongside these advanced genomic tests and non-Invasive Prenatal Diagnosis (NIPD) for Monogenic CHD and single-gene disorders known to cause CHD from maternal blood samples. This is a highly anticipated area that could revolutionize prenatal diagnosis by making it safer and more accessible for genetic screening in high-risk populations, including low birth weight (LBW). Nanomedicine Approaches combine genomic data with proteomic or metabolomic data to identify more comprehensive risk profiles for CHD, aiming for more personalized risk assessment and earlier detection. Further research is needed to elucidate specific epigenetic pathways linking environmental exposures and social determinants to CHD development. Studies should focus on identifying biomarkers of developmental programming that could enable early intervention. Suboptimal maternal health, characterized by factors such as anemia and malnutrition during gestation, is correlated with adverse birth outcomes. Overcoming the financial divide requires comprehensive health financing reforms and targeted infrastructure development to ensure equitable access to specialized services across all geographic and socioeconomic divisions (Vrijheid et al., 2021). The integration of multi-omics approaches with advanced computational methods holds promise for identifying novel pathways. Environmental exposures influence cardiac development, so effective prevention strategies are needed for personalized medical approaches for families at risk (Ananthakumar et al., 2024). However, significant investments in technology development, international collaboration, and adaptation of the regulatory framework will be necessary to fully realize the potential of exposome science in preventing congenital heart disease (Bhuvana et al., 2025).

*Table 3. Recent advancements in preconception and prenatal screening for congenital heart disease (CHD) focus on integrating AI, advanced imaging, and multimodal data analysis.*

| Technology | Description | Impact |
|---|---|---|
| AI-Driven Fetal Echo cardiography | Machine learning algorithms automate the identification of cardiac views and the measurement of anatomical structures in ultrasound images. | Standardizes diagnosis, improves detection rates of critical CHD (CCHD) to 97.59%, and reduces operator dependency. |
| Integrated Data Platforms | Combines maternal health records, genetic data, and imaging results for risk stratification. | Enhances early detection of high-risk pregnancies (maternal diabetes, advanced age) and predicts CHD with 86–92% accuracy. |
| Advanced Genetic Screening | Non-invasive prenatal testing (NIPT) and chromosomal microarray analysis (CMA) for detecting 22q11.2 deletions and trisomies. | Identifies 25.62% of CHD cases linked to chromosomal abnormalities prenatally. |
| Portable Ultrasound Devices | Handheld tools with AI-assisted image interpretation for low-resource settings. | Increases accessibility to early screening, in rural areas. |

## CONCLUSION

The burden of congenital heart disease in low- and middle-income countries (LMICs) is heavily influenced by social determinants of health, including socioeconomic status, geographic access to care, education, insurance availability, maternal age, and health infrastructure. LMICs have the highest global CHD incidence and mortality rates, limited access to advanced diagnostics and care, and are projected to see a sharp increase in disability burden over the coming decades. Addressing

SDOH is essential for improving outcomes and equity in CHD care. The integration of DOHaD and SDOH frameworks provides a comprehensive understanding of CHD development and outcomes that extends beyond traditional biomedical approaches. CHD emerges as a condition fundamentally shaped by complex interactions between early-life environmental programming and multilevel social determinants operating across the life course. Environmental exposures during critical developmental windows, the periconceptional period, significantly influence CHD risk through epigenetic programming mechanisms. Genetic susceptibility interacts with environmental and social factors, suggesting that precision approaches must consider both biological and social risk factors.

Disparities in CHD outcomes reflect broader patterns of social inequity, requiring interventions that address upstream social determinants alongside clinical care. Proposals for improvement include initiatives for local capacity building, outreach care, policy reforms to address socioeconomic disparities, and integration of SDOH screening into clinical pathways. Key gaps remain in universal access, early screening and high-quality care for LMIC children with CHD. Addressing the global burden of CHD requires comprehensive approaches that integrate clinical excellence with social justice, environmental protection, and health equity. Policies addressing the social determinants of health, environmental regulations protecting reproductive health, and healthcare systems designed to provide equitable access to high-quality care across all populations.

## REFERENCES


Ananthakumar, B., Nagaraja, B. G., Umesh, S. M., & Raghavan, R. (2025). Predictive Medicine. *Predictive Algorithms for Rehabilitation and Assistive Systems*, 291–314. https://doi.org/DOI: 10.4018/979-8-3373-0194-5.ch011

Ananthakumar, B., Nanjundeshwara, N., Lakshmaiah, A., & Raghavan, R. (2024). Synthetic Gene Circuits as a Promising Approach in Cancer Immunotherapy. *Critical Developments in Cancer Immunotherapy*, 391–418. https://doi.org/DOI: 10.4018/979-8-3693-3976-3.ch011

Belhadjer, Z., Pontailler, M., Hily, M., Gaudin, R., Raisky, O., Bonnet, D., & Houyel, L. (2025). The particular anatomy of atrioventricular septal defect with a common valvar orifice in patients with Down syndrome: An echocardiographic study. *International Journal of Cardiology*, *423*. Advance online publication. DOI: 10.1016/j.ijcard.2025.133003 PMID: 39892564

Bhuvana, G. N., Umesh, S. M., & Raghavan, R. (2025). Expanding the frontiers of Schistosomiasis Treatment: The promise of Nanoparticle-Based Therapies. *Journal of Vector Borne Diseases, 10*(4103/jvbd.jvbd_180_23). https://doi.org/DOI: 10.4103/jvbd.jvbd_180_23

Biradar, S., Suresh, C., Nanjundeshwara, N., & Raghavan, R. (2025). Spatially Variable Genes. *Spatially Variable Genes in Cancer*, 1–28. https://doi.org/DOI: 10.4018/979-8-3693-7728-4.ch001

Byalahunasishetter, B. I., N., V., P., S., C., M., S., S., & Raghavan, R. (2025). Spatial Omics and Bioprinting. *Innovations in Precision Medicine and Genomics*, 85–110. https://doi.org/DOI: 10.4018/979-8-3693-5787-3.ch003

Choudhury, T. Z., Gilbert, B. L., & Garg, V. (2025). Genetic and Environmental Contributors To Congenital Heart Disease. *Current Treatment Options in Cardiovascular Medicine*, *27*(1), 36. DOI: 10.1007/s11936-025-01091-5 PMID: 40438121

Crook, S., Dragan, K., Woo, J. L., Neidell, M., Nash, K. A., Jiang, P., Zhang, Y., Sanchez, C. M., Cook, S., Hannan, E. L., Newburger, J. W., Jacobs, M. L., Petit, C. J., Goldstone, A., Vincent, R., Walsh-Spoonhower, K., Mosca, R., Kumar, T. K. S., & Devejian, N., … The New York State Congenital Heart Surgery Collaborative for Longitudinal Outcomes & Utilization of Resources (CHS-COLOUR). (2024). Impact of Social Determinants of Health on Predictive Models for Outcomes After Congenital Heart Surgery. *Journal of the American College of Cardiology*, *83*(24), 2440–2454. DOI: 10.1016/j.jacc.2024.03.430 PMID: 38866447

Dolk, H., McCullough, N., Callaghan, S., Casey, F., Craig, B., Given, J., Loane, M., Lagan, B. M., Bunting, B., Boyle, B., & Dabir, T. (2020). Risk factors for congenital heart disease: The Baby Hearts Study, a population-based case-control study. *PLoS One, 15*(2), e0227908. DOI: 10.1371/journal.pone.0227908 PMID: 32092068

Garcia, Y. E., Sjögren, B., & Osei-Owusu, P. (2025). G protein regulation by RGS proteins in the pathophysiology of dilated cardiomyopathy. *American Journal of Physiology. Heart and Circulatory Physiology, 328*(2), H348–H360. DOI: 10.1152/ajpheart.00653.2024 PMID: 39772618

Gupta, R., Joshi, P., Mohan, V., Reddy, K. S., & Yusuf, S. (2008). Social determinants of cardiovascular disease outcomes in Indians: The CREATE registry. *European Heart Journal, 29*(5), 668–675. DOI: 10.1093/eurheartj/ehm635

GVS, A. C., Ananthakumar, B., & Raghavan, R. (2025). Enhancing Assistive Technologies With Neuromorphic Computing. *Revolutionizing AI with Brain-Inspired Technology: Neuromorphic Computing*, 207–232. https://doi.org/DOI: 10.4018/979-8-3693-6303-4.ch009

Hikspoors, J. P. J. M., Kruepunga, N., Mommen, G. M. C., Köhler, S. E., Anderson, R. H., & Lamers, W. H. (2022). A pictorial account of the human embryonic heart between 3.5 and 8 weeks of development. *Communications Biology, 5*(1), 226. DOI: 10.1038/s42003-022-03153-x PMID: 35277594

Izquierdo-Condoy, J. S., Arias-Rodríguez, F. D., Díaz-Chamba, W. I., Mena-Noroña, D. A., Toaquiza, L. C., Espín-Sambache, B., Valdivieso-Andrade, E. J., Cangas-Isacaz, A., García-Cañarte, S., Rubio-Niera, M., & Ortiz-Prado, E. (2025). Epidemiological characterization of congenital heart disease at different altitudes in Ecuador: A four-year retrospective study in a pediatric referral hospital. *Frontiers in Public Health, 13*. Advance online publication. DOI: 10.3389/fpubh.2025.1497253 PMID: 39944066

Jin, S., Yoon, S. Z., Choi, Y. J., Kang, G., & Choi, S. U. (2024). Prenatal exposure to air pollutants and the risk of congenital heart disease: A Korean national health insurance database-based study. *Scientific Reports, 14*(1), 16940. DOI: 10.1038/s41598-024-63150-4 PMID: 39043676

Jonas, R. A. (2025). Twenty-five-year milestone for the ECHSA database: Time to focus on patient survival rather than procedural success. *European Journal of Cardio-Thoracic Surgery, 67*(4), ezaf136. Advance online publication. DOI: 10.1093/ejcts/ezaf136 PMID: 40220325

Kalisch-Smith, J. I., Ved, N., & Sparrow, D. B. (2020). Environmental Risk Factors for Congenital Heart Disease. *Cold Spring Harbor Perspectives in Biology*, *12*(3), a037234. DOI: 10.1101/cshperspect.a037234 PMID: 31548181

Kelly, R. G. (2023). The heart field transcriptional landscape at single-cell resolution. *Developmental Cell*, *58*(4), 257–266. DOI: 10.1016/j.devcel.2023.01.010 PMID: 36809764

Krishnan, U., Dhurandhar, V., & Joshi, S. (2025). Clinical profile and outcome of pediatric heart surgeries at a tertiary care center. *Frontiers in Pediatrics*, *13*, 1543755. DOI: 10.3389/fped.2025.1543755 PMID: 40464041

Kukshal, P., Joshi, R. O., Kumar, A., Ahamad, S., Murthy, P. R., Sathe, Y., Manohar, K., Guhathakurta, S., & Chellappan, S. (2023). Case–control association study of congenital heart disease from a tertiary paediatric cardiac centre from North India. *BMC Pediatrics*, *23*(1), 290. DOI: 10.1186/s12887-023-04095-x PMID: 37322441

Lakshmaiah, A., Korrapati, C., Suresh, C., & Raghavan, R. (2025). Synthetic Biology and AI. *Spatially Variable Genes in Cancer*, 265–290. https://doi.org/DOI: 10.4018/979-8-3693-7728-4.ch010

Nagashri, N., Archana, L., & Raghavan, R. (2024). Microbial Volatile Compounds (MVOCs) in Food Industries and Food Safety Applications. *Innovations, Securities, and Case Studies Across Healthcare, Business, and Technology*, 75–96. https://doi .org/DOI: 10.4018/979-8-3693-1906-2.ch005

Nanjundeshwara, N., Lakshmaiah, A., & Raghavan, R. (2025). Aflatoxigenic Fungi. *Aflatoxigenic Fungi*, 225–239. https://doi.org/DOI: 10.1201/9781003487043-29

Nusrat, A., & Wu, M. (2025). Epicardium-myocardium crosstalk orchestrates heart development. *Frontiers in Cell and Developmental Biology*, *13*. Advance online publication. DOI: 10.3389/fcell.2025.1655878 PMID: 41070347

P., A., D., K. M., M., J., P., S., & Raghavan, R. (2025). The Cancer Exposome. *Cancer Exposomics and Environmental Influences on Carcinogenesis*, 161–192. https://doi.org/DOI: 10.4018/979-8-3373-2165-3.ch004

Raghavan, R., & Ahamad, S. (2025). Developmental Origins of Health and Disease. *Cancer Exposomics and Environmental Influences on Carcinogenesis*, 1–34. https:// doi.org/DOI: 10.4018/979-8-3373-2165-3.ch001

Raghavan, R., Moger, S. S., Umesh, S., & Bhuvana, G. N. (2025). Revolutionizing Pain Management. *Unveiling Technological Advancements and Interdisciplinary Solutions for Pain Care*, 129–164. https://doi.org/DOI: 10.4018/979-8-3693-9501-1.ch005

Ramírez-Fuentes, T. C., Jaime-Cruz, R., Patiño-Morales, C. C., Villavicencio-Guzmán, L., Corona, J. C., Revilla-Monsalve, M. C., Jarillo-Luna, R. A., & Salazar-García, M. (2025). Morphological Alterations of Conal Ridges and Differential Expression of AP2α in the Offspring Hearts of Experimental Diabetic Rats. *International Journal of Molecular Sciences*, *26*(11), 5061. DOI: 10.3390/ijms26115061 PMID: 40507872

S., G. V., C., A., Biradar, S., & Raghavan, R. (2025). Neuroscience-Driven Solutions for Speech Impairment. *Advancing Medical Research Through Neuroscience*, 119–146. https://doi.org/DOI: 10.4018/979-8-3693-5464-3.ch006

Safi-Stibler, S., & Gabory, A. (2020). Epigenetics and the Developmental Origins of Health and Disease: Parental environment signalling to the epigenome, critical time windows and sculpting the adult phenotype. *Seminars in Cell & Developmental Biology*, *97*, 172–180. DOI: 10.1016/j.semcdb.2019.09.008 PMID: 31587964

Soliman, O., Acharya, Y., Gilard, M., Duffy, G., Wijns, W., Kannan, V., & Sultan, S. (2024). Systematic review of cardiovascular neurocristopathy—Contemporary insights and future perspectives. *Frontiers in Cardiovascular Medicine*, *11*. Advance online publication. DOI: 10.3389/fcvm.2024.1333265 PMID: 38660479

Solovieva, T., & Bronner, M. E. (2025). Congenital heart defects differ following left versus right avian cardiac neural crest ablation. *Developmental Biology*, *519*, 30–37. DOI: 10.1016/j.ydbio.2024.12.003 PMID: 39667652

Tran, R., Forman, R., Mossialos, E., Nasir, K., & Kulkarni, A. (2022). Social Determinants of Disparities in Mortality Outcomes in Congenital Heart Disease: A Systematic Review and Meta-Analysis. *Frontiers in Cardiovascular Medicine*, *9*, 829902. DOI: 10.3389/fcvm.2022.829902 PMID: 35369346

Tyagi, R., Verma, S., Dash, N., Attri, S. V., Sankhyan, N., & Rohit, M. K. (2022). Folate deficiency: A possible association with congenital heart defects. *Indian Journal of Pediatrics*, *89*, 1013–1015. DOI: 10.1007/s12098-022-04125-z PMID: 35175552

Vey, C., Melnik, N., Dombrowsky, G., & Hitz, M.-P. (2025). Current and future diagnostics of congenital heart disease (CHD). *Medizinische Genetik : Mitteilungsblatt des Berufsverbandes Medizinische Genetik e.V*, *37*(2), 95–102. DOI: 10.1515/medgen-2025-2008 PMID: 40207043

Vrijheid, M., Martinez, D., Manzanares, S., Dadvand, P., Schembari, A., Rankin, J., & Nieuwenhuijsen, M. (2021). Association between parents' socioeconomic conditions and risk of congenital heart defects in offspring: A systematic review and meta-analysis. *Journal of Epidemiology and Community Health*, *75*(11), 1091–1099. DOI: 10.1136/jech-2020-216034 PMID: 33980719

Wells, B. K., Garramone, G. K., Mahomed, A., & Ezin, M. (2025). Teratogenic Effects of Serotonin Receptor 2B Disruption on the Migration and Cardiac Derivatives of the Cardiac Neural Crest. *Birth Defects Research, 117*(7), e2506. DOI: 10.1002/bdr2.2506 PMID: 40667631

Wen, H., Chandrasekaran, P., Jin, A., Pankin, J., Lu, M., Liberti, D. C., Zepp, J. A., Jain, R., Morrisey, E. E., Michki, S. N., & Frank, D. B. (2025). A spatiotemporal cell atlas of cardiopulmonary progenitor cell allocation during development. *Cell Reports, 44*(4). Advance online publication. DOI: 10.1016/j.celrep.2025.115513 PMID: 40178979

Wolton, M., Davey, M. G., & Dietrich, S. (2025). At early stages of heart development, the first and second heart fields are a continuum of lateral head mesoderm-derived, cardiogenic cells. *Developmental Biology, 520*, 200–223. DOI: 10.1016/j.ydbio.2025.01.009 PMID: 39848483

Xu, J., Li, Q., Deng, L., Xiong, J., Cheng, Z., & Ye, C. (2025). Global, regional, and national epidemiology of congenital heart disease in children from 1990 to 2021. *Frontiers in Cardiovascular Medicine, 12*. Advance online publication. DOI: 10.3389/fcvm.2025.1522644 PMID: 40454242

Yasuhara, J., Bigelow, A. M., & Garg, V. (2025). Genetics of Congenital Heart Disease. *Clinics in Perinatology, 52*(3), 589–608. DOI: 10.1016/j.clp.2025.06.010 PMID: 40850718

Ye, X., Li, M., Meng, Y., Duan, S., Zhang, S., & Zhong, K. (2025). D-tetramethrin induces cardiac looping failure in zebrafish during embryonic development. *Comparative Biochemistry and Physiology. Toxicology & Pharmacology : CBP, 294*, 110193. DOI: 10.1016/j.cbpc.2025.110193 PMID: 40086682

Zachariah, J. P., Jone, P.-N., Agbaje, A. O., Ryan, H. H., Trasande, L., Perng, W., & Farzan, S. F.American Heart Association Council on Lifelong Congenital Heart Disease and Heart Health in the Young; Council on Cardiovascular and Stroke Nursing; Council on Epidemiology and Prevention; Council on Lifestyle and Cardiometabolic Health; and Council on Clinical Cardiology. (2024). Environmental Exposures and Pediatric Cardiology: A Scientific Statement From the American Heart Association. *Circulation, 149*(20), e1165–e1175. DOI: 10.1161/CIR.0000000000001234 PMID: 38618723

Zaidi, A. H., Alberts, A., Chowdhury, D., Beaty, C., Brewer, B., Chen, M. H., & de Ferranti, S. D. (2024). Trends in Gaps of Care for Patients With Congenital Heart Disease: Implications for Social Determinants of Health and Child Opportunity Index. *Journal of the American Heart Association, 13*(20), e034796. DOI: 10.1161/JAHA.124.034796 PMID: 39377195

Zaqout, M., Aslem, E., Abuqamar, M., Wolf, D., & Backer, J. (2021). The impact of oral folic acid supplementation on the prevention of congenital heart defects: A systematic review and meta-analysis. *Nutrients, 13*(11), 4003. DOI: 10.3390/nu13114003 PMID: 34836257

# Chapter 2
# Association of Gene Polymorphisms With Neonatal Anomalies and Tumor Risks in CHD Patients

**Duygu Aygunes Jafari**
https://orcid.org/0000-0003-4756-7365
*Faculty of Medicine, Ege University, Turkey*

## ABSTRACT

*Gene polymorphisms involved in cardiac development are increasingly recognized as key contributors to congenital heart disease (CHD), often co-occurring with neonatal anomalies and malignancy risk. Disruptions in developmental pathways such as RAS/MAPK, Notch, and Wnt not only affect cardiac morphogenesis but also exert pleiotropic effects across multiple organ systems. Syndromic CHDs, including Noonan, Alagille, and 22q11.2 deletion syndromes, demonstrate well-established links between specific genetic variants, structural anomalies, and elevated cancer susceptibility. Non-syndromic CHD genes, such as NKX2-5, GATA4, and TBX20, typically lead to isolated cardiac defects, though emerging evidence suggests subtle associations with oncogenic processes. Polygenic risk, copy number variations, and gene–environment interactions further complicate the genetic landscape. Understanding these interrelated mechanisms supports the integration of genomic data into early diagnosis, clinical management, and personalized surveillance strategies for both cardiac and oncologic outcomes.*

DOI: 10.4018/979-8-3373-3735-7.ch002

# I. INTRODUCTION

Congenital heart disease (CHD) is the most common congenital anomaly, occurring in approximately 0.8;1.2% of live births (Lahm et al., 2021). Advances in medical and surgical care have markedly improved survival, yielding a growing population of adults with repaired CHD. However, CHD often co-occurs with anomalies in other organ systems and neurodevelopmental disorders, reflecting shared developmental pathways. For instance, about 13% of infants with CHD have one or more extra-cardiac congenital anomalies (such as renal, gastrointestinal, or musculoskeletal defects), almost twice the prevalence in infants without CHD (Homsy et al., 2015). These may include "neonatal anomalies" like limb malformations or gastrointestinal atresias that co-present with CHD. Moreover, neurodevelopmental disorders (NDD) (encompassing cognitive, motor, and social impairments) are diagnosed in ~10% of children with CHD overall, and in up to 50% of those with complex CHD requiring neonatal surgery. Such statistics underscore that CHD often represents a broader developmental phenotype rather than an isolated cardiac problem (Homsy et al., 2015).

Genetic factors play a significant etiologic role in CHD, but for the majority of patients the cause is multifactorial. Identifiable genetic mutations or chromosomal abnormalities underlie an estimated 20;30% of CHD cases (Pierpont et al., 2018). Specifically, ~3;5% of CHDs are due to single-gene (Mendelian) mutations and ~8;10% are associated with gross chromosomal aneuploidies or pathogenic copy number variants (CNVs) (Pierpont et al., 2018). The remaining cases are likely caused by a combination of polygenic susceptibilities and gene;environment interactions. Indeed, environmental teratogens and maternal conditions substantially influence CHD risk. Maternal pregestational diabetes mellitus, for instance, confers about a 4-fold increased risk of CHD in the offspring (Øyen et al., 2016). Other maternal factors such as rubella infection, phenylketonuria, obesity, and exposure to certain medications or chemicals (e.g. retinoids or alcohol) are well-established contributors to CHD risk. Importantly, the impact of environmental factors often depends on fetal genotype and the timing of exposure during cardiogenesis. Experimental evidence in animal models demonstrates these gene;environment interactions: for instance, brief gestational hypoxia significantly increased the incidence and severity of cardiac defects in mouse embryos heterozygous for Tbx1 or Fgfr1/2 mutations, and caused embryonic demise in those heterozygous for Nkx2-5, whereas wild-type littermates were relatively unaffected (Moreau et al., 2019). This finding suggests that a genetically susceptible cardiac developmental program can be "unmasked" by environmental stress, providing a mechanistic basis for the multifactorial inheritance models often observed in human CHD.

Tumor risks in CHD patients have historically been less appreciated than developmental anomalies, but emerging data indicate intriguing links between the molecular genetics of heart development and oncogenesis. Certain genetic syndromes and mutations that cause CHD also confer elevated risks of malignancy (e.g. childhood leukemia or solid tumors) due to overlapping pathways in organogenesis and cell proliferation control. Several studies have indicated that survivors of congenital heart disease (CHD), even in the absence of syndromic diagnoses, may face a modestly increased long-term risk of cancer compared with the general population. This excess risk has been attributed to underlying genetic predispositions as well as sequelae of CHD therapies, such as exposure to radiation (Lakshmanan & Gimelli, 2023). The present chapter examines these interconnections in detail. The discussion begins with syndromic forms of CHD, in which single-gene mutations or chromosomal abnormalities generate a spectrum of cardiac and extra-cardiac malformations that often coincide with defined tumor susceptibilities. Attention is then directed to non-syndromic CHD genes, particularly transcription factors and signaling molecules that are critical for cardiac morphogenesis but may also exert subtler pleiotropic effects predisposing to malignancy. Subsequent sections review chromosomal abnormalities and copy number variations (CNVs) frequently associated with CHD, highlighting their links to neonatal anomalies and oncogenic processes. Consideration is also given to polygenic and oligogenic contributions to CHD, including evidence from genome-wide association studies (GWAS), polygenic risk score applications, and models of digenic inheritance. Emerging insights from transcriptomic profiling, including bulk and single-cell RNA sequencing, are summarized to illustrate pathogenic gene expression programs and "fetalization" patterns implicated in CHD. The chapter concludes by addressing the clinical translation of these genomic insights, encompassing improved diagnostic strategies, personalized patient management, surveillance for associated tumor risks, and ethical considerations.

Table 1 provides an overview of several key gene polymorphisms implicated in syndromic CHD, highlighting their cardiac phenotypes, associated neonatal anomalies, and tumor risks.

*Table 1. Syndromic CHD Gene Polymorphisms with Associated Anomalies and Tumor Risks*

| Gene/ Region | Notable Variant | CHD Phenotype | Neonatal Anomalies | Tumor Risks | Relative Risk |
|---|---|---|---|---|---|
| PTPN11 (Noonan syndrome) | c.922A>G, p.Asn308Asp (gain-of-function) | Pulmonary valve stenosis; hypertrophic cardiomyopathy | Short stature, facial dysmorphism, skeletal anomalies | Juvenile myelomonocytic leukemia (JMML); neuroblastoma | ~10;15% lifetime cancer risk in mutation-positive Noonan (Ney et al., 2022) |
| JAG1 (Alagille syndrome) | c.2740C>T, p.Pro914Leu (loss-of-function); also large deletions | Peripheral pulmonary artery stenosis; tetralogy of Fallot | Cholestatic liver disease (bile duct paucity), butterfly vertebrae, characteristic facial features | Hepatocellular carcinoma (HCC) and hepatoblastoma (in context of chronic liver disease | Elevated HCC risk: surveillance recommended by adolescence (Spinner et al., 2000/2024) |
| TBX5 (Holt-Oram syndrome) | Various loss-of-function mutations (haploinsufficiency) | Atrial septal defect (ASD) ± ventricular septal defect; conduction block | Radial ray malformations of upper limbs (thumb aplasia/ hypoplasia) | *No strong cancer predisposition* (isolated case reports of cancers; not statistically elevated) | ; |
| 22q11.2 deletion (DiGeorge syndrome) | 3 Mb hemizygous deletion (de novo or inherited) | Conotruncal defects (e.g. truncus arteriosus, tetralogy of Fallot) | Thymic hypoplasia (immune deficiency), cleft palate, hypocalcemia | T-cell acute lymphoblastic leukemia; thymoma (thymic epithelial tumor) ; rare cases in adulthood (moderate risk elevation) | Standardized incidence ~5;10× for thymic malignancies (data limited) |
| Trisomy 21 (Down syndrome) | Full or mosaic third copy of chr21 | Atrioventricular septal defect (complete AV canal) in ~40%; VSD or ASD in others | Characteristic dysmorphic features, hypotonia; duodenal atresia; hematologic abnormalities (transient leukemia) | Acute lymphoblastic and myeloid leukemias (especially acute megakaryoblastic leukemia in infancy) | ~10;30× increased risk of childhood leukemia; ~1;2% cumulative incidence by age 5 (Linabery et al., 2008 |

Representative syndromic conditions are outlined in Table 1, where single-gene mutations or chromosomal abnormalities give rise to congenital heart disease in combination with systemic features and tumor predispositions. These examples underscore recurring themes developed throughout the chapter: developmental regulators such as transcription factors and signaling molecules, while critical for embryonic heart morphogenesis, also function across multiple tissues, accounting for the broad clinical spectrum. Their disruption not only produces multi-organ phenotypes but may also establish a cellular milieu conducive to oncogenesis, often through pathways such as RAS/MAPK or via inactivation of tumor suppressor mechanisms. The following sections explore these syndromic entities in greater depth.

## II. SYNDROMIC FORMS OF CONGENITAL HEART DISEASE

Syndromic CHD refers to heart defects that occur as part of a broader genetic syndrome, typically caused by pathogenic variants in a single gene or a cytogenetic abnormality. In these conditions, cardiac malformations are one feature among a characteristic constellation of clinical findings (dysmorphic features, organ anomalies, developmental delays, etc.), and importantly, some syndromes carry elevated tumor risks. Below it is discussed that several well-known syndromic CHDs, including Noonan syndrome, Alagille syndrome, Holt-Oram syndrome, and others, illustrating how specific gene polymorphisms produce combined cardiac and extra-cardiac phenotypes.

### Noonan Syndrome (RASopathies)

Noonan syndrome is a prominent example of a syndromic CHD with an identifiable monogenic cause. It is an autosomal dominant condition with an estimated incidence of ~1 in 2,000 live births (Ney et al., 2022). Mutations in genes of the RAS/MAPK signaling pathway underlie Noonan syndrome; most commonly PTPN11 (50% of cases), and less frequently SOS1, RAF1, RIT1, KRAS, among others (Tartaglia et al., 2010). These gain-of-function mutations lead to hyperactivation of RAS signaling, which perturbs embryonic development in multiple organ systems. Cardiac anomalies are present in the majority of individuals with Noonan. The classic heart defect is pulmonary valve stenosis (often with dysplastic pulmonary valve), seen in up to 50;60% of patients, sometimes accompanied by hypertrophic cardiomyopathy (in ~20%). Other cardiac findings can include septal defects or branch pulmonary artery stenosis.

Noonan syndrome patients also exhibit distinctive neonatal anomalies such as short stature, pectus excavatum, and characteristic craniofacial dysmorphisms (hypertelorism, down-slanting palpebral fissures, low-set posteriorly rotated ears). Developmental delays or learning difficulties are observed in a subset. Of particular interest, Noonan syndrome exemplifies the link between developmental pathway mutations and tumorigenesis. Germline RAS pathway mutations confer a modest but significant cancer predisposition. Studies focusing on PTPN11-associated Noonan syndrome found an overall malignancy risk of roughly 8;12%, with especially elevated incidence of juvenile myelomonocytic leukemia (JMML) in early childhood (Ney et al., 2022). This leukemia risk is highest in specific *PTPN11* mutant genotypes (e.g. p.Gly60 or p.Thr73 variants) known to trigger myeloproliferation (Ney et al., 2022). Other reported tumors include neuroblastoma, acute lymphoblastic leukemia (ALL), and certain solid tumors (rhabdomyosarcoma and low-grade brain tumors) (Ney et al., 2022), though these occur less frequently than hematologic malignancies. The RAS/MAPK pathway's central role in cell growth likely explains this spectrum: the same hyperactive signaling that perturbs cardiac morphogenesis also predisposes to uncontrolled proliferation in hematopoietic or neural crest-derived cells (Ney et al., 2022). As a result, clinical management of Noonan and related RASopathies (e.g. Costello, Cardiofaciocutaneous syndromes) now includes tumor surveillance protocols, such as periodic blood counts in infancy and ultrasound screening for neuroblastoma in certain high-risk genotypes (Ney et al., 2022). Noonan syndrome thus illustrates how a gene polymorphism (here, PTPN11 or other RAS-pathway gene mutation) can produce both CHD (via developmental effects on the heart) and increase tumor risk (via oncogenic signaling) in the same patients.

## Alagille Syndrome

Alagille syndrome (ALGS) is an autosomal dominant multisystem disorder caused by heterozygous loss-of-function variants in JAG1 (Jagged1) in ~90% of cases, or less commonly NOTCH2, both genes encoding components of the Notch signaling pathway. Alagille has a prevalence of roughly 1 in 30,000;50,000 live births. The syndrome's primary features include chronic cholestatic liver disease due to bile duct paucity, cardiac defects, characteristic facies, ocular embryotoxon, and vertebral anomalies. Cardiac involvement occurs in up to 94% of Alagille patients (Spinner et al., 2000/2024). The most common lesion is pulmonary artery stenosis, often involving peripheral branches (seen in ~67% (Spinner et al., 2000/2024)). More complex CHDs like tetralogy of Fallot (TOF) occur in 7;16% of patients (Spinner et al., 2000/2024), making Alagille one of the notable single-gene causes of TOF. These cardiac findings reflect the importance of JAG1/Notch signaling in neural crest and second heart field contributions to the outflow tract and arteries.

Beyond the heart, neonatal and childhood anomalies in Alagille syndrome include hepatic insufficiency (cholestasis with jaundice and pruritus), which can lead to cirrhosis, butterfly vertebrae (segmentation defects of the spine), renal dysplasia, growth retardation, and characteristic facial features (prominent forehead, deep-set eyes). The chronic liver injury in Alagille has significant implications for tumor risk: ALGS patients are recognized to have an elevated risk of hepatocellular carcinoma (HCC) and hepatoblastoma in childhood and early adulthood (Spinner et al., 2000/2024). Notably, HCC has been documented even in some young Alagille patients without advanced cirrhosis (Spinner et al., 2000/2024), prompting recommendations for periodic liver ultrasound screening in this population (Kamath *et al.*, 2018). The mechanism is thought to involve the combination of persistent cholestatic injury (driving regenerative proliferation) and haploinsufficiency of JAG1/NOTCH2, which may alter cellular differentiation in the liver. Apart from liver cancer, there is not a strong known association of Alagille syndrome with other malignancies. Nonetheless, the Jagged/Notch pathway is a known oncogenic driver in many tissues, and research is ongoing to determine if subtle cancer risks exist. In summary, Alagille syndrome demonstrates how disruption of a developmental signaling pathway can produce CHD alongside specific end-organ anomalies (liver, skeleton) and how secondary effects (cirrhosis) can translate into increased cancer susceptibility (HCC). Early genetic diagnosis of Alagille is important not only for managing cholestasis and heart lesions but also for anticipating complications like HCC, enabling timely transplant evaluation or surveillance.

## Holt-Oram Syndrome

Holt-Oram syndrome (HOS) exemplifies a heart;hand syndrome, linking upper limb malformations with cardiac septation defects. It is caused by heterozygous loss-of-function mutations in TBX5, a T-box transcription factor crucial for both anterior limb and cardiac development. Holt-Oram is inherited in an autosomal dominant pattern (often new mutations) with an incidence around 1 in 100,000. Cardinal features are skeletal abnormalities of the thumbs and forearms (triphalangeal or absent thumb, radial ray aplasia, short forearm) and CHD, classically an atrial septal defect (ASD) or atrioventricular septal defect. Approximately 75% of HOS patients have an ASD (usually ostium secundum) or VSD, and many also have cardiac conduction disease (e.g. AV block or sinus node dysfunction) due to TBX5's role in the cardiac conduction system (National Organization for Rare Disorders [NORD], 2020). Neonates with Holt-Oram can often be identified by their limb anomalies, prompting cardiac evaluation. Unlike Noonan or Alagille, Holt-Oram syndrome is largely limited to heart and limb phenotypes, with little involvement of other organs. Neurodevelopment is typically normal, and there are no metabolic or hepatic components.

Correspondingly, cancer predisposition is not a recognized feature of Holt-Oram syndrome. TBX5 is not a known tumor suppressor or oncogene in the germline context (though interestingly, somatic TBX5 alterations have been investigated in cancers like acute leukemia). A single case report described a Holt-Oram patient who developed early-onset prostate cancer, speculating on TBX5's role in tumor biology (Aherne et al., 2013), but population data do not indicate any significant increase in malignancy among HOS patients. Thus, Holt-Oram is an example where a gene polymorphism has *highly specific developmental effects* (the upper limb and septal structures) with no broad syndrome or cancer syndrome beyond those systems. In the context of this chapter, HOS serves to contrast with other syndromic CHDs: it underscores that not all CHD genes confer tumor risk; the effects depend on the gene's pathway. TBX5 primarily regulates transcriptional programs in heart and limb morphogenesis (Chen et al., 2021); it does not appear to be implicated in cell-cycle control or DNA repair that would tie it to oncogenesis. Clinically, management of Holt-Oram focuses on orthopedic interventions for limb function and cardiac defect repair or pacemaker placement for conduction block. Genetic counseling is important due to autosomal dominant transmission, but no special tumor surveillance is indicated beyond routine care.

## Other Syndromic CHDs

In addition to Noonan, Alagille, and Holt-Oram, numerous other genetic syndromes feature CHD as part of their phenotype. A few noteworthy examples include:

- Chromosome 22q11.2 Deletion Syndrome (DiGeorge/Velocardiofacial syndrome): A microdeletion of 22q11.2 that causes conotruncal CHD (especially tetralogy of Fallot, interrupted aortic arch) in ~75% of cases, along with thymic aplasia (T-cell immunodeficiency), parathyroid hypoplasia (hypocalcemia), cleft palate, and characteristic facial features. This syndrome is discussed in Section IV below. Of note, adults with 22q11.2 deletion have a slightly elevated incidence of certain cancers, such as thyroid carcinoma and possibly thymomas, thought to be related to immune dysfunction or haploinsufficiency of tumor suppressor genes on 22q (Liu et al., 2024).
- CHARGE Syndrome: Caused by dominant CHD7 mutations, CHARGE includes Coloboma of the eye, Heart defects (often TOF, AVSD), Atresia of choanae, Retarded growth/development, Genital anomalies, Ear abnormalities/deafness. Tumor risk is not significantly elevated in CHARGE, but the multi-system anomalies (especially choanal atresia and ear defects) cause considerable morbidity.
- Williams-Beuren Syndrome: A deletion at 7q11.23 including the ELN gene, leading to supravalvular aortic stenosis and other arterial stenoses, distinctive cognitive/personality traits (over-friendliness, verbal strength), and hypercalcemia. No known increased cancer risk is associated with Williams syndrome, illustrating again that not all developmental genes tie into tumor pathways.
- Rubenstein-Taybi Syndrome: Caused by mutations in CREBBP or EP300 (genes encoding histone acetylase proteins). Patients have CHD (~1/3 of cas-

es, various types), broad thumbs, facial dysmorphism, and intellectual disability. There is an elevated risk of certain tumors (e.g. leukemia and lymphoma) in Rubenstein-Taybi, likely due to the global role of CREBBP/EP300 in transcriptional regulation and cell cycle control.

These examples reinforce that syndromic CHDs arise from mutations that perturb fundamental developmental processes. Depending on the gene's functions, the resulting syndrome may involve a wide spectrum of anomalies and possibly cancer predisposition. In clinical practice, recognizing a syndromic pattern in a newborn with CHD is critical: it should prompt genetic testing (e.g. chromosomal microarray or targeted gene panel) to confirm the diagnosis. Identifying a syndrome can significantly alter management; for instance, in Noonan syndrome one might be vigilant for coagulopathies and leukemia; in 22q11.2 deletion, one must address immunodeficiency and avoid live vaccines; in Alagille, one manages liver disease and screens for HCC. Thus, understanding the genetic polymorphisms behind syndromic CHD has tangible benefits for comprehensive care. The subsequent section addresses non-syndromic CHD, characterized by genetic variants that primarily influence cardiac development without producing a complete syndromic phenotype, although even in this context subtle associations with additional anomalies and disease risks have been documented.

## III. NON-SYNDROMIC CHD GENETICS

Non-syndromic CHD refers to heart defects that occur in isolation (or with only minor extra-cardiac findings), often in otherwise phenotypically normal individuals. In many such cases, CHD can still be traced to specific gene mutations or risk variants, but these genetic changes do not cause broad syndromic effects. Instead, they preferentially disrupt cardiac developmental pathways. Discoveries over the past two decades have identified numerous transcription factors, signaling molecules, and structural proteins as critical for heart formation; pathogenic variants in these genes can lead to CHD in the absence of other major malformations. This section highlights a few key genes frequently implicated in non-syndromic CHD (e.g. NKX2-5, GATA4, TBX20, CTNNB1), their typical inheritance patterns, and any ancillary phenotypic or clinical associations (such as arrhythmia or later health risks).

Table 2 provides a summary of selected non-syndromic CHD genes and their associated cardiac lesions. The subsequent discussion highlights representative examples and evaluates potential connections between these CHD-related genes and tumor biology.

*Table 2. Representative Non-Syndromic CHD Genes and Associated Cardiac/ Clinical Features*

| Gene | Inheritance | Typical CHD Phenotypes | Other Features | Comments |
|---|---|---|---|---|
| NKX2-5 | Autosomal Dominant (familial) | Atrial septal defect (secundum ASD); AV block; sometimes Tetralogy of Fallot | Progressive conduction disease (AV block) in adulthood (Običan & Maggio, 2018) | High penetrance; NKX2-5 mutations often familial with variable severity |
| GATA4 | Autosomal Dominant (haploinsufficient) | Atrial and ventricular septal defects (ASD/ VSD); endocardial cushion defects (AV canal) (Mattapally et al., 2015) | Occasional mild extracardiac anomalies (e.g. renal), but often isolated CHD | GATA4 mutation G296S causes septal defects and pulmonary stenosis; interacts with TBX5 (Misra et al., 2012) |
| TBX20 | Autosomal Dominant (haploinsufficient or dominant-negative) | Diverse CHDs: ASD, VSD, Tetralogy of Fallot, valvular defects (tricuspid regurgitation) (Kirk et al., 2007; Chen et al., 2021) | Some variants associated with dilated cardiomyopathy or arrhythmia (Chen et al., 2021) | Broad role in heart development; regulates chamber growth, septation, valve formation (Chen et al., 2021) |
| CTNNB1 | De novo (usually); Autosomal Dominant if inherited | Ventricular outflow tract defects (e.g. pulmonary atresia with intact septum, conotruncal anomalies); septal defects in some cases (Sinibaldi et al., 2023) | Neurodevelopmental delay, spastic diplegia, and visual impairment (CTNNB1 syndrome) in heterozygous loss-of-function variants (Sinibaldi et al., 2023) | Encodes β-catenin (Wnt signaling). Germline LoF causes CHD + developmental disabilities (Sinibaldi et al., 2023); somatic mutations common in hepatoblastoma, linking Wnt pathway to cancer |
| NOTCH1 | Autosomal Dominant (reduced penetrance) | Bicuspid aortic valve (BAV); calcific aortic stenosis; TOF in rare cases | Some have mild limb anomalies or cleft palate (variable) | Haploinsufficiency of NOTCH1 can cause isolated BAV. Somatic NOTCH1 mutations occur in T-ALL leukemia, but germline NOTCH1-BAV patients do not have greatly increased leukemia incidence |

Non-syndromic CHD genes often encode fundamental cardiac transcriptional regulators. NKX2-5, for instance, is one of the first identified familial CHD genes (scholarly reports date back to the 1990s). *NKX2-5* mutations classically cause ASD with atrioventricular block; affected individuals might present in adulthood with heart block even if the ASD was small and asymptomatic, linking a developmental defect to an adult arrhythmia phenotype. *NKX2-5* exemplifies how some isolated CHD genes can also influence postnatal cardiac function (conduction tissue development) but do not produce wide systemic issues or malignancies.

GATA4 is another paradigmatic CHD gene. GATA4 encodes a zinc-finger transcription factor that, together with TBX5 and others, orchestrates cardiac septation during embryogenesis. Multiple dominant mutations in *GATA4* have been found in humans with septal defects. A landmark discovery by Garg *et al.* (2003) (Garg et al., 2003) showed a *GATA4* missense mutation (p.Gly296Ser) in a family with atrial septal defects and pulmonary valve stenosis; functional studies later confirmed this mutation disrupts GATA4's DNA binding and its physical interaction with TBX5 (Misra et al., 2012). GATA4-related CHD is typically "isolated" to the heart. Patients may have atrial and VSDs, sometimes an AV canal defect (especially when GATA4 mutations co-occur with NKX2-5 or other factors), but they generally do not have the dysmorphic features or growth issues seen in syndromic conditions. There is no strong evidence that *GATA4* heterozygous mutations confer increased cancer risk, the gene is certainly important in cardiac development, and somatic GATA4 alterations can be found in some tumors (e.g. certain gonadal tumors), but individuals with germline GATA4 mutations are not recognized to have a cancer syndrome.

TBX20 is a T-box family transcription factor essential for multiple aspects of heart formation. Unlike TBX5 (which causes Holt-Oram syndrome with limb involvement), *TBX20* mutations usually cause isolated CHD without limb defects. Studies have shown *TBX20* mutations in families and sporadic cases lead to a wide spectrum of CHD: septal defects (both ASD and VSD), outflow tract anomalies like TOF, and valve malformations (e.g. mitral or tricuspid regurgitation due to valve leaflet abnormalities) (Kirk et al., 2007; Chen et al., 2021). Some truncating *TBX20* variants have been linked to adult-onset dilated cardiomyopathy as well, highlighting pleiotropy even within the heart. In general, TBX20-related CHD is isolated (no consistent extra-cardiac features). There is no known tumor predisposition associated with *TBX20* variants. That said, TBX20's broad role (including potential involvement in cardiac cell proliferation) makes it a subject of interest, and research has shown it can modulate pathways that overlap with cancer biology (e.g. interaction with β-catenin), but patients with *TBX20* mutations are not clinically observed to have higher cancer rates.

One fascinating gene at the intersection of CHD and broader developmental processes is CTNNB1, encoding β-catenin. Germline *CTNNB1* loss-of-function mutations cause a syndromic intellectual disability condition (sometimes termed "CTNNB1 syndrome" or NEDSDV: Neurodevelopmental Disorder with Spastic Diplegia and Visual defects) in which congenital heart defects occur more often than expected (Sinibaldi et al., 2023). Though CTNNB1 syndrome includes global developmental delay and spasticity (so one could consider it syndromic), it was not traditionally recognized until recently, and many cases present initially for CHD or hypotonia. The CHDs reported with *CTNNB1* variants include outflow tract abnormalities like absent pulmonary valve, atrioventricular canal defects with arch hypoplasia, and TOF (Sinibaldi et al., 2023). CTNNB1 is a crucial effector of the Wnt signaling pathway and a component of cell adhesion complexes. Notably, somatic activating mutations in *CTNNB1* are very common in certain cancers (over 90% of sporadic hepatoblastomas, a pediatric liver tumor, have Wnt pathway activation, often via CTNNB1 mutations). There is emerging evidence that children with germline *CTNNB1* haploinsufficiency might have an elevated risk of embryonal tumors like hepatoblastoma (Nussbaumer & Benesch, 2022). Indeed, a few cases of hepatoblastoma have been noted in patients with congenital β-catenin related disorders (though often in conjunction with other genetic factors). The hypothesis is that reducing β-catenin levels developmental-ly could create a vulnerability where secondary hits (somatic) drive oncogenesis in the liver or other tissues. While data are limited, CTNNB1 exemplifies a gene where the overlap of CHD genetics and cancer genetics is mechanistically tangible, Wnt/β-catenin signaling must be precisely balanced for normal organ development, and both hypo- and hyper-activation can lead to disease (CHD or cancer, respectively). Clinicians might consider surveillance for liver tumors in young patients with CTNNB1 syndrome, especially since hepatoblastoma generally occurs in infancy/early childhood.

Another non-syndromic CHD gene with an interesting dual role is NOTCH1. Heterozygous NOTCH1 mutations can cause familial bicuspid aortic valve (BAV) and related left ventricular outflow tract defects, often with incomplete penetrance (Garg *et al.*, 2005). These individuals usually have isolated BAV or valve calcification in adulthood, with no syndrome. However, NOTCH1 is notable because somatic mutations in the NOTCH pathway (especially NOTCH1 itself) are a hallmark of T-cell acute lymphoblastic leukemia (T-ALL), occurring in >50% of T-ALL cases. Do germline NOTCH1 mutation carriers (with BAV) have a higher risk of leukemia? Thus far, no clear epidemiologic link has been shown; the germline haploinsufficiency might not predispose to leukemia, possibly because the context and nature of mutations differ (germline loss-of-function vs somatic gain-of-function in T-ALL). It serves as a reminder that gene function can be context-dependent: in heart valve development, half dose of NOTCH1 leads to BAV; in thymocytes, specific activating mutations drive leukemia. From a clinical perspective, a patient with BAV and a known NOTCH1 mutation would not typically undergo cancer surveillance beyond general population guidelines.

In summary, non-syndromic CHD genes highlight the diversity of genetic contributions to heart development. Many are transcription factors (NKX2-5, GATA4, TBX5, TBX20) or signaling pathway components (NOTCH1, signaling mediators) that are heart-enriched in their effects. They usually manifest with isolated cardiac malformations and *minimal* extracardiac involvement; perhaps a subtle anomaly or predisposition (like conduction block or mild dysmorphism), but not the multi-system syndrome seen with chromosomal abnormalities or metabolic disorders. Importantly, while these genes are not classically "cancer genes" in the germline sense, their pathways often overlap with oncogenic processes (e.g. Wnt in CTNNB1, Notch in NOTCH1, T-box factors in cell cycle regulation). Thus, research continues to explore whether there are unappreciated long-term risks for individuals with mutations in these genes, especially as more patients are identified via genetic testing.

Non-syndromic CHD may also arise through polygenic inheritance, reflecting the cumulative effect of multiple common genetic variants rather than a single high-impact mutation, as discussed in Section V (Polygenic Contributions). Even in cases attributed to ostensibly monogenic causes, phenotypic expressivity can be influenced by additional genetic factors, occasionally blurring the distinction between "syndromic" and "non-syndromic" forms. For example, a pathogenic GATA4 variant may be accompanied by additional anomalies due to the presence of a second genetic alteration elsewhere in the genome. This principle provides a conceptual bridge to the subsequent section on chromosomal abnormalities and copy-number variants, which often implicate multiple genes, manifest with combined anomalies, and may confer tumor predisposition.

## IV. CHROMOSOMAL ABNORMALITIES AND COPY NUMBER VARIATIONS IN CHD

Large-scale genetic alterations, including aneuploidies (gain or loss of entire chromosomes) and submicroscopic copy number variations (CNVs), account for a substantial proportion of CHD cases, particularly those accompanied by additional anomalies. These abnormalities frequently involve dozens to hundreds of genes and commonly result in syndromic presentations. The discussion below highlights chromosomal conditions with well-established associations to CHD, along with recurrent CNVs identified in CHD cohorts, and examines how such genomic imbalances contribute to neonatal anomalies and potential tumor susceptibility.

Trisomy 21 (Down Syndrome): Down syndrome is the most common chromosomal cause of CHD. Approximately 40;50% of infants with trisomy 21 have a congenital heart defect (Elmagrpy et al., 2011), most often an atrioventricular septal defect (AVSD, also called endocardial cushion defect) or a ventricular septal defect. The presence of an AVSD in a newborn is highly suggestive of Down syndrome and prompts genetic testing if not already diagnosed. Down syndrome also entails a wide range of anomalies: characteristic facial features, hypotonia, single palmar crease, duodenal atresia, Hirschsprung disease, and intellectual disability, among others. Regarding tumor susceptibility, Down syndrome is characterized by a substantially increased predisposition to leukemia. Children with Down syndrome have a 10-20 fold greater risk of developing acute lymphoblastic leukemia (ALL) or acute myeloid leukemia (especially the megakaryoblastic subtype, AMKL) in childhood (Linabery et al., 2008). For example, the cumulative incidence of leukemia in Down syndrome during childhood is around 2;3%, compared to 0.05% in the general population. This predisposition is thought to result from overexpression of certain chromosome 21 genes in hematopoietic cells (e.g. ERG and ETS2) that cooperate with somatic mutations to drive leukemogenesis. Interestingly, while blood cancers are more frequent, individuals with Down syndrome have *lower* incidences of many solid tumors (possibly due to anti-angiogenic or immune-related effects of trisomy 21). Nonetheless, leukemia is a significant concern and Down syndrome patients with CHD require coordinated care that addresses both cardiopulmonary issues and vigilant monitoring for hematologic signs (e.g. the transient neonatal myeloproliferative disorder unique to Down syndrome). From a cardiac perspective, patients with AVSD and Down syndrome often undergo surgical repair in infancy with good outcomes; having the genetic diagnosis informs perioperative management (for instance, Down syndrome patients are more prone to pulmonary hypertension and require specific anesthetic considerations). Table 3 (below) summarizes key data on Trisomy 21 and other chromosomal causes of CHD.

22q11.2 Deletion Syndrome: A deletion of ~3 million base pairs on chromosome 22q11.2 causes DiGeorge syndrome/velocardiofacial syndrome. This is the most common microdeletion syndrome (occurring in ~1:4,000 live births) and is highly associated with CHD; especially conotruncal defects. About 35% of patients with 22q11.2 deletion have tetralogy of Fallot, and others have truncus arteriosus or interrupted aortic arch. The deleted region contains the TBX1 gene, among others, which is a critical regulator of pharyngeal arch development (hence the cardiac and thymic defects). Beyond CHD, 22q11.2 deletion causes thymic hypoplasia (with immunodeficiency), parathyroid hypoplasia (hypocalcemia), palatal abnormalities (cleft palate or velopharyngeal insufficiency leading to nasal speech), renal anomalies, and an array of neuropsychiatric issues (including a ~25% risk of schizophrenia in adulthood). Given the immune dysfunction, one might expect an increased cancer risk (since T-cell surveillance is affected). Indeed, there is some evidence that individuals with 22q11.2 deletion have a moderately increased risk of cancers, notably non-Hodgkin lymphoma and thyroid carcinoma (possibly 2;3 times general population risk according to some studies) (Liu et al., 2024). Rare cases of thymic carcinoma and lymphoblastic lymphoma have been reported in this syndrome as well (since the thymus is small but not entirely absent, malignant transformation can occur in residual thymic tissue). Overall, however, cancer is not as prominent a concern in 22q11.2 deletion as the developmental and psychiatric issues are. The 22q11.2 deletion illustrates how a CNV can simultaneously cause structural birth defects and longer-term disease vulnerabilities via loss of multiple genes. From a clinical standpoint, any patient with conotruncal CHD (like TOF) should be tested for 22q deletion (e.g. via microarray or FISH), because establishing the diagnosis has implications for calcium monitoring, infection prophylaxis, family recurrence risk (~10% if inherited), and anticipatory guidance for learning difficulties.

Turner Syndrome (45,X): Turner syndrome results from complete or mosaic monosomy X in females (incidence ~1 in 2,500 female births). CHD occurs in 30;50% of individuals with Turner syndrome, making it another major genetic contributor to CHD prevalence. The most frequent cardiac malformations are bicuspid aortic valve and coarctation of the aorta; present in up to 50% of Turner patients on detailed imaging. Other cardiovascular issues include elongation of the transverse aortic arch, hypertension, and a higher risk of aortic root dilation and dissection in adulthood. Neonatal features of Turner syndrome (besides CHD) often include lymphedema (swollen hands/feet or cystic hygroma in utero), webbed neck, kidney anomalies (horseshoe kidney), and short stature; most Turner patients also have primary ovarian failure (streak gonads) leading to infertility. In terms of tumor risk, Turner syndrome has a unique consideration: if any Y chromosome material is present (as in some mosaic Turner variants), there is a high risk of gonadoblastoma developing in the dysgenetic gonads. For pure 45,X individuals without Y material, there isn't a dramatically increased general cancer risk, but some studies suggest a slight increase in childhood brain tumors and perhaps hematologic malignancies (though data are limited and confounded by growth hormone therapy in some cases). The SHOX gene (on the X chromosome pseudoautosomal region) is implicated in Turner skeletal features, and loss of a second SHOX copy contributes to short stature; the role of specific Turner genes in cancer predisposition is less clear. Turner syndrome underscores how sex chromosome anomalies affect cardiovascular development (BAV and coarctation have ~100-fold higher prevalence in Turner than general population) and also how mosaicism can alter risk (necessitating prophylactic gonadectomy if Y material is detected, to prevent gonadoblastoma).

Beyond these, researchers have identified several recurrent CNVs (subchromosomal deletions/duplications) enriched in CHD patients. Notable hotspots include 1q21.1, 8p23.1, and 15q11.2, among others (Ehrlich & Prakash, 2022). For example, a 1.5-Mb duplication at 1q21.1 or deletion at 1q21.1 is found in some patients with Tetralogy of Fallot or other septal defects (Ehrlich & Prakash, 2022). The 8p23.1 deletion (which encompasses part of the GATA4 region) is associated with cardiac defects (due to GATA4 haploinsufficiency) and occasionally developmental delay. These CNVs typically have variable expressivity; not all carriers have CHD; and often they don't cause obvious syndromic facies, so they may be discovered only via genomic testing in a CHD patient. As for tumor associations, most of these CNVs are too rare for large epidemiologic studies, but some insights exist: the 1q21.1 duplication, for instance, has been reported in a few cases of neuroblastoma, raising the question of whether it might subtly increase neuroblastoma risk (given that it includes genes involved in neural crest development). However, concrete evidence is lacking and at present, these CNVs are not regarded as cancer predisposition syndromes.

Table 3 provides a concise overview of major chromosomal abnormalities with their CHD and tumor associations:

*Table 3. Chromosomal Abnormalities and CNVs with Dual CHD and Tumor Implications*

| Chromosomal Abnormality | Key Cardiac Defects | Neonatal Anomalies | Tumor Risk | Relevant Genes | Frequency in CHD |
|---|---|---|---|---|---|
| Trisomy 21 (Down syndrome) | AV canal defect (40%), VSD, ASD | Craniofacial dysmorphism, hypotonia, duodenal atresia, intellectual disability | Leukemia (ALL, AML); ~20× risk (Linabery et al., 2008); transient neonatal leukemoid reaction | DSCAM, DYRK1A, ERG (chr21 dosage-sensitive developmental genes) | ~8;10% of CHD cases |
| 22q11.2 deletion (DiGeorge) | TOF (35%), truncus arteriosus, IAA | Cleft palate, thymic and parathyroid hypoplasia, T-cell immunodeficiency | Thymoma, Non-Hodgkin lymphoma; mild ↑ risk; Thyroid carcinoma ~3× risk (moderate) | TBX1, CRKL (deleted genes affecting pharyngeal arch development) | ~3;5% of CHD cases (high in conotruncal CHD) |
| 45,X (Turner syndrome) | Bicuspid aortic valve (~30%), coarctation (~15;30%) | Lymphedema, webbed neck, streak gonads, renal anomalies, short stature | Gonadoblastoma (if Y mosaicism present); slight ↑ brain tumor risk (uncertain) | SHOX (haploinsufficiency causes short stature); VEGF genes (possibly linked to lymphatics) | ~1;2% of CHD cases (female births) |
| 1q21.1 duplication (recurrent CNV) | Conotruncal defects, septal defects (variable) | Developmental delay (variable penetrance); sometimes macrocephaly | Not well established; occasional neuroblastoma reported (unclear link) | GJA5 (connexin40) and others in region; PRDM16 (involved in cardiogenesis) | ~1% of TOF or other CHD (estimates vary) |
| 8p23.1 deletion (includes GATA4) | Tetralogy of Fallot, AVSD (due to GATA4 deletion) | Facial dysmorphism, developmental delay (variable) | Not known to confer specific tumor risk | GATA4, SOX7 (critical heart development genes in deleted segment) | <1% of CHD; enriched in septal defects (GATA4) |

Table 3 emphasizes that chromosomal disorders like Down syndrome and 22q11.2 deletion contribute a non-trivial share of CHD cases seen clinically (for instance, trisomy 21 accounts for roughly 1 in 10 infants with CHD). It also shows that these conditions often come with predictable co-morbidities; some of which include elevated cancer risks (most strikingly, leukemia in Down syndrome). Therefore, integration of care is vital: a child with CHD due to a chromosomal syndrome should have not only cardiology follow-up but also monitoring or prophylactic measures relevant to their syndrome (e.g. CBC screenings in Down syndrome infants, calcium checks and immune workups in DiGeorge, blood pressure and aortic imaging in Turner, etc.). As genetic testing (like chromosomal microarray) is now standard for infants with moderate or complex CHD, these chromosomal diagnoses are being made earlier, allowing anticipation of associated issues.

Another category worth mentioning is copy number variations identified through genome-wide studies of CHD cohorts. Research has found that de novo CNVs are significantly enriched in CHD patients, especially those with extra-cardiac anomalies (ECA). One large study reported de novo CNVs in ~10% of CHD cases with ECAs vs ~2% in isolated CHD (Zu et al., 2020). These CNVs can be unique (non-recurrent) and individually rare, but collectively they highlight genes and pathways important in cardiac development. For example, CNVs disrupting genes like *CHD7* (in CHARGE), *KMT2D* (in Kabuki syndrome, which can include CHD), or *RAS pathway genes* have been uncovered. Some of these genes are also known cancer genes (KMT2D/MLL2 is a frequent target in lymphomas). Thus, CNV analysis further reinforces the overlap between CHD genetics and oncogenesis: CNVs may simultaneously predispose to CHD and to malignancy if they delete or duplicate dosage-sensitive cancer genes. For instance, a deletion encompassing PTEN could cause a CHD (through developmental effect) and also create a cancer predisposition (PTEN hamartoma syndrome). Though such instances are relatively rare, they exemplify pleiotropy of CNVs.

In summary, chromosomal abnormalities and CNVs underscore a principle that dosage imbalance of multiple genes can lead to CHD accompanied by a spectrum of anomalies, and occasionally, cancer susceptibility. They remind clinicians to maintain a broad outlook when managing CHD patients; if a genetic syndrome or CNV is present, care must extend beyond the heart to the whole patient's spectrum of needs.

## V. POLYGENIC AND OLIGOGENIC CONTRIBUTIONS (COMPLEX GENETICS OF CHD)

While monogenic and chromosomal causes are significant, a large proportion of CHD; particularly isolated defects in otherwise healthy individuals; may result from the aggregate effect of many genetic variants of small effect, rather than one powerful mutation. This polygenic inheritance means that CHD can resemble other common diseases (like diabetes or hypertension) where risk is distributed in the population and influenced by numerous loci. In recent years, researchers have applied genome-wide approaches (GWAS, exome sequencing in large cohorts, etc.) to uncover the complex genetic architecture of CHD. Additionally, evidence has emerged for oligogenic models (where a combination of a few rare variants might be necessary to cause disease in one individual). This section reviews key findings from genome-wide association studies (GWAS) in CHD, the development and application of polygenic risk scores (PRS), and illustrative cases of digenic or oligogenic inheritance. The discussion further considers how these insights align with the concept of gene polymorphisms contributing to subtle anomalies or predisposition to tumor development.

## A. Genome-Wide Association Studies (GWAS)

GWAS interrogate common single-nucleotide polymorphisms (SNPs) across the genome in large cohorts of patients and controls to find variants associated with disease. Early GWAS for CHD faced challenges (CHD is heterogeneous, sample sizes were modest). However, recent consortia with thousands of patients have yielded the first robust loci. For instance, a 2020 GWAS of >4,000 CHD patients identified a genome-wide significant hit on chromosome 5q22.2 near the gene *MSX1*, which was associated with CHD overall and septal defects in particular (Lahm et al., 2021). *MSX1* is a transcription factor involved in outflow tract and palate development, making biological sense. Another locus on chromosome 20p12.1 at the MACROD2 gene was linked specifically to transposition of the great arteries (TGA) (Lahm et al., 2021). A third locus on 17q21.3 near GOSR2 (involved in Golgi transport) was associated with anomalies of the thoracic arteries/veins (Lahm et al., 2021). These findings are notable as some of the first common variant signals for CHD. They also highlight that different CHD subtypes might have distinct genetic signatures; a polygenic locus may predispose strongly to one lesion (e.g., a TGA locus distinct from an ASD locus). Overall, the effect sizes of these SNPs are modest (odds ratios ~1.2;1.5), meaning no single SNP is destiny, but collectively they contribute.

Beyond individual loci, GWAS have shown that CHD risk is indeed polygenic. A study by Spendlove *et al.* (2022) demonstrated that polygenic risk scores (PRS) constructed from multiple common variants can modestly predict CHD risk (Spendlove et al., 2022). By aggregating thousands of SNP effects (weighted by GWAS effect size), the authors found the PRS was significantly elevated in CHD patients compared to controls, though with overlapping distributions. This indicates that common variants captured in CHD GWAS have a modest but significant contribution to CHD expression (Spendlove et al., 2022). In practical terms, while monogenic mutations often show incomplete penetrance (some carriers unaffected), the presence of a high polygenic load might tilt a carrier towards disease manifestation. For example, someone with a pathogenic *TBX5* mutation might only develop an atrial septal defect if they also carry a "riskier" polygenic background for heart defects (which could include variants in pathways of cardiac cushions, cilia, etc.).

One notable angle of polygenic studies is investigating maternal-fetal genotype interactions. Since the intrauterine environment is partly determined by maternal genotype, researchers have done GWAS on mothers of CHD cases as well. An interesting example involves the maternal folate metabolism pathway. Common variants in folate-related genes (e.g. *MTHFR, MTHFD1*) have been studied for association with CHD. A meta-analysis found that the fetal genotype MTHFD1 rs2236225 AA (a variant reducing enzyme efficiency) was associated specifically with increased risk of tetralogy of Fallot, with an odds ratio ~2.8 compared to GG genotype (Yi et al., 2025). This suggests a gene-environment interplay: if the fetus cannot metabolize folate as well (AA genotype) and maternal folate is suboptimal, cardiac neural crest cells may be more prone to outflow tract defects. This finding reinforces the concept that common polymorphisms (here in a metabolic gene) can increase CHD risk modestly, especially in certain nutritional environments. Notably, *MTHFD1* and *MTHFR* variants have also been implicated in neural tube defects, aligning with the idea of a shared folate-sensitive developmental pathway for heart and neural tube (which might explain why a subset of babies with TOF also have spina bifida in some studies).

GWAS and polygenic analyses have so far not uncovered strong links between CHD polygenic risk and tumor risk, and this is probably because the effects are diffuse. However, one intriguing area is the overlap between polygenic signals for cardiac development and those for cancer. For instance, Wnt signaling genes appear in GWAS hits (WNT3 near one of the loci for arterial anomalies (Lahm et al., 2021), and Wnt is a well-known cancer pathway. It is conceivable that a high polygenic burden in certain pathways might predispose to both CHD and later-life cancer; though presently speculative, future studies analyzing the genomes of CHD survivors who develop cancer could shed light on this.

## B. Polygenic Risk Scores and Prediction

As mentioned, a polygenic risk score (PRS) sums the effects of many variants to stratify individuals by genetic risk. In CHD, the clinical utility of PRS is still in early research phase. The diversity of CHD phenotypes complicates matters; a PRS for "any CHD" is less predictive than a PRS tailored to a specific lesion (like a PRS for conotruncal defects). Efforts like the one by Spendlove *et al.* used PRS derived from adult populations (UK Biobank participants with bicuspid valve, etc.) and applied them to pediatric CHD cohorts (Spendlove et al., 2022). They found that PRS was significantly associated with CHD status ($p<0.005$), confirming polygenic inheritance, but the effect size was modest. In practical terms, current PRS might explain only a few percent of CHD variance; not enough for standalone predictive screening. However, as sample sizes increase (international CHD GWAS consortia are growing) and as more variants are discovered, PRS might improve. One could envision in the future that a polygenic score could identify couples at higher risk of having a baby with CHD (especially if both parents carry many risk alleles),or identify CHD survivors who might have higher risk of complications.

Table 4 provides a general comparison of variant types in CHD genetics:

*Table 4. Types of Genetic Variants and their Contributions to CHD Risk*

| Variant Type | Typical Effect Size | Population Frequency | Role in CHD |
|---|---|---|---|
| Common SNPs | Very small (OR ~1.1;1.3 per allele) | High (minor allele >5%) | Contribute polygenically; individually not causal but in aggregate can modulate CHD risk (Spendlove et al., 2022). Useful for PRS research. |
| Low-frequency variants | Modest (OR ~1.5;3.0) | Intermediate (1;5%) | Some show moderate associations in specific CHD subtypes (e.g. certain missense variants in regulatory genes). Rarely identified via GWAS due to frequency. |
| Rare variants (single-gene mutations) | Large effect (OR >3, often causal) | Rare (<1%) | Include most monogenic CHD genes (e.g. *GATA4*, *TBX1*): often *de novo* or familial mutations with high penetrance. Account for ~5% of CHD (Zu et al., 2020). |
| Copy Number Variants (CNVs) | Variable effect (some are high impact like 22q11 del; others lower) | Rare (<0.1% each, collectively a few % of CHD) | Pathogenic CNVs (deletions/duplications) found in 3;10% of CHD cases (Zu et al., 2020). Often cause syndromic CHD. Impact depends on genes within the CNV (e.g. 7q11 deletion causes Williams syndrome with CHD). |

Table 4 illustrates that although rare variants and copy number variations exert strong effects and are more readily associated with CHD in individuals, the more modest polygenic burden from common variants is widespread and cumulatively significant. The interaction between these categories is critical; for instance, the penetrance of a rare CHD-causing mutation may be influenced by an individual's polygenic background. Such complexity helps explain why even in families with seemingly clear Mendelian inheritance, disease expression may skip generations or present with variable severity; a phenomenon referred to as oligogenic inheritance.

## C. Oligogenic Models and Digenic Interactions

Oligogenic inheritance refers to situations where pathogenic variants in two or more genes act in combination to produce disease in an individual, with none of the variants alone being sufficient to cause the condition. In CHD, there have long been hints of this. For example, some mice engineered with a single heterozygous mutation do not develop CHD, but when a second mutation is added, CHD appears (two-hit model). Clinically, there have been reports of families where two siblings with CHD each inherited different "complementary" mutations from their parents, suggesting a multi-hit requirement.

Recent genomic studies have started to systematically search for digenic combinations. A 2025 study by Kars (Kars et al., 2025) analyzed exome sequencing from >3,900 CHD trios and looked for pairs of gene variants that co-occur in CHD patients more than expected (after excluding known monogenic causes). They identified several candidate gene-gene interactions that might contribute to CHD (e.g., damaging variants in gene A and gene B together significantly enriched in cases). While each combination was rare, collectively about 2;3% of CHD patients in the cohort appeared to have a plausible digenic cause. One striking finding was that *14%* of CHD patients harbored a loss-of-function variant in a gene that is also implicated in cancer predisposition (compared to ~7% of controls), suggesting a double-hit scenario where those variants plus others cause CHD. Examples included pairs of variants in interacting proteins of the cytoskeletal and Rho-GTPase pathways (such as *ARHGEF12* and *TCF12*). Individually, heterozygous mutations in *TCF12* can cause craniosynostosis, and *ARHGEF12* is involved in cell migration; together, they might disrupt cardiac neural crest migration leading to outflow defects (this combination was enriched in CHD cases in the study). Interestingly, *TCF12* and related genes have been studied in cancer (e.g., TCF12 translocations in leukemia), hinting that some digenic CHD gene sets involve one or more genes from cancer-related pathways.

Another concrete example of oligogenic inheritance is seen in heterotaxy syndrome (situs ambiguous with complex CHD). Heterotaxy has been associated with mutations in cilia-related genes such as DNAH5, ZNF423, and MKS1. In some cases, patients carry variants in more than one ciliary gene; while a single mutation may be insufficient to produce the phenotype, the combined effect of two defects can result in heterotaxy (Burnicka-Turek et al., 2016). These findings align with the concept of a "cumulative mutational burden": if multiple genes in a developmental network are slightly impaired by variants, the combined effect can cross a threshold to produce malformation.

From the tumor risk perspective, oligogenic models raise an interesting possibility: an individual might carry, say, one mutation in a cardiac development gene and another in a tumor suppressor gene ; the two hits produce CHD but also leave the tumor suppressor gene defective in every cell, perhaps raising long-term cancer risk. There's not clear evidence yet of specific oligogenic combinations causing both CHD and cancer in the same person, but the enrichment of cancer-gene variants in CHD patients (noted above) is provocative. It may suggest that some cancer predisposition genes (like those involved in chromatin regulation or DNA repair) also subtly influence heart development, and when combined with a second hit, cause

CHD. If true, CHD patients with such genetic backgrounds could have hidden cancer risks. This remains a speculative area requiring further study.

In summary, polygenic and oligogenic contributions depict CHD as a complex genetic disorder for a large subset of patients. Unlike a clear Mendelian syndrome, these cases involve multiple gene polymorphisms of varying effect sizes. The upshot for clinicians is that genetic testing in CHD is expanding beyond single-gene tests; whole exome or genome sequencing can reveal multiple candidate variants and interpreting them may require network-based thinking (e.g. two "possibly damaging" variants in related pathways might jointly explain the CHD). It also underscores the importance of studying large populations to derive risk scores and identify at-risk groups (e.g., women of reproductive age with high polygenic risk might benefit from preconception counseling or folate supplementation).

## VI. TRANSCRIPTOMIC SIGNATURES IN CHD (FROM FETAL GENE PROGRAMS TO SINGLE-CELL ANALYSIS)

Understanding gene polymorphisms and mutations provides the static "genetic blueprint" of CHD, but gene expression studies (transcriptomics) offer dynamic insights into how those genetic differences translate into molecular pathways and phenotypes. In recent years, transcriptomic technologies; including bulk RNA sequencing, single-cell RNA sequencing (scRNA-seq), and other high-throughput gene expression assays; have been applied to congenital heart disease. These approaches help characterize the downstream effects of genetic variants, identify dysregulated pathways in diseased cardiac tissue, and sometimes uncover unexpected biomarkers or therapeutic targets. A fascinating concept that has emerged is the "fetalization" of gene expression in diseased hearts; meaning that the gene expression profile in certain CHD or heart failure contexts reverts to a more fetal-like state.

### A. Bulk RNA-SEQ Studies of CHD

Bulk RNA sequencing involves extracting RNA from heart tissues (e.g., an excised cardiac tissue sample during surgery) and sequencing to quantify all expressed genes. Several studies have compared transcriptomes of cardiac tissue from CHD patients (often infants undergoing surgery) to those of non-CHD control hearts. These studies have revealed a broad spectrum of molecular signatures in different CHD types (Odogwu et al., 2023). For example, right ventricular tissue from infants with tetralogy of Fallot shows upregulation of genes involved in hypoxia responses and extracellular matrix remodeling, presumably due to pressure overload from the RV outflow obstruction. In contrast, ventricular tissue from hypoplastic left heart syndrome (HLHS) shows a different pattern, with changes in proliferation and sarcomere genes. Odogwu and Nelson (2023) reviewed many such studies and found no single unifying gene expression change across all CHDs, but rather distinct pathways perturbed in different anatomical defects (Odogwu et al., 2023). This underscores that CHD is mechanistically heterogeneous at the molecular level; an atrial septal defect vs. a conotruncal defect may have different transcriptomic etiologies even if phenotypically both are "CHD."

One recurring theme in bulk transcriptomics is the role of non-coding RNAs. For instance, a study by Jiang *et al.* (2019) found that the long non-coding RNA SNHG6 was highly overexpressed in myocardium of infants with ventricular septal defects compared to controls (Jiang et al., 2019). They further showed that SNHG6 overexpression in cell models inhibited cardiomyocyte proliferation and increased apoptosis, suggesting it contributes to septal malformation (by limiting the growth of the septal myocardium). Such findings highlight how transcriptomics can pinpoint novel molecular players (like lncRNAs or microRNAs) that might not be obvious from DNA studies alone. Other investigations have identified microRNA expression differences; for example, some microRNAs (miR-19b, miR-29c) were found upregulated in cardiac tissue of tetralogy of Fallot patients (Odogwu et al., 2023), and these microRNAs are known to target developmental signaling transcripts.

A particularly interesting transcriptomic signature relates to heart failure in CHD patients. Pediatric hearts with CHD that develop heart failure (or adult hearts with congenital lesions that eventually fail) often show a gene expression shift reminiscent of fetal heart tissue. Akat *et al.* (2014) demonstrated that failing adult hearts (not specific to CHD) re-express certain fetal isoforms of contractile proteins and switch metabolism gene expression back to a fetal pattern (Akat et al., 2014). In CHD, a similar "fetal gene program" activation has been observed in cases of pressure overload (like an unrepaired large VSD causing heart failure). For example, upregulation of fetal isoform genes like *ANP*, *BNP*, and *β-myosin heavy chain* (MYH7) and downregulation of adult isoforms (MYH6) is a classic fetal gene reversion signature. Transcriptomic analyses confirm that failing CHD hearts share many gene expression changes with normal fetal hearts, including patterns in metabolic enzymes and extracellular matrix components (Odogwu et al., 2023). This phenomenon, often termed fetalization, reflects the heart muscle's attempt to revert to a more plastic, proliferative state under stress. While adaptive in some ways, it also is associated with reduced contractile efficiency and arrhythmia propensity.

In sum, bulk RNA-seq has provided a catalog of dysregulated genes and pathways in CHD tissues; from upregulated fibrotic pathways, to downregulated calcium handling genes, to aberrant noncoding RNA expression. Each CHD subtype may have unique signatures, but common to many is evidence of altered developmental programs (some cells stuck in an immature state, others overly stressed).

## B. Single-Cell Transcriptomics

Single-cell RNA sequencing (scRNA-seq) takes transcriptomics to the next level by resolving gene expression at the level of individual cells, rather than an average over a bulk tissue. This is particularly powerful for the heart, which is a complex mix of cardiomyocytes, endothelial cells, smooth muscle, fibroblasts, and immune cells. scRNA-seq allows us to ask: in a CHD-affected heart, which cell types are present and what are their states? Are certain cell populations missing, overabundant, or expressing abnormal genes?

Initial single-cell studies in human cardiac development provided reference atlases of normal heart cell types across developmental stages (Odogwu et al., 2023). Building on that, researchers have begun to apply scRNA-seq to CHD. For example, in a recent study on hearts from fetuses with CHD, scRNA-seq identified disruptions in cellular differentiation trajectories: certain progenitor cell types in CHD hearts failed to transition properly into mature cardiomyocytes, getting "stalled" in an earlier state. Another study examined single-cell profiles in a mouse model of maternal diabetes-induced CHD, finding that maternal diabetes leads to dysregulation of gene expression in second heart field progenitors (which give rise to outflow tract), with excess oxidative stress pathways turned on (Manivannan et al., 2022).

Single-cell analysis has also revealed cell type-specific disease signatures in CHD. For instance, fibroblast-like cells in malformed cardiac valves of patients with bicuspid aortic valve showed elevated expression of extracellular matrix genes and TGF-β pathway genes at the single-cell level, indicating an activated myofibroblast state possibly contributing to early calcification. In another example, scRNA-seq of ventricular tissue from HLHS patients (collected at time of transplant) showed that cardiomyocytes expressed lower levels of contraction genes and higher proliferation markers compared to donor hearts, whereas endothelial cells expressed higher levels of angiogenic factors (possibly an attempt to compensate for hypoxia). These granular insights help in pinpointing which cell compartments are most affected by the genetic mutations of CHD.

Notably, single-cell transcriptomics can also identify rare cell populations that might be important. In one study of CHD, a small subset of cells with a neural crest-like expression profile was found lingering in hearts of TOF patients, suggesting aberrant differentiation of neural crest-derived cells might underlie the outflow tract defect (these cells normally should mature into smooth muscle or undergo apoptosis after contributing to septation). Finding such "misplaced" or persistent progenitor cells is only possible with single-cell resolution.

As scRNA-seq technology improves (especially the ability to analyze nuclei from frozen heart tissue), more studies directly on human CHD tissues are expected. These studies could uncover, for example, if CHD hearts have an increased population of proliferating cells (or conversely too few), or if certain supporting cells (like epicardium-derived cells) failed to populate the heart correctly. Each of these clues helps trace back to developmental mechanisms.

One challenge is obtaining human fetal heart tissue for study; much of the single-cell work may rely on animal models or stem cell-derived organoids to simulate CHD conditions. Nevertheless, even indirect approaches (like differentiating patient-derived induced pluripotent stem cells, iPSCs, into cardiomyocytes and doing single-cell analysis) have been informative. They can reveal differences in gene regulatory networks in cells carrying CHD mutations vs. controls.

## C. "Fetalization" of Gene Expression and Epigenetic Changes

As introduced earlier, the concept of fetal gene reactivation is a hallmark of pathological stress in the heart. In the context of CHD, this often comes into play when considering the long-term physiology of a malformed heart. Many adolescents or adults with CHD (even if repaired) develop heart failure or arrhythmias decades later. A contributing factor is that their cardiomyocytes might retain an immature phenotype. Some pediatric cardiologists describe the myocardium of infants with CHD (especially those with volume overload lesions) as biologically "neonatal" or "fetal-like" even after the normal postnatal transition. Transcriptomic evidence supports this: failing myocardium from CHD patients shows upregulation of genes that are high in fetal heart and downregulation of adult genes (Odogwu et al., 2023). For example, there is persistent expression of *NPPA* (atrial natriuretic peptide) and *ACAN* (aggrecan); genes that are abundant in the fetal heart; in the ventricles of older CHD patients with heart failure, compared to normally developing hearts where those genes would be low after infancy. This fetalization can be viewed as the heart trying to recapitulate the fetal growth program to repair or adapt to stress, but it also means contractile and electrical properties do not mature normally.

Epigenetic analyses (such as chromatin accessibility and DNA methylation studies) complement transcriptomics by explaining *how* gene expression is regulated in CHD. Recent epigenomic work shows that enhancer architecture in diseased human hearts undergoes a fetalization process; developmental enhancers that are normally silenced after birth become reactivated; consistent with a failure of postnatal epigenetic maturation; CHD-linked enhancers also shape cardiomyocyte programs (Armendariz et al., 2023). Additionally, environmental influences (like hypoxia or nutrient deficiencies) could leave epigenetic marks that cause sustained changes in gene expression. A notable example is retinoic acid (vitamin A) signaling: excessive retinoid exposure in utero can cause conotruncal CHD and later neuropsych issues; an epigenetic study showed that retinoid exposure leads to hypermethylation of the RARβ gene enhancer in heart and neural tissue, potentially silencing this receptor and causing maldevelopment. This ties into the earlier discussion (Section I introduction) about teratogen-associated CHD; transcriptomic and epigenomic studies are providing mechanisms for those observations.

To illustrate teratogen effects, Table 5 summarizes some known environmental exposures linked to CHD and any known tumor associations, along with their postulated epigenetic mechanisms (as gleaned from animal and human studies):

*Table 5. Teratogen Exposures, Associated CHD, and Later Tumor Risks*

| **Prenatal Exposure** | **Common Cardiac Defect** | **Other Anomalies** | **Associated Childhood Tumor** | **Proposed Mechanism (Epigenetic)** |
|---|---|---|---|---|
| Maternal Valproate (antiepileptic drug) | Secundum ASD, VSD (OR ~1.5 for CHD overall) | Neural tube defects (spina bifida), craniofacial dysmorphisms (Fetal Valproate Syndrome) | Hepatoblastoma (slight ↑ incidence reported in valproate embryopathy cohorts) | Histone deacetylase (HDAC) inhibition leading to altered acetylation of cardiac gene regulators (e.g. GATA4) |
| Excess Vitamin A / Retinoids (e.g. isotretinoin) | Conotruncal defects (overriding aorta, outflow tract septation defects) (Willhite et al., 1986); also aortic arch hypoplasia | Craniofacial anomalies (microtia, cleft palate), thymic aplasia (much like 22q11.2 syndrome) | Neuroblastoma (some studies suggest slight ↑ risk in offspring of women with high vitamin A intake, though not definitively proven) | Disruption of neural crest migration via retinoic acid receptor signaling; persistent RAR-β hypermethylation and misregulation of Hox genes |
| Diethylstilbestrol (DES) (synthetic estrogen) | Possible ↑ in Coarctation of aorta and other left-sided defects (reports vary) | Müllerian duct anomalies (T-shaped uterus, vaginal adenosis) in female offspring; undescended testes in males | Clear cell adenocarcinoma of vagina/cervix in female offspring (15;30× increased in young adults) | Aberrant estrogen receptor signaling; hypomethylation of ERα target genes leading to persistent developmental changes in reproductive tract. Cardiac effect mechanism not well understood (potentially via vascular remodeling pathways). |

*Sources:* Epidemiological data on malformations; tumor risk data from longitudinal studies (DES Follow-up Study); mechanistic hypotheses from experimental models (Willhite et al., 1986; Jentink et al., 2010).

Teratogen examples (Table 5) illustrate that environmental factors can cause both CHD and later tumor risks through epigenetic reprogramming. Valproate's link to hepatoblastoma, for instance, is attributed to in utero exposure causing genomic changes in the fetal liver that predispose to tumor formation (valproate is a known HDAC inhibitor, so it can globally alter gene expression). This introduces an additional dimension to the discussion: susceptibility arises not only from genetic polymorphisms that predispose to anomalies and tumors, but also from environmentally driven epigenetic alterations, which can function in a similar capacity.

In conclusion, transcriptomic and epigenetic studies give life to the static genome by showing how gene polymorphisms manifest in the molecular phenotype of CHD. Key takeaways are; CHD tissues often exhibit gene expression profiles that reflect both the developmental origin of the defect and the heart's response to abnormal structure or physiology (like fetalization in heart failure). Single-cell approaches are unraveling cellular composition changes in CHD, which will link specific gene mutations to their cellular consequences. And external factors leave molecular signatures that bridge CHD and tumorigenesis (as seen with retinoids or valproate). Integration of transcriptomic data with genomic findings is a next frontier; for example, if a patient's DNA has a variant in a transcription factor, and their heart tissue RNA-seq shows downstream targets misexpressed, that strengthens causal inference and can guide precision therapy (like targeting a dysregulated pathway with drugs). These translational possibilities are examined in the subsequent section.

## VII. CLINICAL TRANSLATION AND PRECISION MEDICINE

The growing understanding of genetic polymorphisms in CHD and their associations with developmental anomalies and tumor susceptibility is increasingly shaping clinical practice. This section examines the translation of these insights into patient care, with particular attention to three domains: (A) genetic testing for CHD patients and their families; (B) precision medicine strategies that individualize management on the basis of genetic findings; and (C) ethical considerations raised by genomic information, including concerns related to privacy and incidental findings.

### A. Genetic Testing in CHD Patients

Given the high proportion of CHD cases due to genetic causes, professional guidelines increasingly recommend genetic evaluation and testing for patients with CHD, especially if one or more of the following are present: additional congenital anomalies, dysmorphic features, developmental delay, or a family history of CHD (Pierpont *et al.*, 2018). In the neonatal intensive care setting, studies have even advocated for routine genomic testing of all critical CHD cases, citing diagnostic yields above 20% when broad tests are applied (Helm & Ware, 2024).

The types of genetic tests include:

- Chromosomal microarray (CMA): First-tier test for CHD with any extra anomalies. CMA can detect aneuploidies and CNVs. It has a yield of ~15;20%

in CHD with extracardiac anomalies (Zu et al., 2020), identifying abnormalities like 22q11.2 deletions, trisomies, etc. Even in isolated CHD, CMA can find pathogenic CNVs in up to ~3;10% of cases, which may have prognostic or management implications (e.g., a 1p36 deletion explaining CHD and guiding neurodevelopmental follow-up).

- Targeted single-gene tests: Used when a specific syndrome is strongly suspected clinically (e.g., *PTPN11* sequencing if classic Noonan features, *TBX5* if Holt-Oram limb defects). However, given overlapping phenotypes, these are often supplanted by panel or exome tests.
- Multigene panels: These test dozens to hundreds of CHD-related genes simultaneously. There are commercial panels focusing on syndromic CHD genes, and others on cardiomyopathy/arrhythmia genes (sometimes relevant in CHD patients). Panel testing can achieve a diagnosis in a significant subset (for example, finding *GATA4*, *NOTCH1*, *FLT4*, *JAG1*, etc. mutations). Panels are cost-effective and have relatively straightforward interpretation, but they miss novel genes and atypical presentations.
- Whole Exome Sequencing (WES) or Whole Genome Sequencing (WGS): These are increasingly utilized for CHD, especially when panel or CMA are negative and suspicion of genetic etiology remains. WES has been shown to diagnose ~10% additional cases beyond CMA/panel in research cohorts (e.g., de novo likely pathogenic variants in novel genes). As sequencing costs fall, some centers are moving directly to WGS for infants with significant CHD, to capture all variant types (including CNVs and non-coding variants) in one test. Notably, rapid WGS can be life-saving in NICU cases by diagnosing syndromes that inform acute management (like finding a metabolic disorder underlying heart failure).

When a pathogenic variant is found in a CHD patient, cascade testing of the family is recommended. This means offering targeted genetic testing to parents and sometimes siblings. For autosomal dominant conditions, determining if the variant was inherited or de novo is crucial for recurrence risk counseling. For example, if a baby's TOF is due to a *TBX1* deletion (22q11.2) and it's found to be inherited from a mildly affected parent, then other at-risk relatives can be tested and the family can be alerted to associated features (speech therapy for velopharyngeal insufficiency, etc.). If a disease-causing variant is identified in one child, prenatal diagnosis or preimplantation genetic testing can be offered in future pregnancies.

Genetic results can directly affect clinical care. A classic case is 22q11.2 deletion: if diagnosed in a newborn with CHD, one must be cautious with live vaccines (due to

T-cell deficits), supplement calcium, and plan early intervention for developmental delays. Similarly, a diagnosis of Williams syndrome (7q11.23 deletion) in a baby with supravalvular aortic stenosis would prompt monitoring for hypercalcemia in infancy and avoiding overly high vitamin D intake.

Cancer surveillance is another aspect: if a CHD patient is found to have a RA-Sopathy mutation (Noonan), the care plan might involve periodic blood counts and abdominal ultrasounds in childhood to screen for JMML or neuroblastoma (Ney et al., 2022). In the case of a CHD patient with a PTEN mutation (leading to Cowden syndrome), one would initiate thyroid ultrasounds and other tumor screenings per PTEN hamartoma syndrome protocols, even though the initial presentation was CHD (there have been reports of PTEN mutations causing CHD like Ebstein anomaly, coupling with macrocephaly and later cancer risks). Thus, genetic testing bridges pediatric cardiology with medical genetics and oncology in some instances.

It must be acknowledged that genetic testing can also yield variants of uncertain significance (VUS). This is where multidisciplinary input, including bioinformatics, is needed to interpret whether a variant contributes to the phenotype. In those scenarios, additional studies (segregation in family, functional assays) might be needed, or one must rely on evolving literature.

Genetic counseling is essential when offering testing. Families need to understand the possible outcomes (positive, negative, VUS) and the implications for other family members. Particularly in the era of WES/WGS, incidental findings can occur (like discovering a BRCA1 mutation unrelated to CHD in the course of exome sequencing a baby). The American College of Medical Genetics (ACMG) has guidelines on reporting a set of medically actionable incidental findings; families can opt in or out of receiving that information. This brings us into the ethical considerations discussed later.

## B. Precision Medicine Approaches

Armed with genetic information, clinicians can sometimes tailor therapies or surveillance; this is the promise of precision medicine in CHD. Some current and future approaches include:

- Targeted Therapies for Pathway Dysfunction: In a few syndromic CHD conditions, understanding the molecular pathway has led to targeted treatments. For example, in Noonan syndrome with hypertrophic cardiomyopathy, there are emerging trials of MEK inhibitors (like trametinib) to reverse or halt cardiomyopathy by dampening the overactive RAS/MAPK signaling (one case report showed improvement in function). In another instance, patients with Costello syndrome (HRAS mutations, high cancer risk) might benefit from experimental RAS pathway inhibitors to treat severe hypertrophic cardiomyopathy or prevent tumors. These targeted treatments are still investigational but highlight a path forward where therapy is based on genotype.

- Pharmacogenomics in CHD Management: Certain genetic polymorphisms can influence response to medications commonly used in CHD patients. For example, warfarin (an anticoagulant often used in patients with mechanical valves or Fontan circulation) has dosing partly determined by VKORC1 and CYP2C9 genotypes. In pediatric CHD patients requiring warfarin, genotyping could help in dosing and preventing clots or bleeds. Another area is β-blockers in Marfan syndrome (FBN1 mutations) vs. Losartan targeting TGF-β pathway; not exactly pharmacogenomics, but genotype (presence of TGFBR mutations in Loeys-Dietz vs FBN1 in Marfan) might influence whether an ARB or β-blocker is more effective for aortic protection.
- Risk Stratification and Monitoring: Knowing a patient's genetic background can refine their risk profile for complications. For instance, long QT syndrome genes (ion channel mutations) have been found in some CHD patients with sudden death. If a CHD patient has a coexisting channelopathy mutation identified, more aggressive arrhythmia surveillance or prophylactic beta blockers/ICD might be warranted. Similarly, recognition of a Muscular dystrophy gene (like DMD) in a boy with CHD (say, if found on exome because of elevated liver enzymes or something) would prompt cardiomyopathy surveillance even if the heart defect was repaired, since DMD causes later cardiomyopathy.
- Preventive Strategies: At the population level, identifying specific polygenic risk profiles or environmental exposures that contribute to CHD provides critical insights for preventive strategies. The prime example is folic acid supplementation, which primarily prevents neural tube defects but also has been associated with a modest reduction in CHD incidence (particularly conotruncal defects). If a woman is known to carry high-risk alleles in folate metabolism genes (like MTHFD1, as discussed, or MTHFR C677T homozygosity), one could argue for ensuring high folate levels preconception and during pregnancy. In the future, polygenic risk profiling might identify couples who could benefit from precise interventions (dietary, lifestyle) to mitigate risk to offspring.
- Personalized Surgery/Catheterization Planning: This is a more speculative angle, but imagine knowing that a child's CHD is due to a certain extracellular matrix gene mutation; a surgeon might choose a different conduit or anticipate tissue fragility. In Marfan (FBN1) patients with aortic aneurysm, surgeons operate earlier on the aorta because the tissue is genetically weaker.

One can extend that concept to other connective tissue gene mutations in CHD affecting valve or vessel quality.

- Regenerative Medicine and Gene Therapy: In severe CHD like single ventricle defects, heart failure can be a late consequence. There is research into cell-based therapies (e.g., injecting stem cell-derived cardiomyocytes). If the genetic cause is known, gene editing therapies might be conceivable in the future (for example, CRISPR correction of a known single-gene mutation causing cardiomyopathy in an induced pluripotent stem cell line, then differentiating and transplanting autologous cells). While not yet reality for structural CHD, these ideas are emerging for cardiomyopathies and could eventually cross over.

It is important to temper expectations: CHD is predominantly managed with interventions like surgery and catheterization, and that will remain the case for the foreseeable future. But genetics provides additional layers of care; anticipating which patients might have arrhythmias, which might not do well with certain medications, which need screening for thyroid or liver issues, etc. It also increasingly influences family counseling (the recurrence risk for CHD in a family can range from 3% up to 50% depending on whether a dominant mutation is found). Thus, precision medicine in CHD often means precision surveillance and counseling rather than a pill to fix the defect.

## C. Ethical and Social Considerations

The integration of extensive genetic information into CHD care raises several ethical issues:

- Genetic Counseling and Informed Consent: When performing genomic testing (like WES) in a child with CHD, consent must cover the possibility of incidental findings (like discovering a BRCA1 mutation or predisposition to adult cancer). Parents need to decide if they want those results, which might predict future disease risk unrelated to the child's current condition. Moreover, results may have familial implications; finding a hereditary mutation in a child essentially tests the parents by proxy. This can raise concerns if, for example, non-paternity is discovered or if one parent is found to carry a pathogenic mutation that could affect their own health (like a cardiomyopathy gene). Genetic counseling is critical to navigate these situations with sensitivity and clarity.
- Privacy and Discrimination: Genetic information, such as predisposition to cancer or other diseases, must be kept confidential. In some countries, laws

like the Genetic Information Nondiscrimination Act (GINA) in the US protect against health insurance or employment discrimination based on genetics. However, these protections are not universal (for example, GINA does not cover life insurance or disability insurance). Families may worry that knowing about a cancer risk (like TP53 mutation) could make it hard to get life insurance. Thus, the care team should advise families on these matters, perhaps even recommending they secure certain insurances *before* undergoing testing if they are concerned. Pediatric genetic testing also raises the question of whether children should be tested for predispositions that typically manifest in adulthood, such as BRCA1-associated cancer risk. Current practice generally discourages such testing until the individual reaches maturity and can make an informed decision, except in situations where early knowledge is required to guide medical management during childhood.

- Reproductive Decision-Making: Discovering a genetic cause for CHD can influence family planning. Parents who learn they carry a dominant mutation causing CHD might opt for prenatal diagnosis in future pregnancies or even preimplantation genetic testing (PGT) with IVF to select an embryo without the mutation. These technologies present ethical questions about selection and the definition of "acceptable risk." Some may question whether selecting against an embryo with a CHD mutation is appropriate, especially if the CHD is surgically treatable. These are personal decisions, but providers should facilitate non-directive counseling. Additionally, if a fetus is diagnosed with a severe CHD (e.g. hypoplastic left heart) and moreover a genetic syndrome portending neurodevelopmental impairment, parents face decisions about continuation of pregnancy or the aggressiveness of postnatal care. Ethics consultations are sometimes utilized in scenarios of complex CHD with additional genetic findings (like trisomy 13) to guide compassionate, family-centered decision-making.
- Data Sharing vs. Privacy: In research, sharing genetic and transcriptomic data from CHD patients accelerates discovery (as larger datasets are crucial for complex genetics). However, participants must trust that their data will be de-identified and used responsibly. Ongoing debates about how much to share genomic data (like depositing sequences in public databases) reflect the tension between collective benefit and individual privacy. Families should be informed if their genomic data will be shared broadly (even if de-identified, one day full genomes might be theoretically re-identifiable).
- Psychosocial Impact: Learning that one carries a genetic mutation can cause anxiety or alter self-image. Parents sometimes experience guilt (unfounded or otherwise) for having "passed on" a mutation to their child. Psychological support should be provided as part of genetic counseling to help families

process this information. Conversely, some parents feel relief or empowerment knowing the cause of their child's CHD, as it ends diagnostic odysseys and gives them knowledge to act on (such as screening siblings or taking preventive measures). Ensuring families have accurate expectations is part of the ethical practice; e.g., clarifying that finding a mutation in a child's DNA won't magically cure the heart defect, but it can inform care.

- Equity and Access: As genomic medicine becomes more prevalent, a concern is that not all populations have equal access. Genetic testing and advanced therapies may be less available in low-resource settings, even though CHD birth prevalence is consistent worldwide. This could exacerbate health disparities. There are efforts to create more affordable testing and to include diverse populations in CHD genetic studies (since historically, European-ancestry populations have been over-represented, which may bias discovery of risk variants). Ethically, the field must strive for inclusivity so that the benefits of genetic advances reach all groups.

In practice, many pediatric cardiology programs now operate in close collaboration with geneticists and genetic counselors, creating a multidisciplinary approach to CHD management. This ensures that the ethical aspects are considered alongside medical ones at each step (from obtaining consent for a genetic test to communicating results responsibly).

One illustrative scenario: a newborn is diagnosed with truncus arteriosus (a CHD). Genetic testing finds a 22q11.2 deletion. The team informs the family not only about the heart surgery plan but also about DiGeorge syndrome and its implications. They test the parents and find the mother has the deletion mosaic in some cells (very mild features). They then discuss with the parents the 50% chance any future child could inherit it, and options like prenatal testing. They also emphasize that the child will need immunologic and developmental follow-up. The mother, hearing about schizophrenia risk in adulthood, becomes anxious; here the team must provide balanced counseling that not every person with the deletion develops that, and environment plays a role, etc. This scenario touches on many points: multi-system care, familial implications, and psychosocial impact. With careful communication and support, the family can navigate these challenges, which showcases the importance of ethical, patient-centered care in the era of genomics.

## VIII. CONCLUSION

### A. Summary of Key Points:

This chapter has outlined how genetic polymorphisms; ranging from single nucleotide variants to whole-chromosome abnormalities;are implicated in congenital heart disease (CHD) and its broader manifestations. CHD, which affects approximately 1% of live births (Lahm et al., 2021), frequently arises from a complex interplay between genetic and environmental influences. Around one-third of affected individuals present with additional birth defects or developmental disorders (Homsy et al., 2015), underscoring the existence of shared developmental pathways.

Syndromic forms of CHD illustrate the consequences of highly penetrant mutations in single genes (e.g., PTPN11 in Noonan syndrome, JAG1 in Alagille syndrome, TBX5 in Holt-Oram syndrome) or chromosomal aberrations (such as trisomy 21 and 22q11.2 deletion), which produce characteristic clusters of anomalies. These conditions exemplify how disruption of pivotal developmental signaling cascades;including RAS/MAPK, Notch, and transcriptional regulatory networks;can produce multi-organ effects. Importantly, several syndromes also confer heightened tumor risks, such as the markedly increased incidence of leukemia in Down syndrome (10;20-fold; Linabery et al., 2008) or the predisposition to myeloproliferative disorders observed in Noonan syndrome (Ney et al., 2022).

Non-syndromic CHD genes, including NKX2-5, GATA4, TBX20, and CTNNB1, typically give rise to isolated cardiac malformations but also demonstrate subtler extra-cardiac consequences. For example, NKX2-5 mutations are associated with conduction system disease, and CTNNB1 variants with neurodevelopmental impairment. These genes highlight both the broader systemic implications of ostensibly cardiac-restricted mutations and the convergence of CHD pathways with oncogenesis (e.g., β-catenin/CTNNB1 in hepatoblastoma; NOTCH1 in hematologic malignancies).

Chromosomal abnormalities and recurrent CNVs further underscore the genetic complexity of CHD, with conditions such as Down syndrome alone accounting for an estimated 8% of cases. These large-scale genomic alterations not only contribute to structural cardiac defects but also predispose to subsequent health challenges, including malignancies and metabolic disorders.

The exploration of *polygenic and oligogenic factors* revealed CHD as a complex trait in many cases: common variants cumulatively impact risk (Spendlove et al., 2022), and occasionally two or more rare mutations interact in one patient to cause CHD. This complex genetics concept is crucial for future research and possibly for personalized risk prediction. The transcriptomics section then added a functional dimension; showing how genetic variants reshape gene expression programs in the heart, in some cases reverting cells to a fetal-like state (Odogwu et al., 2023). It is striking that the "fetal gene program" re-emerges in diseased or stressed hearts, underlining the continuum between development and disease. Single-cell transcriptomics further allowed us to pinpoint which cell types and pathways are deranged in CHD, offering insight into pathogenesis that pure genetics alone might miss (for instance, identifying lingering neural crest cells or aberrant proliferative signals in CHD hearts). Throughout these sections, one theme is clear: the genes that build the heart often play roles in fundamental cellular processes (proliferation, differentiation, migration), so disturbances can have far-reaching consequences, including oncogenesis. Conversely, some oncogenes/tumor suppressors, when germline mutated, can manifest as CHD among other issues. This bidirectional link between CHD and tumor biology is a cutting-edge area that blends developmental biology with cancer research.

Clinically, these insights have tangible impacts. Genetic testing is now a standard part of CHD care, enabling precise diagnoses that inform management beyond the heart (e.g., endocrine surveillance in DiGeorge, cancer screening in RASopathies). The concept of precision medicine in CHD is in its infancy but growing; whether it's using genotype to guide therapy (as in MEK inhibitors for Noonan-related cardiomyopathy) or employing polygenic risk scores to identify high-risk families for preventive interventions. From an ethical perspective, genomic testing introduces new complexities, as information derived from a single test may influence life planning for an entire family and raises critical questions regarding consent, privacy, and equity.

## B. Future Research Directions:

The field of CHD genetics and genomics is rapidly evolving. One priority is to discover the remaining genetic factors underlying CHD, especially for the ~70-80% of cases still without a definitive genetic explanation. This will likely involve larger GWAS (potentially pan-ethnic to capture diverse risk alleles), deep sequencing of noncoding regions (searching for regulatory mutations affecting heart enhancers), and advanced bioinformatic approaches to detect gene-gene interactions. Moreover, integrating multi-omics data (genomics, transcriptomics, epigenomics, proteomics) through computational models could illuminate how a particular genotype leads to a phenotype; for instance, constructing gene regulatory networks for normal vs. CHD hearts.

Another burgeoning area is the study of somatic mutations in CHD. Recent evidence suggests that some CHDs, particularly mosaic conditions like vascular tumors or even isolated CHDs, might result from somatic mutations arising during embryogenesis (e.g., a mosaic NOTCH1 mutation confined to heart tissue). Investigating heart tissue directly for somatic variants might explain some sporadic CHD cases, an approach parallel to cancer genomics.

On the tumor risk side, more epidemiologic research is needed to quantify long-term cancer incidence in CHD cohorts, especially as surgical survivors live longer. Is the slight increased cancer risk in adult CHD due to shared genetics, or due to treatment exposures (like X-rays, cardiopulmonary bypass oxidative stress)? Cohort studies linking genetic data with outcomes could parse this. If, for instance, adult CHD patients with certain polymorphisms show a 5% cancer incidence by age 50 compared to 3% in those without, that could inform screening guidelines for CHD survivors.

Gene therapy and genome editing represent a future horizon. An emerging ethical and translational question concerns whether CHD could one day be prevented through correction of pathogenic mutations in utero. It sounds like science fiction, but with CRISPR being used in vivo for some conditions and fetal surgeries already done for structural anomalies (like spina bifida repair in utero), one can envision a time where a pathogenic variant causing a lethal CHD might be edited in fetal cardiac cells to improve outcome. That will require leaps in safe delivery methods and precise targeting, and it raises profound ethical questions; but the groundwork (like base editors, prime editing) is being laid in research labs now.

## C. Clinical and Public Health Impact:

As research progresses, the impacts will be felt from the clinic to the broader public health sphere. For clinicians, a deeper genetic understanding of CHD means more accurate prognosis and personalized care plans. For instance, recognition that a patient's CHD occurs within the context of a cancer-predisposition syndrome enables coordinated care with oncology specialists and facilitates timely preventive or therapeutic interventions. In some cases, it might influence reproductive counseling; if a family has a dominantly inherited CHD gene, public health initiatives might ensure they have access to genetic counseling and options to reduce recurrence (which also reduces healthcare burden of severe CHD in the next generation). From a public health perspective, reducing exposure to known teratogens (like better regulation of medications in pregnancy, folate fortification of foods which has already shown reductions in CHD rates) is a direct outcome of understanding gene-environment interactions.

Additionally, creating registries that link genetic data with outcomes can help healthcare systems allocate resources; for instance, knowing how many CHD survivors might develop certain complications can guide screening programs. Public health screening might one day include not just echocardiograms for high-risk pregnancies but also genetic screening panels for couples (as part of expanded carrier screening) that include CHD-associated genes. However, this must be done thoughtfully to avoid causing alarm for variants of uncertain significance.

In conclusion, the genomics of CHD is illuminating the fundamental biology of how hearts form and fail, while simultaneously bridging to other fields like oncology and endocrinology. It paints a picture of developmental pathways that, when perturbed, yield both structural anomalies in infancy and potential disease vulnerabilities later in life. The ultimate goal of this knowledge is to improve patient outcomes; by enabling earlier diagnosis (sometimes even prenatal), guiding interventions (medical, surgical, or lifestyle), and anticipating complications (like tumors) before they manifest. CHD has gone from being seen purely as a structural plumbing problem to a systemic genetic condition for many patients. The long-term expectation is that continued research, combined with equitable implementation of genomic medicine, will not only improve surgical outcomes for CHD but also support lifelong, integrated care addressing the broad spectrum of challenges experienced by patients and their families.

## REFERENCES


Aherne, N. J., Rangaswamy, G., & Thirion, P. (2013). Prostate cancer in a male with Holt-Oram syndrome: First clinical association of the TBX5 mutation. *Case Reports in Urology, 405343*. Advance online publication. DOI: 10.1155/2013/405343 PMID: 23984174

Akat, K. M., Moore-McGriff, D., Morozov, P., Brown, M., Gogakos, T., Correa Da Rosa, J., Mihailovic, A., Sauer, M., Ji, R., Ramarathnam, A., Totary-Jain, H., Williams, Z., Tuschl, T., & Schulze, P. C. (2014). Comparative RNA-sequencing analysis of myocardial and circulating small RNAs in human heart failure and their utility as biomarkers. *Proceedings of the National Academy of Sciences of the United States of America, 111*(30), 11151–11156. DOI: 10.1073/pnas.1401724111 PMID: 25012294

Armendariz, D. A., Goetsch, S. C., Sundarrajan, A., Sivakumar, S., Wang, Y., Xie, S., Munshi, N. V., & Hon, G. C. (2023). CHD-associated enhancers shape human cardiomyocyte lineage commitment. *eLife*, *12*, e86206. DOI: 10.7554/eLife.86206 PMID: 37096669

Burnicka-Turek, O., Steimle, J. D., Huang, W., Felker, L., Kamp, A., Kweon, J., Peterson, M., Reeves, R. H., Maslen, C. L., Gruber, P. J., Yang, X. H., Shendure, J., & Moskowitz, I. P. (2016). Cilia gene mutations cause atrioventricular septal defects by multiple mechanisms. *Human Molecular Genetics*, *25*(14), 3011–3028. DOI: 10.1093/hmg/ddw155 PMID: 27340223

Chen, Y., Xiao, D., Zhang, L., Cai, C. L., Li, B. Y., & Liu, Y. (2021). The Role of Tbx20 in Cardiovascular Development and Function. *Frontiers in Cell and Developmental Biology*, *9*, 638542. DOI: 10.3389/fcell.2021.638542 PMID: 33585493

Ehrlich, L., & Prakash, S. K. (2022). Copy-number variation in congenital heart disease. *Current Opinion in Genetics & Development*, *77*, 101986. DOI: 10.1016/j.gde.2022.101986 PMID: 36202051

Elmagrpy, Z., Rayani, A., Shah, A., Habas, E., & Aburawi, E. H. (2011). Down syndrome and congenital heart disease: Why the regional difference as observed in the Libyan experience? *Cardiovascular Journal of Africa*, *22*(6), 306–309. DOI: 10.5830/CVJA-2010-072 PMID: 22159317

Garg, V., Kathiriya, I. S., Barnes, R., Schluterman, M. K., King, I. N., Butler, C. A., Rothrock, C. R., Eapen, R. S., Hirayama-Yamada, K., Joo, K., Matsuoka, R., Cohen, J. C., & Srivastava, D. (2003). GATA4 mutations cause human congenital heart defects and reveal an interaction with TBX5. *Nature*, *424*(6947), 443–447. DOI: 10.1038/nature01827 PMID: 12845333

Garg, V., Muth, A. N., Ransom, J. F., Schluterman, M. K., Barnes, R., King, I. N., Grossfeld, P. D., & Srivastava, D. (2005). Mutations in NOTCH1 cause aortic valve disease. *Nature*, *437*(7056), 270–274. DOI: 10.1038/nature03940 PMID: 16025100

Helm, B. M., & Ware, S. M. (2024). Clinical Decision Analysis of Genetic Evaluation and Testing in 1013 Intensive Care Unit Infants with Congenital Heart Defects Supports Universal Genetic Testing. *Genes*, *15*(4), 505. DOI: 10.3390/genes15040505 PMID: 38674439

Homsy, J., Zaidi, S., Shen, Y., Ware, J. S., Samocha, K. E., Karczewski, K. J., DePalma, S. R., McKean, D., Wakimoto, H., Gorham, J., Jin, S. C., Deanfield, J., Giardini, A., Porter, G. A.Jr, Kim, R., Bilguvar, K., López-Giráldez, F., Tikhonova, I., Mane, S., & Chung, W. K. (2015). De novo mutations in congenital heart disease with neurodevelopmental and other congenital anomalies. *Science*, *350*(6265), 1262–1266. DOI: 10.1126/science.aac9396 PMID: 26785492

Jentink, J., Loane, M. A., Dolk, H., Barisic, I., Garne, E., Morris, J. K., & de Jong-van den Berg, L. T.EUROCAT Antiepileptic Study Working Group. (2010). Valproic acid monotherapy in pregnancy and major congenital malformations. *The New England Journal of Medicine*, *362*(23), 2185–2193. DOI: 10.1056/NEJMoa0907328 PMID: 20558369

Jiang, Y., Zhuang, J., Lin, Y., Wang, X., Chen, J., & Han, F. (2019). Long noncoding RNA SNHG6 contributes to ventricular septal defect formation via negative regulation of miR-101 and activation of Wnt/β-catenin pathway. *Die Pharmazie*, *74*(1), 23–28. DOI: 10.1691/ph.2019.8736 PMID: 30782246

Kamath, B. M., Baker, A., Houwen, R., Todorova, L., & Kerkar, N. (2018). Systematic review: The epidemiology, natural history, and burden of Alagille syndrome. *Journal of Pediatric Gastroenterology and Nutrition*, *67*(2), 148–156. DOI: 10.1097/MPG.0000000000001958 PMID: 29543694

Kars, M. E., Stein, D., Stenson, P. D., Cooper, D. N., Chung, W. K., Gruber, P. J., Seidman, C. E., Shen, Y., Tristani-Firouzi, M., Gelb, B. D., & Itan, Y. (2025). Deciphering the digenic architecture of congenital heart disease using trio exome sequencing data. *American Journal of Human Genetics*, *112*(3), 583–598. DOI: 10.1016/j.ajhg.2025.01.024 PMID: 39983722

Kirk, E. P., Sunde, M., Costa, M. W., Rankin, S. A., Wolstein, O., Castro, M. L., Butler, T. L., Hyun, C., Guo, G., Otway, R., Mackay, J. P., Waddell, L. B., Cole, A. D., Hayward, C., Keogh, A., Macdonald, P., Griffiths, L., Fatkin, D., Sholler, G. F., & Harvey, R. P. (2007). Mutations in cardiac T-box factor gene TBX20 are associated with diverse cardiac pathologies, including defects of septation and valvulogenesis and cardiomyopathy. *American Journal of Human Genetics, 81*(2), 280–291. DOI: 10.1086/519530 PMID: 17668378

Lahm, H., Jia, M., Dreßen, M., Wirth, F., Puluca, N., Gilsbach, R., Keavney, B. D., Cleuziou, J., Beck, N., Bondareva, O., Dzilic, E., Burri, M., König, K. C., Ziegelmüller, J. A., Abou-Ajram, C., Neb, I., Zhang, Z., Doppler, S. A., Mastantuono, E., & Krane, M. (2021). Congenital heart disease risk loci identified by genome-wide association study in European patients. *The Journal of Clinical Investigation, 131*(2), e141837. DOI: 10.1172/JCI141837 PMID: 33201861

Lakshmanan, S., & Gimelli, A. (2023). Cancer risk in adult congenital heart disease. *International Journal of Cardiology: Congenital Heart Disease, 12*, 100441. 10.1016/j.ijcchd.2023.100441

Linabery, A. M., Blair, C. K., Gamis, A. S., Olshan, A. F., Heerema, N. A., & Ross, J. A. (2008). Congenital abnormalities and acute leukemia among children with Down syndrome: A Children's Oncology Group study. *Cancer Epidemiology, Biomarkers & Prevention, 17*(10), 2572–2577. DOI: 10.1158/1055-9965.EPI-08-0284 PMID: 18829445

Liu, B., Lu, Y., Wang, Q., Dai, Y., & Liu, L. (2024). Cancer in 22q11.2 deletion syndrome: A case report and literature review. *European Journal of Medical Genetics, 70*, 104959. DOI: 10.1016/j.ejmg.2024.104959 PMID: 38969060

Manivannan, S., Mansfield, C., & Zhang, X.. (2022). Single-cell transcriptomic profiling unveils dysregulation of cardiac progenitor cells and cardiomyocytes in a mouse model of maternal hyperglycemia. *Communications Biology, 5*, 820. DOI: 10.1038/s42003-022-03779-x PMID: 35970860

Mattapally, S., Nizamuddin, S., & Murthy, K. S.. (2015). c.620C>T mutation in GATA4 is associated with congenital heart disease in South India. *BMC Medical Genetics, 16*, 7. DOI: 10.1186/s12881-015-0152-7 PMID: 25928801

Misra, C., Sachan, N., McNally, C. R., Koenig, S. N., Nichols, H. A., Guggilam, A., Lucchesi, P. A., Pu, W. T., Srivastava, D., & Garg, V. (2012). Congenital heart disease–causing Gata4 mutation displays functional deficits in vivo. *PLOS Genetics, 8*(5), e1002690. DOI: 10.1371/journal.pgen.1002690 PMID: 22589735

Moreau, J. L. M., Kesteven, S., Martin, E. M. M. A., Lau, K. S., Yam, M. X., O'Reilly, V. C., del Monte-Nieto, G., Baldini, A., Feneley, M. P., Moon, A. M., Harvey, R. P., Sparrow, D. B., Chapman, G., & Dunwoodie, S. L. (2019). Gene-environment interaction impacts on heart development and embryo survival. *Development, 146*(4), dev172957. Advance online publication. DOI: 10.1242/dev.172957 PMID: 30787001

National Organization for Rare Disorders. (2020). Holt-Oram syndrome. In *NORD Rare Disease Database.* https://rarediseases.org/rare-diseases/holt-oram-syndrome/

Ney, G., Gross, A., Livinski, A., Kratz, C. P., & Stewart, D. R. (2022). Cancer incidence and surveillance strategies in individuals with RASopathies. *American Journal of Medical Genetics. Part C, Seminars in Medical Genetics, 190*(4), 530–540. DOI: 10.1002/ajmg.c.32018 PMID: 36533693

Nussbaumer, G., & Benesch, M. (2022). Hepatoblastoma in molecularly defined, congenital diseases. *American Journal of Medical Genetics. Part A, 188*(9), 2527–2535. DOI: 10.1002/ajmg.a.62767 PMID: 35478319

S.Običan, L. Maggio, Holt-oram Syndrome. Obstetric Imaging: Fetal Diagnosis and Care, 2018, pp. 557–559, https://doi.org/DOI: 10.1016/B978-0-323-44548-1.00132-7

Odogwu, N. M., Hagen, C., & Nelson, T. J. (2023). Transcriptome studies of congenital heart diseases: Identifying current gaps and therapeutic frontiers. *Frontiers in Genetics, 14*, 1278747. DOI: 10.3389/fgene.2023.1278747 PMID: 38152655

Øyen, N., Diaz, L. J., Leirgul, E., Boyd, H. A., Priest, J., Mathiesen, E. R., Quertermous, T., Wohlfahrt, J., & Melbye, M. (2016). Prepregnancy Diabetes and Offspring Risk of Congenital Heart Disease: A Nationwide Cohort Study. *Circulation, 133*(23), 2243–2253. DOI: 10.1161/CIRCULATIONAHA.115.017465 PMID: 27166384

Pierpont, M. E., Brueckner, M., Chung, W. K., Garg, V., Lacro, R. V., McGuire, A. L., Mital, S., Priest, J. R., Pu, W. T., Roberts, A., Ware, S. M., Gelb, B. D., & Russell, M. W., American Heart Association Council on Cardiovascular Disease in the Young, Council on Cardiovascular and Stroke Nursing, & Council on Genomic and Precision Medicine. (2018). Genetic basis for congenital heart disease: Revisited: A scientific statement from the American Heart Association. *Circulation, 138*(21), e653–e711. DOI: 10.1161/CIR.0000000000000606 PMID: 30571578

Sinibaldi, L., Garone, G., Mandarino, A., Iarossi, G., Chioma, L., Dentici, M. L., Merla, G., Agolini, E., Micalizzi, A., Mancini, C., Niceta, M., Macchiaiolo, M., Diodato, D., Onesimo, R., Blandino, R., Delogu, A. B., De Rosa, G., Trevisan, V., Iademarco, M., & Calcagni, G. (2023). Congenital heart defects in CTNNB1 syndrome: Raising clinical awareness. *Clinical Genetics, 104*(5), 528–541. DOI: 10.1111/cge.14404 PMID: 37455656

Spendlove, S. J., Bondhus, L., Lluri, G., Sul, J. H., & Arboleda, V. A. (2022). Polygenic risk scores of endo-phenotypes identify the effect of genetic background in congenital heart disease. *HGG Advances*, *3*(3), 100112. DOI: 10.1016/j.xhgg.2022.100112 PMID: 35599848

Spinner, N. B., Loomes, K. M., Krantz, I. D., Adam, M. P., Feldman, J., & Mirzaa, G. M. (2000). Alagille syndrome. In M. P. Adam, J. Feldman, G. M. Mirzaa, et al. (Eds.), *GeneReviews®* [Internet]. University of Washington, Seattle. (Updated 2024, January 4). https://www.ncbi.nlm.nih.gov/books/NBK1273/

Tartaglia, M., Zampino, G., & Gelb, B. D. (2010). Noonan syndrome: Clinical aspects and molecular pathogenesis. *Molecular Syndromology*, *1*(1), 2–26. DOI: 10.1159/000276766 PMID: 20648242

Willhite, C. C., Hill, R. M., & Irving, D. W. (1986). Isotretinoin-induced craniofacial malformations in humans and hamsters. *Journal of Craniofacial Genetics and Developmental Biology. Supplement*, *2*, 193–20. PMID: 3491113

Yi, K., He, S. E., Guo, T., Wang, Z. Q., Zhang, X., Xu, J. G., Zhang, H. Y., Liu, W. G., & You, T. (2025). Association of MTHFD1 G1958A (rs2236225) gene polymorphism with the risk of congenital heart disease: A systematic review and meta-analysis. *BMC Medical Genomics*, *18*(1), 20. DOI: 10.1186/s12920-024-02052-w PMID: 39871280

Zu, B., Zheng, Z., & Fu, Q. (2020). Molecular diagnostics for congenital heart disease: A narrative review of the current technologies and applications. *Journal of Bio-X Research*, *3*, 92–96. DOI: 10.1097/JBR.0000000000000068

# Chapter 3
# Risk of Congenital Heart Disease in Assisted Reproductive Pregnancies:
## Mechanisms, Evidence, and Clinical Implications

**Shadab Ahamad**
https://orcid.org/0000-0003-0788-4817
*Sri Sathya Sai Sanjeevani Research Foundation, India*

**Ramya Raghavan**
https://orcid.org/0000-0002-9953-543X
*Sri Sathya Sai University for Human Excellence, India*

## ABSTRACT

*Congenital heart disease (CHD) is the most common congenital anomaly worldwide, affecting 8–12 per 1,000 live births and contributing significantly to infant morbidity and mortality. Concurrently, assisted reproductive technologies (ART), including in vitro fertilization (IVF) and intracytoplasmic sperm injection (ICSI), have become increasingly prevalent, resulting in over 8 million births globally. Evidence indicates a modest but consistent elevation in CHD risk among ART-conceived offspring, particularly non-syndromic ventricular septal defects, atrial septal defects, and conotruncal anomalies such as tetralogy of Fallot. Population-based registries report a 1.3–2.0-fold increased relative risk, with ICSI and multiple gestations conferring higher susceptibility. Mechanistic studies suggest multifactorial pathways involving*

DOI: 10.4018/979-8-3373-3735-7.ch003

*ART-related interventions, maternal factors (advanced age, metabolic disorders), pregnancy complications (multiple gestations, preterm birth), and epigenetic dysregulation during critical windows of cardiac development.*

## 1. INTRODUCTION

Congenital heart disease (CHD) is the most prevalent congenital anomaly worldwide, accounting for approximately one-third of all major birth defects and affecting an estimated 8–12 per 1,000 live births. Recent meta-analyses estimate that over 1.35 million children are born with CHD annually, underscoring its profound impact on global child health and survival. Although advances in diagnostic and therapeutic modalities have significantly improved outcomes in high-income countries, stark disparities persist. In low- and middle-income regions, underdiagnosis, limited access to care, and higher fertility rates contribute to a disproportionate burden of CHD, which remains a leading cause of infant morbidity and mortality (Xu et al., 2025). Additionally, CHD is more prevalent in infants, indicating shared biological vulnerabilities (Palma et al., 2023). The etiopathogenesis of CHD is multifactorial, arising from a complex interplay of genetic, epigenetic, and environmental determinants that influence cardiac morphogenesis during early embryogenesis (Choudhary et al., 2025). The most commonly reported lesions include ventricular septal defects (20-30%) and atrial septal defects (15-20%), while cyanotic heart diseases account for ~30% of cases (Saxena et al., 2019). Despite increasing understanding of genetic and developmental pathways, many cases remain idiopathic, highlighting the need to explore novel risk factors and emerging exposures.

## 2. ASSISTED REPRODUCTIVE TECHNOLOGIES (ARTS): AN OVERVIEW

Assisted reproductive technology (ART) included medical interventions that manipulate gametes or embryos to achieve pregnancy, such as in vitro fertilization (IVF), intracytoplasmic sperm injection (ICSI), gamete or embryo donation, cryopreservation, and gestational surrogacy. Since the first successful IVF birth in 1978, ART has transformed infertility management, evolving through several technological milestones:

- IVF (1970s–1980s): Fertilization of oocytes with sperm in vitro.
- ICSI (1990s): Direct injection of a single sperm into an oocyte, enabling conception in severe male-factor infertility.

- Cryopreservation and Frozen Embryo Transfer (2000s): Vitrification improved embryo survival and allowed deferred transfer, reducing ovarian hyperstimulation risk.
- Preimplantation Genetic Testing (2010s–present): Allows chromosomal screening, indirectly influencing embryo selection and implantation success.

The global ART market is expanding rapidly and is projected to reach nearly $45 billion by 2026, driven by technological progress and growing demand (Kashyap and Tripathi, 2023). The International Committee for Monitoring Assisted Reproductive Technologies (ICMART) reported more than 5 million ART by 2018 across 83 countries, resulting in approximately 671,000–728,000 live births annually (Baker et al., 2025). ART utilization is highest in Europe, North America, and East Asia, where ART births now comprise 3–7% of all deliveries (Pinborg et al., 2023). However, access to ART remains limited in many regions due to high costs, limited infrastructure, and social stigma, resulting in significant disparities in utilization and outcomes.

*Figure 1. ART pregnancies exhibit prevalence of CHD as shown in Table 2. Multiple Studies report Relative risks (RR) and odds ratios (OR) of CHD in ART pregnancies as shown in Table 2 and Table 4.*

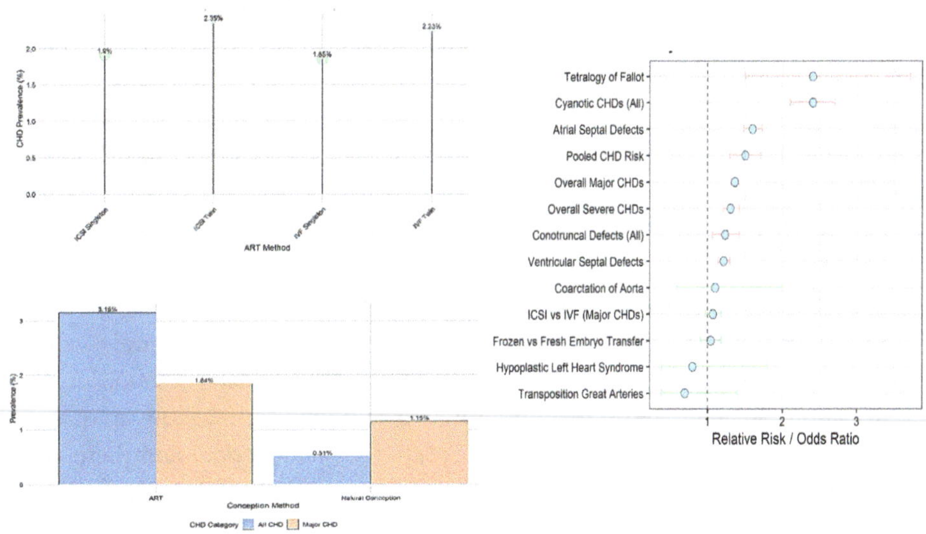

## 3. RATIONALE FOR INVESTIGATING THE ASSOCIATION BETWEEN ART AND CHD RISK

In parallel with the global burden of CHD, the use of assisted reproductive technologies has expanded dramatically over the past four decades. More than 8 million births have resulted from ART procedures worldwide (Pinborg et al., 2023) Although ART has revolutionized infertility management, emerging evidence indicates a modest but consistent elevation in the risk of congenital anomalies—particularly cardiovascular malformations—in ART-conceived offspring compared to those conceived spontaneously (Figure 1 and 2).

A comprehensive meta-analysis including 113 studies and 768,929 ART-conceived children compared with 40,709,337 spontaneously conceived children demonstrated a marginal but significant higher risk of congenital anomalies among ART offspring. Subgroup analyses revealed higher risk for children conceived via ICSI, Day 3 embryo transfer, and fresh embryo transfer (FET), compared to IVF, Day 5 transfer, or FET (Bhat et al., 2025).

Further risk stratification indicates that the highest risk is seen in ICSI-conceived multiples, followed by ICSI singletons. Tararbit et al. (2013) reported a 2·4-fold increased risk of tetralogy of Fallot (adjusted OR 2·4, 95% CI 1·5-3·7), with ICSI specifically associated with an adjusted OR of 3·0 (95%CI 1·0–8·9). Although IVF-conceived singletons show a more moderate risk, the difference in absolute risk (1.8% vs 1.2%) still warrants clinical attention (Potiris et al., 2024). Subsequent meta-analyses have reinforced these findings, demonstrating a 70% increased risk of CHD in ART pregnancies (RR 1.71, 95% CI 1.25-2.34) (Gullo et al., 2023) and nearly two-fold increase in severe CHDs (OR 1.98, 95% CI 1.30-3.02) (Lemieux et al., 2024).

Despite growing evidence, critical gaps remain. Most data are derived from high-income countries, limiting the generalizability of results to developing regions where ART protocols, genetic backgrounds, environmental exposures, and healthcare systems differ substantially. Moreover, ART registries in low- and middle-income countries are incomplete or absent, leading to potential underestimation or misclassification. Standardized screening protocols and long-term follow-up data are lacking. Mechanistic pathways remain incompletely understood, and there is no consensus on targeted cardiac screening for ART-conceived children, especially in resource-limited settings.

In response to these gaps, this chapter aims to provide a comprehensive synthesis of current knowledge at the interface of ART and CHD. Specifically, the objectives are: (1) to synthesize current epidemiological data on the prevalence and risk of CHD in ART-conceived offspring, with a focus on global and developing country contexts; (2) to critically examine the biological mechanisms that may underlie

ART-associated cardiac anomalies; (3) to review current clinical guidelines and best practices for cardiac screening and management in ART-conceived children; and (4) to identify key research gaps and propose priorities for future investigation. By integrating these domains, this chapter aims to inform evidence-based policy, guide clinical practice, and catalyze research that addresses the unique needs of ART-conceived children worldwide.

## 4. EPIDEMIOLOGY OF CHD IN ART PREGNANCIES: EVIDENCE FROM KEY COHORT AND REGISTRY STUDIES

Over the past two decades, epidemiological research has consistently demonstrated a modest but clinically meaningful increase in the risk of CHD among children conceived through ART compared to those conceived naturally. Across multiple population-based registries and meta-analyses, the relative increase in CHD risk ranges from 36% and 71%, although the absolute risk remains relatively low. Large-scale datasets have been particularly informative, as they permit stratification by ART technique, plurality, defect type, and severity.

### Major International Registries and Cohort Studies

Key registry and surveillance systems across Europe, North America, and Asia have generated robust, longitudinal data on ART-conceived births and congenital anomalies. Representative registries are summarized in Table 1 & 2.

*Table 1. Registry Studies*

| Registry/Study Name | Geographic Coverage | Study Period |
|---|---|---|
| Nordic CoNARTaS | Denmark, Finland, Norway, Sweden | 1984-2015 |
| EUROCAT Network | 23 European countries | 2008-2015 (CHD data) |
| EPICARD (Paris) | Paris metropolitan area | 1987-2009, 2005-2008 |
| DANBIO (Denmark) | Denmark nationwide | Ongoing since 2000 |
| ROB-FIN (Finland) | Finland nationwide | Ongoing since 1999 |
| NOR-DMARD (Norway) | Norway nationwide | Ongoing since 2000 |
| SRQ-ARTIS (Sweden) | Sweden nationwide | Ongoing since 1999 |
| Copenhagen Baby Heart Study | Copenhagen region | Specific cohort study |
| US National ART Surveillance | United States nationwide | Ongoing |
| Australian ART Registry | Australia and New Zealand | Ongoing since 1979 |

## Nordic Registry Evidence: The Gold Standard

The Nordic CoNARTaS Registry is widely regarded as the most methodologically rigorous dataset evaluating ART-related risks. It includes 7.7 million live births across Denmark, Finland, Norway, and Sweden, of which 171,735 were ART-conceived. Major CHDs were recorded in 1.84% of ART-conceived children versus 1.15% of spontaneously conceived children (adjusted OR 1.36; 95% CI 1.31–1.41), and severe CHDs were observed in 0.35% versus 0.26%, respectively (adjusted OR 1.30; 95% CI 1.20–1.42) (Sargisian et al., 2024; Wennerholm et al., 2013). The large sample size, high-quality registries, and uniform healthcare systems strengthen the validity of these findings and establish ART as an independent risk factor for both total and major CHDs.

## EPICARD Paris Registry: Insights into Defect Patterns

The EPICARD registry, a specialized CHD surveillance program in the Paris metropolitan area, enables detailed analysis of specific cardiac phenotypes. Among 1,583 CHD cases, ART—particularly ICSI—was strongly associated with conotruncal anomalies. Tetralogy of Fallot demonstrated an OR of 2.4 (95% CI 1.5–3.7), while ICSI-specific risk reached OR of 3.0 (95% CI 1.0–8.9) (Tararbit et al., 2013). Subsequent meta-analyses validate this pattern. A meta-analysis of 8 cohort studies encompassing 25,856 ART-conceived children demonstrated a 45% increased risk (OR 1.45, 95% CI: 1.20-1.76) (Giorgione et al., 2018), while Pinborg et al. (2023) reported a pooled relative risk (RR) of 1.71 (95% CI: 1.25–2.34) for CHD in ART pregnancies, a finding reaffirmed by the most recent comprehensive review by Bhat et al. (2025), which included over 768,000 ART-conceived offspring.

These results support clinical recommendations that IVF should remain the preferred first-line ART method for non-severe male infertility, with ICSI reserved for severe male factor cases, due to its higher association with CHDs.

Additionally, the French National Surveillance Program (Bourdon et al., 2024) identified medically assisted reproduction and prematurity as independent predictors of CHD, with an overall prevalence close to 1% in the general population.

## Other High-Income Registries Evidence

Multiple national registries corroborate the ART-CHD association. In North America, the U.S. National ART Surveillance System (NASS) identified a twofold higher prevalence of acyanotic CHD, particularly VSD and ASD, among ART-conceived neonates (Appiah et al., 2024). The Australian ART Registry (Hansen et al., 2013) reported similar trends, with 2.7% of ART-conceived infants affected versus 1.4% in spontaneous conceptions (RR 2.5, 95% CI: 1.5–4.0). The Norwegian national cohort covering two decades (1994–2014) documented a CHD prevalence of 144.6 per 10,000 live births, demonstrating declining rates of severe lesions but a persistent excess of septal defects among ART pregnancies (Leirgul et al., 2025).

CHD registry in Québec that automatically identifies individuals with CHD and extracts their cardiac anatomy from clinical data (Watelle et al., 2024). A notable 2.3% of cases having records from multiple institutions, indicating that patients with more complex CHD are more likely to receive care from multiple facilities.

## Evidence from Asia: Emerging but Consistent Patterns

Although high-quality data from Asia remain limited, emerging registries in Sri Lanka, Pakistan, and Bangladesh report CHD prevalence of 2.8–3.1% among ART-conceived infants, primarily driven by ventricular and atrial septal defects. Relative risks range from 2.0 to 2.3, closely mirroring Western data. Despite variations in healthcare infrastructure and registry completeness, the consistency of risk elevation across diverse populations supports the biological plausibility and global relevance of ART-associated CHD risk.

*Table 2. International Cohort Studies and Registries on CHD Prevalence in ART Pregnancies*

| Study/ Registry | ART Type | CHD Prevalence (%) | Main CHD Subtypes Reported | Relative Risk (RR) / Odds Ratio (OR) | Reference |
|---|---|---|---|---|---|
| CoNARTaS Copenhagen Cohort | IVF, ICSI, Egg Donation | 2.5% in ART vs 1.3% in natural conception | Septal defects, conotruncal defects (tetralogy of Fallot) | RR = 1.9 (CI 1.2–2.9) | (Sargisian et al., 2024) |
| USA NAAS | IVF, ICSI | 3.0% in ART vs 1.4% in spontaneous conception | Acyanotic CHD, ventricular septal defects (VSD), atrial septal defects (ASD) | OR = 2.1 (CI 1.5–3.0) | (Appiah et al., 2024) |
| Nordic Subset | IVF, ICSI | 2.3% in ART vs 1.5% in spontaneous conception | Conotruncal defects, left-sided defects (hypoplastic left heart syndrome) | RR = 1.8 (CI 1.1–3.0) | (Wennerholm et al., 2013) |
| Norway national | IVF, ICSI, Ovulation Induction | 2.8% in ART vs 1.6% in natural conception | Acyanotic CHD (ASD, VSD), Conotruncal defects | OR = 2.3 (CI 1.7–3.1) | (Leirgul et al., 2025) |
| Australian ART Registry (2021) | IVF, ICSI | 2.7% in ART vs 1.4% in spontaneous conception | Syndromic CHD, including DiGeorge syndrome and Down syndrome | RR = 2.5 (CI 1.5–4.0) | (Hansen et al., 2013) |
| France | Medically assisted reproduction (MAR) | 1.9% in MAR | All CHD subtypes | OR = 1.2 (CI 1.1-1.5) | (Bourdon et al., 2024) |
| Sri Lanka, national ART cohort | IVF, ICSI | 2.9% | VSD, ASD, and rare conotruncal defects | OR = 2.0 (CI 1.4-3.0) | (Registry, 2021) |

continued on following page

*Table 2. Continued*

| Study/ Registry | ART Type | CHD Prevalence (%) | Main CHD Subtypes Reported | Relative Risk (RR) / Odds Ratio (OR) | Reference |
|---|---|---|---|---|---|
| Pakistan, single-center study | IVF, ICSI | 2.8% | Acyanotic CHD (ASD, VSD), Conotruncal defects | OR = 2.3 (CI 1.7-3.1) | (Ali, 2020) |
| Bangladesh, multi-center cohort | IVF, ICSI | 3.1% | Septal defects, Acyanotic CHD, Conotruncal defects | RR = 2.2 (CI 1.6-3.5) | (Ahmed, 2019) |

Collectively, these registries demonstrate (Figure 1):

- ART is associated with a 1.3–2.0-fold increase in risk of total and major CHDs.
- The association is strongest for non-syndromic septal and conotruncal defects, supporting a developmental/epigenetic rather than chromosomal pathway.
- ICSI and multiple gestations confer the highest risk.
- IVF-only pregnancies show a lower but still elevated risk.
- Parental age, prematurity, and subfertility partially mediate this association but do not fully explain it.

Importantly, the observed associations are largely driven by non-syndromic defects, implying that epigenetic and developmental rather than chromosomal mechanisms may be responsible (Paternostro et al., 2023).

## Evidence from Indian and Regional Context

India's rapidly growing ART market mirrors a demographic shift toward delayed parenthood, urban infertility, and higher socioeconomic participation of women. Yet, registry completeness and birth-defect surveillance remain limited (Table 3 & 4). According to the Indian Council of Medical Research (ICMR) ART Registry Report (2023), India performs over 200,000 cycles annually, making it one of the world's largest ART providers. National ART adoption has surged due to delayed childbearing, urbanization, and improved access. However, systematic birth-defect surveillance remains limited.

*Table 3.Current Status of ART Use and Registry Data in India*

| Registry/Study | ART Use in India | Key Findings |
|---|---|---|
| Indian ART Registry (2021) | India's first national ART registry | National ART usage has increased dramatically over the last decade. |
| Indian Society of Assisted Reproduction (ISAR) 2020 Report | National registry of ART outcomes in India | ART pregnancies tend to have slightly higher complication rates, including CHD. |
| Dr. Rathi ART Center Cohort Study (2018) | Mumbai, urban cohort of ART pregnancies | Cohort found a 2.5% CHD rate in ART-conceived infants, with common defects being VSD, ASD, and conotruncal anomalies. |

Despite high ART volume, India lacks a comprehensive ART–CHD linkage registry. The implementation of the ART Regulation Act (2021) and Surrogacy Regulation Act (2021), alongside the ICMR ART Registry Report (2023), provides an opportunity to integrate congenital anomaly surveillance and improve data quality.

The success rate of ART in India is around 30-40%, which is comparable to international standards. A cohort from the Indian subcontinent (n = 2,444 births) found 29 birth defects, but sample size was small, limiting statistical power. It emphasized the need for robust ART registries and longer-term follow-up (Banker et al., 2019).

*Table 4. Regional Studies on CHD in ART-conceived Infants in India.*

| Population | ART Techniques | Prevalence of CHD | CHD Subtypes Reported | Relative Risk (RR) / Odds Ratio (OR) | Ref |
|---|---|---|---|---|---|
| North India, multi-center cohort | IVF, ICSI | 3.20% | Acyanotic defects (VSD, ASD), Conotruncal defects (Tetralogy of Fallot) | OR = 2.5 (CI 1.5-4.0) | (Kumar, 2020) |
| Mumbai, single-center cohort | IVF, ICSI | 2.50% | Acyanotic defects, especially ASD and VSD | RR = 1.8 (CI 1.1-2.9) | (Rathi, 2018) |
| Delhi, single-center cohort | IVF | 2.90% | Acyanotic CHD (ASD, VSD), Syndromic CHD (Down syndrome) | RR = 2.0 (CI 1.4-3.0) | (Sharma, 2019) |
| South India, multi-center study | IVF, ICSI, Egg donation | 2.70% | Acyanotic CHD (VSD, ASD), Conotruncal defects | OR = 2.2 (CI 1.6-3.5) | (Verma, 2021) |
| Pune, retrospective cohort | IVF, ICSI, Ovulation Induction | 3.00% | Conotruncal defects, Acyanotic CHD (ASD, VSD) | RR = 2.3 (CI 1.8-4.0) | (Singh, 2022) |

## 5. BIOLOGICAL AND PATHOPHYSIOLOGICAL MECHANISMS: MECHANISTIC CONSIDERATIONS AND RISK FACTORS

Understanding why ART-conceived children have a higher risk of CHD requires an integrated view of parental characteristics, ART-related procedures, and pregnancy-specific influences. The developing heart is highly vulnerable to disturbances in gene regulation, cellular signaling, and placental function during the first weeks of embryogenesis. ART-related interventions often coincide with these critical developmental windows. Although no single mechanism fully explains the association, converging evidence from clinical, epigenetic, and experimental studies supports a multifactorial model involving three domains: (1) direct effects of ART procedures, (2) parental and maternal factors, and (3) pregnancy-level complications, including multiple gestations (Bi et al., 2022). These domains interact to modify the intrauterine environment, disrupt cardiogenic pathways, and increase susceptibility to structural cardiac anomalies.

### Direct ART effects

ART procedures—including ovarian stimulation, in vitro manipulation of gametes and embryos, and embryo transfer—can influence developmental signaling at the molecular level. Variations in culture media composition, oxygen concentration, pH, and temperature have been shown to alter gene expression and cardiac developmental pathways. Experimental models confirm that ART-exposed embryos demonstrate dysregulation in genes essential for cardiac looping and septation, suggesting that even subtle deviations in laboratory conditions may have lasting developmental consequences.

Furthermore, the method of conception matters. A large population-based study analyzing 57,681 pregnancies compared ART to ovulation induction (OI), untreated subfertile, and fertile conceptions, indicating small but notable differences in teratogenic exposures. While Category D/X medication use was relatively low across all groups (<1%), ART and OI pregnancies still carried higher exposure rates than fertile pregnancies (Kemp-Casey et al., 2025). These findings underscore that procedural and medical interventions surrounding ART may contribute to risk beyond underlying infertility alone.

Importantly, not all infertility types confer the same risk. Pregnancies resulting from male-factor infertility appear to have lower rates of adverse outcomes than those due to female-factor infertility, suggesting that intrinsic maternal reproductive conditions—and not ART per se—may be significant drivers of risk. This distinction highlights the complexity of attributing risk solely to ART procedures and underscores the need for mechanism-based stratification in future research.

## Maternal factors

ART pregnancies often occur in individuals with underlying infertility conditions, advanced maternal age, or metabolic disturbances—all of which independently affect cardiac development.

- Advanced maternal age increases the risk of chromosomal nondisjunction, altered oocyte quality, and placental insufficiency.
- Metabolic disorders such as PCOS, endometriosis, and insulin resistance create a pro-inflammatory and hyperinsulinemic environment disruptive to cardiogenesis.
- Socioeconomic adversity adds an additional biological layer: Lemieux et al. (2024) reported that maternal material deprivation significantly increases CHD risk, while higher neighborhood ethnic concentration appeared protective, suggesting social determinants may mediate biological stress pathways.

From a genetic standpoint, cardiac development relies on precise expression of transcription factors such as NKX2-5, GATA4, TBX5, ISL1, MEF2C, and HAND1/2, which orchestrate mesoderm specification, heart tube formation, and chamber morphogenesis. Disruptions in these pathways underpin many forms of non-syndromic CHD.

Notably, syndromic causes such as 22q11.2 deletion syndrome do not fully account for the elevated CHD rates seen in ART cohorts. Paternostro et al. (2023) argue that maternal age and infertility-related factors, rather than ART itself, may be responsible for a substantial portion of the observed risk—reinforcing the importance of careful confounder adjustment in epidemiological studies.

## Epigenetic Dysregulation

One of the most compelling mechanistic explanations linking ART to CHD is epigenetic modification. ART involves manipulation during the period of epigenetic reprogramming, when DNA methylation patterns and histone modifications are reset. Interference during this vulnerable window can lead to persistent alterations in gene expression at cardiogenic loci.

- ART has been associated with aberrant DNA methylation, histone modification, and altered chromatin accessibility.
- Li et al. (2024) demonstrated that ART-conceived offspring exhibit epigenetically mediated impairments in cardiovascular function, with potential long-term health implications.

- Placental epigenomic profiling by Voros et al. (2025) revealed dysregulated imprinted and developmental genes specific to cardiac pathways in ART pregnancies, suggesting that the placenta—not just the embryo—is a critical target of ART-related epigenetic stress.

These findings provide biological plausibility for ART-related cardiac anomalies and indicate that optimization of laboratory conditions and embryo culture media could reduce risk.

## Confounding Factors and Multiple pregnancy effects

Pregnancy complications are major contributors to CHD risk, and ART significantly increases the likelihood of multiple gestations. Twin and triplet pregnancies are associated with:

- Hemodynamic imbalance
- Placental vascular dysfunction
- Twin–twin transfusion syndrome
- Chronic hypoxic stress

These processes interfere with cell proliferation, myocardial compaction, and cardiac septation during critical developmental periods. Thus, multiple gestations are not merely coincidental but pathophysiologically relevant confounders.

Evidence supports this: ART-conceived multiples and ICSI singletons show the highest rates of CHD. Henningsen et al. (2023) reported:

- Major malformations in 6.0% of fresh ICSI-conceived children vs 5.3% in IVF
- A specific excess of hypospadias in ICSI offspring, possibly due to paternal genetic/epigenetic defects
- Shifting indications for ICSI (beyond male infertility) may alter risk profiles over time

In addition, maternal medication exposure plays a role. Lemieux et al. (2024) found modest but significant associations between CHD and antidepressant use (OR 1.23) and antihypertensives (OR 2.07). ART and OI pregnancies had higher Category D medication exposure in the first trimester (ART 4.9% vs fertile 0.6%) (Kemp-Casey et al., 2025), suggesting increased medicalization of ART pregnancies contributes to cardiac risk.

## 6. CHD SUBTYPES REPORTED IN ART PREGNANCIES: PATTERNS, SPECIFIC RISKS, AND CLINICAL IMPLICATIONS

The relationship between ART and CHD is not uniform across all cardiac malformations. Instead, specific CHD subtypes show varying strengths of association, reflecting differences in embryologic origins, vulnerability to ART-related perturbations, and patterns of clinical detection. Understanding these subtype-specific trends is critical for accurate risk stratification, counseling, and neonatal screening in ART-conceived infants.

### Evolving Patterns of CHD in the General Population and ART Cohorts

Population-based data from Norway (1994–2014) demonstrate a decline in severe CHD, but a continued rise in septal defects, with an overall CHD prevalence of 144.6 per 10,000 live births (Leirgul et al., 2025). These secular trends reflect improved prenatal diagnosis and survival but also highlight a real increase in milder defects—consistent with findings in ART cohorts.

Prospective comparisons of ART infants vs. naturally conceived controls show a higher frequency of minor anomalies—such as patent foramen ovale (PFO), atrial septal defect (ASD), and ventricular septal defect (VSD)—even when differences are not statistically significant, ART infants experience more neonatal complications (Zhou et al., 2014). Large-scale studies confirm this pattern: ART pregnancies are linked to higher rates of chromosomal anomalies, male genital defects, and cardiac malformations (Potiris et al., 2024).

A recent study reported major CHD prevalence of 1.84% in ART vs 1.15% in spontaneous conception, with greater risk in multiple gestations (Sargisian et al., 2024). Notably, although the absolute risk is modest, the relative risk is consistently elevated, justifying targeted screening.

### Acyanotic vs Cyanotic CHD: Differential Associations

Acyanotic defects, which constitute 89–91% of all CHD, display the strongest and most reproducible association with ART.

- Septal defects: 14.2% in ART vs 7.5% in controls (Rasouli et al., 2024)
- VSD: consistently elevated risk OR 1.3–1.6 across studies (Galdini et al., 2021)

These defects are more likely to be detected due to intensified prenatal and postnatal monitoring in ART pregnancies, suggesting both true biological risk and surveillance bias.

Cyanotic lesions (Tetralogy of Fallot, Transposition of the Great Arteries) represent severe conotruncal malformations with distinct embryologic origins. Findings are variable:

- Increased prevalence of cyanotic CHD in ART and non-ART infertility treatments (Appiah et al., 2024)
- Conflicting data for TGA, with some studies suggesting decreased risk (Tararbit et al., 2013)

Thus, cyanotic CHDs show selective rather than universal association with ART.

## Conotruncal Defects: The Most Strongly Linked to ART

Conotruncal defects (TOF, TGA, IAA) arise from abnormal neural crest migration and are among the most severe forms of CHD. They account for 25–30% of nonsyndromic CHD.

The strongest and most consistent ART-specific association is with Tetralogy of Fallot (TOF):

- OR 2.4–3.0 (Tararbit et al., 2014)
- ART exposure in TOF cases: 6.6% vs 3.5% in controls (p=0.002) (Sargisian et al., 2024)

This robust association suggests that ART-related mechanisms—possibly epigenetic and placental—selectively disrupt conotruncal development.

## Syndromic vs Non-syndromic CHD

A key concern has been whether ART simply increases syndromic or chromosomal abnormalities. However, evidence suggests otherwise.

- Non-syndromic CHD is the primary driver of the ART–CHD association (Paternostro et al., 2023).
- Rates of aneuploidy and 22q11.2 deletion (present in ~10% of TOF) do not fully explain the excess risk.
- Appiah et al. (2024) reported OR 2.06 for cyanotic CHD in ART even after adjusting for syndromes.

ART does not merely increase syndromic defects; it appears to influence isolated cardiac malformations, reinforcing the role of epigenetic and placental mechanisms (Table 5).

*Table 5. Clinical Presentation of Syndromic CHDs*

| CHD Category | Associated Features | CHD Types |
|---|---|---|
| Syndromic CHDs (All) | Extra-cardiac anomalies, dysmorphic features | Variable depending on syndrome |
| 22q11.2 Deletion Syndrome | Conotruncal defects, immunodeficiency | TOF, TGA, IAA, VSD |
| Down Syndrome (Trisomy 21) | AV canal defects, intellectual disability | AVSD, VSD, ASD |
| Turner Syndrome | Left-sided obstructive lesions | CoA, HLHS, BAV |
| DiGeorge Syndrome | Conotruncal defects, thymic aplasia | TOF, IAA, TGA |
| Noonan Syndrome | Pulmonary stenosis, facial features | Pulmonary stenosis, HCM |
| CHARGE Syndrome | Multiple congenital anomalies | TOF, VSD, ASD |

## 7. ART METHOD-SPECIFIC RISK ANALYSIS

### ICSI vs IVF

Assisted reproductive technology method–specific analyses reveal that the type of procedure, stage of embryo transfer, and pregnancy plurality profoundly influence the risk profile for congenital anomalies, particularly CHDs. Among ART modalities, ICSI consistently shows a higher risk than conventional IVF. While ART-conceived infants overall display elevated risk of major congenital anomalies compared to naturally conceived infants (OR 1.67, 95% CI 1.59–1.76), ICSI confers an additional 9% increase in anomalies compared to IVF, with notable elevations in urogenital and musculoskeletal defects (Veeramani et al., 2024). Importantly, the risk of cardiac, gastrointestinal, and neurological malformations persists even after adjusting for parental and perinatal factors, highlighting a potential biological impact of micromanipulation during fertilization. Specifically, ICSI has been strongly associated with Tetralogy of Fallot, with an odds ratio of 3.0 (1.0–8.9), suggesting an enhanced susceptibility of conotruncal development to ART-related perturbations (Tararbit et al., 2013). Beyond procedure type, several perinatal determinants—such as infant sex, gestational age, birth weight, and etiology of infertility—modulate CHD risk and are more frequently altered in ART conceptions, particularly in IVF offspring where circulatory anomalies are most common.

## Fresh vs Frozen Embryo Transfer

Embryo transfer protocol further modulates anomaly risk. Although letrozole-stimulated frozen-thawed embryo transfer (FET) improves live birth rates and reduces the risk of pregnancy loss, hypertensive disorders of pregnancy, and large-for-gestational-age infants, artificial-cycle FET offers no significant protection against gestational diabetes. Despite these obstetric benefits, congenital anomaly risk appears minimally influenced by transfer method alone. The Nordic registry reported no significant difference in CHD risk between fresh and frozen embryo transfers (Wennerholm et al., 2013). However, when stratified by ART type and transfer stage, more nuanced patterns emerge. Day 3 embryo transfer and fresh transfer protocols exhibit slightly higher congenital anomaly rates compared to Day 5 (blastocyst) transfer or frozen embryo cycles, particularly when combined with ICSI (Bhat et al., 2025). These findings suggest that early-stage embryos may be more vulnerable to suboptimal uterine environments or epigenetic disruption, whereas blastocyst-stage selection may offer a protective effect. Nonetheless, ART-conceived children, regardless of protocol, consistently show a marginally higher overall risk of congenital anomalies than those conceived spontaneously (Sargisian et al., 2024), indicating that intrinsic factors related to infertility, laboratory manipulation, or embryonic development contribute to risk beyond transfer technique.

## Multiple vs Singleton Gestations

Multiple gestations represent a critical amplifier of ART-associated CHD risk. ART markedly increases the likelihood of twins and higher-order pregnancies, and multiplicity itself is a well-established independent risk factor for congenital anomalies. Tararbit et al. (2014) demonstrated that multiple pregnancies significantly elevate CHD risk, particularly when associated with Day 3 embryo transfer, fresh transfer cycles, or donor conception. Population data show that congenital anomalies occur in 18.8% of ART pregnancies compared to 8.1% in spontaneous pregnancies, with heart defects specifically reported in 16.3% versus 6.2% (p=0.005). Zdanowicz et al. (2024) reported a cumulative effect of ART on CHD in monochorionic twins, even in the absence of differences in gestational age or neonatal outcomes, indicating that the combined impact of ART and shared placental circulation may exacerbate developmental vulnerability. Consistent with this, Sargisian et al. (2024) found CHD prevalence of 2.47% in ART multiples compared to 1.62% in ART singletons, confirming multiplicity as a robust and recurrent risk enhancer across studies.

## Clinical Classification: Major vs Minor CHD

When classified by clinical severity, ART shows a stronger association with minor (non-surgical) CHDs than with major surgical defects. Meta-analytic evidence demonstrates that minor CHDs have a relative risk of 1.71 (1.25–2.34), compared to 1.36 (1.31–1.41) for major CHDs (Gullo et al., 2023). Critical CHDs, though less frequent in absolute terms, exhibit the highest relative risk (RR 1.98, 1.30–3.02) (Lemieux et al., 2024). This gradient suggests a potential surveillance bias, as ART pregnancies undergo more intensive prenatal monitoring, increasing the detection of minor anomalies that might otherwise go unnoticed in spontaneous pregnancies. However, the persistence of elevated risk across both minor and major categories—and the particularly strong associations with ICSI, conotruncal defects, and multiple gestations—indicates that biological mechanisms also contribute.

# 8. DIAGNOSTIC CONSIDERATIONS, CLINICAL IMPLICATIONS AND RECOMMENDATIONS

The consistent evidence of a modest but clinically meaningful increase in congenital heart disease (CHD) among pregnancies conceived through assisted reproductive technology (ART) has strengthened the rationale for enhanced diagnostic vigilance and standardized prenatal surveillance protocols. Although the absolute risk of CHD in ART-conceived offspring remains relatively low, early and accurate detection is critical for optimizing perinatal outcomes, facilitating timely interventions, and enabling informed reproductive counseling. Advances in fetal imaging, non-invasive genetic testing, and multidisciplinary fetal cardiac care now allow earlier identification of structural heart defects, improving both prognosis and parental preparedness.

## Screening Protocols: Role of fetal echocardiography in ART pregnancies

Fetal echocardiography, the gold standard for prenatal cardiac diagnosis, is increasingly recommended for ART pregnancies regardless of the presence of additional risk factors. Professional organizations such as the American Heart Association (AHA) and the International Society of Ultrasound in Obstetrics and Gynecology (ISUOG) classify ART conception as a moderate-risk indication warranting targeted fetal cardiac evaluation (Carvalho et al., 2023). The optimal timing for detailed fetal echocardiography is 18–22 weeks' gestation; however, in higher-risk ART scenarios—such as intracytoplasmic sperm injection (ICSI) conceptions, monochorionic twin pregnancies, increased nuchal translucency, or parental congenital disease—early first-trimester scans (11–13 weeks) using high-resolution transvaginal ultrasonography may detect major anomalies such as conotruncal or atrioventricular septal defects. Subsequent mid-trimester re-evaluation enhances diagnostic accuracy and allows refinement of initial findings.

Emerging evidence supports the value of structured, multi-stage cardiac surveillance in ART pregnancies. Tertiary fetal medicine units increasingly implement three-step protocols comprising an early first-trimester screening, a comprehensive second-trimester fetal echocardiogram, and a third-trimester assessment of cardiac growth, function, and rhythm. Advanced modalities such as color Doppler, M-mode imaging, and 3D/4D echocardiography have improved detection of subtle lesions, including small septal defects and outflow-tract abnormalities—defects disproportionately reported in ART conceptions (Rasouli et al., 2024; Yang et al., 2025). Early screening is particularly valuable for identifying cyanotic lesions. Lemieux et al. (2024) demonstrated that severe CHD detected in the first trimester is often prognostically significant and may be missed without targeted surveillance. Population-based data from over 9.6 million singleton live births in the United States revealed that cyanotic CHD prevalence was more than double in infants conceived via infertility treatments compared to spontaneous conceptions (1.2 vs. 0.5 per 1,000 live births), with infertility treatment utilization increasing from 1.9% to 3.1% over the study period (Appiah et al., 2024). These findings underscore not only the rising global reliance on ART but also the importance of integrating fetal echocardiography, genetic counseling, and chromosomal analysis—particularly for conotruncal defects—into routine ART prenatal care. Linked population databases and long-term ART registries are crucial for evaluating the safety of newer laboratory and transfer techniques, supporting evidence-based pre-treatment counseling and policy formulation

## Ethical and Psychosocial Considerations

The increasing use of assisted reproductive technologies has brought profound ethical and psychosocial challenges that extend beyond clinical outcomes. As ART-conceived pregnancies carry a modestly higher risk of CHD and other structural anomalies, ethical obligations in reproductive medicine now encompass not only achieving conception but also ensuring informed choice, equitable access, and holistic care for families. The interplay of hope, vulnerability, and medical complexity that defines ART demands sensitive, transparent, and ethically sound clinical communication supported by psychosocial guidance.

Informed consent is paramount; couples must be counseled not only about the benefits of ART but also about the potential risks, including the modestly increased risk of CHD in offspring. This process should be transparent, evidence-based, and tailored to the couple's values and circumstances.

Clinicians must also ensure that consent extends beyond procedural aspects to include the long-term implications for offspring health. According to the Indian Council of Medical Research (ICMR) ART Guidelines (2023) and the International Federation of Fertility Societies (IFFS) Consensus (2024), consent discussions should explicitly address:

- The small but measurable increase in congenital anomaly risk (including CHD);
- The role of parental factors such as age and comorbidities;
- The potential need for prenatal genetic testing or fetal echocardiography;
- Options for single-embryo transfer to minimize multiple gestation risk;
- Long-term follow-up and registry participation for outcome monitoring.

Parental anxiety is a significant concern, particularly regarding the risk of malformations. Studies highlight that parents of children with CHD often experience heightened stress, uncertainty, and psychological burden, which can be exacerbated by the knowledge that ART may increase these risks. Interventions such as psychological support, peer counseling, and the use of 3D models to explain CHD can help mitigate anxiety and empower families.

The ethical principles of beneficence ("to do good") and non-maleficence ("to do no harm") acquire special significance in ART, where clinicians intervene at the earliest stages of human development. While the primary goal of ART is to overcome infertility, it must not compromise the long-term health of offspring. Procedural optimization—such as limiting ovarian hyperstimulation, minimizing embryo manipulation, and adopting evidence-based culture media—represents a practical embodiment of these principles. Balancing the benefits of ART—such as fulfilling the desire for parenthood—against potential risks requires nuanced, individualized counseling. Clinicians must foster a supportive environment where couples can make informed choices, fully aware of both the possibilities and limitations of current knowledge

The principle of justice demands equitable access to safe and regulated ART services. In low- and middle-income countries, cost barriers and limited access to accredited fertility centers often push couples toward unregulated clinics lacking adequate monitoring and counseling infrastructure. This disparity heightens the risk of poor outcomes and ethical lapses.

National health authorities should therefore ensure equitable ART access through public–private partnerships, insurance coverage for infertility care, and mandatory adherence to ethical and clinical standards. In the Indian context, the expansion of

ART services must be matched by ethical governance, transparency in pricing, and integration of congenital anomaly screening as part of the standard ART package.

## 9. FUTURE DIRECTIONS

The future of CHD management in the context of assisted reproductive technologies ART is shaped by rapid advancements in imaging, genomics, artificial intelligence, and long-term outcome research. As scientific understanding deepens, these innovations have the potential not only to improve early diagnosis and personalized care but also to clarify the mechanisms linking ART to cardiac malformations. Among the most transformative developments are 3D technologies—including 3D printing, virtual reality (VR), and high-resolution imaging—that allow clinicians to visualize complex cardiac anatomy with remarkable precision. These tools enable surgical planning and simulation, improve coordination among multidisciplinary teams, and enhance transparency in clinical decision-making. Importantly, the use of 3D-printed models in parental counseling has been shown to reduce anxiety and foster informed consent by providing a tangible understanding of their child's condition. This shift from traditional two-dimensional imaging to immersive, patient-specific modeling signals a new era of individualized CHD care in ART-conceived offspring.

Artificial intelligence (AI) and machine learning further accelerate this transformation. Automated interpretation of fetal and neonatal echocardiograms can increase diagnostic accuracy and reduce operator dependency, enabling earlier detection of subtle cardiac defects that may be overlooked by conventional methods. AI-driven risk prediction models integrating parental factors, ART procedures, and embryological data may allow stratification of ART pregnancies into low- and high-risk categories, guiding personalized surveillance strategies. Such approaches are particularly relevant for procedures like intracytoplasmic sperm injection (ICSI) and frozen embryo transfer, which have been associated with higher rates of CHD. As these technologies mature, AI-enhanced screening could become a standard component of prenatal care for ART pregnancies.

Simultaneously, genomic and epigenomic research is uncovering the biological pathways that may connect ART procedures to altered cardiac development. Next-generation sequencing, single-cell transcriptomics, and methylation profiling are beginning to reveal subtle gene expression changes and epigenetic dysregulation associated with embryo manipulation, culture conditions, and parental infertility. These discoveries raise the possibility of identifying high-risk subgroups and designing targeted preventive strategies. For example, understanding the role of imprinting disorders, oxidative stress, or placental signaling pathways may allow refinement of ART protocols to reduce epigenetic disruption. Ultimately, integrating molecular insights with clinical data will pave the way for precision reproductive medicine, where ART protocols are tailored to optimize both conception success and offspring cardiovascular health.

However, major knowledge gaps remain. Longitudinal cohort studies of ART-conceived individuals into adolescence and adulthood are urgently needed to clarify the true magnitude and trajectory of CHD risk. Most current evidence is limited to neonatal or early childhood outcomes, leaving uncertainties about late-onset cardiac dysfunction, arrhythmias, or the interaction between ART-related cardiac anomalies and adult cardiovascular risk factors. These studies must use standardized CHD definitions, consistent diagnostic criteria, and harmonized follow-up protocols to overcome heterogeneity that currently hampers comparisons across populations. Large-scale, multi-ethnic registries linking ART procedures, genetic data, pregnancy outcomes, and long-term cardiovascular health could provide the high-quality evidence required to inform clinical guidelines and policy decisions.

Standardization of research methodologies is equally critical to address limitations in the literature. Variability in CHD classification across studies contributes to inconsistent risk estimates, while increased surveillance in ART pregnancies may inflate apparent CHD rates due to ascertainment bias. Differences in national registry practices and follow-up durations further complicate data interpretation, and residual confounding from underlying infertility or parental health behaviors remains difficult to eliminate. Future investigations must adopt rigorous designs, adjust for key confounders, and incorporate biologically plausible mechanisms to strengthen causal inference. Priorities for future research include mechanistic studies to elucidate biological pathways, long-term follow-up of ART-conceived individuals with and without CHD, evaluation of prevention strategies through optimized ART protocols, and economic analyses assessing the cost-effectiveness of enhanced screening and surveillance.

## 10. CONCLUSIONS

Congenital heart disease (CHD) is a major global health issue, particularly affecting infant mortality rates in low and middle-income countries (LMICs) such as India. Key challenges in addressing CHD include low awareness, delayed diagnosis and referral, and the availability, inaccessibility, and unaffordability of essential medical care. Present research highlights the lack of dedicated research and the impact of widespread malnutrition on the management of CHD. Private NGO initiatives, such as the Sri Sathya Sai Sanjeevani Research Centre in India, provide free cardiac interventions, emphasizing the need to bridge healthcare access gaps for CHD (Ahamad & Kukshal, 2025). Congenital heart disease (CHD) is the most common congenital anomaly worldwide, affecting 8–12 per 1,000 live births and contributing significantly to infant morbidity and mortality. Concurrently, assisted reproductive technologies (ART), including in vitro fertilization (IVF) and intracytoplasmic sperm injection (ICSI), have become increasingly prevalent, resulting in over 8 million births globally. Evidence indicates a modest but consistent elevation in CHD risk among ART-conceived offspring, particularly non-syndromic ventricular septal defects, atrial septal defects, and conotruncal anomalies such as tetralogy of Fallot. Population-based registries—including Nordic CoNARTaS, EPICARD, U.S. National ART Surveillance, and Australian ART Registry—report a 1.3–2.0-fold increased relative risk, with ICSI and multiple gestations conferring higher susceptibility. Mechanistic studies suggest multifactorial pathways involving ART-related interventions, maternal factors (advanced age, metabolic disorders), pregnancy complications (multiple gestations, preterm birth), and epigenetic dysregulation during critical windows of cardiac development (Raghavan & Ahamad, 2025). ART procedures may alter gene expression, DNA methylation, and placental signaling, disrupting cardiogenesis and increasing structural defect risk. The CHD genetic associations involving CRELD1, MYH6, and MYH7 genes show consistent replication across Indian populations. The genetic mechanisms underlying CHD are complex and not fully understood, with various genetic abnormalities contributing to its development (Kukshal et al., 2023). Despite this, absolute CHD risk remains low, and most ART-conceived children are unaffected. Clinical implications include targeted prenatal cardiac screening, particularly fetal echocardiography at 18–22 weeks, and counseling regarding parental age, comorbidities, and multiplicity. Ethical considerations emphasize informed consent, psychosocial support, equitable ART access, and procedural optimization. Future research should focus on precision reproductive medicine, integrating genomics, imaging, and artificial intelligence for individualized risk assessment and early detection. Harmonized registry data and multi-ethnic cohort studies are essential to clarify long-term cardiovascular outcomes, refine ART protocols, and guide evidence-based recommendations. These findings underscore the need for multidisciplinary approaches that balance reproductive success with offspring cardiovascular health, advancing clinical practice and research at the interface of ART and pediatric cardiology (Kukshal et al., 2023).

In summary, current evidence consistently demonstrates a modest but meaningful increase in CHD risk among ART-conceived pregnancies, with the highest-quality data—such as the Nordic registry of 7.7 million births—showing a 36–71% relative risk increase. This association is driven primarily by non-syndromic CHD, particularly ventricular septal defects and tetralogy of Fallot. ICSI is associated with higher risk than conventional IVF, and multiple gestations further amplify this burden. Despite this elevated relative risk, the absolute risk remains low, with major CHD affecting 1.84% of ART pregnancies compared to 1.15% of spontaneous conceptions.

These findings justify enhanced prenatal cardiac screening and vigilant postnatal follow-up while providing reassurance that most ART-conceived children will not develop CHD. At the same time, they highlight the need for balanced counseling that integrates clinical evidence with empathy and ethical responsibility.

The intersection of ART and CHD stands at the cutting edge of reproductive and pediatric medicine. Technological innovations offer unprecedented opportunities for early diagnosis, precision treatment, and improved outcomes, yet they also raise complex ethical, psychosocial, and research challenges. The future lies in multidisciplinary collaboration that bridges reproductive medicine, fetal cardiology, genetics, bioethics, and health policy. By combining robust scientific inquiry with compassionate clinical practice, we can ensure that ART continues to advance not only the possibility of parenthood but also the lifelong health and well-being of future generations.

## REFERENCES


Ahamad, S., & Kukshal, P. (2025). Summary of initiatives for treating congenital heart disease: Enhancing quality of life and bridging the knowledge gap. *Annals of the National Academy of Medical Sciences (India)*, *61*(1), 40–44. DOI: 10.25259/ANAMS_242_2024

Ahmed, F. (2019). Congenital Heart Defects in ART-conceived Infants: A Study from Bangladesh. *Journal of Obstetrics and Gynaecology Bangladesh*, *34*(1), 45–49. DOI: 10.3329/jogb.v34i1.41985

Ali, Z. (2020). Congenital Heart Disease in ART Babies: A Single-center Study from Pakistan. *Pakistan Journal of Medical Sciences*, *36*(5), 890–894. DOI: 10.12669/pjms.36.5.2559 PMID: 32704258

Appiah, D., Sang, J., Olayemi, O. E., Broni, E. K., Baykoca-Arslan, B., Ebong, I. A., & Kim, C. (2024). Infertility treatments and cyanotic congenital heart defects among livebirths in the USA: Findings from a contemporary cohort. *Human Reproduction (Oxford, England)*, *39*(9), 2115–2123. DOI: 10.1093/humrep/deae161 PMID: 39008825

Baker, V. L., Dyer, S., Chambers, G. M., Keller, E., Banker, M., de Mouzon, J., Elgindy, E., Bai, F. M., Ishihara, O., Jwa, S. C., Kupka, M. S., Zegers-Hochschild, F., & Adamson, G. D. (2025). International Committee for Monitoring Assisted Reproductive Technologies (ICMART): World report for cycles conducted in 2017-2018. *Human Reproduction (Oxford, England)*, *40*(6), 1110–1126. DOI: 10.1093/humrep/deaf049 PMID: 40239109

Banker, M., Arora, P., Banker, J., Benani, H., Shah, S., & Lalitkumar, P. G. L. (2019). Prevalence of structural birth defects in IVF-ICSI pregnancies resulting from autologous and donor oocytes in Indian sub-continent: Results from 2444 births. *Acta Obstetricia et Gynecologica Scandinavica*, *98*(6), 715–721. DOI: 10.1111/aogs.13541 PMID: 30663773

Bhat, P., Dhyani, V. S., Lakshmi, V., Uppangala, S., Adiga, S. K., Adiga, P., Kumar, P., & Gupta, A. (2025). Congenital anomalies observed in children conceived through assisted reproductive technology—A systematic review and meta-analysis. *Journal of Assisted Reproduction and Genetics*, *42*(5), 1547–1565. DOI: 10.1007/s10815-025-03454-0 PMID: 40163274

Bi, W., Xiao, Y., Wang, X., Cui, L., Song, G., Yang, Z., Zhang, Y., & Ren, W. (2022). The association between assisted reproductive technology and cardiac remodeling in fetuses and early infants: A prospective cohort study. *BMC Medicine, 20*(1), 104. DOI: 10.1186/s12916-022-02303-6 PMID: 35361200

Bourdon, G., Lenne, X., Godart, F., Storme, L., Theis, D., Subtil, D., Bruandet, A., & Rakza, T. (2024). Epidemiology of congenital heart defects in France from 2013 to 2022 using the PMSI-MCO (French Medical Information System Program in Medicine, Surgery, and Obstetrics) database. *PLoS One, 19*(4), e0298234. DOI: 10.1371/journal.pone.0298234 PMID: 38626139

Carvalho, J. S., Axt-Fliedner, R., Chaoui, R., Copel, J. A., Cuneo, B. F., Goff, D., Gordin Kopylov, L., Hecher, K., Lee, W., Moon-Grady, A. J., Mousa, H. A., Munoz, H., Paladini, D., Prefumo, F., Quarello, E., Rychik, J., Tutschek, B., Wiechec, M., & Yagel, S. (2023). ISUOG Practice Guidelines (updated): Fetal cardiac screening. *Ultrasound in Obstetrics & Gynecology, 61*(6), 788–803. DOI: 10.1002/uog.26224 PMID: 37267096

Galdini, A., Fesslova, V. M. E., Gaeta, G., Candiani, M., Pozzoni, M., Chiarello, C., & Cavoretto, P. I. (2021). Prevalence of Congenital Heart Defects in Pregnancies Conceived by Assisted Reproductive Technology: A Cohort Study. *Journal of Clinical Medicine, 10*(22), 5363. DOI: 10.3390/jcm10225363 PMID: 34830645

Giorgione, V., Parazzini, F., Fesslova, V., Cipriani, S., Candiani, M., Inversetti, A., Sigismondi, C., Tiberio, F., & Cavoretto, P. (2018). Congenital heart defects in IVF/ICSI pregnancy: Systematic review and meta-analysis. *Ultrasound in Obstetrics & Gynecology, 51*(1), 33–42. DOI: 10.1002/uog.18932 PMID: 29164811

Gullo, G., Scaglione, M., Laganà, A. S., Perino, A., Andrisani, A., Chiantera, V., Cucinella, G., Gitas, G., Barra, F., & Riemma, G. (2023). Assisted Reproductive Techniques and Risk of Congenital Heart Diseases in Children: A Systematic Review and Meta-analysis. *Reproductive Sciences (Thousand Oaks, Calif.), 30*(10), 2896–2906. DOI: 10.1007/s43032-023-01252-6 PMID: 37145300

Hansen, M., Kurinczuk, J. J., Klerk, N., Burton, P., & Bower, C. (2013). Assisted reproductive technology and major birth defects in Western Australia. *Obstetrics and Gynecology, 121*(4), 852–863. DOI: 10.1097/AOG.0b013e31828738e5 PMID: 22996103

Henningsen, A.-K. A., Opdahl, S., Wennerholm, U.-B., Tiitinen, A., Rasmussen, S., Romundstad, L. B., Bergh, C., Gissler, M., Forman, J. L., & Pinborg, A. (2023). Risk of congenital malformations in live-born singletons conceived after intracytoplasmic sperm injection: A Nordic study from the CoNARTaS group. *Fertility and Sterility, 120*(5), 1033–1041. DOI: 10.1016/j.fertnstert.2023.07.003 PMID: 37442533

Kashyap, S., & Tripathi, P. (2023). Assisted Reproductive Technology (Regulation) Act 2021: Critique and Contestations. *Asian Bioethics Review, 16*(2), 149–164. DOI: 10.1007/s41649-023-00253-6 PMID: 38586570

Kemp-Casey, A., Hart, R., Milne, E., Bower, C., Walls, M. L., Yovich, J. L., Burton, P., Liu, Y., Barblett, H., & Hansen, M. (2025). Are assisted reproductive technology pregnancies more likely to be exposed to teratogenic medication? A whole-population study. *Australian and New Zealand Journal of Obstetrics and Gynaecology, 65*(3), 390–397. DOI: 10.1111/ajo.13911 PMID: 39651600

Kukshal, P., Joshi, R. O., Kumar, A., Ahamad, S., Murthy, P. R., Sathe, Y., Manohar, K., Guhathakurta, S., & Chellappan, S. (2023). Case–control association study of congenital heart disease from a tertiary paediatric cardiac centre from North India. *BMC Pediatrics, 23*(1), 290. DOI: 10.1186/s12887-023-04095-x PMID: 37322441

Kumar, S. (2020). Prevalence of Congenital Heart Disease in ART-conceived Infants: A North India Cohort Study. *Indian Journal of Pediatrics, 87*(3), 207–212. DOI: 10.1007/s12098-019-03125-2 PMID: 31900850

Leirgul, E., Fomina, T., Greve, G., Tell, G. S., Sandberg, M., & Øyen, N. (2025). Trends in Birth Prevalence of Congenital Heart Defects in Norway—A Population Study 1994–2014. *Acta Paediatrica, n/a*(n/a). https://doi.org/DOI: 10.1111/apa.70235

Lemieux, A., Khalilipalandi, S., Lauzon-Schnittka, J., Taillefer, V., Tousignant, A., Perreault, L., Rego, K., Dubois, M., Watelle, L., Roy, L.-O., & Dallaire, F. (2024). Meta-Analysis of Risk Factors for Congenital Heart Disease: Part 2, Maternal Medication, Reproductive Technologies, and Familial and Fetal Factors. *The Canadian Journal of Cardiology, 40*(12), 2496–2511. DOI: 10.1016/j.cjca.2024.09.011 PMID: 39288833

Li, J., Liu, Y., Huang, H., & Jin, L. (2024). Cardiovascular health of offspring conceived by assisted reproduction technology: A comprehensive review. *Frontiers in Cardiovascular Medicine, 11*. Advance online publication. DOI: 10.3389/fcvm.2024.1287060 PMID: 38292241

Palma, A., Morais, S., Silva, P. V., & Pires, A. (2023). Congenital heart defects and preterm birth: Outcomes from a referral center. *Revista Portuguesa de Cardiologia, 42*(5), 403–410. DOI: 10.1016/j.repc.2022.05.009 PMID: 36828187

Paternostro, C., Springer, S., Kasprian, G., Yerlikaya-Schatten, G., & Reischer, T. (2023). Clinical Course and Outcome of Prenatally Detected 22q11.2 Deletion Syndrome—A Retrospective Analysis. *Diagnostics (Basel)*, *13*(13), 2244. DOI: 10.3390/diagnostics13132244 PMID: 37443638

Pinborg, A., Wennerholm, U. B., & Bergh, C. (2023). Long-term outcomes for children conceived by assisted reproductive technology. *Fertility and Sterility*, *120*(3 Pt 1), 449–456. DOI: 10.1016/j.fertnstert.2023.04.022 PMID: 37086833

Potiris, A., Perros, P., Drakaki, E., Mavrogianni, D., Machairiotis, N., Sfakianakis, A., Karampitsakos, T., Vrachnis, D., Antonakopoulos, N., Panagopoulos, P., Drakakis, P., & Stavros, S. (2024). Investigating the Association of Assisted Reproduction Techniques and Adverse Perinatal Outcomes. *Journal of Clinical Medicine*, *13*(2), 328. DOI: 10.3390/jcm13020328 PMID: 38256462

Raghavan, R., & Ahamad, S. (2025). Developmental Origins of Health and Disease. *Cancer Exposomics and Environmental Influences on Carcinogenesis*, 1–34. https://doi.org/DOI: 10.4018/979-8-3373-2165-3.ch001

Rasouli, S., Radgoodarzi, M., Azarbad, R., Ghazvini, A., Sotoudeheian, M., Taghizadeh, M., & Dakkali, M. S. (2024). Congenital Heart Defects in Pregnancies Conceived by Assisted Reproductive Technology: Comparing Functional and Structural Defects. *Cureus*, *16*(2), e54810. DOI: 10.7759/cureus.54810 PMID: 38529454

Rathi, A. (2018). Incidence of Congenital Heart Defects in ART Pregnancies in Mumbai: A Retrospective Study. *Journal of Obstetrics and Gynaecology of India*, *68*(5), 363–367. DOI: 10.1007/s13224-018-1134-3

Registry, S. L. A. R. T. (2021). Congenital Heart Disease and ART Pregnancy Outcomes: A National Cohort Study. *Sri Lanka Journal of Obstetrics and Gynaecology*, *43*(2), 123–128. DOI: 10.4038/sljog.v43i2.808

Sargisian, N., Petzold, M., Furenäs, E., Gissler, M., Spangmose, A. L., Malchau Lauesgaard, S., Opdahl, S., Pinborg, A., Henningsen, A.-K. A., Westvik-Johari, K., Rönö, K., Bergh, C., & Wennerholm, U.-B. (2024). Congenital heart defects in children born after assisted reproductive technology: A CoNARTaS study. *European Heart Journal*, *45*(45), 4840–4858. DOI: 10.1093/eurheartj/ehae572 PMID: 39326528

Saxena, A., Relan, J., Agarwal, R., Awasthy, N., Azad, S., Chakrabarty, M., Dagar, K. S., Devagourou, V., Dharan, B. S., Gupta, S. K., Iyer, K. S., Jayranganath, M., Joshi, R., Kannan, B., Katewa, A., Kohli, V., Kothari, S. S., Krishnamoorthy, K. M., Kulkarni, S., & Vijaykumar, R. (2019). Indian guidelines for indications and timing of intervention for common congenital heart diseases: Revised and updated consensus statement of the Working group on management of congenital heart diseases. *Annals of Pediatric Cardiology*, *12*(3), 254–286. DOI: 10.4103/apc.APC_32_19 PMID: 31516283

Sharma, P. (2019). Congenital Heart Disease in IVF Pregnancies: An Institutional Experience from Delhi. *Indian Heart Journal*, *71*(2), 119–124. DOI: 10.1016/j.ihj.2019.02.019

Singh, R. (2022). Congenital Heart Disease in ART Babies: A Study from Pune. *Heart Asia*, *14*(1), 23. DOI: 10.1136/heartasia-2021-010524

Tararbit, K., Houyel, L., Bonnet, D., Vigan, C., Lelong, N., Goffinet, F., & Khoshnood, B. (2013). The risk for four specific congenital heart defects associated with assisted reproductive techniques: A population-based evaluation. *Human Reproduction (Oxford, England)*, *28*(2), 367–374. DOI: 10.1093/humrep/des400 PMID: 23178272

Tararbit, K., Lelong, N., Thieulin, A. C., Houyel, L., Bonnet, D., Goffinet, F., & Khoshnood, B. (2014). Assessing the role of multiple pregnancies in the association between tetralogy of Fallot and assisted reproductive techniques: A path-analysis approach. *Orphanet Journal of Rare Diseases*, *9*, 27. DOI: 10.1186/1750-1172-9-27 PMID: 24555734

Veeramani, M., Balachandren, N., Hong, Y. H., Lee, J., Corno, A. F., Mavrelos, D., & Kastora, S. L. (2024). Assisted reproduction and congenital malformations: A systematic review and meta-analysis. *Congenital Anomalies*, *64*(3), 107–115. DOI: 10.1111/cga.12561 PMID: 38577728

Verma, S. (2021). Congenital Heart Defects in ART Pregnancies: A South Indian Perspective. *The Indian Journal of Medical Research*, *153*(3), 354–359. DOI: 10.4103/ijmr.IJMR_652_20

Voros, C., Papadimas, G., Theodora, M., Mavrogianni, D., Athanasiou, D., Sapantzoglou, I., Bananis, K., Athanasiou, A., Athanasiou, A., Tsimpoukelis, C., Papapanagiotou, I., Vaitsis, D., Koulakmanidis, A.-M., Daskalaki, M. A., Topalis, V., Thomakos, N., Antsaklis, P., Chatzinikolaou, F., Loutradis, D., & Daskalakis, G. (2025). From Petri Dish to Primitive Heart: How IVF Alters Early Cardiac Gene Networks and Epigenetic Landscapes. *Biomedicines*, *13*(8), 2044. DOI: 10.3390/biomedicines13082044 PMID: 40868294

Watelle, L., Roy, L.-O., Lauzon-Schnitka, J., Newell, G., Dumas, A., Nadeau, A., Xiong, W. T., Rego, K., Beaulieu, C., Groulx-Boivin, E., Roy-Lacroix, M.-È., Vaujois, L., Drolet, C., Dancea, A., Dahdah, N., Bigras, J.-L., & Dallaire, F. (2024). The Quebec Congenital Heart Disease Registry: A Model of Prospective Databank to Facilitate Research in Congenital Cardiology. *CJC Pediatric and Congenital Heart Disease*, *3*(2), 57–66. DOI: 10.1016/j.cjcpc.2023.12.001 PMID: 38774679

Wennerholm, U. B., Henningsen, A. K., Romundstad, L. B., Bergh, C., Pinborg, A., Skjaerven, R., & Gissler, M. (2013). Perinatal outcomes of children born after frozen-thawed embryo transfer: A Nordic cohort study from the CoNARTaS group. *Human Reproduction (Oxford, England)*, *28*(9), 2545–2553. DOI: 10.1093/humrep/det272 PMID: 23832793

Xu, J., Li, Q., Deng, L., Xiong, J., Cheng, Z., & Ye, C. (2025). Global, regional, and national epidemiology of congenital heart disease in children from 1990 to 2021. *Frontiers in Cardiovascular Medicine*, *12*, 1522644. DOI: 10.3389/fcvm.2025.1522644 PMID: 40454242

Yang, S., Qin, G., He, G., Liang, M., Liang, Y., Luo, S., Yang, Z., Pang, Y., Long, F., & Tang, Y. (2025). Evaluation of first-trimester ultrasound screening strategy for fetal congenital heart disease. *Ultrasound in Obstetrics & Gynecology*, *65*(4), 478–486. DOI: 10.1002/uog.29186 PMID: 40019943

Zdanowicz, J. A., Yildrim, G., Fonseca, A., Hecher, K., & de Sousa, M. T. (2024). Is There a Cumulative Effect for Congenital Heart Defects in Monochorionic Twins after Assisted Reproduction? – A Retrospective Analysis at a Tertiary Referral Center. *Geburtshilfe und Frauenheilkunde*, *84*(03), 274–281. DOI: 10.1055/a-2238-3181 PMID: 38455999

Zhou, J., Liu, H., Gu, H., Cui, Y., Zhao, N., Chen, J., Gao, L., Zhang, Y., & Liu, J. (2014). Association of Cardiac Development with Assisted Reproductive Technology in Childhood: A Prospective Single-Blind Pilot Study. *Cellular Physiology and Biochemistry*, *34*(3), 988–1000. DOI: 10.1159/000366315 PMID: 25201231

Warnick, [illegible] Nguyen, C., [illegible] A., [illegible] LeRoy, R., Bemiller, C., [illegible] (2024). [illegible] Heart Disease Reporting [illegible]

W[illegible] M. (2014). [illegible]

[illegible]

[illegible]

[illegible]

[illegible]

Chapter 4
# The Paternal Link to Congenital Heart Disease:
## Phthalate Exposure Alters Sperm Gene Expression and Increases Offspring Cardiac Risk

**Shanthagoud P. Biradar**
https://orcid.org/0009-0001-9080-2300
*Sri Sathya Sai University for Human Excellence, India*

**Ramya Raghavan**
https://orcid.org/0000-0002-9953-543X
*Sri Sathya Sai University for Human Excellence, India*

## ABSTRACT

*Endocrine disrupting chemicals (EDCs) such as Dibutyl Phthalate exposure affects the expression of male germ cell genes expression associated with cardiac development pathways. Phthalates exposure, in males affects spermatogenesis, increasing offspring's susceptibility to congenital heart disease (CHD). In silico analysis confirmed that phthalates induce gene changes in cardiomyopathy, aortic aneurysms, and septal hypertrophy pathways, suggesting the intergenerational transmission of congenital heart disease risk. The Gene Ontology of MYBPC3, TNNI3, and KLF4 represent the strongest direct associations with CHD, particularly in cardiomyopathies. Despite the continuous turnover of spermatogonia, the risk of congenital heart conditions linked to germline transmission remains. Pathway analysis showed genes PDX1, KLF4, DES, ERCC2, MYBPC3, NDUFV2, PHYH, TNNI3, and FLI1 associated with embryonic, morphogenesis and cardiogenesis defects. Our work show sperm germ cells are susceptible to environmental toxicants, which can compromise offspring's heart development and function.*

DOI: 10.4018/979-8-3373-3735-7.ch004

## INTRODUCTION

Adult male germline stem cells, or spermatogonia, undergo mitotic proliferation and, post-puberty, develop into spermatocytes that enter meiosis, ultimately yielding haploid spermatozoa. Exposure to di-butyl phthalate (DBP) from medications alters the RNA of human sperm. The RNA elements required more than one spermatogenic cycle to resolve. (Estill et al., 2019). Notably, the incidence of congenital heart conditions linked to male germline transmission remains underreported (Mariana & Cairrao, 2020).

Our hypothesis focuses on the effects of paternal preconception exposure to phthalic acid esters and their links to congenital heart diseases (CHD) and birth outcomes. We identified differentially expressed genes (DEGs) between the cohorts with non-DBP and background levels of exposure and the High-DBP sample cohort (GSE129216, 2019) using the limma R package. The GSEA plot displays a significant p-value (0.002) and a negative NES (-1.68), indicating that the gene set is significantly downregulated in the experimental High DBP samples compared to the non-DBP controls. Notably, the downregulated genes in sperm were associated with cardiac pathways and cardiomyopathy (Figure 1). Our findings support the hypothesis of an association between paternal DBP exposure and cardiovascular issues in offspring.

Cardiomyopathy and CHD share overlapping molecular pathways, including genes involved in heart structure, function, and development. The genes PDX1, KLF4, DES, ERCC2, MYBPC3, NDUFV2, PHYH, TNNI3, and FLI1 play roles in transcription regulation and structural integrity related to cardiogenesis. Differential expressed genes are also involved in molecular mechanisms in heart development and function. Transcription factors PDX1, KLF4, and FLI1 are essential regulators during embryonic and cardiac morphogenesis (Table 1). For example, mutations in transcription factors cause cardiac malformations and arrhythmias. The oxidative stress induced by DBP can activate pro-inflammatory pathways, further exacerbating tissue damage. DES (desmin), TNNI3 (troponin I), and MYBPC3 (myosin-binding protein C) encode structural proteins essential for maintaining the integrity and function of cardiac muscle (Table 2). We further propose a framework that delineates male germ cell genes associated with congenital heart disease (CHD) pathology. Mutations in CHD genes or cardiomyopathies often overlap with other congenital disabilities due to shared developmental pathways.

*Figure 1. Male germ cells are susceptible to environmental toxicants, such as phthalates, which can lead to mutations and increase the risk of CHD in the offspring.*

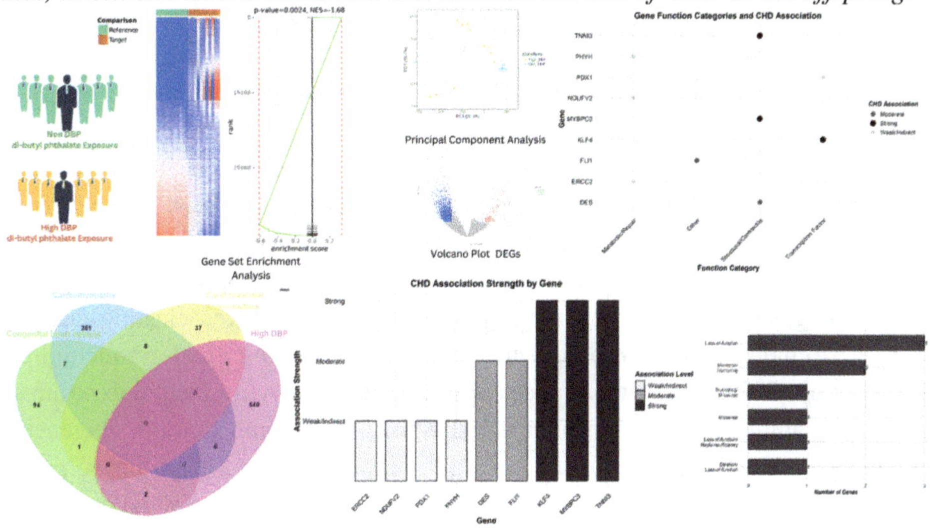


*Table 1. The top differentially expressed genes from the GSE129216 dataset include bulk RNA-seq raw data from baseline and high di-butyl phthalate (DBP) exposure in human sperm samples (GSE129216, 2019).*

| Gene | Molecular Mechanism | Cardiac Impact |
|---|---|---|
| PDX1 | Transcriptional regulation of pancreatic genes | Indirect via metabolic effects |
| ERCC2 | DNA repair via nucleotide excision repair | Indirect via DNA damage |
| KLF4 | Transcriptional regulation of cardiac genes | 1-2% of hypertrophic cardiomyopathy cases, Heart failure, arrhythmias |
| FLI1 | Cardiac development regulation, ETS transcription factor activity | Jacobsen syndrome congenital anomalies |
| DES | Structural cardiac protein, Intermediate filament assembly | 1-2% of dilated Cardiomyopathy, conduction defects |
| MYBPC3 | Sarcomeric protein regulation ventricular growth, contractility | Hypertrophic Cardiomyopathy |
| NDUFV2 | Electron transport complex I mitochondrial function | Mitochondrial energy production, oxidative stress |
| PHYH | Fatty acid alpha-oxidation | Secondary cardiac toxicity, Cardiomyopathy, arrhythmias |
| TNNI3 | Troponin complex regulation | Direct contractile regulation, dilated Cardiomyopathy |

## EXPOSOMICS ASSOCIATION TO CONGENITAL HEART DEFECTS

The exposomics approach to congenital heart disease (CHD) represents the totality of environmental exposures that influence cardiac development during paternal gametogenesis. Reproductive toxicological studies in exposomics integrate sperm related biological mechanisms influenced by social, household, occupational, and environmental factors that contribute to the pathogenesis of CHD. The scope of paternal exposome effects extends beyond immediate offspring to impact subsequent generations. F2 and F3 generation effects have been documented in animal models, suggesting that paternal environmental exposures can create lasting changes in the germline that affect subsequent generations, including great-grandchildren (Juarez et al., 2020). Recent evidence suggests paternal environmental exposures, particularly phthalates, may influence CHD risk in offspring through epigenetic and genetic mechanisms. A CHD association between paternal exposure to pesticides and alkyl phenolic compounds is reported. The development of patent ductus arteriosus in offspring suggests that paternal toxicity may increase the risk of congenital heart disease (Vince Fazekas-Pongor et al., 2020). Phthalate esters may contribute to CHD due to their role as endocrine disruptors (Justin P. Zachariah et al., 2024). Endocrine-disrupting chemicals contribute to infertility, may lead to epigenetic transgenerational inheritance. In vitro studies have shown that mono-n-butyl phthalate (MBP) can inhibit sperm motility and capacitation by suppressing tyrosine phosphorylation (Xie et al., 2019).

Phthalates have been linked to the development of abnormal subintestinal vessels, indicating a direct impact on angiogenesis during development (Peng et al., 2024). The paternal contribution to CHD risk through environmental exposures has gained increasing recognition, with mounting evidence suggesting that sperm-mediated transmission of environmental damage can significantly influence embryonic development. Unlike maternal exposures that directly affect the developing fetus, paternal exposures exert their effects through alterations in sperm quality, genetic integrity, and epigenetic programming that persist through fertilization and early embryogenesis (Raghavan & Ahamad, 2025). Population-level implications of transgenerational paternal effects suggest that current CHD rates may partly reflect historical environmental exposures experienced by previous generations. The transgenerational effects perspective emphasizes the importance of comprehensive exposome assessment that considers multigenerational exposure histories rather than focusing solely on immediate periconceptional factors.

So, we obtained gene expression data from the Gene Expression Omnibus (GEO) database at the National Center for Biotechnology Information (NCBI). The GSE129216 dataset includes bulk RNA-seq raw data from baseline and high di-butyl phthalate (DBP) exposure from human sperm samples (GSE129216, 2019). The study participants initially received a non-DBP mesalamine treatment, then transitioned to a high-DBP mesalamine treatment in subsequent visits. The MARS study was designed to conduct a longitudinal assessment (4-6 months) of semen quality in human males in relation to high exposure to di-butyl phthalate (DBP). The identification of statistically significant DEGs associated with Cardiomyopathy suggests paternal germline transmission altered by High DBP exposure for a few months could still contribute to increased risk of CHD in the offspring.

Endocrine-disrupting chemicals (EDCs), such as phthalate exposure, in males during critical perinatal stages, increase offspring's susceptibility to congenital heart disease (CHD). Disruptions in cardiac development also affect energy metabolism and/ or genomic stability. The genetic basis of congenital heart disease (CHD) involves complex interactions between multiple genes affecting cardiac development, structure, and function. The genes PDX1, ERCC2, KLF4, FLI1, DES, MYBPC3, NDUFV2, PHYH, and TNNI3 demonstrate strong associations with cardiac abnormalities. MYBPC3, TNNI3, and KLF4 represent the strongest direct associations with CHD, particularly in cardiomyopathies. Genes such as PDX1, ERCC2, NDUFV2, and PHYH exhibit weaker or indirect connections to the cardiac pathway. The ERCC2, involved in DNA repair, and NDUFV2, a component of the mitochondrial respiratory chain, as well as PHYH, are critical for normal cellular function. Present evidence suggests that paternal exposure to phthalate esters may be associated with cardiovascular disease in neonates, which warrants further research.

More details are provided in Figure 1, which includes gene set enrichment analysis and the identification of genes altered at both base-level and high-level exposure to di-butyl phthalate (DBP) in human sperm RNA. Sarcomeric proteins (MYBPC3, TNNI3) cause direct contractile dysfunction by disrupting protein-protein interactions and altering calcium sensitivity. Transcription factors (KLF4, FLI1) affect cardiac gene expression and developmental programs. Structural proteins (DES) cause cytoskeletal abnormalities leading to mechanical dysfunction. Metabolic enzymes (PHYH, NDUFV2) cause secondary cardiac effects through cellular energy dysfunction or toxin accumulation. Phthalate esters are widely used as plasticizers, leading to inevitable human exposure and posing a risk to sperm health and germline transmission (Casciaro et al., 2024). A positive association between paternal exposure to pesticides and alkylphenolic compounds and the development of patent ductus arteriosus in offspring suggests that paternal toxicity may increase the risk of congenital heart disease (Vince Fazekas-Pongor et al., 2020).

*Table 2. High di-butyl phthalate (DBP) exposure effects on human sperm (GSE129216, 2019). In silico analysis of dibutyl phthalate impacts on human sperm, from MARS data available at the Gene Expression Omnibus (GEO) database at the National Center for Biotechnology Information (NCBI).*

| Gene Symbol | Differentially Expressed Genes | Primary Function Reported |
|---|---|---|
| PDX1 | Pancreatic and Duodenal Homeobox 1 | Transcription factor for pancreatic development |
| ERCC2 | Excision Repair Cross-Complementation Group 2 | DNA repair enzyme in nucleotide excision repair |
| KLF4 | Kruppel-Like Factor 4 | Transcription factor regulating cell differentiation |
| FLI1 | Friend Leukemia Integration 1 Transcription Factor | ETS family transcription factor |
| DES | Desmin | Intermediate filament protein |
| MYBPC3 | Myosin Binding Protein C3 | Cardiac myosin binding protein |
| NDUFV2 | NADH Ubiquinone Oxidoreductase Core Subunit V2 | Mitochondrial complex I subunit |
| PHYH | Phytanoyl-CoA 2-Hydroxylase | Peroxisomal enzyme for fatty acid oxidation |
| TNNI3 | Troponin I3 Cardiac Type | Cardiac troponin inhibitory subunit |

Previous investigation on the impact of di-butyl phthalate (DBP) exposure from medications on human sperm RNA in men revealed that changes in sperm RNA elements require more than one spermatogenic cycle to resolve. (Estill et al., 2019). From the Japan Environment and Children's Study on infants diagnosed with CHDs, various paternal exposures to substances such as photo copying machines, laser printers, and soluble paints were found to be associated with increased risks of CHDs in the offspring. Periconceptional paternal occupational exposure could be a risk factor for CHDs, highlighting the need for further research, including studies utilizing biomarkers to better understand this association (Hayama-Terada et al., 2023). The phthalate raises concerns about fetal development and long-term cardiovascular health. DBP toxicity to sperm as a causative factor for CHD needs longitudinal studies to show causation. Male germ cells are susceptible to environmental toxicants, such as phthalates, and compromise our ecosystems. Notably, despite the continuous turnover of spermatogonia, pollutants, and toxic exposures to occupational hazards such as those from photocopying machines, laser printers, and soluble paints were found to be associated with an increased risk of CHD.

## DEVELOPMENTAL ORIGINS OF HEALTH AND CHD

The intersection of parental exposure to environmental chemicals and the health of offspring is a critical area of research. Understanding the long-term effects of reproductive toxicantss deoffspring velopment and disease susceptibility can benefit from ininilico approaches. Computational models to predict the effects of chemical exposures can be effectively linked to stem cells in offspring. The combinatorial in vitro screening strategies can enhance our understanding of how parental exposures influence future generations and cardiotoxicity effects. Parental exposure to environmental chemicals, such as pesticides, heavy metals, and endocrine disruptors, can have profound effects on reproductive health and fetal development. Environmental, household, or occupational exposures can lead to epigenetic changes, genetic mutations, and alterations in gene expression that may predispose individuals to cardiac conditions.

Developmental origins of health and disease advocates for the prevention of CHD, especially when data show that the association between paternal DBP exposure increases risk for CHD. While maternal exposures have been widely studied, recent research has highlighted paternal factors in the germline burden of CHD (Hojat Dehghanbanadaki et al., 2024). The focus on males' health is critical, as paternal factors are increasingly recognized as influential in the health of offspring and the occurrence of congenital anomalies. There is a link between congenital heart defects (CHDs) and paternal exposure to EDCs such as phthalates during the periconceptional period. More evidence is needed to reposition the paternal perinatal phthalate exposure not merely as an alteration of the male germline but as a potential epigenetic driver of the risk of CHD.

In congenitally malformed hearts, the conduction system may exhibit anatomical variants, such as dual SA or AV nodes, which can complicate surgical interventions. CHD involves structural heart malformations. The most straightforward congenitally malformed hearts that pediatric cardiologists encounter are dysplasia of a single valve or an isolated septal defect. One of the most well-studied congenital lesions is Tetralogy of Fallot, where long-term prognosis is significantly altered when the pulmonary valve cannot be preserved during initial surgery, creating varying degrees of pulmonary insufficiency. Surgical corrections for congenital heart lesions involve patching, conduit placement, and advanced techniques to reshape the malformed heart. Many techniques require cardiac bypass, and foreign material inserted into the heart can form boundaries of future macroreentrant circuits. Coronary artery translocation during surgeries like transposition of the great arteries can lead to coronary stenosis and aortic root dilation, increasing the risk of tachyarrhythmias.

*Table 3. Developmental origins of CHD*

| Cellular Field | Primary Contribution | Biological Mechanisms Affected | Associated CHD Outcomes |
|---|---|---|---|
| First Heart Field (FHF) | Primarily, the Left Ventricular Myocardium. | Retinoic acid signaling and BMP inhibition. | LV hypoplasia or altered conduction properties. |
| Second Heart Field (SHF) | Right Ventricle, Outflow Tract, and part of the Atria. | Endocrine disruptors, BPA, phthalates, and teratogens. | Outflow tract malformations and double outlet right ventricle. |
| Cardiac Neural Crest Cells (cNCCs) | Aorticopulmonary septation, aortic arch patterning, and valve formation. | Oxidative stress, hypoxia, viral infections. | Conotruncal anomalies, Truncus arteriosus, Tetralogy of Fallot |

Genetic disorders such as Holt-Oram syndrome and DiGeorge syndrome can modify the risk of arrhythmia in congenitally malformed hearts. Furthermore, genetic variants, including aneuploidies (trisomy 21) and Copy Number Variants (CNVs) at hotspots like 22q11.2, can contribute to syndromic forms of CHD associated with extracardiac anomalies, developmental disorders, and increased susceptibility to infections. The complex regulatory disruptions caused by these genetic alterations can impair cell-cell communication, signaling pathways, and structural maturation, thereby exacerbating both primary and secondary complications. As a result, there is an increased susceptibility to congenital diseases, including cardiovascular conditions.

Genetic variants disrupt the regulation of cell-cell communication, which is essential for heart development. Aneuploidies are the first identified genetic cause of CHD and are commonly diagnosed in patients with sCHD. Comparative genomic hybridisation arrays (CGH-array) or chromosomal microarrays (CMA) lead to the identification of CNVs in patients with sCHD and nsCHD. Genetic factors play a significant role in influencing the spectrum of complications observed in CHD patients through several mechanisms. Variations in specific genes, such as those involved in critical cardiac developmental pathways (GATA4, TBX5, NOTCH1), can affect the structural integrity and functional maturation of the heart. Heterotaxy, the abnormal arrangement of organs, can trigger arrhythmias due to the presence of dual SA or AV nodes or the absence of an SA node. Several genetic alterations may predispose patients to primary cardiac issues and secondary complications like arrhythmias and heart failure. Here, we demonstrate the use of a literature review and an in-silico study of paternal exposure, which can be further developed to test offspring stem cells or to explore combinatorial in vitro screening approaches in the future.

## PHTHALATE-ASSOCIATED REPRODUCTIVE TOXICITY

Phthalates, ubiquitous industrial chemicals used as plasticizers in consumer products, represent a major environmental health concern due to their endocrine-disrupting properties and widespread human exposure. Toxic chemicals can disrupt normal cardiac development by interfering with hormonal signaling pathways, inducing oxidative stress, and causing epigenetic modifications. Dibutyl phthalate (DBP), a widely used plasticizer, has been shown to have significant negative impacts on sperm quality and function. An increase in morphologically abnormal sperm. DBP exposure leads to a significant decrease in sperm count and motility. The abnormalities in sperm morphology and function have been observed in both animal models and human epidemiological studies (J. Wang et al., 2021). In vitro studies have demonstrated that DBP and its metabolite, mono-n-butyl phthalate (MBP), can inhibit sperm motility and capacitation by suppressing tyrosine phosphorylation, a crucial process for normal sperm function (Xie et al., 2019). DBP interacts with peroxisome proliferator-activated receptors (PPAR) and other xenobiotic sensors, disrupting the hormonal balance necessary for spermatogenesis. Industrialization has introduced phthalates as environmental risk factors for congenital heart disease (CHD). Phthalate esters pose a risk to sperm health and germline transmission, suggesting that the effects can persist across generations (Casciaro et al., 2024).

Dibutyl phthalate (DBP) has been linked to CHD and sperm quality and function. DBP exposure leads to a significant decrease in sperm count and motility in animal models and human epidemiological studies (J. Wang et al., 2021). Multiple cohort studies, systematic reviews, and meta-analyses have consistently identified relationships between prenatal phthalate exposure, including DBP, and adverse birth outcomes (Trasande et al., 2024). However, male germline transmission of CHD needs to account for exposure to phthalates or DBP. The phthalate esters could be major contributors due to their role as endocrine disruptors (Justin P. Zachariah et al., 2024).

*Figure 2. Odds Ratios For Different CHD Subtypes Associated With Paternal Chemical Exposures Reported In The Literature.*

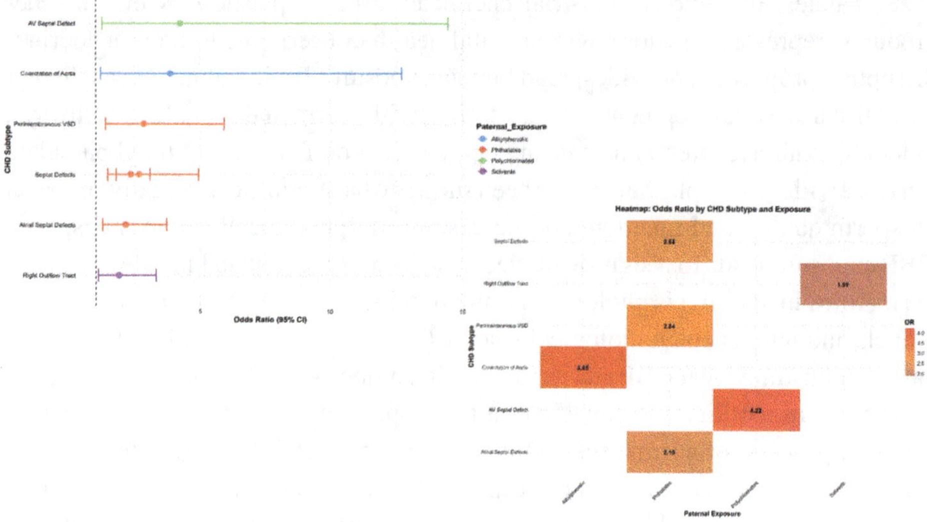


Our work focuses on the effects of paternal preconception exposure to phthalic acid esters and their links to birth outcomes. Here, we propose the role of phthalates in the etiology of CHD via male germline transmission. Analysis by CHD subtypes revealed differential risks associated with paternal exposure to chemicals. Figure 3 illustrates that atrioventricular septal defects showed the highest risk (OR = 4.22), followed by coarctation of the aorta (OR = 3.85) and perimembranous ventricular septal defects (OR = 2.84). Notably, phthalate exposures are consistently associated with septal defects across multiple studies. Subtype-specific analysis identified septal defects as the most frequently studied outcome, with consistent positive associations across studies. The mean odds ratio for septal defects was 2.51, indicating a more than 2-fold increased risk associated with paternal phthalate exposure. There is substantial evidence suggesting an association between paternal DBP exposure and cardiovascular diseases in offspring. The exact mechanisms are complex and multifaceted. Many of the genes implicated in cardiomyopathy are known to play crucial roles in cardiac morphogenesis. DBP exposure affects myocardial integrity, increasing susceptibility to congenital heart defects. Endocrine disruption, oxidative stress, genetic and epigenetic modifications, and interference predispose to CHD. Further research is needed to fully elucidate the effects of phthalates and their implications for perinatal exposure.

*Figure 3. Phthalates Disrupt Leydig And Sertoli Cells and Germline Signaling Pathways*

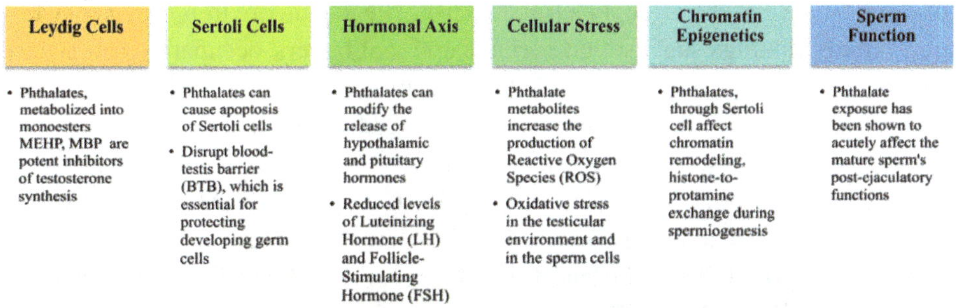


## PROPOSED MECHANISMS OF TOXICITY

Paternal smoking demonstrates dose-dependent relationships with CHD risk, particularly affecting specific cardiac structures. The mechanisms involve carbon monoxide and nicotine inducing endothelial dysfunction, reducing placental blood flow, and interfering with cardiac angiogenesis. Smoking-related oxidative stress damages sperm DNA and alters epigenetic programming, which is critical for cardiac development (Nowak et al., 2024). Literature suggests phthalate environmental exposures has reproductive toxicities which could influence developmental pathways. Congenital heart disease during critical periods of gamete development, DBP can then alter gene expression and increase CHD susceptibility in the offspring (Mo et al., 2022). Human-induced pluripotent stem cell-derived cardiomyocytes (hiPSC-CMs) are recognized as a powerful technology that can better represent human cardiomyocyte responses in drug screening. The ToxPi, or Toxicological Prioritization Index, framework is discussed as a tool for integrating multiple sources of evidence to improve decision-making in toxicology. Phthalate esters have been shown to impair calcium handling and increase susceptibility to arrhythmia (Mariana & Cairrao, 2020). It can lead to thinning of the ventricular wall, hypoplastic septa, and abnormal chamber pressure profiles in late gestation.

### Occupational Exposure

Phthalate esters are widely used as plasticizers, leading to risk to sperm health and germline transmission (Casciaro et al., 2024). Paternal exposures before conception associate ventricular septal defects with phthalates and other environmental toxicants (Kim P.J. Wijnands et al., 2014). A positive association between paternal exposure to pesticides and alkylphenolic compounds and the development of patent ductus arteriosus in offspring, suggesting a paternal risk factor for congenital heart disease (Vince Fazekas-Pongor et al., 2020). The Japan Environment and Children's Study findings suggest that periconceptional fathers' occupational exposure is linked to a higher risk of infant CHDs (Hayama-Terada et al., 2023). The Japan Environment and Children's Study, examining 28,866 participants, demonstrated that fathers exposed to photocopying machines/laser printers regularly had a 38% increased risk of infant CHDs (OR = 1.38, 95%CI: 1.00-1.91). More dramatically, occasional exposure to lead-containing solder increased CHD risk by 203% (OR = 2.03, 95%CI: 1.06-3.88), while lead-free solder exposure showed an even higher risk increase of 245% (OR = 3.45, 95%CI: 1.85-6.43 Paternal exposures to substances such as photocopying machines, laser printers, and soluble paints were found to be associated with increased risks of CHDs (Fazekas-Pongor et al., 2021).

## Animal Studies

Preconception exposure to di(2-ethylhexyl) phthalate (DEHP) in male mice significantly alters sperm methylation. It affects gene expression in developing embryos (Vince Fazekas-Pongor et al., 2020). Gene ontology analyses revealed that DEHP exposure affects developmental genes, including those involved in embryonic development and morphogenesis. (Oluwayiose et al., 2021). The findings suggest that periconceptional paternal occupational exposure to phthalates increases the risk of CHDs in children, as compromised sperm structural and functional integrity is reported (Stefano Raffaele Giannubilo et al., 2024). For instance, prenatal exposure to phthalates has been shown to disrupt the expression of cell cycle regulators and could potentially affect cardiovascular development. Furthermore, CHD-related NKX2.5 and TBX5 genes are altered by DBP exposure in zebrafish models.

*Table 4. Paternal Association With Congenital Heart Diseases*

| Paternal Factor | Mechanism/Description | Relevance to CHD | Reference |
|---|---|---|---|
| De Novo Mutations (in sperm) | Mutations in critical cardiac genes, Transcription Factors, and structural proteins that arise during spermatogenesis. | A significant cause of sporadic CHD; risk increases with advanced paternal age. | (Nowak et al., 2024) |
| Altered Sperm Epigenome | Changes in DNA methylation or histone modifications in sperm due to paternal exposures (diet, smoking, toxicants). | It can lead to altered gene expression in the embryo, potentially affecting developmental pathways. | (Breton et al., 2021) (Lismer et al., 2020) |
| Paternal Toxicant Exposure | Exposure to environmental toxins, lifestyle factors (smoking, high-fat diet), or occupational hazards that damage sperm DNA or its epigenetic profile. | Increased rates of chromosomal aberrations and single-gene mutations in offspring. | (Juarez et al., 2020) |

continued on following page

*Table 4. Continued*

| Paternal Factor | Mechanism/Description | Relevance to CHD | Reference |
|---|---|---|---|
| Paternal occupational phthalate exposure | Phthalates alter the sperm methylome (DNA methylation) and sperm small non-coding RNAs (sncRNAs), thus changing the epigenetic programming inherited by the embryo. | Altered gene expression of developmental gene families<br>Increased risk of Ventricular Septal Defect (VSD) and Pulmonary Stenosis (PS). | (Fazekas-Pongor et al., 2021) |
| Endocrine-Disrupting Chemicals (EDCs): Phthalates, Dioxins Bisphenol A (BPA) Dioxin (TCDD) | Interfere with hormonal regulation of gene transcription via estrogen, androgen, and thyroid hormone receptors. | Modulates estrogen receptor α and β activity in fetal cardiomyocytes | (Kaltsas et al., 2025)<br>(Baker et al., 2023) |

## Metabolic Effects

The effects of parental DBP exposure can manifest as health issues in offspring. Prenatal exposure to DBP has been linked to reproductive system malformations, such as hypospadias and cryptorchidism, in male offspring (J. Wang et al., 2021). There is a challenge in effectively identifying potential hazards that may affect various organs in the body. Neurodevelopmental issues, such as language delays and other cognitive impairments, are reported. Animal studies have shown that DBP exposure can lead to obesity and dyslipidemia in offspring (Breton et al., 2021). Alcohol exposure damages cardiac neural crest cells and increases apoptosis during critical stages of cardiac development. The toxic effects extend beyond direct cellular damage to include epigenetic modifications that persist across generations (Zhang et al., 2022). Key gaps include the inability to identify hazards across multiple target organs, predict, and assess drug safety liabilities. Organic solvents exhibit differential effects based on CHD subtype, with paternal solvent exposure being significantly associated with atrial septal defects and right ventricular outflow tract obstructions. The mechanisms involve disruption of cardiac neural crest cell development and interference with normal cardiac morphogenesis during critical developmental windows.

## Oxidative Stress

Advanced paternal age represents a well-established risk factor for CHDs through accumulated de novo mutations in sperm. Fathers aged 35-39 years show a 14% increased CHD risk (OR = 1.14, 95%CI: 1.09-1.19), while those ≥40 years demonstrate a 27% increased risk (OR = 1.27, 95%CI: 1.14-1.42). The most significant association is observed in fathers over 45 years, who exhibit a 69% increased risk of patent ductus arteriosus specifically (HR = 1.69, 95% CI: 1.17-2.43). DBP exposure increases oxidative stress levels, inflammation, and damage to cardiovascular tissues. In zebrafish, DBP exposure can affect cardiac transcription factors such as NKX2.5

and TBX5 with cardiotoxic effects, including altered heart rate and pericardial edema (Sun & Li, 2019). The spermiotoxic effects of various phthalate esters in mice highlight poor sperm parameters, pro-oxidant antioxidant ratios in spermatozoa, sperm numbers, and the phosphorylation of protein kinase A substrates, which are crucial for capacitation (Oluwayiose et al., 2021). Air pollutants and industrial chemicals induce oxidative stress markers associated with outflow tract defects. Microbial volatiles and pollutants can be transported from paternal residential areas to affect fetal development through multiple pathways (Nagashri et al., 2024).

The timing of exposure during the periconceptional period is particularly critical, as cardiac development begins within the first weeks after fertilization. The development of three-dimensional (3D) culture systems using stem cells can better mimic the in vivo environment, enhance the physiological relevance of the models, and improve the understanding of drug interactions and toxicities. Heavy metals, including chromium, arsenic, cadmium, and mercury, exhibit specific associations with CHD through multiple toxic mechanisms. Metal ions can replace essential cofactors in enzymatic reactions, generate reactive oxygen species that bind to DNA, causing genomic defects. Mercury exposure, though affecting only 0.5% of fathers, demonstrates particularly high potency for developmental toxicity.

Furthermore, environmental chemicals, with multiple exposures to pesticides and industrial pollutants, have been implicated in the development of CHD. Given the complexity of cardiac physiology, there is an urgent need for augmentative human-computing interfaces (S. et al., 2025). Organic solvents affect cardiac development by disrupting cellular membrane integrity and interfering with signal transduction pathways. Exposure to solvents during spermatogenesis can alter the composition of the sperm membrane and impact fertilization mechanisms. In contrast, exposure to residual solvents can have a direct impact on early embryonic development. Several classes of environmental chemicals, including organotins, bisphenol-like chemicals, pesticides, and quaternary ammonium compounds, exhibited strong bioactivity against CHD targets (Qian et al., 2020).

## SPERM DNA FRAGMENTATION AND GENETIC INTEGRITY

The mechanism involves increased mutation rates in sperm due to the continuous mitotic divisions of spermatogonia throughout a man's lifetime. Each sperm cell division introduces approximately two new mutations. By age 40, sperm carry roughly 65 new mutations compared to those from 20-year-old fathers. However, the direct causal effect of paternal age-related de novo mutations on CHD risk is relatively modest, with delayed paternity from mid-20s to mid-40s increasing offspring CHD risk by only about 20%. There is a growing demand for hazard and risk assessment that exceeds the capacity to produce necessary toxicity data, often relying on traditional animal models with limited human relevance (Nowak et al., 2024).

Sperm DNA fragmentation (SDF) results from multiple toxic exposures, including heat, radiation, oxidative stress, and abnormal apoptosis. Unlike oocytes, mature sperm lack DNA repair activity, making them particularly vulnerable to environmental damage (Voros et al., 2025). When SDF exceeds the oocyte's repair threshold, damaged DNA is transferred to the embryo, increasing the risk of chromosomal aneuploidy and potentially affecting cardiac development. Clinical evidence demonstrates that elevated paternal SDF correlates with increased aneuploidy rates in miscarried conceptuses. The sperm DNA damage contributes to early embryonic abnormalities that may include cardiac malformations. SDF mechanism is particularly relevant for CHD development given the critical timing of cardiac morphogenesis during early embryogenesis (Bhat et al., 2025).

Cardiac morphogenesis at weeks 2-8 of embryonic development creates critical vulnerability windows. Paternally transmitted factors can interact with maternal environmental exposures to influence cardiac development outcomes. Nanotechnology-based assays can detect developmental and exposure windows for CHD subtypes associated with paternal exposures (Bhuvana et al., 2025). Social determinants for environmental chemicals, with predicted human exposure, showed activity-to-exposure ratios between modeled blood concentrations and in vitro bioactivity of one to five orders of magnitude. High-resolution detection and diagnosis indicate that even at low environmental exposure levels, phthalates have significant effects on cardiac function (Xie et al., 2019).

## Endocrine Disruption

Paternal exposures alter sperm epigenetic profiles, including DNA methylation, histone modifications, and non-coding RNA expression, which can persist through embryonic reprogramming and affect cardiac development. Animal studies identified numerous differentially methylated regions in both sperm and embryonic tissues. Di(2-ethylhexyl) phthalate (DEHP) is a significant environmental pollutant linked to CHD, acting as a risk factor (Rachel Nicoll, 2018).

Agricultural workers face exposure to pesticides and herbicides that demonstrate significant CHD associations. Insecticide exposure affects 17.0% of fathers, while herbicide exposure occurs in 5.7% of the study population. Agricultural and food industry chemicals can disrupt the food chain and endocrine signaling pathways, which are critical for cardiac development. They induce epigenetic changes that persist across generations. Paternal exposure to phthalates and polychlorinated compounds is associated with an increased risk of various types of CHDs (Claudia A. Snijder et al., 2012). Endocrine disruptors and plasticizers disrupt critical developmental windows, thereby affecting the migration and differentiation of cardiac neural crest cells.

The interaction between paternal exposure timing and genetic susceptibility creates critical windows of vulnerability. Periconceptional exposure, from 3 months before conception through early pregnancy, represents the most critical period. Sperm development takes approximately 74 days, and environmental exposures during the critical developmental window can directly affect the sperm that will fertilize the egg. Altered histone H3 lysine four trimethylation (H3K4me3) in sperm can escape embryonic reprogramming and contribute to transgenerational phenotypes. Sperm with abnormal H3K4me3 patterns show evidence of impaired fertility and offspring with severe birth defects, potentially including cardiac abnormalities. The mechanism involves transmission of aberrant epigenetic signals that disrupt normal gene expression patterns during cardiac morphogenesis. Discussion of histone deacetylase (HDAC) inhibitors as anticancer agents and their association with delayed cardiac repolarization and potential lethal arrhythmias (Lismer et al., 2020).

*Table 5. Phthalate Compounds and Their Toxicity and Health Effects*

| Compound | Common uses | Reproductive Toxicity<br>Proposed Health Impacts |
|---|---|---|
| Diethyl phthalate (DEP) | Personal care products (fragrances, deodorants), plastics | Low toxicity, skin and eye irritation; endocrine disruptor. |
| Dimethyl phthalate (DMP) | Insect repellents, plastics, and perfumes | Mild toxicity, developmental and reproductive toxicity. |
| Di-n-butyl phthalate (DBP) | Adhesives, paints, coatings, and plastics | Endocrine disruptor, liver damage, and reproductive toxicity. |
| Di-n-octyl phthalate (DNOP) | Flexible plastics (PVC), adhesives, and coatings | Toxic to aquatic life, liver and kidney damage with prolonged exposure. |
| Diisobutyl phthalate (DIBP) | Adhesives, sealants, and coatings | endocrine disruptor, developmental toxicity. |
| Benzyl butyl phthalate (BBP) | Plastics (PVC), flooring, and adhesives | Associated with developmental and reproductive toxicity. |
| Di(2-ethylhexyl) phthalate (DEHP) | PVC plastics (medical devices, flooring, cables) | High toxicity, endocrine disruption, developmental and reproductive toxicity, and carcinogenic. |
| Diisononyl phthalate (DINP) | Plasticizers, medical devices, and toys | Potential carcinogen, toxic to the liver and kidneys, suspected endocrine disruptor. |
| Di(2-propylheptyl) phthalate (DPHP) | Plastics (PVC), flooring, and adhesives | Reproductive toxicity, endocrine disruption. |
| Diethylene glycol dibenzoate (DEGDB) | Plasticizers and coatings | Low toxicity but may cause skin irritation; not extensively studied. |

continued on following page

*Table 5. Continued*

| Compound | Common uses | Reproductive Toxicity Proposed Health Impacts |
|---|---|---|
| Dipropyl phthalate (DPP) | Perfumes, cosmetics, and plastics | skin irritation, suspected endocrine disruption. |
| Tert-butylphthalate (TBP) | Plastics, adhesives, and coatings | contain carcinogens and endocrine disruptors. |
| Isodecyl phthalate (IDP) | Plastics, paints, and coatings | Reproductive and developmental toxicity. |
| Cyclohexyl phthalate (CHP) | Plasticizers and as a solvent | Toxicity to the liver and kidneys, suspected carcinogen. |
| Dibutyl benzyl phthalate (DBBP) | Flexible PVC, adhesives, and sealants | Reproductive and developmental toxicity. |
| Butyl benzyl phthalate (BBzP) | Plastics, adhesives, and paints | Endocrine disruptor, developmental toxicity, and carcinogenic properties. |
| Di(2-ethylhexyl) adipate (DEHA) | Flexible plastics and as a solvent | Low toxicity, but a potential irritant; used as a substitute for DEHP. |

## PATERNAL EXPOSURE AND ITS IMPLICATIONS FOR CONGENITAL ABNORMALITIES

Emerging evidence reveals that paternal environmental exposures significantly influence the risk of congenital heart defects (CHDs) in offspring, challenging the traditional focus on maternal factors alone. Studies using TCDD (dioxin) exposure demonstrate transgenerational reductions in sperm quality and increased preterm birth risk in unexposed partners. Dose-response analysis revealed significant trends for exposure frequency and CHD risk. The Hayama-Terada study demonstrated a significant dose-response relationship (p for trend = 0.018), with regular occupational exposures associated with higher risks compared to occasional exposures. Factory workers, janitors, painters, and plywood mill workers show increased associations with various CHD subtypes. The mechanisms involve chronic exposure to industrial solvents, adhesives, paints, and formaldehyde that can cross-link DNA, disrupt cellular metabolism, and alter gene expression patterns (Table 3).

Similarly, the Snijder study found increasing risk with higher exposure probabilities (p for trend = 0.002). Industrial chemicals and pollutants generate reactive oxygen species that overwhelm sperm antioxidant defenses, leading to DNA strand breaks, membrane damage, and altered protein function. Healthcare workers exposed to sterilizing disinfectants, formaldehyde, and radiation show specific risk patterns. Medical sterilizing disinfectant exposure affects 14.3% of exposed fathers, while exposure to radiation and radioactive substances occurs in 5.3%. Radioactive or chemotherapeutic exposures can directly damage sperm DNA and alter epigenetic programming through mutagenic mechanisms. DNA damage effects are particularly pronounced in sperm due to their high DNA compaction and limited repair mechanisms. The resulting cellular damage can affect both fertilization capacity and the genetic and epigenetic pathways (Ananthakumar et al., 2024).

The paternal exposome encompasses complex interactions between occupational chemicals, lifestyle factors, age-related mutations, and epigenetic mechanisms that collectively contribute to CHD development through multiple pathways affecting sperm quality, genetic integrity, and transgenerational inheritance. Chromatin modifications in sperm provide a stable mechanism for storing and transmitting environmental information. Unlike DNA methylation, which undergoes extensive reprogramming during embryogenesis, certain histone modifications can persist and influence embryonic gene expression. Biological persistence enables environmental exposures experienced by fathers to have lasting effects on offspring development, including an increased risk of cardiac malformation (Juarez et al., 2020).

The effects of parental DBP exposure can manifest in various health issues in offspring. Prenatal exposure to DBP has been linked to reproductive system malformations, such as hypospadias and cryptorchidism, in male offspring (J. Wang et al., 2021). Neurodevelopmental issues, such as language delays and other cognitive impairments, are commonly observed in children. Animal studies have shown that DBP exposure can lead to obesity and dyslipidemia in offspring, as evidenced by increased body weight and altered lipid metabolism (Breton et al., 2021).

Congenital heart defects are common anomalies, whose phenotyping, environmental, and genetic causes are essential for predicting prognosis and recurrence risk. There are now more adults than children living with CHD, with a majority of adults being female. Long-term outcomes for females with CHD are influenced by sex-specific differences (Lindley, 2025). The CHD is a multifactorial disease caused by environmental factors and genetics, including aneuploidies, CNVs, SNVs, and InDels. The HPO term "Abnormal heart morphology" (HP:0001627) is associated with more than 1559 genes, many of which do not show sufficient evidence for an association with human CHD. Congenitally malformed hearts carry a greater burden of right ventricular pressure, volume loading, and dysfunction compared to acquired heart disease. Differences in ion channel balance and handling in the remodeling right ventricle can predispose the congenitally malformed heart to a higher incidence of ventricular arrhythmias (Leirgul et al., 2025). Conduction heterogeneity, indicated by a fragmented QRS pattern, correlates with the risk of future sudden cardiac arrest. Further, the risk of acquired neonatal significant brain injury, specifically white matter injury, during the perinatal transition in newborns with congenital heart disease is common. In the transposition of the great arteries (TGA), after surgical intervention, affected children continue to experience significant neurodevelopmental impairments. The CHD-related prenatal and neonatal physiological factors may have lasting effects on fetal predictors of neurodevelopmental and congenital heart disease (CHD) outcomes (Wolfe & Peyvandi, 2025).

## FUTURE DIRECTIONS

The increasing number of chemicals in consumer and industrial markets poses significant challenges for regulatory programs in assessing potential risks to human and ecological health. The introduction of long-read sequencing (lrGS) might offer the detection of previously undetectable variants. Morphological and physiological cardiac changes can be studied using in vivo and in vitro models of CHD, most often utilising stem cell-derived cardiomyocytes. Machine learning algorithms and quantitative structure-activity relationship (QSAR) models are commonly used in silico screening (Ananthakumar, Nanjundeshwara, et al., 2025). ML and AI models analyze existing data to establish correlations between chemical structures and their biological effects, allowing for the prediction of cardiotoxicity for untested compounds (Vey et al., 2025). CRISPRCas13 therapy has successfully prevented cardiac hypertrophy in a humanized mouse model of a specific subtype of HCM. The role of NOTCH1 hypomorphic mutations in cardiomyocytes derived from induced pluripotent stem cells (iPSCs) in patients with hypoplastic left heart syndrome. The effects of inflammatory cytokines on cardiac tissues and cardiomyocytes can be utilized with gene-editing technology (Lakshmaiah et al., 2025).

A comprehensive exposomics analysis is crucial for understanding the genetic factors and environmental influences on CHD. Social determinants information can enhance prognosis prediction and recurrence risk assessment in families. Currently, thorough genetic workups are only available to a minority of patients with CHD, highlighting the need for improved diagnostic methods and frameworks (P. et al., 2025). Many novel candidate genes have been identified through genomic studies. Require experimental validation to confirm their causative roles in CHD. The role of hiPSC technology in cardiovascular disease modeling and drug development, emphasizing its importance in precision medicine. By using iPSC-derived cardiomyocytes from different donors, researchers can characterize inter-individual variability in drug responses. Evaluation of a combinatorial in vitro, in silico screening approach for cardiotoxicity profiling of environmental hazards using a library of chemicals (Byalahunasishetter et al., 2025).

The care for female patients with CHD is a lifelong continuum that encompasses cumulative health exposures and experiences, highlighting the need for ongoing care optimization and research into the impacts of pregnancy and other health-related factors on their quality of life and survival (Lindley, 2025). Systems such as the ImageXpress Micro and FLIPR Tetra are used to automate the measurement of cardiomyocyte responses to pharmacological compounds. Improving the understanding of how genetic variants influence specific clinical outcomes and complications remains an ongoing challenge. Many drugs can induce cardiotoxicity, which complicates the drug development process and increases the risk of late-stage failures. High-content live cell imaging technology provides an advanced platform for the real-time observation of cardiomyocyte behavior and function. Live cell imaging is an innovative technique that enables researchers to monitor critical physiological parameters, such as contractility and calcium flux, which are essential for muscle contraction and relaxation. By capturing dynamic (Biradar et al., 2025).

## Gene-environment interactions

Neurodevelopmental impairments are the most common comorbidity in individuals with congenital heart disease. Various risk factors for neurodevelopmental impairments have been identified, including prenatal factors, genetic abnormalities, cardiovascular physiology, environmental influences, social determinants of health, and mental health issues (Wolfe & Peyvandi, 2025). Several environmental factors, combined with genetic predispositions, contribute to CHD development and progression, warranting further research.

The spectrum of congenital heart disease varies widely, ranging from simple septal defects to complex conditions like heterotaxy with multiple heart malformations. Despite advancements in surgical repair since the introduction of the B-T-T shunt, individuals with congenital heart disease still experience a higher rate of sudden cardiac arrest compared to the general population. Recent developments in pacing and cardioversion have been made to manage bradyarrhythmias and tachyarrhythmias adverse effects and limitations (Han, 2025). The unique challenges of monitoring cardiovascular health in autistic patients include atypical sensory profiles, altered autonomic regulation, and communication difficulties. The computational strategies for continuous monitoring and predictive care (Ananthakumar, Nagaraja, et al., 2025). Most studies are based on limited populations, highlighting the need for more diverse datasets to improve diagnostic and predictive accuracy across different ethnic groups.

The emerging field of paternal exposomics reveals significant contributions of paternal environmental exposures to CHD risk in offspring. The impact of prenatal exposure to PM2.5 air pollution led to adverse birth outcomes. An increase in PM2.5 exposure during pregnancy was associated with a higher risk of preterm birth, with an odds ratio of 1.17 for an interquartile range increase in exposure (Trasande et al., 2024) (Byun et al., 2025). The components of PM2.5, such as elemental carbon and secondary inorganic aerosols, were found to have complex mechanisms involving genetic mutations, epigenetic inheritance, sperm DNA damage, and gene-environment interactions (Nowak et al., 2024).

The clinical implications necessitate expanded preconceptional care that addresses paternal health optimization. Pollutants PM2.5 constituents, particularly organic matter and black carbon, significantly increase CHD risk, calling for occupational safety improvements and personalized risk assessment (Li et al., 2025). susceptibility. Unlike the traditional focus on maternal factors, evidence demonstrates that paternal occupational chemical exposures, lifestyle factors, and age-related changes substantially influence cardiac development outcomes (Breton et al., 2021). The transgenerational nature of some paternal effects emphasizes the importance of population-level prevention strategies that consider multigenerational health impacts.

Future research priorities on chemicals, toxicological pathways, and longitudinal studies to document transgenerational effects. In the future, intervention trials can demonstrate the efficacy of prevention. The integration of advanced exposure assessment methods with multi-omics approaches offers promising avenues for precision medicine applications in CHD prevention (Bhuvana et al., 2025).

## Broad Gene Testing and Advanced Sequencing Techniques

Non-coding RNAs (ncRNAs) play a crucial role in regulating gene expression, influencing both embryonic development and the pathogenesis of diseases, particularly congenital heart disease (CHD) and placental development. The fetal heart-placenta axis is a critical bidirectional signaling network that is modulated by non-coding RNAs (ncRNAs). Non coding RNA through epigenetic and post-transcriptional mechanisms regulate cardiogenesis and placental morphogenesis. Dysregulation of ncRNAs can disrupt key developmental processes such as cardiac cell differentiation, angiogenesis, and trophoblast invasion, contributing to the pathogenesis of CHD and highlighting their potential as biomarkers (H. Wang et al., 2026). The implementation of comprehensive genetic panels and the integration of long-read genome sequencing (lrGS) can enhance the detection of complex variants, structural variants, and repetitive sequences. Combining genomic data, environmental factors, improve diagnosis, treatment strategies. Significant associations were found between congenital anomalies and factors such as maternal age, high-altitude exposure, preeclampsia, and consanguinity, with high altitude specifically linked to increased risks for patent ductus arteriosus and anorectal anomalies (Linares et al., 2025).

The findings emphasize the importance of considering environmental factors in clinical management and surveillance of high-risk populations. Preventive strategies for congenital anomalies in newborns with Down syndrome, and hypotheses around environmental chemicals linked to adverse cardiovascular outcomes. The Tox21 or

ToxCast high-throughput screening (HTS) data, as well as bulk and single-cell transcriptomic and epigenomic datasets, can aid in identifying disease variants (Zachariah et al., 2024). The offspring iPSCs can be subjected to combinatorial endpoints, such as contractility, electrophysiological properties, and cellular signaling pathways.

*Table 6. Summary of Genes linked to phthalates from biological and embryological studies*

| Gene | Gene Symbol | Role in Embryology | Effect of Phthalate Exposure |
|---|---|---|---|
| Aryl Hydrocarbon Receptor | AHR | Regulates the body's response to environmental toxins and regulates gene expression in development. | Phthalates, especially DEHP, can activate AHR, influencing early development. |
| Peroxisome Proliferator-Activated Receptor Gamma | PPARG | Involved in adipocyte differentiation and regulation of metabolic processes. | Phthalate esters, DEHP can activate PPARG, influencing adipogenesis and metabolic processes. |
| Estrogen Receptor Alpha | ESR1 | Essential for normal reproductive development and function. | Act as endocrine disruptors, mimicking estrogen and binding to ESR1. |
| Retinoic Acid Receptor Alpha | RARA | Involved in regulating embryonic development, particularly in the nervous system and limb patterning. | Phthalates can alter the expression of RARA, affecting embryonic development, especially in the central nervous system. |
| Cytochrome P450 1A1 | CYP1A1 | Involved in the metabolism of xenobiotics, including phthalates and other environmental toxins. | Phthalates can induce the expression of CYP1A1, leading to altered metabolic detoxification pathways. |
| Androgen Receptor | AR | Mediates the effects of androgens in sexual differentiation and development. | DBP and DEHP are anti-androgenic, reducing AR signaling. |
| Superoxide Dismutase 1 | SOD1 | Protects cells from oxidative stress and is involved in cellular defense mechanisms. | Phthalates can induce oxidative stress, SOD1 expression |
| Transforming Growth Factor Beta Receptor | TGFBR | Plays a crucial role in cell growth, differentiation, and embryogenesis. | Phthalates can affect TGFBR signaling, disrupting normal cell differentiation and growth during development. |
| Folate Receptor Alpha | FOLR1 | Essential for folate transport in embryonic development, particularly in neural development. | Phthalates may interfere with folate metabolism, affecting FOLR1 and its role in neurodevelopment. |
| Glutathione S-Transferase Pi 1 | GSTP1 | Detoxifies reactive metabolites and plays a role in cellular defense against toxins. | Phthalates can reduce GSTP1 activity, leading to impaired detoxification. |
| Nuclear Receptor Subfamily 4 Group A Member 1 | NR4A1 | Involved in regulating cell growth, differentiation, and apoptosis. | Phthalates may interfere with NR4A1 activity, altering cell differentiation and apoptosis. |
| Homeobox A1 | HOXA1 | Plays a role in regulating early embryonic development and patterning, particularly in the central nervous system and craniofacial development. | Phthalates can disrupt HOXA1 expression, affecting embryonic patterning. |
| Wnt Family Member 3A | WNT3A | Key regulator of cell fate determination, embryonic development, and stem cell maintenance. | Phthalates may influence WNT3A expression, disrupting cell signaling pathways involved in embryogenesis. |
| Vascular Endothelial Growth Factor | VEGF | Regulates blood vessel formation during development (angiogenesis). | Phthalates can affect VEGF expression, potentially disrupting angiogenesis. |
| Sonic Hedgehog | SHH | Critical in establishing body patterning, especially in limb and brain development. | Phthalates can alter SHH expression, impacting developmental signaling pathways. |
| Fibroblast Growth Factor 2 | FGF2 | Plays a role in embryonic development, including neurogenesis and organogenesis. | Phthalates can influence FGF2 signaling, affecting cell growth and differentiation. |

## Epigenetic Marker Evaluation (Epi-signatures)

Phthalates affect developmental pathways and contribute to cardiovascular effects. The hypothesis gains its strength due to endocrine disruption, oxidative stress, genetic and epigenetic modifications, which alter cardiogenesis (Xu et al., 2025). Notably, phthalate-induced changes in transcription factor expression and methylation suggest potential etiological mechanisms of CHD.

Utilizing DNA methylation signatures (DNAm epi-signatures) offers a valuable approach for diagnostic screening and reclassification of ambiguous genetic findings, such as syndromes associated with CHD (Williams–Beuren and Velocardiofacial syndromes). Further developing experimental approaches, validating new candidate genes identified through genomic studies, and ensuring their causative role in CHD (Choudhury et al., 2025). Some drugs with known cardiotoxic effects, including estrogenic modulators (clomiphene, raloxifene), anti-arrhythmic drugs (amiodarone, haloperidol), and antipsychotic drugs (chlorpromazine), need further investigation. The computational models and iPSCs are used to assess these risks, drug development. The ECHSA-CCDB is the second-largest congenital cardiac database in the world, documenting over 25 years, from 1999 to August 2024. The overall 30-day mortality (30d-M) and hospital mortality (HM) rates were reported as 3.65% and 4.09%, respectively, with significant variations based on age groups. Mortality rates for neonates were notably higher at 8.71% (30d-M) and 10.28% (HM), while rates for infants, children, and adults were lower, indicating a trend of reduced mortality with increasing age. A documented decrease in mortality rates over time across all age groups and quality improvement in congenital heart surgery. The public health approach is critical in understanding of intergenerational health impacts to prevent the risks associated with CHD (Protopapas et al., 2025).

## CHD variants of unknown significance (VUS)

Periconceptional paternal phthalate exposure is a risk factor for CHDs, highlighting the need for biomarkers for therapeutic applications (Hayama-Terada et al., 2023). Given the widespread use of phthalates in various products, including medications, the findings from this work have significant public health implications. Understanding the risks associated with paternal exposure supports the hypothesis based on evidence from molecular biology, male reproductive physiology, environmental medicine, and toxicology (Patel et al., 2025).

The heterogeneity of CHD and broad gene testing panels leads to frequent detection of VUS, complicating genetic diagnosis and counseling. Emerging technologies for measuring cardiomyocyte physiology, including high-content imaging, calcium-sensitive dyes, and automated imaging systems (Biradar et al., 2025). Innovative technologies enable the study of cardiac responses to drugs and environmental chemicals. The long-term goal of this research is to manipulate molecular pathways regulated by NOTCH1, GATA5, and NOS3 to develop pharmacological therapies. Ongoing research investigates epigenetic markers, including DNA methylation, the effects of hyperglycemia on chromatin accessibility, the Nos3 locus, nitric oxide, and the Notch1 regulator Jarid2, to assess the impact of chromatin regulatory gene alterations. Congenital heart defects, their clinical utility, and integration with genomic data are still in development (Yasuhara et al., 2025). There is an urgent need to integrate human-relevant platforms and approaches into drug development to better predict cardiovascular safety. Advanced exposure assessment methods, including wearable sensors, biomarker panels, and environmental monitoring technologies, could enhance exposure characterization, facilitate more precise risk assessment, and mitigate liabilities associated with new therapeutic agents (GVS et al., 2025). Overall, future research must aim to address current limitations in genetic diagnostics of CHD by improving variant detection and validation. Public health policies can facilitate more precise and personalized preventive measures.

## CONCLUSION

In conclusion, this study clearly demonstrates that male germ cells are highly susceptible to environmental toxicants such as phthalates, leading to mutations and jeopardizing genome integrity. Furthermore, despite the constant turnover of spermatogonia, the differentially expressed genes (DEGs) are directly associated with cardiomyopathy and congenital heart disease (CHD). Given the widespread use of phthalates in various products, including medications, the findings from this work have significant public health implications. The risks associated with paternal exposure can inform guidelines and interventions aimed at reducing exposure and protecting reproductive health.

## DECLARATION OF COMPETING INTEREST

The authors declare that they have no known competing financial interests or personal relationships that could have appeared to influence the work reported in this paper.

## REFERENCES


Ananthakumar, B., Nagaraja, B. G., Umesh, S. M., & Raghavan, R. (2025). Predictive Medicine. *Predictive Algorithms for Rehabilitation and Assistive Systems*, 291–314. https://doi.org/DOI: 10.4018/979-8-3373-0194-5.ch011

Ananthakumar, B., Nanjundeshwara, N., Lakshmaiah, A., & Raghavan, R. (2024). Synthetic Gene Circuits as a Promising Approach in Cancer Immunotherapy. *Critical Developments in Cancer Immunotherapy*, 391–418. https://doi.org/DOI: 10.4018/979-8-3693-3976-3.ch011

Ananthakumar, B., Nanjundeshwara, N., Lakshmaiah, A., & Raghavan, R. (2025). Nanocarriers for Delivering Nucleic Acids in Plants. *Nanocarriers in Plant Science and Agriculture*, 207–234. https://doi.org/DOI: 10.4018/979-8-3693-9869-2.ch008

Baker, B. H., Zhang, S., Simon, J. M., McLarnan, S. M., Chung, W. K., & Pearson, B. L. (2023). Environmental carcinogens disproportionally mutate genes implicated in neurodevelopmental disorders. *Frontiers in Neuroscience*, *17*. Advance online publication. DOI: 10.3389/fnins.2023.1106573 PMID: 37599994

Bhat, P., Dhyani, V. S., Lakshmi, V., Uppangala, S., Adiga, S. K., Adiga, P., Kumar, P., & Gupta, A. (2025). Congenital anomalies observed in children conceived through assisted reproductive technology—A systematic review and meta-analysis. *Journal of Assisted Reproduction and Genetics*, *42*(5), 1547–1565. DOI: 10.1007/s10815-025-03454-0 PMID: 40163274

Bhuvana, G. N., Umesh, S. M., & Raghavan, R. (2025). Expanding the frontiers of Schistosomiasis Treatment: The promise of Nanoparticle-Based Therapies. *Journal of Vector Borne Diseases, 10*(4103/jvbd.jvbd_180_23). https://doi.org/DOI: 10.4103/jvbd.jvbd_180_23

Biradar, S., Suresh, C., Nanjundeshwara, N., & Raghavan, R. (2025). Spatially Variable Genes. *Spatially Variable Genes in Cancer*, 1–28. https://doi.org/DOI: 10.4018/979-8-3693-7728-4.ch001

Breton, C. V., Landon, R., Kahn, L. G., Enlow, M. B., Peterson, A. K., Bastain, T., Braun, J., Comstock, S. S., Duarte, C. S., Hipwell, A., Ji, H., LaSalle, J. M., Miller, R. L., Musci, R., Posner, J., Schmidt, R., Suglia, S. F., Tung, I., Weisenberger, D., & Fry, R. (2021). Exploring the evidence for epigenetic regulation of environmental influences on child health across generations. *Communications Biology*, *4*(1), 1–15. DOI: 10.1038/s42003-021-02316-6 PMID: 34158610

Byalahunasishetter, B. I., N., V., P., S., C., M., S., S., & Raghavan, R. (2025). Spatial Omics and Bioprinting. *Innovations in Precision Medicine and Genomics*, 85–110. https://doi.org/DOI: 10.4018/979-8-3693-5787-3.ch003

Byun, G., Choi, Y., Lee, J.-T., & Bell, M. L. (2025). Effects of Prenatal Exposure to PM2.5 Chemical Components on Adverse Birth Outcomes and Under-5 Mortality in South Korea. *Epidemiology (Cambridge, Mass.)*, *36*(4), 531. DOI: 10.1097/EDE.0000000000001868 PMID: 40257114

Casciaro, C., Hamada, H., Bloise, E., & Matthews, S. G. (2024). The paternal contribution to shaping the health of future generations. *Trends in Endocrinology and Metabolism*, *0*(0). Advance online publication. DOI: 10.1016/j.tem.2024.10.007 PMID: 39562264

Choudhury, T. Z., Gilbert, B. L., & Garg, V. (2025). Genetic and Environmental Contributors To Congenital Heart Disease. *Current Treatment Options in Cardiovascular Medicine*, *27*(1), 36. DOI: 10.1007/s11936-025-01091-5 PMID: 40438121

Dehghanbanadaki, H., Jimbo, M., Fendereski, K., Kunisaki, J., Horns, J. J., Ramsay, J. M., & Hotaling, J. M. (2025). Transgenerational effects of paternal exposures: The role of germline de novo mutations. *Andrology*, *13*(1), 101–118.

Estill, M., Hauser, R., Nassan, F. L., Moss, A., & Krawetz, S. A. (2019). The effects of di-butyl phthalate exposure from medications on human sperm RNA among men. *Scientific Reports*, *9*(1), 12397. DOI: 10.1038/s41598-019-48441-5 PMID: 31455814

Fazekas-Pongor, V., Csáky-Szunyogh, M., Fekete, M., Mészáros, Á., Cseh, K., & Pénzes, M. (2020). Congenital heart diseases and parental occupational exposure in a Hungarian case-control study in 1997 to 2002. *Congenital Anomalies*, *61*(2), 55–62. DOI: 10.1111/cga.12401 PMID: 33140474

Fazekas-Pongor, V., Fekete, M., Csáky-Szunyogh, M., Cseh, K., & Pénzes, M. (2021). Parental occupational exposure and congenital heart diseases in a Hungarian case–control study. *International Archives of Occupational and Environmental Health*, *94*(3), 515–527. DOI: 10.1007/s00420-020-01589-4 PMID: 33170344

Giannubilo, S. R., Marzioni, D., Tossetta, G., Montironi, R., Meccariello, M. L., & Ciavattini, A. (2024). The "Bad Father": Paternal Role in Biology of Pregnancy and in Birth Outcome. *Biology (Basel), 13*(3), 165. DOI: 10.3390/biology13030165 PMID: 38534435

*GSE129216*. (2019). https://www.ncbi.nlm.nih.gov/geo/query/acc.cgi?acc=GSE129216

GVS, A. C., Ananthakumar, B., & Raghavan, R. (2025). Enhancing Assistive Technologies With Neuromorphic Computing. *Revolutionizing AI with Brain-Inspired Technology: Neuromorphic Computing*, 207–232. https://doi.org/DOI: 10.4018/979-8-3693-6303-4.ch009

Han, F. (2025). Sudden cardiac death in congenital heart disease—A narrative review and update. *Frontiers in Cardiovascular Medicine, 12*. Advance online publication. DOI: 10.3389/fcvm.2025.1539958 PMID: 40371062

Hayama-Terada, M., Aochi, Y., Ikehara, S., Kimura, T., Yamagishi, K., Sato, T., & Iso, H. (2023). Paternal occupational exposures and infant congenital heart defects in the Japan Environment and Children's Study. *Environmental Health and Preventive Medicine, 28*, 12–12. DOI: 10.1265/ehpm.22-00202 PMID: 36740268

Juarez, P. D., Hood, D. B., Song, M.-A., & Ramesh, A. (2020). Use of an Exposome Approach to Understand the Effects of Exposures From the Natural, Built, and Social Environments on Cardio-Vascular Disease Onset, Progression, and Outcomes. *Frontiers in Public Health, 8*, 379. DOI: 10.3389/fpubh.2020.00379 PMID: 32903514

Kaltsas, A., Markou, E., Kyrgiafini, M.-A., Zikopoulos, A., Symeonidis, E. N., Dimitriadis, F., Zachariou, A., Sofikitis, N., & Chrisofos, M. (2025). Oxidative-Stress-Mediated Epigenetic Dysregulation in Spermatogenesis: Implications for Male Infertility and Offspring Health. *Genes, 16*(1), 1. Advance online publication. DOI: 10.3390/genes16010093 PMID: 39858640

Lakshmaiah, A., Korrapati, C., Suresh, C., & Raghavan, R. (2025). Synthetic Biology and AI. *Spatially Variable Genes in Cancer*, 265–290. https://doi.org/DOI: 10.4018/979-8-3693-7728-4.ch010

Leirgul, E., Fomina, T., Greve, G., Tell, G. S., Sandberg, M., & Øyen, N. (2025). Trends in Birth Prevalence of Congenital Heart Defects in Norway—A Population Study 1994–2014. *Acta Paediatrica, n/a*(n/a). https://doi.org/DOI: 10.1111/apa.70235

Li, D., Li, T., Wang, Y., Pan, F., Chen, J., Ruan, J., & Xu, W. (2025). Greenness exposure mitigate PM2.5-associated congenital heart defects in China: A mediation analysis of chemical composition and seasonal-spatial vulnerability. *International Journal of Hygiene and Environmental Health*, *269*, 114624. DOI: 10.1016/j.ijheh.2025.114624 PMID: 40684539

Linares, D., Luna, B., Loayza, E., del Callejo, A., Garcia-Sejas, M., Erostegui, C., & Taboada, G. (2025). High altitude exposure and the birth prevalence of congenital anomalies in newborns with Down syndrome. *Early Human Development*, *205*, 106270. DOI: 10.1016/j.earlhumdev.2025.106270 PMID: 40280041

Lindley, K. J. (2025). Introduction to the Compendium on Lifelong Care in Women: Applying a Sex- and Gender-Lens to Practice. *Circulation Research*, *136*(6), 551–552. DOI: 10.1161/CIRCRESAHA.125.326335 PMID: 40080537

Lismer, A., Siklenka, K., Lafleur, C., Dumeaux, V., & Kimmins, S. (2020). Sperm histone H3 lysine 4 trimethylation is altered in a genetic mouse model of transgenerational epigenetic inheritance. *Nucleic Acids Research*, *48*(20), 11380–11393. DOI: 10.1093/nar/gkaa712 PMID: 33068438

Mariana, M., & Cairrao, E. (2020). Phthalates Implications in the Cardiovascular System. *Journal of Cardiovascular Development and Disease*, *7*(3), 26. DOI: 10.3390/jcdd7030026 PMID: 32707888

Mo, J., Liu, X., Huang, Y., He, R., Zhang, Y., & Huang, H. (2022). Developmental origins of adult diseases. *Medical Review (Berlin, Germany)*, *2*(5), 450–470. DOI: 10.1515/mr-2022-0027 PMID: 37724166

Nagashri, N., Archana, L., & Raghavan, R. (2024). Microbial Volatile Compounds (MVOCs) in Food Industries and Food Safety Applications. *Innovations, Securities, and Case Studies Across Healthcare, Business, and Technology*, 75–96. https://doi.org/DOI: 10.4018/979-8-3693-1906-2.ch005

Nicoll, R. (2018). Environmental Contaminants and Congenital Heart Defects: A Re-Evaluation of the Evidence. *International Journal of Environmental Research and Public Health*, *15*(10), 2096. DOI: 10.3390/ijerph15102096 PMID: 30257432

Nowak, K., Oluwayiose, O. A., Houle, E., Maxwell, D. L., Sawant, S., Paskavitz, A., Ford, J. B., Minguez-Alarcon, L., Calafat, A. M., Hauser, R., & Pilsner, J. R. (2024). Urinary concentrations of phthalate and phthalate alternative metabolites and sperm DNA methylation: A multi-cohort and *meta*-analysis of men in preconception studies. *Environment International*, *192*, 109049. DOI: 10.1016/j.envint.2024.109049 PMID: 39393261

Oluwayiose, O. A., Marcho, C., Wu, H., Houle, E., Krawetz, S. A., Suvorov, A., Mager, J., & Richard Pilsner, J. (2021). Paternal preconception phthalate exposure alters sperm methylome and embryonic programming. *Environment International*, *155*, 106693. DOI: 10.1016/j.envint.2021.106693 PMID: 34120004

P., A., D., K. M., M., J., P., S., & Raghavan, R. (2025). The Cancer Exposome. *Cancer Exposomics and Environmental Influences on Carcinogenesis*, 161–192. https://doi.org/DOI: 10.4018/979-8-3373-2165-3.ch004

Patel, A., Sharma, R., & Kumar, S. (2025). Risk factor profiling in congenital heart disease: Maternal and environmental determinants. *Medical Science Journal*, *15*(5), 234–241.

Peng, W., Yi, X., Peng, Y., Lu, H., & Liu, H. (2024). Developmental toxicity and mechanism of dibutyl phthalate on the development of subintestinal vessels in zebrafish. *Scientific Reports*, *14*(1), 28464. DOI: 10.1038/s41598-024-80088-9 PMID: 39558027

Protopapas, E., Padalino, M., Tobota, Z., Ebels, T., Speggiorin, S., Horer, J., Kansy, A., Jacobs, J. P., Fragata, J., Maruszewski, B., Vida, V., & Sarris, G. (2025). The European Congenital Heart Surgeons Association congenital cardiac database: A 25-year summary of congenital heart surgery outcomes†. *European Journal of Cardio-Thoracic Surgery*, *67*(4), ezaf119. Advance online publication. DOI: 10.1093/ejcts/ezaf119 PMID: 40193525

Qian, Y., Shao, H., Ying, X., Huang, W., & Hua, Y. (2020). The Endocrine Disruption of Prenatal Phthalate Exposure in Mother and Offspring. *Frontiers in Public Health*, *8*. Advance online publication. DOI: 10.3389/fpubh.2020.00366 PMID: 32984231

Raghavan, R., & Ahamad, S. (2025). Developmental Origins of Health and Disease. *Cancer Exposomics and Environmental Influences on Carcinogenesis*, 1–34. https://doi.org/DOI: 10.4018/979-8-3373-2165-3.ch001

Snijder, C. A., Vlot, I. J., Burdorf, A., Obermann-Borst, S. A., Helbing, W. A., Wildhagen, M. F., Steegers, E. A. P., & Steegers-Theunissen, R. P. M. (2012). Congenital heart defects and parental occupational exposure to chemicals. *Human Reproduction (Oxford, England)*, *27*(5), 1510–1517. DOI: 10.1093/humrep/des043 PMID: 22357765

Sun, G., & Li, Y. (2019). Exposure to DBP induces the toxicity in early development and adverse effects on cardiac development in zebrafish (*Danio rerio*). *Chemosphere*, *218*, 76–82. DOI: 10.1016/j.chemosphere.2018.11.095 PMID: 30469006

Trasande, L., Nelson, M. E., Alshawabkeh, A., Barrett, E. S., Buckley, J. P., Dabelea, D., Dunlop, A. L., Herbstman, J. B., Meeker, J. D., Naidu, M., Newschaffer, C., Padula, A. M., Romano, M. E., Ruden, D. M., Sathyanarayana, S., Schantz, S. L., Starling, A. P., Hamra, G. B., Smith, P. B., & Karr, C. (2024). Prenatal phthalate exposure and adverse birth outcomes in the USA: A prospective analysis of births and estimates of attributable burden and costs. *The Lancet. Planetary Health, 8*(2), e74–e85. DOI: 10.1016/S2542-5196(23)00270-X PMID: 38331533

Vey, C., Melnik, N., Dombrowsky, G., & Hitz, M.-P. (2025). Current and future diagnostics of congenital heart disease (CHD). *Medizinische Genetik : Mitteilungsblatt des Berufsverbandes Medizinische Genetik e.V, 37*(2), 95–102. DOI: 10.1515/medgen-2025-2008 PMID: 40207043

Voros, C., Papadimas, G., Theodora, M., Mavrogianni, D., Athanasiou, D., Sapantzoglou, I., Bananis, K., Athanasiou, A., Athanasiou, A., Tsimpoukelis, C., Papapanagiotou, I., Vaitsis, D., Koulakmanidis, A.-M., Daskalaki, M. A., Topalis, V., Thomakos, N., Antsaklis, P., Chatzinikolaou, F., Loutradis, D., & Daskalakis, G. (2025). From Petri Dish to Primitive Heart: How IVF Alters Early Cardiac Gene Networks and Epigenetic Landscapes. *Biomedicines, 13*(8), 2044. DOI: 10.3390/biomedicines13082044 PMID: 40868294

Wang, H., Chen, X., Li, Y., Xiao, S., Teng, T., Yang, S., Wang, K., & Zhang, M. (2026). Non-coding RNAs in congenital heart disease and placental development: Bridging molecular mechanisms to clinical biomarkers and therapies. *Non-Coding RNA Research, 16*, 1–20. DOI: 10.1016/j.ncrna.2025.08.006 PMID: 41080762

Wang, J., Zhang, X., Li, Y., Liu, Y., & Tao, L. (2021). Exposure to Dibutyl Phthalate and Reproductive-Related Outcomes in Animal Models: Evidence From Rodents Study. *Frontiers in Physiology, 12*. Advance online publication. DOI: 10.3389/fphys.2021.684532 PMID: 34955869

Wijnands, K. P. J., Zeilmaker, G. A., Meijer, W. M., Helbing, W. A., & Steegers-Theunissen, R. P. M. (2014). Periconceptional parental conditions and perimembranous ventricular septal defects in the offspring. *Birth Defects Research. Part A, Clinical and Molecular Teratology, 100*(12), 944–950. DOI: 10.1002/bdra.23265 PMID: 25196200

Wolfe, K., & Peyvandi, S. (2025). Neurodevelopmental outcomes in congenital heart disease: Modifiable and nonmodifiable substrates. *Current Opinion in Cardiology, 40*(4), 259. DOI: 10.1097/HCO.0000000000001218 PMID: 40401446

Xie, F., Chen, X., Weng, S., Xia, T., Sun, X., Luo, T., & Li, P. (2019). Effects of two environmental endocrine disruptors di-*n*-butyl phthalate (DBP) and mono-*n*-butyl phthalate (MBP) on human sperm functions in vitro. *Reproductive Toxicology (Elmsford, N.Y.)*, *83*, 1–7. DOI: 10.1016/j.reprotox.2018.10.011 PMID: 30391722

Xu, J., Li, Q., Deng, L., Xiong, J., Cheng, Z., & Ye, C. (2025). Global, regional, and national epidemiology of congenital heart disease in children from 1990 to 2021. *Frontiers in Cardiovascular Medicine*, *12*. Advance online publication. DOI: 10.3389/fcvm.2025.1522644 PMID: 40454242

Yasuhara, J., Bigelow, A. M., & Garg, V. (2025). Genetics of Congenital Heart Disease. *Clinics in Perinatology*, *52*(3), 589–608. DOI: 10.1016/j.clp.2025.06.010 PMID: 40850718

Zachariah, J. P., Jone, P. N., Agbaje, A. O., Ryan, H. H., Trasande, L., Perng, W., & Farzan, S. F. (2024). Environmental exposures and pediatric cardiology: A scientific statement from the American heart association. *Circulation*, *149*(20), e1165–e1175.

Zhang, M., Sun, Y., Zhao, X., Liu, R., Yang, B.-Y., Chen, G., Zhang, W., Dong, G.-H., Yin, C., & Yue, W. (2022). How Parental Predictors Jointly Affect the Risk of Offspring Congenital Heart Disease: A Nationwide Multicenter Study Based on the China Birth Cohort. *Frontiers in Cardiovascular Medicine*, *9*. Advance online publication. DOI: 10.3389/fcvm.2022.860600 PMID: 35722125

# Chapter 5
# Integrating Exposomics with Genomics and Epigenomics:
## A Holistic Approach to Unraveling the Etiology of Congenital Heart Disease

**Tarun Kumar Patel**
https://orcid.org/0009-0003-3002-8100
*Department of Biotechnology, Sant Guru Ghasidas Government P.G. College, Kurud, India*

## ABSTRACT

*This chapter explores the etiology of congenital heart disease (CHD), affecting newborns globally, through integrated genomics, epigenomics, and exposomics to advance diagnostics and prevention. It examines how multi-omics approaches uncover molecular mechanisms driving CHD and inform personalized interventions. Genomics identifies variants in NOTCH1 and VEGFA, linked to defects like tetralogy of Fallot, addressing variability. Epigenomics reveals DNA methylation, histone modifications, and non-coding RNAs mediating gene-environment interactions, with studies linking maternal exposures to altered cardiac gene expression. Exposomics quantifies environmental influences using metabolomics, sensors, and biomarkers to assess pollutants and lifestyle factors. Multi-omics integration, using ML and network analysis, enhances biomarker discovery and risk prediction. Challenges include data harmonization, privacy, and equitable technology access. Future directions emphasize collaboration, funding, and causal inference for preventive strategies to reduce CHD burden via precision medicine.*

DOI: 10.4018/979-8-3373-3735-7.ch005

## INTRODUCTION

Congenital heart disease (CHD) represents a spectrum of structural cardiac anomalies present at birth, affecting approximately 1% of newborns globally (van der Linde et al., 2011). As a multifactorial condition, CHD arises from intricate interplay among genetic, epigenetic, and environmental factors. The advent of multi-omics approaches integrating genomics, epigenomics, and exposomics offers a transformative framework to unravel CHD's complex etiology, paving the way for improved diagnostics and preventive strategies.

Genomics focuses on the study of an organism's complete set of DNA, identifying genetic variants associated with CHD. Key genes, such as NOTCH1 and VEGF, have been implicated in cardiac morphogenesis, with mutations contributing to conditions like tetralogy of Fallot and hypoplastic left heart syndrome (Page et al., 2019). However, genomics alone explains only a fraction of CHD cases, as de novo mutations and polygenic risk scores highlight the variability in phenotypic expression (Zaidi & Brueckner, 2017). While genomics identifies predispositions, epigenomics bridges these to environmental factors, as explored next. Epigenomics examines heritable changes in gene expression without altering DNA sequence, acting as a bridge between genetic predisposition and environmental influences. Epigenetic mechanisms, including DNA methylation and histone modifications, regulate cardiac development and are sensitive to environmental exposures like maternal smoking or folate deficiency (Linglart & Bonnet, 2022). Epigenome-wide association studies (EWAS) have begun to uncover CHD-associated epigenetic signatures, offering insights into how environmental factors modulate gene expression during critical developmental windows. Exposomics, the systematic study of the exposome, captures the totality of environmental exposures across an individual's lifespan. This includes chemical (e.g., pollutants, teratogens), physical (e.g., radiation), and lifestyle factors (e.g., diet, stress) that may influence CHD risk (Motairek et al., 2023). Advanced methods like metabolomics and wearable sensors enable comprehensive exposome profiling, revealing how maternal factors, such as diabetes or air pollution exposure, contribute to CHD pathogenesis (Helbig et al., 2021).

The integration of these omics disciplines aims to construct a holistic model of CHD etiology (Figure 1). By combining genomic predisposition, epigenetic regulation, and environmental exposures, researchers can better understand the molecular mechanisms driving CHD and identify novel biomarkers for risk prediction. This multi-omics approach also holds promise for personalized medicine, enabling tailored interventions to mitigate CHD risk based on individual genetic and environmental profiles. The objectives of this integration are threefold: to elucidate the causal pathways of CHD, to enhance risk stratification for early intervention, and to inform preventive strategies that address both genetic and environmental determinants. This chapter explores the synergy of genomics, epigenomics, and exposomics in CHD research, highlighting methodologies, challenges, and future directions for translating multi-omics insights into clinical practice. Gene-environment interactions in CHD are exemplified by how genetic variants in folate metabolism genes (e.g., MTHFR) interact with maternal folate deficiency, altering DNA methylation and increasing risk of defects like tetralogy of Fallot. The chapter targets students, researchers, and clinicians by highlighting personalized medicine, e.g., exposome-informed prevention to reduce CHD incidence.

## THE GENOMIC LANDSCAPE OF CHD

### Key Genetic Variants and Pathways in CHD

The genomic landscape of CHD is shaped by a complex interplay of genetic variants and signaling pathways critical for cardiac development. Key genes, such as *NOTCH1* and *VEGF*, are pivotal in CHD pathogenesis due to their roles in cardiogenesis. *NOTCH1*, a transmembrane receptor, regulates cell fate decisions during cardiac development. Mutations in *NOTCH1* disrupt valve formation and ventricular septation, contributing to conditions like bicuspid aortic valve and tetralogy of Fallot (Xiang et al., 2025). Whole-exome sequencing studies have identified rare *NOTCH1* variants in sporadic CHD cases, emphasizing its significance (Page et al., 2019). Key genetic variants and their associated CHD phenotypes with functional impact is briefly summarized in Table 1.

*Figure 1. Graphical Abstract: Integrating Genomics, Epigenomics, and Exposomics for Understanding CHD Etiology. [A multitude of environmental factors (Exposome) interact with an individual's genetic blueprint (Genomics), dynamically altering its function (Epigenomics) within the holistic human system, leading to and being influenced by the development of Coronary Heart Disease]*

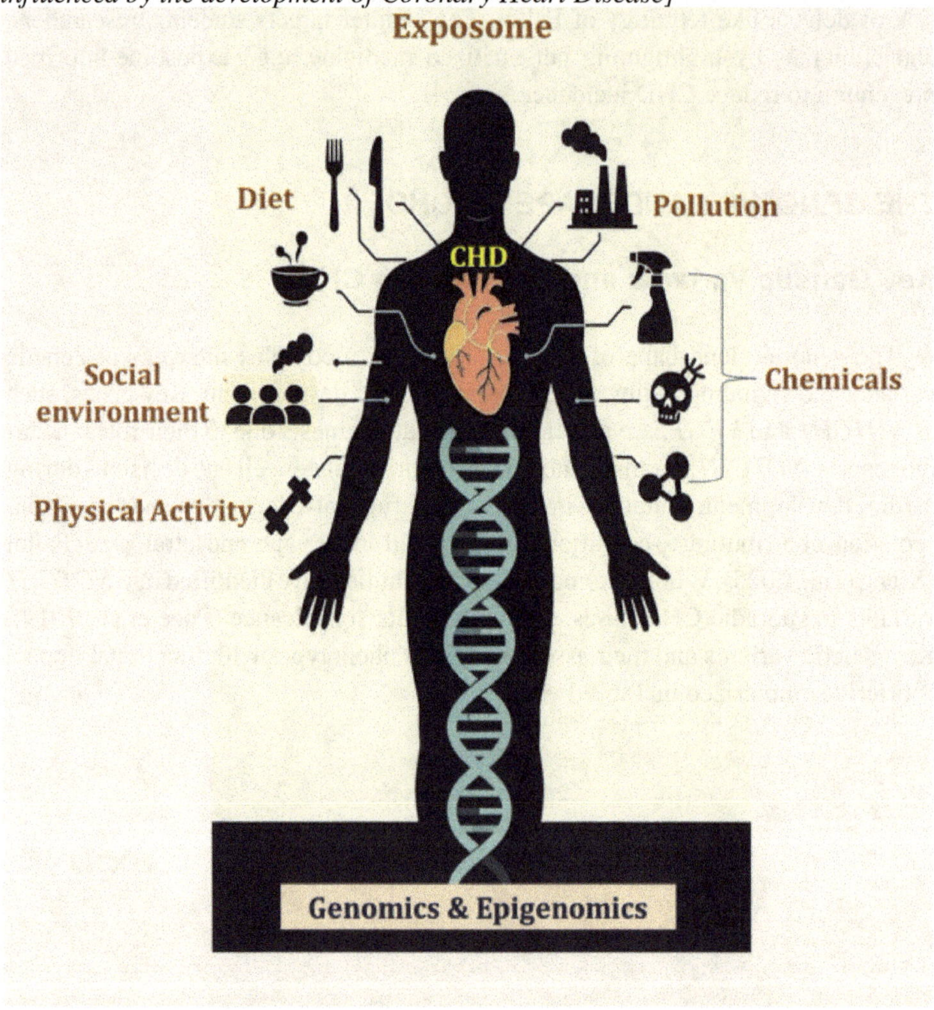


*VEGF* (vascular endothelial growth factor) is essential for angiogenesis and cardiac morphogenesis. Variants in *VEGFA* and its receptors impair vascular development, leading to defects such as pulmonary atresia and septal defects. Polymorphisms in *VEGFA* increase CHD risk by altering gene expression (Hăşmăşanu et al., 2023). Beyond these, pathways like Wnt/β-catenin and TGF-β are implicated in CHD. Wnt signaling governs cardiac progenitor cell differentiation, and its dysregulation is linked to conotruncal defects (Azhdari et al., 2025). Similarly, TGF-β pathway variants disrupt extracellular matrix formation, contributing to aortic anomalies (Tingting et al., 2020).

*Table 1. Key Genetic Variants and Their Associated CHD Phenotypes with Functional Impact*

| Gene | Variant Type | CHD Phenotype | Functional Impact | Reference |
|---|---|---|---|---|
| NOTCH1 | Missense, de novo | Bicuspid aortic valve, Tetralogy of Fallot | Disrupts valve formation, impairs ventricular septation | Wang et al., 2021 |
| VEGFA | Polymorphism | Pulmonary atresia, Septal defects | Alters angiogenesis, reduces cardiac morphogenesis | Hăşmăşanu et al., 2023 |
| CHD7 | De novo | Hypoplastic left heart syndrome | Impairs chromatin remodeling, affects cardiac looping | Yan et al., 2020 |
| GATA4 | De novo, deletion | Atrial septal defects | Reduces cardiogenic differentiation | Fan et al., 2021 |
| TBX5 | Missense | Ventricular septal defects | Disrupts transcription factor activity | Rivera-Madera et al., 2025 |

Polygenic risk scores, integrating common variants across these pathways, enhance CHD risk prediction, though rare de novo mutations often drive severe phenotypes (O'Sullivan et al., 2022). These findings underscore the genetic heterogeneity of CHD, necessitating integrative approaches to fully elucidate its genomic basis.

## Limitations of Genomics Alone in Explaining CHD Variability

While genomics has advanced our understanding of CHD, it alone cannot fully explain the condition's phenotypic variability. Genetic variants, such as those in *NOTCH1* or *VEGFA*, account only for a fraction of CHD cases, leaving a significant proportion unexplained (Ashiq et al., 2023; Xiang et al., 2025). Rare de novo mutations, identified through whole-exome sequencing, contribute to severe CHD phenotypes but are insufficient to capture the full spectrum of disease heterogeneity (Sierant et al., 2025). Polygenic risk scores, aggregating common variants, improve risk prediction but struggle with low penetrance and variable expressivity, where identical mutations yield diverse outcomes (Spendlove et al., 2022).

Environmental factors, unaddressed by genomics, significantly influence CHD. Maternal exposures like diabetes or pollutants alter gene expression, modulating disease risk (Choudhury et al., 2025). Epigenetic modifications, such as DNA methylation, further complicate the genomic landscape by mediating gene-environment interactions, which genomics alone cannot capture (Linglart & Bonnet, 2022). Additionally, non-coding regions, often overlooked in genomic studies, regulate cardiac development, and their variants contribute to CHD variability (Penaloza et al., 2025).

Technical limitations also hinder genomic approaches. Current sequencing technologies may miss low-frequency variants or complex structural rearrangements (Chen et al., 2025). Moreover, the multifactorial nature of CHD demands integration with other omics layers, such as epigenomics and exposomics, to elucidate how genetic predisposition interacts with environmental triggers. These gaps highlight the need for multi-omics approaches to comprehensively address CHD's complex etiology.

## Role of De Novo Mutations and Polygenic Risk Scores in CHD

De novo mutations and polygenic risk scores (PRS) are critical in understanding the genomic basis of CHD. De novo mutations, spontaneous genetic alterations not inherited from parents, significantly contribute to severe CHD phenotypes. Whole-exome sequencing studies reveal that 8% of sporadic CHD cases involve de novo mutations in genes like *NOTCH1*, *CHD7*, and *GATA6*, disrupting cardiac development processes such as valve formation and septation (Sevim Bayrak et al., 2020). These mutations, often in coding regions, have high penetrance and are linked to complex defects like tetralogy of Fallot and hypoplastic left heart syndrome (Yasuhara & Garg, 2021). However, their rarity limits their explanatory power across diverse CHD populations.

Polygenic risk scores, aggregating the effects of multiple common genetic variants, address CHD's genetic heterogeneity. Polygenic risk score (PRS) analysis in a pediatric population identified genetic variants in GATA4, SMAD7, VEGF, MTRR, and ISL1 associated with ventricular septal defects (VSDs), enhancing risk stratification for congenital heart disease. Further refinement of PRS models is necessary to improve their predictive accuracy for VSD and other congenital heart conditions (Sarwar et al., 2025). PRS, when integrated with clinical data, enhance the ability to predict CHD and its associated comorbidities, facilitating improved risk assessment and management for affected individuals (Thompson et al., 2025). PRS face challenges in capturing the complex interplay of rare and de novo genetic variants, often underperforming in predictive accuracy due to their limited ability to incorporate nonlinear effects and regulatory mechanisms. The Epi-PRS framework addresses these limitations by leveraging large language models to impute cell-type-specific epigenomic signals, significantly enhancing PRS performance in predicting genetic risk for diseases like breast cancer and type 2 diabetes (Zeng et al., 2025). The interplay of de novo mutations and PRS highlights CHD's multifactorial nature, necessitating integration with epigenomics and exposomics for comprehensive risk assessment. While the genomic landscape of CHD reveals critical genetic drivers, the dynamic interplay between genes and environmental factors, mediated by epigenomics, further elucidates the complex etiology of congenital heart disease.

## EPIGENOMICS: THE BRIDGE BETWEEN GENES AND ENVIRONMENT

### Mechanisms of Epigenetic Regulation in Cardiac Development

Epigenetic regulation plays a pivotal role in cardiac development, orchestrating gene expression without altering DNA sequence, and serves as a critical link between genetic predisposition and environmental influences in CHD. Key mechanisms include DNA methylation, histone modifications, and non-coding RNA activity, each modulating cardiac morphogenesis during embryogenesis.

*DNA methylation*, the addition of methyl groups to cytosine bases, regulates gene silencing and activation in cardiac progenitor cells. Hypermethylation of promoter regions in genes like *NKX2-5* and *GATA4* suppresses their expression, disrupting cardiogenic differentiation and leading to defects such as septal anomalies (Linglart & Bonnet, 2022). DNA methylation, particularly at CpG sites, regulates gene expression critical for embryonic development, including cardiogenesis, and its deregulation, involving genes like APOA5 and PCSK9, is linked to CHD such as aortic valve stenosis. Altered methylation patterns, influenced by DNA methyltransferases (DNMT3A, DNMT3B) and ten-eleven translocation enzymes (TETs), mediate demethylation. Exposure-sensitive pathways alter TET activity at loci like LMNA, linked to structural defects and may contribute to CHD pathogenesis by disrupting precise gene expression (Rodríguez-Pérez et al., 2025; Romanò et al., 2025).

*Histone modifications*, including acetylation and methylation, alter chromatin structure to control gene accessibility. Histone acetyltransferases (HATs) like p300 enhance *GATA4* expression, promoting cardiac cell differentiation, while histone deacetylases (HDACs) repress cardiogenic genes, potentially causing ventricular septal defects (Funamoto et al., 2023). Histone H3K27 trimethylation, mediated by the Polycomb complex, silences cardiac-specific genes during early development, and its dysregulation is linked to conotruncal defects (Wang et al., 2022).

*Non-coding RNAs*, particularly microRNAs (miRNAs) and long non-coding RNAs (lncRNAs), fine-tune cardiac gene expression. miR-1 and miR-133 regulate cardiac muscle differentiation by targeting *Notch* signaling, and their aberrant expression is associated with outflow tract defects (Mannarino et al., 2025). LncRNAs, such as *ANRIL*, promotes alteration of the vascular smooth muscle cell phenotype, with disruptions implicated in CHD (Xie et al., 2025).

*Table 2. Epigenetic Mechanisms and Environmental Exposures in CHD*

| Epigenetic Mechanism | Environmental Exposure | Affected Gene/ Pathway | CHD Outcome | Mitigation Strategy | Reference |
|---|---|---|---|---|---|
| DNA methylation (hypermethylation) | Maternal smoking | *GATA4, NKX2-5* | Ventricular septal defects | Smoking cessation programs | Rodríguez-Pérez et al., 2025 |
| DNA methylation (hypomethylation) | Folate deficiency | *MTHFR, TBX20, TBX1* | Tetralogy of Fallot | Folate supplementation | González-Peña et al., 2021 |
| Histone acetylation | Air pollutants (PM2.5) | *H3K9* | cardiac hypertrophy | Air purifiers, pollution control | Sun et al., 2021 |
| Hypomethylation | Nitrogen dioxide ($NO_2$) | *SIVA1* and *MDM2* | Ventricular Septal Defect (VSD), Pulmonary Valve Stenosis (PVS), and Coarctation of the Aorta (COA) | Exposure monitoring, urban planning | Stingone et al., 2017 |
| DNA methylation (hypomethylation) | Inadequate maternal nutrition during pregnancy | IGF2 | Cardiovascular Disease (CVD) | Appropriate maternal nutrition | Joshi et al., 2020 |

These mechanisms are highly sensitive to environmental cues, such as maternal smoking or folate deficiency, which alter methylation patterns or miRNA expression, impacting cardiac development (Karas Kuželički & Doljak, 2024). Epigenome-wide association studies (EWAS) have revealed CHD-specific epigenetic signatures, underscoring the need to integrate these mechanisms with genomic and exposomic data to fully understand CHD etiology.

## Gene-Environment Etiologies in CHD

Genetic predispositions, such as variants in NOTCH1, interplay with exposures like maternal diabetes, leading to hypermethylation of IGF2 and increased CHD risk (Li et al., 2024). This holistic view reveals complex interactions driving pathogenesis. Epigenetic mechanisms play a pivotal role in linking maternal diabetes, particularly gestational diabetes mellitus (GDM), to cardiac diseases in offspring by establishing long-term cellular memory through alterations in gene expression without changing the DNA sequence. During fetal development, exposure to a hyperglycemic intrauterine environment modulates cardiomyocyte metabolism and mitochondrial function, influencing the production of metabolites like acetyl-CoA and S-adenosyl methionine, which regulate epigenetic modifiers such as histone acetyltransferases, DNA methyltransferases, and demethylases. This mito-nuclear communication creates a feedback loop where mitochondrial-derived signals affect epigenetic patterns, and vice versa, predisposing the offspring to cardiovascular dysfunction. For instance, in offspring of GDM mothers, differential methylation at CpG sites in genes like MEST and IGF2 in circulating DNA correlates with macrosomia and growth dysregulation, while placental studies show decreased PGC-1α levels linked to H3K27 acetylation and promoter methylation, effects potentially mitigated by metformin via AMPK activation. Additionally, upregulated miR-101 in cord blood reduces EZH2 expression, altering histone H3 trimethylation at lysine 27, further contributing to cardiac programming. These changes can persist into adulthood, exacerbating mitochondrial oxidative stress and inflammation, and may even propagate intergenerationally through germ cell epigenetics, increasing CVD risk in subsequent generations (Tocantins et al., 2022). Building on epigenetic mechanisms, we now examine environmental exposure risks in the next section.

## Evidence Linking Environmental Exposures to Epigenetic Changes in CHD

Environmental exposures significantly influence CHD through epigenetic modifications, altering gene expression without changing DNA sequence. Maternal smoking and folate deficiency, among other exposures, are strongly linked to epigenetic changes that disrupt cardiac development, contributing to CHD pathogenesis.

Maternal smoking during pregnancy is a well-documented risk factor for CHD, inducing epigenetic alterations like DNA methylation changes. Tobacco smoke exposure hypermethylates promoter regions of cardiac genes such as *GATA4* and *NKX2-5*, suppressing their expression and impairing cardiogenesis (Jiang et al., 2017). A epigenome-wide association study (EWAS) identified differential methylation among offspring of smoking mothers, correlating with ventricular septal defects (Joubert et al., 2016; Jiang et al., 2017). Cigarette smoking induces increased histone acetylation mainly by decreasing the activity and expression of HDAC components, affecting cardiac cell differentiation (Qin et al., 2021; Zong et al., 2019).

Folate deficiency, critical for one-carbon metabolism, alters DNA methylation patterns, increasing CHD risk. Folate deficiency, particularly when linked to genetic variations in the folate/methionine cycle genes such as MTHFR, MTR, and MTRR, is associated with an increased risk of CHD by disrupting DNA methylation and homocysteine metabolism, which are critical for cardiac development. These genetic changes can impair folate metabolism, potentially leading to structural heart defects in the fetus (Karas Kuželički & Doljak, 2024). Major genes associated with Tetralogy of Fallot (TOF), including NOTCH1, FLT4, GATA4, NKX2-5, TBX1, JAG1, MYH6, and LBX1, play critical roles in cardiac and vascular development, with mutations disrupting signaling pathways, transcription regulation, and myocyte function, leading to structural heart defects. These genes contribute to both syndromic and non-syndromic TOF, with approximately 20% of cases linked to chromosomal anomalies like 22q11.2 deletion (Horenstein et al., 2024). Supplementation trials have shown that adequate folate intake mitigates these epigenetic disruptions, reducing CHD incidence (Linglart & Bonnet, 2022).

Other exposures, such as air pollutants (e.g., PM2.5) and maternal diabetes, also drive epigenetic changes. The dysregulation of miRNAs like miR-1 and miR-133 by PM2.5 exposure, disrupts gene expression networks critical for cardiogenesis, potentially leading to structural cardiac abnormalities such as ventricular septal defects, atrial septal defects, or valve malformations, and functional cardiac abnormalities like impaired cardiac contractility, arrhythmias, or altered cardiac conduction. These disruptions can contribute to congenital heart diseases and long-term cardiac dysfunction (Meng et al., 2024). Maternal diabetes, particularly gestational diabetes mellitus (GDM), induces hypermethylation of genes such as IGF2 and H19 in offspring tissues, which is associated with an increased risk of cardiac diseases like CHD and impaired cardiac function recovery post-ischemia. These epigenetic changes, driven by intrauterine hyperglycemia, may predispose offspring to long-term cardiovascular complications through altered gene expression in pathways critical for heart development and function (Li et al., 2024). These findings, supported by EWAS and animal models, highlight how environmental factors reshape the epigenome, amplifying CHD susceptibility are discussed further.

## Techniques like EWAS and Their Application to CHD

EWAS are powerful tools for identifying epigenetic modifications associated with CHD, offering insights into how environmental factors influence gene expression during cardiac development. Unlike genome-wide association studies (GWAS), which focus on genetic variants, EWAS analyze epigenetic marks-primarily DNA methylation-across the genome to uncover CHD-related epigenetic signatures.

EWAS typically employ high-throughput technologies, such as Illumina's Infinium MethylationEPIC BeadChip, to assess methylation at millions of CpG sites. In CHD research, EWAS have identified differential DNA methylation patterns in 84 genes, including ABCG1, SREBF1, and TNNT1, associated with coronary heart disease and atherosclerosis, implicating their roles in lipid metabolism and vascular inflammation. These methylation changes serve as potential biomarkers for CHD risk and progression, though further validation is needed for clinical application (Fernández-Sanlés et al., 2017). EWAS to detect hypermethylation in *GATA4* promoters in tetralogy of Fallot cases, correlating with reduced gene expression and impaired cardiac differentiation (Linglart & Bonnet, 2022). These findings highlight EWAS's ability to pinpoint epigenetic alterations driving CHD phenotypes.

Beyond methylation, EWAS integrate with other techniques like chromatin immunoprecipitation sequencing (ChIP-seq) to study histone modifications. The study by Spurrell et al. (2022) employed ChIP-seq to investigate enhancer architecture in heart disease, revealing a genome-wide fetalization of enhancer landscapes in CHD that indicates altered epigenetic regulation. Specifically, ChIP-seq analysis highlighted changes in histone modifications, such as H3K27ac, associated with dysregulated gene expression contributing to CHD pathogenesis. Additionally, assay for transposase-accessible chromatin sequencing (ATAC-seq) was used to profile open chromatin regions during heart development, revealing developmental pathways and non-coding mutations linked to CHD. The technique identified accessible regulatory elements and highlighted epigenetic changes that contribute to abnormal gene expression involved in CHD pathogenesis (Ameen et al., 2022). These methods complement EWAS by providing a multi-layered view of epigenetic regulation. Validated findings from cohorts like the Pediatric Cardiac Genomics Consortium use ENCODE for annotation, confirming methylation at cardiac enhancers in independent studies (Spurrell et al., 2022).

EWAS applications in CHD face challenges, including the need for large, well-characterized cohorts and robust statistical methods to account for confounding factors like maternal exposures. Integrating EWAS with machine learning improves the detection of coronary heart disease and associated methylation patterns influenced by smoking (Dogan et al., 2021). Such integrative approaches enhance EWAS's utility in linking environmental exposures to epigenetic changes, paving the way for personalized CHD risk prediction and prevention strategies. Building on the epigenetic mechanisms that mediate gene-environment interactions in CHD, the next section on exposomics will explore methods to comprehensively quantify environmental factors driving these epigenetic changes and their role in CHD pathogenesis.

## EXPOSOMICS: CAPTURING THE ENVIRONMENTAL DIMENSION

The exposome encompasses the totality of environmental exposures an individual encounters from conception to death, capturing their cumulative impact on health outcomes like CHD. The term and concept of exposome is introduced by Christopher Paul Wild in 2012 and refined in recent studies, the exposome includes external factors (e.g., air pollutants, diet, smoking), internal biological responses (e.g., metabolites, oxidative stress), and lifestyle influences (e.g., stress, physical activity) (Wild, 2012). In CHD research, the exposome provides a framework to investigate how environmental factors interact with genetic and epigenetic mechanisms to drive disease.

The scope of the exposome is vast, spanning chemical exposures (e.g., heavy metals, endocrine disruptors), physical factors (e.g., radiation), and socio-behavioral elements (e.g., maternal stress). For CHD, key exposures include maternal smoking, which alters fetal cardiac development, and air pollutants like PM2.5, linked to septal defects (Li et al., 2025). Advanced exposome profiling, using metabolomics and wearable sensors, quantifies these exposures. For instance, metabolomics identifies biomarkers of pollutant exposure, while sensors track real-time environmental data (Doherty et al., 2021). These tools enable precise measurement of exposures during critical developmental windows.

The exposome's dynamic nature requires longitudinal studies to capture temporal variations, particularly during pregnancy when CHD risk is highest (Helbig et al., 2021). By integrating exposomic data with genomics and epigenomics, researchers can elucidate how environmental exposures modify gene expression, contributing to CHD etiology. This holistic approach enhances risk prediction and informs preventive strategies.

## Methods for Exposome Profiling

Exposome profiling quantifies the totality of environmental exposures to elucidate their role in CHD. Advanced methods like metabolomics, wearable sensors, and biomarker analyses provide comprehensive tools to capture external and internal exposures, enabling precise assessment of their impact on CHD pathogenesis.

*Metabolomics* involves the high-throughput analysis of small molecules (metabolites) in biological samples, reflecting the interplay of environmental exposures and physiological responses. Liquid chromatography-mass spectrometry (LC-MS) and gas chromatography-mass spectrometry (GC-MS) are widely used to detect metabolites associated with CHD-relevant exposures, such as air pollutants (e.g., PM2.5) and maternal diet. Fetal exposure to maternal smoking, which includes polycyclic aromatic hydrocarbons, was associated with altered lipid and amino acid profiles in umbilical cord blood, potentially contributing to congenital heart diseases and septal defects due to disrupted metabolic pathways. These changes in metabolites, such as increased levels of specific lipids and amino acids, may reflect underlying mechanisms linking environmental exposures to cardiac developmental abnormalities (Cajachagua-Torres et al., 2022). Untargeted metabolomics, which surveys multiple metabolites, has revealed biomarkers of maternal smoking and folate deficiency, offering insights into their role in disrupting cardio-metabolic health (Cajachagua-Torres et al., 2022). Targeted metabolomics further quantifies specific compounds, like oxidative stress markers, to assess exposure-related damage during embryogenesis (Liu et al., 2011).

*Wearable sensors* provide real-time, longitudinal data on environmental and lifestyle exposures. Devices equipped with GPS, accelerometers, and air quality monitors track maternal exposure to pollutants, physical activity, and stress levels, all linked to CHD risk. Wearable sensors were used to monitor PM2.5 exposure in pregnant women, correlating higher levels with epigenetic changes in cardiac genes like *GATA4* (Helbig et al., 2021). Wearable technology also captures physiological data, such as heart rate variability, reflecting maternal stress responses that may influence fetal cardiac development (Liu et al., 2024). These sensors enable dynamic exposure assessment during critical developmental windows, overcoming limitations of retrospective questionnaires.

*Biomarker analyses*, including proteomics and adductomics, complement metabolomics by identifying protein and DNA adducts formed by environmental toxicants. Adductomics, the comprehensive study of DNA, protein, and other macromolecular adducts formed by environmental exposures, provides critical insights into the molecular mechanisms underlying heart defects and diseases. Research, including Pereira and Antunes (2019) and Lockridge (2023), highlights how adductomics identifies chemical modifications from environmental toxicants like polycyclic aromatic hydrocarbons (PAHs), which can disrupt cellular processes and contribute to cardiovascular pathogenesis. Zhang and Schmidlin (2024) emphasize the integration of adductomics with metabolomics in systems biology, revealing how adducts alter lipid and amino acid metabolism, potentially leading to congenital heart defects or adult-onset cardiovascular diseases. Cooke et al. (2018) and Imani et al. (2025) further demonstrate that adducts from air pollution and oxidative stress, detectable in biological samples, are linked to metabolic dysregulation and redox imbalances, which may exacerbate cardiac developmental abnormalities or disease progression by interfering with critical signaling pathways. Thus, adductomics serves as a powerful tool to elucidate the environmental and metabolic contributors to heart defects and diseases. Proteomics studies have identified altered protein expression in response to maternal diabetes, a known CHD risk factor (Lin et al., 2024). These methods provide molecular evidence of exposure effects, bridging external factors to biological outcomes.

*Challenges and Advances*: Exposome profiling faces challenges like data integration and variability in exposure measurements. A machine learning model using administrative data to predict congenital heart defects, demonstrating high accuracy in identifying at-risk infants based on maternal and neonatal characteristics (Shi et al., 2023). This approach highlights the potential of machine learning to enhance early detection and intervention for congenital heart disease by leveraging large-scale health data. Standardization of protocols and large-scale cohort studies enhance reproducibility. Combining these methods with genomics and epigenomics offers a holistic view of CHD etiology, informing preventive strategies.

# INTEGRATION STRATEGIES AND METHODOLOGIES

## Multi-omics Data Integration Tools

Multi-omics data integration tools, such as machine learning (ML) and network analysis, are pivotal for synthesizing genomic, epigenomic, and exposomic data to elucidate CHD etiology. These tools address the complexity and heterogeneity of multi-omics datasets, enhancing biomarker discovery and risk prediction. Some of the multi-omics integration tools and their applications in CHD are summarized in Table 3.

*Machine Learning (ML)*: ML algorithms, including random forests and deep neural networks, integrate diverse omics layers for CHD research. Machine learning models, including GPS-mult, random forests, and support vector machines (SVMs), could be applied in predicting CHD risk through the integration of multi-omics data such as genomics, proteomics, and metabolomics. The GPS-mult model, a gradient-based predictive system, is particularly significant for its ability to capture complex, synergistic interactions across heterogeneous omics datasets, enabling precise identification of at-risk individuals for CHD. Random forests enhance prediction by aggregating decision trees to handle high-dimensional data, offering robustness against overfitting and high accuracy in detecting congenital heart defects. Similarly, SVMs contribute by optimizing decision boundaries to classify patients effectively based on multi-omics features, ensuring high sensitivity. The superior integrative capacity of GPS-mult compared to random forests and SVMs underscores its potential to advance personalized risk assessment and early intervention for CHD in clinical practice, driving translational research forward (Lin et al., 2025). Unsupervised machine learning models, such as clustering and dimensionality reduction techniques, in CHD to identify hidden patterns in complex datasets without predefined labels. These models aid in stratifying patient risk and uncovering novel CHD-associated biomarkers by analyzing diverse clinical and imaging data, enhancing diagnostic and prognostic capabilities (Toscano & Moras, 2024). These models handle high-dimensional data, capturing non-linear interactions critical for CHD.

*Table 3. Multi-Omics Integration Tools and Their Applications in CHD*

| Tool/Method | Omics Layers Integrated | Application in CHD | Computational Requirements | Scalability | Reference |
|---|---|---|---|---|---|
| Random Forest | Genomics, proteomics, exposomics | Predicts CHD risk | Moderate; standard GPU | High | Pal & Parija, 2021 |
| Similarity Network Fusion (SNF) | Epigenomics, exposomics | Identifies GATA4 methylation networks | High; large memory | Moderate | Miranda et al., 2023 |
| MOGONET | Genomics, epigenomics | Detects gene-environment interactions | High; GPU clusters | Moderate | Wang et al., 2021 |
| IntegrAO | All omics | Optimizes CHD biomarker discovery | Very high; cloud computing | Low | Ma et al., 2025 |
| Deep Neural Networks | Genomics, exposomics | Classifies CHD subtypes | Very high; specialized hardware | Moderate | Cheng et al., 2024 |

*Network Analysis*: Network-based approaches, like Similarity Network Fusion (SNF), construct patient similarity networks from individual omics datasets, integrating them to identify CHD-associated molecular interactions (Miranda et al., 2023). Graph convolutional networks, such as MOGONET, leverage multi-omics data to predict clinical outcomes, identifying biomarkers like methylation (Sahoo & Sundararajan, 2024). These methods model complex gene-environment interactions, revealing regulatory networks disrupted in CHD.

Challenges include data heterogeneity and computational complexity, addressed by tools like IntegrAO, which optimizes multi-omics integration for CHD (Ma et al., 2025). These tools enhance precision medicine by linking molecular profiles to CHD phenotypes.

## Successful Integrative Studies in Other Diseases

Integrative multi-omics studies in diseases like cancer and asthma provide valuable frameworks for CHD research. These studies combine genomics, epigenomics, and exposomics to uncover disease mechanisms and inform precision medicine.

The study by Fountzilas et al. (2025) discusses multiple machine learning techniques for cancer detection, including supervised learning (e.g., random forests, support vector machines), deep learning (e.g., convolutional neural networks for imaging), and integrative multiomic models combining genomic, proteomic, and radiomic data. Specific accuracy metrics vary by application, but the study highlights that ensemble method and deep learning model often achieve diagnostic accuracies exceeding 85–95% in tasks like tumor classification and early detection across cancers such as breast, lung, and colorectal, depending on the dataset and model optimization (Ahmad et al., 2025). Network-based approaches for integrating multi-omics data to understand gene-environment interactions in noncommunicable diseases include Gene Regulatory Networks (GRNs), which model interactions between genes, transcription factors, and regulatory elements using transcriptomic and epigenomic data to identify regulatory hubs; Protein-Protein Interaction (PPI) Networks, which integrate proteomic data to map protein interactions and reveal functional modules altered in diseases like cancer; Metabolic Networks, which combine metabolomic and proteomic data to model metabolic pathways affected by environmental exposures; Co-expression Networks, which use transcriptomic data to identify co-expressed gene clusters linked to disease states; and Similarity Network Fusion (SNF), a powerful method that constructs similarity networks for each omics dataset (e.g., genomic, proteomic) and iteratively fuses them into a unified network to capture shared patterns across data types, enhancing the identification of robust biomarkers and molecular signatures. These approaches collectively integrate genomic, epigenomic, transcriptomic, and proteomic data to construct comprehensive models of biological systems, improving the detection of disease-specific molecular signatures and biomarkers for early diagnosis and personalized treatment of noncommunicable diseases, though specific biomarkers depend on the disease and dataset analyzed (Alemu et al., 2025). These approaches highlight the power of multi-omics in identifying actionable therapeutic targets.

In asthma, integrative studies have elucidated gene-environment interactions. The genome-wide association studies (GWAS), epigenome-wide association studies (EWAS), and metabolomics collectively link PM2.5 exposure to epigenetic changes, such as DNA methylation alterations, which contribute to asthma exacerbations by modulating immune responses and airway inflammation. These multi-omics approaches reveal how environmental pollutants like PM2.5 interact with genetic and epigenetic factors to influence asthma severity and susceptibility (Kabesch & Tost, 2020). Similarly, deep learning could be used to integrate genomic and exposomic data, identifying volatile organic compound-related biomarkers for pediatric asthma (Gautam et al., 2022). These studies demonstrate how multi-omics can capture complex environmental influences on disease.

These successes offer blueprints for CHD research, where similar tools can integrate genetic variants (e.g., *NOTCH1*), epigenetic marks, and exposures like maternal smoking to predict risk and guide interventions.

## Proposed Workflows for CHD Research

Proposed workflows for CHD research integrate genomic, epigenomic, and exposomic data to elucidate disease etiology and enhance risk prediction. A structured multi-omics pipeline begins with data collection. Genomic data, including whole-exome sequencing, identify variants like *NOTCH1* mutations, while epigenomic data from EWAS capture methylation patterns (e.g., *GATA4*). Exposomic data, gathered via metabolomics and wearable sensors, quantify environmental exposures like PM2.5.

Preprocessing and harmonization follow, addressing data heterogeneity. Tools like ComBat normalize batch effects across omics datasets, ensuring compatibility (Voß et al., 2022). Integration employs ML and network analysis. Random forest models integrate omics layers to predict CHD risk with high accuracy, while CHDmap, a Patient Similarity Network (PSN) developed by integrating clinical and echocardiographic data from CHD surgeries using natural language processing and machine learning, could be used for personalized prediction of postoperative outcomes such as complications and mechanical ventilation duration. By employing a k-nearest neighbor algorithm and structure-mapping theory, CHDmap identifies similar patient groups to support clinical decision-making, achieving competitive performance in predicting complications and ventilation duration compared to clinical experts, thereby enhancing individualized care in CHD management (Li et al., 2024; Sumwiza et al., 2023).

Standardized protocols are essential to minimize bias, while validated tools, such as quality-of-life questionnaires or NYHA classifications, ensure reliable outcome measurement. Data privacy must be maintained in compliance with regulations like HIPAA or GDPR. For genetic studies, whole-exome sequencing or public databases (e.g., ClinVar, gnomAD) provide critical insights, while environmental or patient-reported data may be gathered through surveys or exposure databases. The result is a curated, secure dataset ready for analysis.

Data analysis involves both quantitative and advanced computational approaches. Descriptive and inferential statistics (e.g., t-tests, regression models) are used to test hypotheses, while survival analysis (e.g., Kaplan-Meier curves) is valuable for longitudinal outcomes. Genetic studies may employ variant calling, pathway analysis (using tools like DAVID or KEGG), or machine learning for predictive modeling of CHD risk or imaging-based anomaly detection. Software such as R, Python, or specialized platforms like Galaxy facilitate these analyses. Results are then interpreted in the context of existing literature, with validation through replication in independent cohorts or sensitivity analyses to ensure robustness. Limitations, such as sample size or confounding factors, must be carefully addressed to strengthen the findings.

Disseminating results is essential to maximize the impact of CHD research. Findings should be prepared as manuscripts for submission to peer-reviewed journals (e.g., Circulation, Journal of the American College of Cardiology) or presented at conferences like those hosted by the American Heart Association or European Society of Cardiology. Engaging patients and families through accessible summaries, blogs, or advocacy groups (e.g., Mended Hearts) ensures broader outreach. Data sharing in repositories like dbGaP or Zenodo aligns with open science principles and funder requirements. Translating findings into clinical practice is a critical next step, involving collaboration with clinicians to develop diagnostic tools, treatment guidelines, or novel therapies, such as gene-based interventions or advanced imaging technologies. Policy advocacy, such as promoting screening programs, can further amplify public health impact.

Finally, CHD research is an iterative process that requires planning for future directions. Unanswered questions or new hypotheses generated from the study should guide subsequent investigations. Securing funding from organizations like the NIH, American Heart Association, or Children's Heart Foundation, and fostering multicenter collaborations, enhances the generalizability and impact of future studies. By integrating cutting-edge technologies, patient-centered perspectives, and global considerations, researchers can contribute to a deeper understanding of CHD and improved outcomes for affected individuals.

While integration strategies and methodologies provide powerful tools to unravel CHD's complex etiology, the next section on challenges and concerns addresses critical technical, ethical, and scientific hurdles that must be overcome to fully realize their potential.

## CHALLENGES AND CONCERNS

### Technical: Data Harmonization, Exposure Measurement Accuracy

Integrating multi-omics data for CHD research faces significant technical challenges, particularly in data harmonization and exposure measurement accuracy. Data harmonization involves aligning heterogeneous datasets from genomics, epigenomics, and exposomics, which differ in scale, format, and collection methods. Batch effects, platform variability, and missing data complicate integration.

*Exposure measurement accuracy* poses another hurdle. Exposomic data, collected via metabolomics or wearable sensors, often suffer from temporal and spatial variability. Longitudinal sampling and high-resolution sensors improve accuracy but increase costs and complexity. Addressing these challenges requires robust computational tools and standardized methodologies to ensure reliable multi-omics integration for CHD research.

## Ethical: Privacy in Exposome Data, Equity in Access to Multi-Omics Technologies

Ethical challenges in CHD multi-omics research include privacy concerns in exposome data and equitable access to advanced technologies. Privacy in exposome data is critical due to the sensitive nature of environmental and lifestyle data collected via wearable sensors and metabolomics. These datasets, capturing maternal exposures like diet or stress, risk re-identification when linked with genomic profiles, potentially breaching confidentiality (Bradley et al., 2022). Unencrypted exposome data from wearable devices increase privacy risks in CHD cohorts. Robust encryption, anonymization, and strict data-sharing protocols are essential to protect participant privacy while enabling research (Hughes et al., 2023).

Equity in access to multi-omics technologies poses another challenge. High-cost sequencing and exposome profiling tools, like LC-MS for metabolomics, are often inaccessible in low-resource settings, exacerbating health disparities in CHD diagnosis and prevention. This inequity restricts the global application of personalized CHD interventions. Strategies like cost-effective platforms and international collaborations are needed to democratize access (Hoagland & Kipping, 2024).

Translating genomic insights from CHD biobanks into clinical practice faces significant challenges, particularly in safeguarding privacy during data linkage and ensuring equitable access in low- and middle-income countries (LMICs). As demonstrated in the study linking CHD biobank data with administrative health records in New South Wales, Australia, privacy concerns are paramount; the use of de-identified data, probabilistic linkage via specialized centers like CHeReL, and adherence to data-separation principles are essential to protect participant confidentiality while enabling large-scale genomic analyses for identifying cardiovascular outcomes (Lain et al., 2023). However, extending such approaches to LMICs introduces barriers like limited infrastructure for biobanking, insufficient funding for genomic sequencing, and inadequate administrative data systems, which hinder the identification of genetic variants associated with post-surgical variability in CHD outcomes. These disparities exacerbate global inequities, as high-income settings can leverage standardized care and ethical frameworks to inform prevention strategies, whereas LMICs struggle with basic access to surgical interventions and genetic testing, potentially delaying the translation of findings into personalized care for at-risk CHD patients worldwide (Lain et al., 2023). Addressing these ethical concerns ensures responsible and inclusive multi-omics research for CHD.

## Scientific: Causality vs. Correlation in Complex Datasets

Distinguishing causality from correlation in multi-omics datasets for CHD research is a significant scientific challenge. The integration of genomic, epigenomic, and exposomic data generates complex, high-dimensional datasets where associations, such as between PM2.5 exposure and *GATA4* methylation, may reflect correlation rather than causation (Romanò et al., 2025). This distinction is critical for identifying true CHD drivers.

Complex datasets often reveal strong associations, but confounding factors like maternal lifestyle or genetic background obscure causal relationships. A recent study specifically investigates the MTHFR c.1286A>C polymorphism in CAD patients, finding a significant association with methylation disorders and low serum 5-MTHF (active folate) levels. It establishes a correlation with CHD but notes that dietary folate intake and bioavailability are critical confounders, as low folate levels exacerbate hypomethylation but causality remains unconfirmed due to these factors (Pietruszyńska-Reszetarska et al., 2024).

Statistical methods like Mendelian randomization help infer causality by using genetic variants as instrumental variables, but their application in CHD is limited (de Ruiter et al., 2025). Machine learning models, while adept at detecting patterns, often overfit to correlations, misattributing environmental exposures as causal (Komatsu et al., 2021).

Longitudinal cohort studies and experimental models, such as CRISPR-edited organoids, are essential to validate causal pathways (Zaidi & Brueckner., 2017). However, these approaches are resource-intensive and challenging to scale. Advanced causal inference tools, like Bayesian networks, show promise in disentangling gene-environment interactions in CHD but require robust validation (Ruan et al., 2021). Addressing this challenge is crucial for translating multi-omics findings into reliable CHD interventions.

Despite the technical, ethical, and scientific challenges in multi-omics research for CHD, the next section on future directions and clinical implications explores how overcoming these hurdles can advance personalized risk prediction and preventive strategies.

# FUTURE DIRECTIONS AND CLINICAL IMPLICATIONS

## Potential for Personalized CHD Risk Prediction

Personalized risk prediction for CHD leverages multi-omics integration to tailor preventive and diagnostic strategies. By combining genomic variants, epigenomic profiles, and exposomic data, machine learning models like random forests achieve high predictive accuracy for CHD risk (Vitorino 2024). Polygenic risk scores (PRS) are significant in congenital heart disease (CHD) as they aggregate the effects of multiple genetic variants to quantify an individual's genetic predisposition, improving risk stratification and prediction of CHD, particularly for specific subtypes like septal defects. By integrating PRS with endophenotype data, such as heart valve issues or murmurs, they provide insights into the complex genetic architecture of CHD, enabling better identification of at-risk individuals and potentially guiding personalized preventive or therapeutic strategies, though further validation is needed for clinical translation (Spendlove et al., 2022). Wearable sensors further enhance predictions by capturing real-time environmental exposures, enabling dynamic risk assessment during pregnancy (Liu et al., 2024). These approaches allow for early identification of at-risk fetuses, facilitating targeted interventions like folate supplementation to mitigate epigenetic disruptions. Future advancements in causal inference and standardized multi-omics platforms will refine personalized CHD risk models, supporting precision medicine.

## Multi-omics for Identification of Vulnerable Populations, Discovery of Actionable Biomarkers

Multi-omics approaches, encompassing the integration of genomics, epigenomics, proteomics, and metabolomics, represent a transformative strategy for congenital heart disease (CHD) by enabling the precise identification of vulnerable populations, the discovery of actionable biomarkers, and the implementation of early interventions to mitigate disease progression (Nordestgaard et al., 2025). Drawing parallels from atherosclerotic cardiovascular disease (ASCVD), where genome-wide association studies (GWAS) pinpoint genetic variants (e.g., near LDLR and PCSK9) that stratify high-risk groups through polygenic risk scores modulated by epigenetic factors like DNA methylation, multi-omics in CHD can similarly delineate at-risk cohorts—such as fetuses with NKX2-5 or GATA4 mutations exposed to environmental stressors-by layering genomic predispositions with proteomic signatures of plaque-like instability and metabolomic indicators of oxidative stress or endothelial dysfunction (Maiorino & Loscalzo, 2023; Nordestgaard et al., 2025). In heart failure (HF) contexts, which often complicate adult CHD outcomes, multi-omics-driven subtyping via transcriptomic and proteomic profiling reveals circulating biomarkers like enhanced-sensitivity troponins or natriuretic peptides that forecast subclinical cardiac remodeling, allowing for targeted pharmacotherapy in vulnerable subgroups; extending this to CHD, such integration could uncover novel metabolites or histone modifications as early harbingers of structural defects, guiding preemptive interventions like metabolic modulators or gene therapies during critical developmental windows to avert lifelong complications (Bastos et al., 2025). Multi-omics integration identifies vulnerable populations (e.g., via PRS + exposome profiling) and biomarkers like altered miR-133 for early intervention in high-risk pregnancies (Pi et al., 2025). By leveraging computational tools like network analysis and machine learning for holistic data fusion, these approaches not only enhance risk stratification in genetically or environmentally susceptible populations but also empower precision medicine paradigms, such as exposome-informed screening in high-risk pregnancies, ultimately reducing CHD incidence and severity through timely, personalized preventive measures (Fang et al., 2025; Chu et al., 2020).

## Preventive Strategies Informed by Exposome-Genome-Epigenome Interactions

Preventive strategies for CHD leverage exposome-genome-epigenome interactions to mitigate risk through targeted interventions. Multi-omics integration identifies actionable pathways, enabling personalized prevention. For instance, genomic variants like *NOTCH1* mutations, combined with exposomic data on maternal smoking, reveal epigenetic changes that increase CHD risk (Plusquin et al., 2018). A 2023 study showed that folate supplementation in mothers with *MTHFR* variants restored methylation patterns, reduces septal defect risk (González-Peña et al., 2021). Wearable sensors monitoring PM2.5 exposure guide environmental interventions, such as air purifiers, to lower pollutant-driven epigenetic disruptions (Krismanuel, 2025). Machine learning models integrating these omics layers predict high-risk pregnancies with high accuracy, enabling early interventions like dietary adjustments or stress management (Pi et al., 2025). Maternal diabetes, linked to *IGF2* hypermethylation, can be managed through glycemic control to prevent cardiovascular disease (Thornton et al., 2024). These multi-omics-informed strategies advance CHD prevention through precision medicine, focusing on personalized environmental and lifestyle interventions.

## Call for Interdisciplinary Collaboration and Funding

Advancing CHD research through multi-omics requires robust interdisciplinary collaboration and sustained funding. Integrating genomics, epigenomics, and exposomics demands expertise from geneticists, bioinformaticians, environmental scientists, and clinicians to address complex datasets and translate findings into clinical practice. Collaborative efforts, such as the Pediatric Cardiac Genomics Consortium, has significantly advanced the understanding of congenital heart disease by integrating large-scale genomic data with clinical insights, facilitating the identification of genetic and environmental factors contributing to the condition. Their collaborative efforts have enabled comprehensive studies that enhance diagnostic and therapeutic strategies for congenital heart disease (Choudhury et al., 2025). Interdisciplinary teams can develop standardized protocols for data harmonization and causal inference, overcoming technical barriers like batch effects.

Funding is critical to support large-scale cohort studies, advanced technologies (e.g., LC-MS for metabolomics), and computational infrastructure for machine learning models like MOGONET. Recent study highlighted that underfunding limits multi-omics research in low-resource settings, exacerbating global health disparities (Alemu et al., 2025). Increased investment from public and private sectors can accelerate biomarker discovery and personalized interventions, such as folate supplementation to mitigate epigenetic risks. Global consortia and funding agencies must prioritize CHD multi-omics to drive equitable, impactful research.

## CONCLUSION

Congenital heart disease presents a complex interplay of genetic, epigenetic, and environmental factors, necessitating a multi-omics approach to unravel its etiology. Genomics identifies key variants like *NOTCH1* and *VEGFA*, yet its limitations in capturing phenotypic variability underscore the need for broader perspectives. Epigenomics reveals how DNA methylation, histone modifications, and non-coding RNAs mediate gene-environment interactions, linking exposures like maternal smoking to CHD phenotypes (Linglart & Bonnet, 2022). Exposomics quantifies environmental influences, from pollutants to maternal factors, using tools like metabolomics and wearable sensors to pinpoint their role in cardiac development.

Integrating these omics layers through machine learning and network analysis offers a holistic view of CHD, enabling precise risk prediction and personalized interventions. Successful multi-omics strategies in cancer and asthma provide blueprints for CHD, demonstrating how tools like Similarity Network Fusion can uncover molecular pathways. Proposed workflows, leveraging standardized data harmonization and cohort validation, pave the way for biomarker discovery and preventive strategies, such as folate supplementation to mitigate epigenetic disruptions.

However, challenges persist. Data harmonization and exposure measurement accuracy require advanced algorithms, while privacy concerns and inequitable access to technologies demand ethical solutions. Exposomics raises concerns on data privacy, discrimination, and equitable access, especially in LMICs. Distinguishing causality from correlation remains critical to ensure reliable findings. Future directions emphasize interdisciplinary collaboration, robust funding, and causal inference to translate multi-omics insights into clinical practice, offering hope for reducing CHD burden through tailored prevention and early intervention.

## REFERENCES


Ahmad, S., Zafar, I., Shafiq, S., Sehar, L., Khalil, H., Matloob, N., Hina, M., Muntaha, S. T., Khan, H., Khan, N. U., Rana, S., Unar, A., Azmat, M., Shafiq, M., Jardan, Y. A. B., Dauelbait, M., & Bourhia, M. (2025). Deep learning-based computational approach for predicting ncRNAs-disease associations in metaplastic breast cancer diagnosis. *BMC Cancer, 25*(1), 830. DOI: 10.1186/s12885-025-14113-z PMID: 40329245

Alemu, R., Sharew, N. T., Arsano, Y. Y., Ahmed, M., Tekola-Ayele, F., Mersha, T. B., & Amare, A. T. (2025). Multi-omics approaches for understanding gene-environment interactions in noncommunicable diseases: Techniques, translation, and equity issues. *Human Genomics, 19*(1), 8. DOI: 10.1186/s40246-025-00718-9 PMID: 39891174

Ameen, M., Sundaram, L., Shen, M., Banerjee, A., Kundu, S., Nair, S., Shcherbina, A., Gu, M., Wilson, K. D., Varadarajan, A., Vadgama, N., Balsubramani, A., Wu, J. C., Engreitz, J. M., Farh, K., Karakikes, I., Wang, K. C., Quertermous, T., Greenleaf, W. J., & Kundaje, A. (2022). Integrative single-cell analysis of cardiogenesis identifies developmental trajectories and non-coding mutations in congenital heart disease. *Cell, 185*(26), 4937–4953.e23. DOI: 10.1016/j.cell.2022.11.028 PMID: 36563664

Ashiq, S., Hyder, S. N., Ashiq, K., & Sabar, M. F. (2023). Role of Vascular Endothelial Growth Factor as a Potential Biomarker in Congenital Heart Defects: A Systematic Review. *The journal of Tehran Heart Center, 18*(4), 237–243. https://doi.org/DOI: 10.18502/jthc.v18i4.14822

Azhdari, M., & zur Hausen, A. (2025). Wnt/β-catenin and notch signaling pathways in cardiovascular disease: Mechanisms and therapeutics approaches. *Pharmacological Research, 211*, 107565. DOI: 10.1016/j.phrs.2024.107565 PMID: 39725339

Bastos, J. M., Colaço, B., Baptista, R., Gavina, C., & Vitorino, R. (2025). Innovations in heart failure management: The role of cutting-edge biomarkers and multi-omics integration. *Journal of Molecular and Cellular Cardiology Plus, 11*, 100290. DOI: 10.1016/j.jmccpl.2025.100290 PMID: 40129519

Bradley, E. A., Khan, A., McNeal, D. M., Bravo-Jaimes, K., Khanna, A., Cook, S., Opotowsky, A. R., John, A., Lee, M., Pasquali, S., Daniels, C. J., Pernick, M., Kirkpatrick, J. N., & Gurvitz, M. (2022). Operational and Ethical Considerations for a National Adult Congenital Heart Disease Database. *Journal of the American Heart Association, 11*(7), e022338. DOI: 10.1161/JAHA.121.022338 PMID: 35301853

Cajachagua-Torres, K. N., Blaauwendraad, S. M., El Marroun, H., Demmelmair, H., Koletzko, B., Gaillard, R., & Jaddoe, V. W. V. (2022). Fetal Exposure to Maternal Smoking and Neonatal Metabolite Profiles. *Metabolites*, *12*(11), 1101. DOI: 10.3390/metabo12111101 PMID: 36422240

Chen, H. H., & Stewart, A. F. R. (2025). Identifying Structural Variants and Their Contribution to Cardiovascular Disease Risk: The Long and the Short of It. *Journal of the American Heart Association*, *14*(4), e039948. DOI: 10.1161/JAHA.124.039948 PMID: 39950435

Cheng, M., Wang, J., Liu, X., Wang, Y., Wu, Q., Wang, F., Li, P., Wang, B., Zhang, X., & Xie, W. (2024). Development and Validation of a Deep-Learning Network for Detecting Congenital Heart Disease from Multi-View Multi-Modal Transthoracic Echocardiograms. *Research (Washington, D.C.)*, *7*, 0319. https://doi.org/DOI: 10.34133/research.0319

Choudhury, T. Z., Gilbert, B. L., & Garg, V. (2025). Genetic and Environmental Contributors To Congenital Heart Disease. *Current Treatment Options in Cardiovascular Medicine*, *27*(1), 36. DOI: 10.1007/s11936-025-01091-5 PMID: 40438121

Chu, R., Chen, W., Song, G., Yao, S., Xie, L., Song, L., Zhang, Y., Chen, L., Zhang, X., Ma, Y., Luo, X., Liu, Y., Sun, P., Zhang, S., Fang, Y., Dong, T., Zhang, Q., Peng, J., Zhang, L., & Kong, B. (2020). Predicting the Risk of Adverse Events in Pregnant Women With Congenital Heart Disease. *Journal of the American Heart Association*, *9*(14). Advance online publication. DOI: 10.1161/jaha.120.016371 PMID: 32662348

Cooke, M. S., Hu, C.-W., Chang, Y.-J., & Chao, M.-R. (2018). Urinary DNA adductomics – A novel approach for exposomics. *Environment International*, *121*, 1033–1038. DOI: 10.1016/j.envint.2018.10.041 PMID: 30392940

de Ruiter, S. C., Tschiderer, L., Grobbee, D. E., Willeit, P., den Ruijter, H. M., Schmidt, A. F., & Peters, S. A. E. (2025). Mendelian Randomisation: Concepts, Opportunities, Challenges, and Future Directions. *Global Heart*, *20*(1). Advance online publication. DOI: 10.5334/gh.1438 PMID: 40547872

Dogan, M. V., Knight, S., Dogan, T. K., Knowlton, K. U., & Philibert, R. (2021). External validation of integrated genetic-epigenetic biomarkers for predicting incident coronary heart disease. *Epigenomics*, *13*(14), 1095–1112. DOI: 10.2217/epi-2021-0123 PMID: 34148365

Doherty, B. T., Koelmel, J. P., Lin, E. Z., Romano, M. E., & Godri Pollitt, K. J. (2021). Use of Exposomic Methods Incorporating Sensors in Environmental Epidemiology. *Current Environmental Health Reports*, *8*(1), 34–41. DOI: 10.1007/s40572-021-00306-8 PMID: 33569731

Fan, D., Pang, S., Chen, J., Shan, J., Cheng, Q., & Yan, B. (2021). Identification and functional study of GATA4 gene regulatory variants in atrial septal defects. *BMC Cardiovascular Disorders*, *21*(1), 321. DOI: 10.1186/s12872-021-02136-w PMID: 34193080

Fang, Q., Fan, H., Li, Q., Zhang, M., Zhou, Z., Du, J., & Huang, J. (2025). Multi-Omic Insight Into the Molecular Networks in the Pathogenesis of Coronary Artery Disease. *Journal of the American Heart Association*. Advance online publication. DOI: 10.1161/jaha.124.037203 PMID: 40135555

Fernández-Sanlés, A., Sayols-Baixeras, S., Subirana, I., Degano, I. R., & Elosua, R. (2017). Association between DNA methylation and coronary heart disease or other atherosclerotic events: A systematic review. *Atherosclerosis*, *263*, 325–333. DOI: 10.1016/j.atherosclerosis.2017.05.022 PMID: 28577936

Fountzilas, E., Pearce, T., Baysal, M. A., Chakraborty, A., & Tsimberidou, A. M. (2025). Convergence of evolving artificial intelligence and machine learning techniques in precision oncology. *NPJ Digital Medicine*, *8*(1). Advance online publication. DOI: 10.1038/s41746-025-01471-y PMID: 39890986

Funamoto, M., Imanishi, M., Tsuchiya, K., & Ikeda, Y. (2023). Roles of histone acetylation sites in cardiac hypertrophy and heart failure. *Frontiers in Cardiovascular Medicine*, *10*, 1133611. DOI: 10.3389/fcvm.2023.1133611 PMID: 37008337

Gautam, Y., Johansson, E., & Mersha, T. B. (2022). Multi-Omics Profiling Approach to Asthma: An Evolving Paradigm. *Journal of Personalized Medicine*, *12*(1), 66. DOI: 10.3390/jpm12010066 PMID: 35055381

González-Peña, S. M., Calvo-Anguiano, G., Martínez-de-Villarreal, L. E., Ancer-Rodríguez, P. R., Lugo-Trampe, J. J., Saldivar-Rodríguez, D., Hernández-Almaguer, M. D., Calzada-Dávila, M., Guerrero-Orjuela, L. S., & Campos-Acevedo, L. D. (2021). Maternal Folic Acid Intake and Methylation Status of Genes Associated with Ventricular Septal Defects in Children: Case-Control Study. *Nutrients*, *13*(6), 2071. DOI: 10.3390/nu13062071 PMID: 34204335

Hăşmăşanu, M. G., Procopciuc, L. M., Matyas, M., Zonda, G. I., & Zaharie, G. C. (2023). Genetic Polymorphisms of Vascular Endothelial Growth Factor in Neonatal Pathologies: A Systematic Search and Narrative Synthesis of the Literature. *Children (Basel, Switzerland)*, *10*(4), 744. DOI: 10.3390/children10040744 PMID: 37189993

Helbig, C., Ueberham, M., Becker, A. M., Schlink, U., & Kraemer, U. (2021). Wearable sensors for human environmental exposure in urban settings. *Current Pollution Reports*, *7*(4), 417–433. DOI: 10.1007/s40726-021-00186-4

Hoagland, A., & Kipping, S. (2024). Challenges in Promoting Health Equity and Reducing Disparities in Access Across New and Established Technologies. *The Canadian Journal of Cardiology, 40*(6), 1154–1167. DOI: 10.1016/j.cjca.2024.02.014 PMID: 38417572

Horenstein, M. S., Diaz-Frias, J., & Guillaume, M. (2024). Tetralogy of Fallot. In *StatPearls*. StatPearls Publishing., https://www.ncbi.nlm.nih.gov/books/NBK513288/

Hughes, A., Shandhi, M. M. H., Master, H., Dunn, J., & Brittain, E. (2023). Wearable Devices in Cardiovascular Medicine. *Circulation Research, 132*(5), 652–670. DOI: 10.1161/CIRCRESAHA.122.322389 PMID: 36862812

Imani, P., Grigoryan, H., Dudoit, S., Shu, X.-O., Wong, J., Zhang, L., Zhang, J., Hu, W., Cai, Q., Gao, Y., Blechter, B., Rahman, M., Zheng, W., Rothman, N., Lan, Q., & Rappaport, S. M. (2025). HSA Adductomics in the Shanghai Women's Health Study Links Lung Cancer in Never-Smokers with Air Pollution, Redox Biology, and One-Carbon Metabolism. *Antioxidants, 14*(3), 335. DOI: 10.3390/antiox14030335 PMID: 40227422

Jiang, X.-Y., Feng, Y.-L., Ye, L.-T., Li, X.-H., Feng, J., Zhang, M.-Z., Shelat, H. S., Wassler, M., Li, Y., Geng, Y.-J., & Yu, X.-Y. (2017). Inhibition of Gata4 and Tbx5 by Nicotine-Mediated DNA Methylation in Myocardial Differentiation. *Stem Cell Reports, 8*(2), 290–304. DOI: 10.1016/j.stemcr.2016.12.016 PMID: 28111280

Joshi, R. O., Chellappan, S., & Kukshal, P. (2020). Exploring the Role of Maternal Nutritional Epigenetics in Congenital Heart Disease. *Current Developments in Nutrition, 4*(11), nzaa166. Advance online publication. DOI: 10.1093/cdn/nzaa166 PMID: 33294766

Joubert, B. R., Felix, J. F., Yousefi, P., Bakulski, K. M., Just, A. C., Breton, C., Reese, S. E., Markunas, C. A., Richmond, R. C., Xu, C. J., Küpers, L. K., Oh, S. S., Hoyo, C., Gruzieva, O., Söderhäll, C., Salas, L. A., Baïz, N., Zhang, H., Lepeule, J., & London, S. J. (2016). DNA Methylation in Newborns and Maternal Smoking in Pregnancy: Genome-wide Consortium Meta-analysis. *American Journal of Human Genetics, 98*(4), 680–696. DOI: 10.1016/j.ajhg.2016.02.019 PMID: 27040690

Kabesch, M., & Tost, J. (2020). Recent findings in the genetics and epigenetics of asthma and allergy. *Seminars in Immunopathology, 42*(1), 43–60. DOI: 10.1007/s00281-019-00777-w PMID: 32060620

Karas Kuželički, N., & Doljak, B. (2024). Congenital Heart Disease and Genetic Changes in Folate/Methionine Cycles. *Genes, 15*(7), 872. DOI: 10.3390/genes15070872 PMID: 39062651

Komatsu, M., Sakai, A., Komatsu, R., Matsuoka, R., Yasutomi, S., Shozu, K., Dozen, A., Machino, H., Hidaka, H., Arakaki, T., Asada, K., Kaneko, S., Sekizawa, A., & Hamamoto, R. (2021). Detection of Cardiac Structural Abnormalities in Fetal Ultrasound Videos Using Deep Learning. *Applied Sciences (Basel, Switzerland)*, *11*(1), 371. DOI: 10.3390/app11010371

Krismanuel, H. (2025). Air pollution and cardiovascular diseases: Mechanisms, evidence, and mitigation strategies. *Journal of Medicine and Life*, *18*(5), 411–427. DOI: 10.25122/jml-2025-0018 PMID: 40599138

Li, H., Zhou, M., Sun, Y., Yang, J., Zeng, X., Qiu, Y., Xia, Y., Zheng, Z., Yu, J., Feng, Y., Shi, Z., Huang, T., Tan, L., Lin, R., Li, J., Fan, X., Ye, J., Duan, H., Shi, S., & Shu, Q. (2024). A Patient Similarity Network (CHDmap) to Predict Outcomes After Congenital Heart Surgery: Development and Validation Study. *JMIR Medical Informatics*, *12*, e49138. DOI: 10.2196/49138 PMID: 38297829

Li, Z., Wang, D., Jin, L., Zhang, J., Xue, T., & Jin, L. (2025). Maternal exposure to fine particulate matter in the air and risk for fetal congenital heart defects: A case-control study. *Reproductive Toxicology (Elmsford, N.Y.)*, *132*, 108816. DOI: 10.1016/j.reprotox.2024.108816 PMID: 39638263

Lin, J., Zhao, D., Liang, Y., Liang, Z., Wang, M., Tang, X., Zhuang, H., Wang, H., Yin, X., Huang, Y., Yin, L., & Shen, L. (2024). Proteomic analysis of plasma total exosomes and placenta-derived exosomes in patients with gestational diabetes mellitus in the first and second trimesters. *BMC Pregnancy and Childbirth*, *24*(1). Advance online publication. DOI: 10.1186/s12884-024-06919-9 PMID: 39478498

Lin, M., Guo, J., Gu, Z., Tang, W., Tao, H., You, S., Jia, D., Sun, Y., & Jia, P. (2025). Machine learning and multi-omics integration: Advancing cardiovascular translational research and clinical practice. *Journal of Translational Medicine*, *23*(1), 388. DOI: 10.1186/s12967-025-06425-2 PMID: 40176068

Linglart, L., & Bonnet, D. (2022). Epigenetics and Congenital Heart Diseases. *Journal of Cardiovascular Development and Disease*, *9*(6), 185. DOI: 10.3390/jcdd9060185 PMID: 35735814

Liu, J., Litt, L., Segal, M. R., Kelly, M. J., Pelton, J. G., & Kim, M. (2011). Metabolomics of oxidative stress in recent studies of endogenous and exogenously administered intermediate metabolites. *International Journal of Molecular Sciences*, *12*(10), 6469–6501. DOI: 10.3390/ijms12106469 PMID: 22072900

Liu, L., Pu, Y., Fan, J., Yan, Y., Liu, W., Luo, K., Wang, Y., Zhao, G., Chen, T., Puiu, P. D., & Huang, H. (2024). Wearable Sensors, Data Processing, and Artificial Intelligence in Pregnancy Monitoring: A Review. *Sensors (Basel)*, *24*(19), 6426. DOI: 10.3390/s24196426 PMID: 39409471

Lockridge, O. (2023). Overview of Adductomics in Toxicology. *Current Protocols*, *3*(2), e672. DOI: 10.1002/cpz1.672 PMID: 36799690

Ma, S., Zeng, A. G. X., Haibe-Kains, B., Goldenberg, A., Dick, J. E., & Wang, B. (2025). Moving towards genome-wide data integration for patient stratification with Integrate Any Omics. *Nature Machine Intelligence*, *7*(1), 29–42. DOI: 10.1038/s42256-024-00942-3

Maiorino, E., & Loscalzo, J. (2023). Phenomics and Robust Multiomics Data for Cardiovascular Disease Subtyping. *Arteriosclerosis, Thrombosis, and Vascular Biology*, *43*(7), 1111–1123. DOI: 10.1161/ATVBAHA.122.318892 PMID: 37226730

Mannarino, S., Calcaterra, V., Puricelli, F., Cecconi, G., Chillemi, C., Raso, I., Cordaro, E., & Zuccotti, G. (2025). The Role of miRNA Expression in Congenital Heart Disease: Insights into the Mechanisms and Biomarker Potential. *Children (Basel, Switzerland)*, *12*(5), 611. DOI: 10.3390/children12050611 PMID: 40426790

Meng, X., Du, W., & Sun, Z. (2024). Fine particulate matter-induced cardiac developmental toxicity [Review]. *Experimental and Therapeutic Medicine*, *29*(1), 6. DOI: 10.3892/etm.2024.12756 PMID: 39534282

Miranda, J., Paules, C., Noell, G., Youssef, L., Paternina-Caicedo, A., Crovetto, F., Cañellas, N., Garcia-Martín, M. L., Amigó, N., Eixarch, E., Faner, R., Figueras, F., Simões, R. V., Crispi, F., & Gratacós, E. (2023). Similarity network fusion to identify phenotypes of small-for-gestational-age fetuses. *iScience*, *26*(9), 107620. DOI: 10.1016/j.isci.2023.107620 PMID: 37694157

Motairek, I., Makhlouf, M. H. E., Rajagopalan, S., & Al-Kindi, S. (2023). The Exposome and Cardiovascular Health. *The Canadian Journal of Cardiology*, *39*(9), 1191–1203. DOI: 10.1016/j.cjca.2023.05.020 PMID: 37290538

Nordestgaard, L. T., Wolford, B. N., de Gonzalo-Calvo, D., Sopić, M., Devaux, Y., Matic, L., Wettinger, S. B., Schmid, J. A., Amigó, N., Masana, L., Catapano, A. L., Kardassis, D., & Magni, P. (2025). Multiomics in atherosclerotic cardiovascular disease. *Atherosclerosis*, *408*, 120414. DOI: 10.1016/j.atherosclerosis.2025.120414 PMID: 40663987

O'Sullivan, J. W., Raghavan, S., Marquez-Luna, C., Luzum, J. A., Damrauer, S. M., Ashley, E. A., O'Donnell, C. J., Willer, C. J., & Natarajan, P., & American Heart Association Council on Genomic and Precision Medicine; Council on Clinical Cardiology; Council on Arteriosclerosis, Thrombosis and Vascular Biology; Council on Cardiovascular Radiology and Intervention; Council on Lifestyle and Cardiometabolic Health; and Council on Peripheral Vascular Disease. (2022). Polygenic Risk Scores for Cardiovascular Disease: A Scientific Statement From the American Heart Association. *Circulation*, *146*(8), e93–e118. DOI: 10.1161/CIR.0000000000001077 PMID: 35862132

Page, D. J., Miossec, M. J., Williams, S. G., Monaghan, R. M., Fotiou, E., Cordell, H. J., Sutcliffe, L., Topf, A., Bourgey, M., Bourque, G., Eveleigh, R., Dunwoodie, S. L., Winlaw, D. S., Bhattacharya, S., Breckpot, J., Devriendt, K., Gewillig, M., Brook, J. D., & Setchfield, K. J., Bu'Lock, F. A., … Keavney, B. D. (2019). Whole Exome Sequencing Reveals the Major Genetic Contributors to Nonsyndromic Tetralogy of Fallot. *Circulation Research*, *124*(4), 553–563. DOI: 10.1161/CIRCRESAHA.118.313250 PMID: 30582441

Pal, M., & Parija, S. (2021). Prediction of Heart Diseases using Random Forest. *Journal of Physics: Conference Series*, *1817*(1), 012009. DOI: 10.1088/1742-6596/1817/1/012009

Penaloza, J. S., Moreland, B., Gaither, J. B., Landis, B. J., Ware, S. M., McBride, K. L., & White, P.CCVM Consortium. (2025). Identification of Long Noncoding RNA Candidate Disease Genes Associated With Clinically Reported Copy Number Variants in Congenital Heart Disease. *Journal of the American Heart Association*, *14*(6), e039177. DOI: 10.1161/JAHA.124.039177 PMID: 40079339

Pereira, S. A., & Antunes, A. M. M. (2019). Special Issue "Adductomics: Elucidating the Environmental Causes of Disease.". *High-Throughput*, *8*(3), 17. DOI: 10.3390/ht8030017 PMID: 31370290

Pi, X., Wang, J., Chu, L., Zhang, G., & Zhang, W. (2025). Prediction of high-risk pregnancy based on machine learning algorithms. *Scientific Reports*, *15*(1), 15561. DOI: 10.1038/s41598-025-00450-3 PMID: 40319080

Pietruszyńska-Reszetarska, A., Pietruszyński, R., Majsterek, I., Popławski, T., Skrzypek, M., Kolesińska, B., Waśko, J., Kapusta, J., Watała, C., & Irzmański, R. (2024). Coronary Artery Disease Is Related to Methylation Disorders Caused by the c.1286A>C *MTHFR* Polymorphism and to Low Serum 5-MTHF and Folic Acid Concentrations—Preliminary Results. *Reports*, *7*(1), 6. DOI: 10.3390/reports7010006 PMID: 40729255

Plusquin, M., Chadeau-Hyam, M., Ghantous, A., Alfano, R., Bustamante, M., Chatzi, L., Cuenin, C., Gulliver, J., Herceg, Z., Kogevinas, M., Nawrot, T. S., Pizzi, C., Porta, D., Relton, C. L., Richiardi, L., Robinson, O., Sunyer, J., Vermeulen, R., Vriens, A., & Vineis, P. (2018). DNA methylome marks of exposure to particulate matter at three time points in early life. *Environmental Science & Technology*, *52*(9), 5427–5437. DOI: 10.1021/acs.est.7b06447 PMID: 29597345

Qin, J., Guo, N., Tong, J., & Wang, Z. (2021). Function of histone methylation and acetylation modifiers in cardiac hypertrophy. *Journal of Molecular and Cellular Cardiology*, *159*, 120–129. DOI: 10.1016/j.yjmcc.2021.06.011 PMID: 34175302

Rivera-Madera, A., Peña-Martínez, E. G., Messon-Bird, J. L., Pomales-Matos, D. A., Echevarría-Bonilla, O. L., Sanabria-Alberto, L., Peterson-Peguero, E. A., & Rodríguez-Martínez, J. A. (2025). Congenital heart disease missense mutations in the TBX5 DNA-binding domain alter thermal stability and DNA-binding affinity. https://doi.org/DOI: 10.1101/2025.05.16.654568

Rodríguez-Pérez, J. M., Ortega-Zhindón, D. B., Villamil-Castañeda, C., Lara-Ortiz, J. S., Borgonio-Cuadra, V. M., Cervantes-Salazar, J. L., Calderón-Colmenero, J., Escalante-Ruiz, Z. N., Retama-Méndez, E., Hernández-García, Y. C., & Pérez-Hernández, N. (2025). Congenital Heart Diseases: Recent Insights into Epigenetic Mechanisms. *Cells*, *14*(11), 820. DOI: 10.3390/cells14110820 PMID: 40497996

Romanò, A., Pagiatakis, C., Gornati, R., Bernardini, G., & Papait, R. (2025). Epigenetics: A link between toxicants and diseases. *iScience*, *28*(6), 112613. DOI: 10.1016/j.isci.2025.112613 PMID: 40487436

Ruan, Y., Liu, X., Zhu, H., Lu, Y., Liu, X., Han, J., Sun, L., Zhang, Y., Gu, X., Zhao, Y., Li, L., Ran, S., Chen, J., Yu, Q., Xu, Y., Xia, H., & He, Y. (2021). Noninherited Factors in Fetal Congenital Heart Diseases Based on Bayesian Network: A Large Multicenter Study. *Congenital Heart Disease*, *16*(6), 529–549. DOI: 10.32604/chd.2021.015862

Sahoo, K., & Sundararajan, V. (2024). Methods in DNA methylation array dataset analysis: A review. *Computational and Structural Biotechnology Journal*, *23*, 2304–2325. DOI: 10.1016/j.csbj.2024.05.015 PMID: 38845821

Sarwar, S., Aslam, S., Khalid, H., Hameed, M. A., & Khan, J., & Shabana. (2025). Polygenic risk score (PRS) analysis of genetic variants in a pediatric Pakistani population with ventricular septal defects (VSDs). *The Egyptian Journal of Medical Human Genetics*, *26*(1). Advance online publication. DOI: 10.1186/s43042-025-00661-3

Sevim Bayrak, C., Zhang, P., Tristani-Firouzi, M., Gelb, B. D., & Itan, Y. (2020). De novo variants in exomes of congenital heart disease patients identify risk genes and pathways. *Genome Medicine, 12*(1). Advance online publication. DOI: 10.1186/s13073-019-0709-8 PMID: 31941532

Shi, H., Book, W., Raskind-Hood, C., Downing, K. F., Farr, S. L., Bell, M. N., Sameni, R., Rodriguez, F. H.III, & Kamaleswaran, R. (2023). A machine learning model for predicting congenital heart defects from administrative data. *Birth Defects Research, 115*(18), 1693–1707. DOI: 10.1002/bdr2.2245 PMID: 37681293

Sierant, M. C., Jin, S. C., Bilguvar, K., Morton, S. U., Dong, W., Jiang, W., Lu, Z., Li, B., López-Giráldez, F., Tikhonova, I., Zeng, X., Lu, Q., Choi, J., Zhang, J., Nelson-Williams, C., Knight, J. R., Zhao, H., Cao, J., Mane, S., & Lifton, R. P. (2025). Genomic analysis of 11,555 probands identifies 60 dominant congenital heart disease genes. *Proceedings of the National Academy of Sciences of the United States of America, 122*(13), e2420343122. Advance online publication. DOI: 10.1073/pnas.2420343122 PMID: 40127276

Spendlove, S. J., Bondhus, L., Lluri, G., Sul, J. H., & Arboleda, V. A. (2022). Polygenic risk scores of endo-phenotypes identify the effect of genetic background in congenital heart disease. *Human Genetics and Genomics Advances, 3*(3), 100112. DOI: 10.1016/j.xhgg.2022.100112 PMID: 35599848

Spurrell, C. H., Barozzi, I., Kosicki, M., Mannion, B. J., Blow, M. J., Fukuda-Yuzawa, Y., Slaven, N., Afzal, S. Y., Akiyama, J. A., Afzal, V., Tran, S., Plajzer-Frick, I., Novak, C. S., Kato, M., Lee, E. A., Garvin, T. H., Pham, Q. T., Kronshage, A. N., Lisgo, S., & Visel, A. (2022). Genome-wide fetalization of enhancer architecture in heart disease. *Cell Reports, 40*(12), 111400. DOI: 10.1016/j.celrep.2022.111400 PMID: 36130500

Stingone, J. A., Luben, T. J., Carmichael, S. L., Aylsworth, A. S., Botto, L. D., Correa, A., Gilboa, S. M., Langlois, P. H., Nembhard, W. N., Richmond-Bryant, J., Shaw, G. M., & Olshan, A. F., & National Birth Defects Prevention Study. (2017). Maternal Exposure to Nitrogen Dioxide, Intake of Methyl Nutrients, and Congenital Heart Defects in Offspring. *American Journal of Epidemiology, 186*(6), 719–729. DOI: 10.1093/aje/kwx139 PMID: 28520847

Sumwiza, K., Twizere, C., Rushingabigwi, G., Bakunzibake, P., & Bamurigire, P. (2023). Enhanced cardiovascular disease prediction model using random forest algorithm. *Informatics in Medicine Unlocked, 41*, 101316. DOI: 10.1016/j.imu.2023.101316

Sun, Q., Ren, X., Sun, Z., & Duan, J. (2021). The critical role of epigenetic mechanism in $PM_{2.5}$-induced cardiovascular diseases. *Genes and Environment : the Official Journal of the Japanese Environmental Mutagen Society, 43*(1), 47. DOI: 10.1186/s41021-021-00219-w PMID: 34654488

Thompson, J.-L. M., Tarr, I. S., Rath, E. M., Troup, M., Ip, E. K. K., Dunwoodie, S. L., Winlaw, D., Giannoulatoudslo, E., Nassar, N., Kirk, E., Chapman, G., Blue, G., Sholler, G., Lain, S., Blue, G. M., Winlaw, D. S., Dunwoodie, S. L., & Giannoulatou, E. (2025). Polygenic Inheritance for Common Comorbidities Associated With Congenital Heart Disease. *JACC Advances, 4*(4), 101673. DOI: 10.1016/j.jacadv.2025.101673 PMID: 40120216

Thornton, J. M., Shah, N. M., Lillycrop, K. A., Cui, W., Johnson, M. R., & Singh, N. (2024). Multigenerational diabetes mellitus. *Frontiers in Endocrinology, 14*. Advance online publication. DOI: 10.3389/fendo.2023.1245899 PMID: 38288471

Tingting, T., Wenjing, F., Qian, Z., Hengquan, W., Simin, Z., Zhisheng, J., & Shunlin, Q. (2020). The TGF-β pathway plays a key role in aortic aneurysms. *Clinica Chimica Acta, 501*, 222–228. DOI: 10.1016/j.cca.2019.10.042 PMID: 31707165

Tocantins, C., Diniz, M. S., Grilo, L. F., & Pereira, S. P. (2022). The birth of cardiac disease: Mechanisms linking gestational diabetes mellitus and early onset of cardiovascular disease in offspring. *WIREs Mechanisms of Disease, 14*(4), e1555. DOI: 10.1002/wsbm.1555 PMID: 35304833

Toscano, A., & Moras, P. (2024). Artificial intelligence in congenital heart disease. *Intelligence-Based Cardiology and Cardiac Surgery*, 279–284. https://doi.org/DOI: 10.1016/b978-0-323-90534-3.00042-1

van der Linde, D., Konings, E. E., Slager, M. A., Witsenburg, M., Helbing, W. A., Takkenberg, J. J., & Roos-Hesselink, J. W. (2011). Birth prevalence of congenital heart disease worldwide: A systematic review and meta-analysis. *Journal of the American College of Cardiology, 58*(21), 2241–2247. DOI: 10.1016/j.jacc.2011.08.025 PMID: 22078432

Vitorino, R. (2024). Transforming Clinical Research: The Power of High-Throughput Omics Integration. *Proteomes, 12*(3), 25. DOI: 10.3390/proteomes12030025 PMID: 39311198

Voß, H., Schlumbohm, S., Barwikowski, P., Wurlitzer, M., Dottermusch, M., Neumann, P., Schlüter, H., Neumann, J. E., & Krisp, C. (2022). HarmonizR enables data harmonization across independent proteomic datasets with appropriate handling of missing values. *Nature Communications, 13*(1). Advance online publication. DOI: 10.1038/s41467-022-31007-x PMID: 35725563

Wang, G., Wang, B., & Yang, P. (2022). Epigenetics in Congenital Heart Disease. *Journal of the American Heart Association, 11*(7), e025163. DOI: 10.1161/JAHA.121.025163 PMID: 35348004

Wang, Y., Fang, Y., Lu, P., Wu, B., & Zhou, B. (2021). NOTCH Signaling in Aortic Valve Development and Calcific Aortic Valve Disease. *Frontiers in Cardiovascular Medicine, 8*, 682298. DOI: 10.3389/fcvm.2021.682298 PMID: 34239905

Wild, C. P. (2012). The exposome: From concept to utility. *International Journal of Epidemiology, 41*(1), 24–32. DOI: 10.1093/ije/dyr236 PMID: 22296988

Xiang, H., Zhuang, J., Bao, L., & Shi, Y. (2025). Variants and molecular mechanism of NOTCH1 in congenital heart disease. *Congenital Heart Disease, 20*(2), 245–263. DOI: 10.32604/chd.2025.064366

Xie, X., Huang, M., Ma, S., Xin, Q., Wang, Y., Hu, L., Zhao, H., Li, P., Liu, M., Yuan, R., Miao, Y., Zhu, Y., & Cong, W. (2025). The role of long non-coding RNAs in cardiovascular diseases: A comprehensive review. *Non-Coding RNA Research, 11*, 158–187. DOI: 10.1016/j.ncrna.2024.12.009 PMID: 39896344

Yan, S., Thienthanasit, R., Chen, D., Engelen, E., Brühl, J., Crossman, D. K., Kesterson, R., Wang, Q., Bouazoune, K., & Jiao, K. (2020). CHD7 regulates cardiovascular development through ATP-dependent and -independent activities. *Proceedings of the National Academy of Sciences of the United States of America, 117*(46), 28847–28858. DOI: 10.1073/pnas.2005222117 PMID: 33127760

Yasuhara, J., & Garg, V. (2021). Genetics of congenital heart disease: A narrative review of recent advances and clinical implications. *Translational Pediatrics, 10*(9), 2366–2386. DOI: 10.21037/tp-21-297 PMID: 34733677

Zaidi, S., & Brueckner, M. (2017). Genetics and genomics of congenital heart disease. *Circulation Research, 120*(6), 923–940. DOI: 10.1161/CIRCRESAHA.116.309140 PMID: 28302740

Zeng, W., Guo, H., Liu, Q., & Wong, W. H. (2025). Improving polygenic prediction from whole-genome sequencing data by leveraging predicted epigenomic features. *Proceedings of the National Academy of Sciences of the United States of America, 122*(24), e2419202122. DOI: 10.1073/pnas.2419202122 PMID: 40504151

Zhang, B., & Schmidlin, T. (2024). Recent advances in cardiovascular disease research driven by metabolomics technologies in the context of systems biology. *NPJ Metabolic Health and Disease, 2*(1). Advance online publication. DOI: 10.1038/s44324-024-00028-z PMID: 40603608

Zong, D., Liu, X., Li, J., Ouyang, R., & Chen, P. (2019). The role of cigarette smoke-induced epigenetic alterations in inflammation. *Epigenetics & amp. Chromatin*, *12*(1). Advance online publication. DOI: 10.1186/s13072-019-0311-8 PMID: 31711545

## KEY TERMS AND DEFINITIONS

**Adductomics:** It is the study of all covalent modifications called adducts that occur when reactive chemicals (from environmental pollutants, diet, drugs, or even normal metabolism) bind to biological molecules like DNA, RNA, or proteins.

# Chapter 6
# Polygenic and Oligogenic Risk in Congenital Heart Disease:
## A Systems View of Multifactorial Etiology

**Priya Sharma**
https://orcid.org/0000-0002-3942-6346
*School of Pharmacy and Emerging Sciences, Baddi University of Emerging Sciences and Technology, India*

**Ravinesh Mishra**
https://orcid.org/0000-0003-4559-1994
*School of Pharmacy and Emerging Sciences, Baddi University of Emerging Sciences and Technology, India*

**Bhartendu Sharma**
*School of Pharmacy and Emerging Sciences, Baddi University of Emerging Sciences and Technology, India*

**Archana Kumari**
*School of Pharmacy and Emerging Sciences, Baddi University of Emerging Sciences and Technology, India*

**Versha Sharma**
*Himachal Pharmacy College, Maganpura, India*

DOI: 10.4018/979-8-3373-3735-7.ch006

## ABSTRACT

*Congenital heart disease (CHD) is the most prevalent birth defect, resulting from complex interactions among genetic, environmental, and developmental factors. While monogenic causes explain a minority of cases, growing evidence supports the role of polygenic and oligogenic contributions in shaping CHD risk. This chapter explores the multifactorial etiology of CHD through a systems biology lens, integrating insights from genomics, teratology, and exposomics. It highlights gene-gene and gene-environment interactions, the utility of polygenic risk scores, and the influence of environmental exposures and epigenetic regulation on cardiac development. By examining emerging methodologies and data integration strategies, the chapter aims to advance understanding of CHD pathogenesis and inform precision medicine approaches for early diagnosis, risk assessment, and prevention.*

## 1. INTRODUCTION

Congenital heart disease (CHD) is the most common structural birth defect, affecting 8–10 per 1,000 live births worldwide. While syndromic cases may arise from well-defined chromosomal abnormalities or high-penetrance single-gene mutations, the majority of CHD is now recognized as multifactorial in origin, shaped by the interplay of numerous genetic variants, epigenetic modifications, and environmental exposures. Recent advances in genome-wide association studies, whole-exome and whole-genome sequencing, and systems biology approaches have revealed that polygenic risk (the cumulative effect of many small-effect variants), oligogenic inheritance (interacting rare variants), and regulatory non-coding changes together contribute significantly to disease susceptibility. At the same time, maternal teratogens and environmental factors can alter fetal epigenetic landscapes, further modifying cardiac gene expression and phenotype. Despite these insights, a unifying framework that integrates polygenic and oligogenic risk with environmental and epigenomic influences remains underdeveloped. This chapter addresses this gap by synthesizing emerging genetic, epigenetic, and exposomic evidence into a systems biology perspective, offering a comprehensive view of CHD etiology that is directly relevant to risk prediction, prevention, and personalized care (Liu et al., 2019). This is opposed to the classical Mendelian system in that; it takes one defective gene to manifest the phenotype. In CHD, genetic risk can be derived through polygenic risk (additive contribution of many common variants) and can be in turn conferred by any one independently interacting with environmental factors including maternal diabetes, drug-induced teratogen, and malnutrition (Li et al., 2024).

Epidemiological studies underscore the multifactorial nature of CHD. While certain syndromic forms of CHD can be traced to well-defined chromosomal abnormalities or single-gene defects (e.g., Down syndrome, 22q11.2 deletion syndrome, NKX2-5 mutations), the majority of cases are classified as sporadic with no obvious Mendelian inheritance. Findings on a higher concordance rate in monozygotic twins than the dizygotic twins as well as the high recurrence risk amongst sibling in the twin and family studies indicate a genetic involvement. However, incomplete concordance even among identical twins' points to the influence of non-genetic factors. Translational science leading to sophistication in genomics, transcriptomics, and bioinformatics has started to unravel the sophisticated genetic architecture of CHD. GWAS have revealed several loci with modest effects on CHD risk, rare coding variants in critical developmental genes have been identified with exome sequencing, and whole-genome sequencing has been used to identify novel genes and mechanisms linking genotype to disease phenotype in CHD. Integrative systems biology approaches are now being applied to map genetic interactions, model network perturbations, and predict phenotypic outcomes based on combined polygenic and oligogenic profiles. These approaches also facilitate the incorporation of epigenetic and environmental data, allowing for a more holistic understanding of CHD pathogenesis (Safdar et al., 2024).

## 2. OVERVIEW OF GENETIC CONTRIBUTIONS TO CONGENITAL HEART DISEASE

The genetic component of the congenital heart disease (CHD) is central in the predisposition and expression of the disease. Although CHD represents a wide array of structural anomalies involving various clinical presentations, a growing amount of evidence suggests that genome modification on a single-nucleotide level to complex chromosomal rearrangements may have severe impacts on tightly controlled mechanisms of cardiac morphogenesis. The unfolding of these genetic contributions plays an imperative role in disease insight understanding, improvement of the precision of diagnosis, and direction of interventions that target such regulations (Shabana et al., 2020).

### 2.1. The Spectrum of Genetic Variation in CHD

The genetic architecture of CHD is heterogeneous, encompassing:

- **Single-gene (monogenic) mutations**: Rare, high-penetrance variants that directly disrupt the function of a key developmental gene. Examples include mutations in *NKX2-5*, *GATA4*, and *TBX5*, which are linked to atrial septal defects, ventricular septal defects, and Holt–Oram syndrome.
- **Oligogenic inheritance**: The combined effect of pathogenic variants in two or more genes, each contributing partially to disease risk but producing a phenotype only when present together.
- **Polygenic risk**: The cumulative impact of numerous common variants with small individual effects, identified through genome-wide association studies (GWAS).
- **Chromosomal abnormalities**: Numerical or structural changes, such as trisomy 21 (Down syndrome), 22q11.2 deletion (DiGeorge syndrome), and Turner syndrome, which often involve complex cardiac defects.
- **Copy number variations (CNVs)**: Sub microscopic deletions or duplications that disrupt dosage-sensitive genes involved in heart development (Patel and Natarajan, 2019).

## 2.2. Monogenic Forms versus Multifactorial Cases

Congenital heart disease (CHD) can arise from both monogenic and multifactorial mechanisms, and distinguishing between these categories is critical for diagnosis, genetic counselling, and management. Monogenic forms of CHD result from pathogenic variants in a single gene with a large effect size, often inherited in Mendelian patterns such as autosomal dominant, autosomal recessive, or X-linked. These cases are typically associated with high penetrance and may present as part of well-characterized syndromes for example, *TBX5* mutations in Holt–Oram syndrome or *NOTCH1* mutations in bicuspid aortic valve disease. In contrast, multifactorial cases emerge from the combined influence of numerous genetic variants, both common and rare, interacting with environmental exposures such as maternal diabetes, teratogens, nutritional deficiencies, or hypoxia during pregnancy. While monogenic CHD can often be identified through targeted gene panels or whole-exome sequencing, multifactorial CHD requires a broader systems-level approach that incorporates polygenic risk scores, oligogenic variant analysis, and environmental risk modeling. Importantly, the clinical presentation of multifactorial CHD is highly variable, with incomplete penetrance and variable expressivity even among individuals sharing similar genetic backgrounds. Recognizing the distinction between monogenic and multifactorial origins not only guides the choice of genetic testing but also shapes patient management strategies, from targeted interventions in monogenic disorders to broader preventive measures in multifactorial cases (Farhan and Hegele, 2013).

## 2.3. Developmental Gene Networks in Cardiac Morphogenesis

Developmental gene networks orchestrate the precise and sequential events of cardiac morphogenesis, integrating multiple signalling pathways, transcriptional regulators, and structural genes to ensure correct heart formation. These networks operate as interconnected modules, where core transcription factors such as NKX2-5, GATA4, TBX5, MEF2C, and HAND family members interact with signalling pathways like Notch, Wnt/β-catenin, BMP, Hedgehog, and FGF to guide processes including cardiac progenitor cell specification, chamber formation, septation, valve development, and conduction system maturation. Each component of the network communicates via feedback and feedforward loops, ensuring robustness against developmental perturbations while maintaining flexibility for adaptive responses. Disruption of a single node whether by monogenic mutation, rare variant combinations, or polygenic burden can propagate through the network, leading to structural defects such as septal anomalies, outflow tract malformations, or abnormal valve architecture. Network redundancy and cross-pathway compensation often mitigate small perturbations, but simultaneous disruptions in multiple interacting genes (oligogenic effects) can exceed the system's buffering capacity. From a systems biology perspective, these networks resemble scale-free architectures with highly connected hub genes whose dysfunction disproportionately impacts developmental outcomes. Recent advances in single-cell RNA sequencing, CRISPR-based perturbation mapping, and computational network inference are enabling detailed reconstruction of these gene networks in human and model systems. Understanding these complex regulatory architectures not only clarifies the molecular etiology of congenital heart disease (CHD) but also opens avenues for targeted molecular therapies that restore or modulate critical developmental programs (Olson, 2006).

## 2.4. Insights from Genomic Technologies

### 2.4.1. Non-Coding Variants in CHD:

Recent research has highlighted that a considerable share of unexplained CHD heritability resides in rare non-coding variants. Unlike protein-coding mutations, these variants often alter regulatory elements such as enhancers, promoters, and non-coding RNAs, thereby influencing transcriptional programs critical for cardiac morphogenesis. For instance, variants affecting enhancer elements near TBX5 and NKX2-5 have been shown to disrupt normal temporal expression, leading to a trial and ventricular septal defect. Similarly, alterations in 3D chromatin architecture—such as disrupted topologically associating domains (TADs)—can decouple promoters from their enhancers, producing cardiac malformations without coding mutations.

Ongoing integrative studies combining whole-genome sequencing, ATAC-seq, and Hi-C chromatin conformation data are beginning to map these non-coding landscapes. This emerging focus on regulatory genomics underscores the importance of moving beyond coding sequences to capture the full genetic spectrum of CHD (Zaidi et al., 2021).

The last two decades have witnessed remarkable progress in identifying genetic contributors to CHD through advanced genomic tools:

- **GWAS** have uncovered common variants in loci such as *MYH6* and *PITX2* associated with atrial septal defects and other anomalies.
- **Whole-exome sequencing (WES)** has revealed rare, damaging variants in genes such as *CHD7*, *SMAD6*, and *NOTCH1* (Richter et al., 2022).
- **Whole-genome sequencing (WGS)** has expanded discovery beyond coding regions, highlighting the importance of non-coding regulatory elements.
- **Chromosomal microarray analysis** has improved detection of pathogenic CNVs, now recognized as a significant cause of both syndromic and non-syndromic CHD (Blue et al., 2017).

## 2.5. Variable Expressivity and Incomplete Penetrance

Two basic genetic principles variable expressivity and incomplete penetration are at the core to clinical diversity of congenital heart disease (CHD). Variable expressivity is the criteria and level extent of clinical manifestation in people carrying the identical pathogenic variant. As an illustration, a defect in a cardiac transcription factor gene can lead to a gross abnormal malformation in one patient, a minor defect of the valve in another, and virtually no detectable defect in a third patient all within the same family. The modifier genes, epigenetic alterations, environmental exposure as well as stochastic developmental events can change this variability. Incomplete penetrance, on the other hand, occurs when individuals who carry a disease-causing mutation do not exhibit any signs or symptoms of the condition. In CHD, this means that some genetic carriers remain phenotypically normal throughout life despite harboring variants known to be pathogenic. Incomplete penetrance poses significant challenges for genetic counselling, as predicting disease risk in carriers becomes more uncertain. Both phenomena highlight the complexity of CHD's genetic architecture, where genotype–phenotype correlations are often blurred. Understanding these mechanisms is crucial for accurate interpretation of genetic test results, refinement of polygenic and oligogenic risk models, and the development of personalized monitoring strategies that account for both genetic predisposition and the modifying influences that shape clinical outcomes (Russell et al., 2018).

Several studies illustrate how distinct genetic alterations can converge on similar CHD phenotypes, while modifier genes shape severity and penetrance. For example, mutations in NKX2-5, TBX5, and GATA4, though molecularly distinct, can all result in atrial septal defects by perturbing overlapping transcriptional networks. Similarly, both ciliary gene mutations and Hedgehog pathway variants have been linked to outflow tract malformations, highlighting convergence of mechanistically different factors on a common phenotype. Importantly, genetic modifiers can modulate disease expression: carriers of GATA4 mutations may range from severe atrioventricular septal defects to nearly normal cardiac anatomy depending on the presence of additional rare variants or protective alleles. This variability underscores the complexity of CHD inheritance and emphasizes the need for oligogenic models that account for interactions between primary mutations and secondary modifiers.

## 2.6. Integrating Genetic Data into Clinical Practice

The incorporation of genetic information into clinical care of congenital heart disease (CHD) is the landmark in the path to precision cardiology and provides the enhanced ability to diagnose, estimate and predict risks, and support personalized treatment of the patients. Recent innovations in genome technologies, including next-generation sequencing (NGS), whole-exome sequencing (WES), and whole-genome sequencing (WGS), have opened the possibility of identifying common and rare variants underlying CHD. When combined with tools like polygenic risk scores (PRS) and oligogenic variant analysis, clinicians can move beyond a binary "mutation present or absent" framework toward a more nuanced risk stratification model. This integration requires careful interpretation of genetic results in the context of clinical findings, family history, and environmental exposures, as not all identified variants have clear pathogenic significance. Multidisciplinary teams comprising cardiologists, geneticists, bioinformaticians, and genetic counsellors play a central role in translating genomic findings into actionable insights. Practical applications include prenatal screening for high-risk pregnancies, guiding surgical or interventional planning based on predicted disease severity, and tailoring long-term follow-up schedules to individual genetic profiles. However, challenges remain, including the need for standardized variant classification, ensuring equitable access to genetic testing, and addressing ethical concerns related to incidental findings and genetic privacy. Ultimately, the effective integration of genetic data into CHD care holds the potential to transform outcomes by enabling earlier detection, targeted intervention, and truly personalized treatment strategies (Sethi et al., 2023).

## 2.7. Towards a Systems Perspective

Moving towards a systems view of congenital heart disease (CHD) means abandoning a single-gene (or single-pathway) model in favour of a more holistic model in which genetic, epigenetic, environmental, and developmental interactions are taken into consideration. Rather than examining each risk component in isolation, systems biology aims to model how multiple layers of biological information genomic sequences, transcriptomic profiles, protein networks, metabolic pathways, and environmental influences interact to shape cardiac development and disease susceptibility. It is especially relevant to CHD, in which the influence of polygenic factors is often coupled with the impacts of oligogenic factors, maternal health, in-utero exposures, and stochastic mechanisms of development. The use of network-based models and pathways can be used to unveil major regulatory nodes and pathways that can be used as convergence points to various genetic variants as new drug targets. Combining multi-omics dataset and high type of computational modeling enables clinicians and researchers to more precisely predict the course of the disease and define the patients at the greatest risk and design interventions as needed. Systems view also enables transfer of research findings to effective population health approaches by considering genetic heterogeneity and environmental exposures of the populations. In the end, this strategy can help to narrow the knowledge-practice gap between molecular scientific and clinical delivery of CHD and eventually assist in achieving more predictive, precise and preventive care in persons with or at risk of CHD (Sperling, 2011).

# 3. POLYGENIC RISK: CUMULATIVE EFFECTS OF COMMON VARIANTS

Polygenic risk is a condition that is determined by multiple genetic variants and each usually has a small impact on an individual and the chances of a person developing a specific disease. Polygenic risk applies in congenital heart disease (CHD), wherein the notion of a specific mutation causing and preventing a disease or illness is replaced by the additive or interactive effect of numerous frequent alleles of the genome (Crouch and Bodmer, 2020). Such variants, typically found by genome-wide association studies (GWAS); do not on their own have enough impact on disease but accumulating them has a significant effect on developmental pathways as a whole, enough to cause a shift towards cardiac malformation with the addition of environmental, or epigenetic factors.

## 3.1. Nature of Common Variants in CHD

Common examples of such polygenic risk variants are likely to be single-nucleotide polymorphisms (SNPs) with distributions of the minor allele frequency (MAF) of least 5 percent in the population. The majority of these changes occur in non-coding regions of the genome and may have an impact on gene translation by altering enhancer action, promoter-targeting or alternative spliçing, and not by changing the tertiary structure of proteins directly. Fewer are located inside coding regions and result in subtle alterations of amino acids that have modest functional influences. In CHD, such variants often affect genes involved in developmental signalling pathways (e.g., Notch, Wnt, BMP) or transcriptional regulators essential for heart morphogenesis. For example, GWAS have implicated loci near *MYH6* in atrial septal defects and *PITX2* in atrial septal and conduction system abnormalities (Kido et al., 2018).

## 3.2. Additive and Interactive Effects

In congenital heart disease (CHD), genetic risk often arises not from a single causative variant but from the combined influence of multiple variants and environmental exposures. Additive effects occur when the contributions of different genetic variants sum together to increase overall disease risk, even if each variant individually exerts only a modest influence. For example, several common variants in cardiac developmental genes may each slightly perturb gene regulation, but together they can cross a threshold that disrupts normal heart morphogenesis. Interactive effects, by contrast, arise when the presence of one variant modifies the impact of another a phenomenon often referred to as epistasis. In such cases, the overall outcome may be more (synergistic) or less (antagonistic) than the combined effects (Domingo et al., 2019). Such interactions may not be between genes and genes alone but also between genes and the environment, e.g. an inherited vulnerability to vascular abnormalities of the outflow tract may be enhanced by maternal smoking or dietary insufficiencies during pregnancy. The relative importance of additive and interactive effects should be considered essential in construction of functional polygenic and oligogenic risk models since their omission may result to underestimates or diversion of the risks. Capturing these complexities in statistical and computational models increases our capacity to forecast the occurrence of CHD, inform our preventive guidance, and reveal new molecular pathways, which grow out of the interaction of numerous contributing factors (Sharma et., 2025).

### 3.3. Polygenic Risk Scores (PRS) in CHD Research

A novel emerging technique, polygenic risk score (PRS), is beginning to feature prominently in the study of congenital heart disease (CHD) since it is a quantitative measure of the heritable number of common risk variants of a person, based upon a count of risk alleles, weighted by the effect size of each as reported in genome-wide association studies (GWAS). APPLYING PRS In CHD, PRS seek to reflect the effects of many small-influence single-nucleotide polymorphisms (SNPs) that when added together may have a large impact on cardiac developmental pathways (Inouye et al., 2021). Despite its prevalence elsewhere in other complex diseases (coronary artery disease, type 2 diabetes, and breast cancer), the application of PRS in CHD is still in an early stage of deployment owing to the small number of large multi-ethnic GWAS data used in the field. Preliminary studies suggest that PRS could eventually assist in stratifying individuals by genetic susceptibility, enabling targeted screening in families with a history of CHD or in pregnancies identified as high risk through fetal imaging (Musunuru et al., 2021). However, several challenges limit immediate clinical translation, including modest predictive power, potential bias due to population-specific allele frequencies, and the difficulty of integrating PRS with other risk determinants such as rare variants, environmental exposures, and epigenetic modifications. Future advances in genomic data integration, functional validation, and machine learning–based modeling may enhance the utility of PRS, paving the way for their incorporation into precision medicine approaches for CHD (Tcheandjieu et al., 2022; Giudicessi et al., 2021).

### 3.4. Biological Mechanisms Linking Common Variants to CHD

Common genetic changes that have been linked to congenital heart disease (CHD) have small individual effects, but on a biological scale can have devastating effects when considered collectively using the concept of developmental systems biology. A large proportion of these forms lie in non-coding sequences of the genome, affecting the regulation of transcription as opposed to the structure of the proteins themselves. These variants may have subtle effects by altering enhancer activity, binding region of promoters, or three-dimensional chromatin structure, thus changing the expression of key cardiac developmental genes at critical windows of embryonic development (Khurana et al., 2016). This breakdown of developmental buffering or canalization increases the susceptibility to morphological defects when other risk factors, such as rare variants, environmental exposures, or stochastic developmental events, are present. Moreover, common variants can influence the function of transcription factor networks (e.g., *GATA*, *NKX2-5*, *TBX* families) and microRNA-mediated post-transcriptional regulation, further compounding subtle developmental imbalances. Thus, while each common variant may have negligible pathogenicity on its own, their combined regulatory effects can erode the stability of complex genetic networks, creating a developmental landscape more prone to structural anomalies in the heart.

## 3.5. Clinical Implications of Polygenic Risk in CHD

Clinical implications The main clinical implications of polygenic risk in congenital heart disease (CHD) are the potential to improve early detection and risk stratification as well as to drive prevention. The polygenic risk scores (PRS) might be used to assess the total risk of rare genetic variants, to determine in advance which individuals or families are at high risk, making closer monitoring through advanced fetal echocardiography during pregnancy or postnatal screening, or later cardiovascular monitoring possible. For couples with a family history of CHD, PRS combined with rare variant analysis and environmental risk assessment may inform reproductive counselling and personalized prenatal care strategies aimed at reducing modifiable risks, such as maternal smoking, poorly controlled diabetes, or exposure to teratogens. In the future, integration of PRS into electronic health records, alongside environmental and lifestyle data, could support predictive models that guide individualized prevention plans. However, the probabilistic nature of polygenic risk means that a high PRS does not guarantee disease occurrence, and a low PRS does not exclude it. Therefore, PRS should be interpreted as part of a broader multifactorial framework rather than as a standalone diagnostic tool. Translating polygenic risk into clinical practice will require larger, multi-ethnic genomic studies, robust validation of predictive models, and clear communication strategies to ensure patients and families understand the meaning and limitations of genetic risk information (Pierpont et al., 2018).

# 4. OLIGOGENIC RISK: INTERACTIONS OF MULTIPLE RARE VARIANTS

Oligogenic risk in congenital heart disease (CHD) refers to the scenario in which two or more rare, functionally significant genetic variants each insufficient on its own to cause disease interact to produce a pathogenic outcome. Unlike monogenic inheritance, where a single high-penetrance mutation is the primary driver of disease, oligogenic inheritance reflects a combined effect model in which multiple variants, often in genes within the same developmental pathway or molecular complex, act together to disrupt cardiac morphogenesis. This interaction may be additive, where each variant independently contributes to the overall pathogenic threshold, or synergistic, where the combined effect is greater than the sum of individual effects due to pathway-level amplification or compensatory mechanism failure (Kalisch-Smith et al., 2020).

Oligogenic risk in CHD tends to be found when the variants affect genes that physically or functionally interact (including networks of transcription factors, NKX2-5, GATA4, TBX5) or structural constituents of the cardiac cytoskeleton. Take the case of a patient with heterozygous variant GATA4 variant and the NKX2-5 variant; they can have more severe or complex defects compared to a patient with any variant. Likewise, mutations in the Notch signalling pathway components or sarcomeric gene products collectively may work to undermine development strength, predisposing to structural malformations, including a conotruncal defect or atrioventricular septal defect (Gifford et al., 2019). This principle has been confirmed in model organisms through experimental trials with two hypomorphic alleles in different cardiac genes able to introduce a defect not observed by either of the mutations when using only a single allele. Improved NGS technologies (both whole-exome sequencing (WES) and whole-genome sequencing (WGS) and bioinformatic tools being optimized to identify combinations of variants based on gene-gene interaction, co-expression profiles and protein-protein interaction networks have enabled the identification of the oligogenic inheritance (Szot et al., 2020).

Clinically, recognizing oligogenic risk has important implications for genetic counselling and patient management. Families with oligogenic inheritance patterns may not display traditional Mendelian segregation, and recurrence risks can be more difficult to estimate (Berliner and Fay, 2007).

The interplay of polygenic and oligogenic mechanisms is increasingly recognized in the clinical manifestation of CHD. For example, a patient harboring rare variants in NKX2-5 and GATA4 may present with complex atrioventricular defects, whereas either variant alone produces no detectable phenotype, illustrating oligogenic synergy. Conversely, polygenic risk scores (PRS) capture the additive effects of numerous common variants with small effect sizes, stratifying risk at the population level. However, PRS accuracy is often limited by the underrepresentation of non-European populations in genome-wide association studies. Future progress lies in combining PRS with oligogenic variant analysis and exposomic data, thereby creating integrative models that account for both inherited and environmental contributions. Clinically, such combined models could refine prenatal counseling, improve family risk assessment, and identify pregnancies requiring intensified surveillance (Priest et al., 2022).

## 5. EPISTASIS AND GENE–GENE INTERACTIONS IN CARDIAC DEVELOPMENT

Epistasis is the interaction between two or more genes where the presence or absence of one or more genes changes the influence of one gene upon a phenotype. With the examples of congenital heart disease (CHD), epistasis highlights the fact that genetic regulation during development of cardiac processes is complicated by multiple genes acting in parallel pathways and molecular networks. These interactions may also both predispose the probability of developing a defect, as well as determine its severity, its anatomical pattern, and extracardiac manifestations. Learning the concept of epistasis is hence fundamental in explaining the genetic architecture of CHD, especially the multifactorial and oligogenic variants that have multiple genetic variants that determine susceptibility to the disease (Vecoli et al., 2014). A highly organized set of cellular and molecular events that activate transcription factors, signal transduction molecules, structural and metabolic regulators control cardiac morphogenesis. The most important transcriptional regulators that include NKX2-5, GATA4, and TBX5 will tend to cooperate, and such cooperation may take place as multi-protein complexes that attach to cardiac gene promoters and enhancers to define whether there is an activation or repression of transcription.

Epistatic effects in CHD are not limited to protein–protein interactions but also include regulatory gene networks and non-coding RNAs. For example, a variant in a transcription factor may have a more pronounced effect if a co-regulated microRNA that normally buffers its downstream targets is also altered. Furthermore, modifier genes that do not cause CHD on their own but modulate the expressivity and penetrance of primary disease-causing mutations are a well-recognized epistatic element (Akanda et al., 2025). Experimental validation has also been carried out in animal models including double knockout or compound heterozygote studies and has clearly demonstrated that some gene-gene combinations result in cardiac malformations not observed in single-mutant counterparts. In clinical practice, epistasis is of importance in genetic counselling of CHD and risk prediction. When more than one interacting variant is observed an increase in the risk of recurrence can be larger than the observed effect of individual variants would suggest (Chaix et al., 2016). This also extends to personalized medicine where the therapy or preventative procedures could possibly have to work on more than one molecular pathway to reinstate developmental harmony. The ultimate impact of including epistasis in genetic models is to shift genetics toward more complex models of genotype-by genotype associations, that are more mechanistic and more appropriate in perspective with the complex interaction of many genetic factors in the same cardiac outcome.

## 6. MOLECULAR PATHWAYS IMPLICATED IN CHD

The development of the human heart is coordinated by a molecular pathway network controlling cell specification, cell proliferation, cell migration, cell differentiation, and tissue remodelling. Interference with these pathways either at the genetic, epigenetic, or environmental level may lead to structural cardiac malformations which in aggregate are called congenital heart disease (CHD). Although hundreds of different genes have been associated with CHD, these genes ultimately share relatively few developmental pathways, a reflection of the principle that phenotypically similar outcomes can be produced by a wide variety of genetic lesions when they act within common core biological processes (MacGrogan et al., 2018).

### 6.1. Notch Signalling Pathway

The key signalling pathway in management of cardiac development is the Notch signalling pathway that influences the cell fate, differentiation, proliferation and heart morphogenesis. Under the background of CHD, defects in Notch signalling either because of rare pathogenic mutations, common regulatory variants, or due to aberrant epigenetic perturbations may disturb the fine orchestration of events involved in a normal heart formation. The pathway is initiated when Notch receptors (NOTCH1–4) on the cell surface interact with transmembrane ligands such as Jagged (JAG1, JAG2) and Delta-like proteins (DLL1, DLL3, DLL4) from neighbouring cells. The ensuing proteolytic events cleave the ligand-bound receptor, liberating the Notch intracellular domain (NICD) that translocates into the nucleus and controls the transcription of such downstream target genes as HES and HEY family members. The outflow tract formation, definite valve morphogenesis and ventricular chamber specification, in particular, require dramatic notch signalling (MacGrogan et al., 2018).

### 6.2. Wnt/β-Catenin Signalling Pathway

The Wnt/β-catenin signalling pathway plays a key role as a central regulator of embryonic heart development, cell proliferation, differentiation, polarity, and patterning of the heart. In canonical pathway, surface localization of secreted Wnt ligands and Frizzled receptors together with low-density lipoprotein receptor related proteins (LRP5/6) on the cell surface results in suppression of the β-catenin destruction complex, a complex made up of APC, Axin and glycogen synthase kinase (GSK-3β). This suppression feeds the accumulation of β-catenin in the cytoplasm and its translocation into the nucleus to combine with TCF/LEF transcription factors to drive the activation of gene-expression programs that specify cardiac mesoderm identity, organise chambers, and develop valves. The temporal and spatial regulation of Wnt signalling is critical: early activation promotes mesoderm induction, whereas later suppression is necessary for proper cardiac differentiation (Ozhan and Weidinger, 2015).

## 6.3. Bone Morphogenetic Protein (BMP) Pathway

Bone Morphogenetic Protein (BMP) pathway is a significant regulator of heart development, which controls essential processes in early heart development, chamber differentiation and valve morphogenesis and septation. The BMPs belong to transforming growth factor-beta (TGF-beta) superfamily of secreted growth factors. During embryogenesis, they bind the BMP2, BMP4, and BMP10 by the ligands of BMP into a heteromeric complex of type I (BMPR1A, BMPR1B) and type II (BMPR2) serine/threonine kinase receptors on the target cell. This interaction activates intracellular SMAD proteins (SMAD1, SMAD5, SMAD8), which form complexes with SMAD4 and translocate to the nucleus to regulate transcription of downstream genes involved in myocardial differentiation, endocardial cushion formation, and outflow tract remodelling. The BMP signalling is both dose and time dependent and extra or low levels of activation causes tasks related heart malformations like atrioventricular septal defects, ventricular malformations, and hypoplastic ventricular malformations. The potent cause of pulmonary arterial hypertension, which may be among the comorbidities of CHD, is mutations in BMPR2 and other components of the pathway. Importantly, BMP signalling is integrated with other developmental pathways, including Wnt, Notch, and FGF, to ensure precise morphogenetic patterning. Disruption of this crosstalk can exacerbate developmental errors (Morrell et al., 2016).

## 6.4. Hedgehog Signalling Pathway

The important controller of heart development during embryogenesis is the Hedgehog (Hh) signalling pathway, which modulates cell proliferation, differentiation, left-right patterning, and outflow tract/ heart chamber morphogenesis. When secreted Hedgehog ligands of the form Sonic Hedgehog (SHH), Indian Hedgehog (IHH), or Desert Hedgehog (DHH) bind the transmembrane receptor Patched (PTCH1), this pathway and its downstream signaling chain are activated. Without a ligand, PTCH1 represses Smoothened (SMO), one of the activators of signalling. Ligand binding relieves this inhibition, allowing SMO to activate downstream transcription factors of the GLI family (GLI1, GLI2, GLI3), which then regulate the expression of target genes critical for cardiac progenitor cell specification, ventricular septation, and arterial pole alignment (Fitzsimons *et al.*, 2022). Disruption of the pathway through mutations in SHH, PTCH1, SMO, or GLI genes, or through environmental insults affecting ciliary function (given the pathway's reliance on primary cilia) has been linked to congenital heart defects including tetralogy of Fallot, atrioventricular septal defects, and pulmonary atresia (Malta et al., 2023).

## 6.5. Fibroblast Growth Factor (FGF) Pathway

The Fibroblast Growth Factor (FGF) signalling pathway plays a pivotal role in multiple stages of cardiac development, including mesoderm induction, proliferation and migration of cardiac progenitor cells, myocardial differentiation, and morphogenesis of the outflow tract and valves. FGFs are a family of secreted proteins (e.g., FGF2, FGF8, FGF10, FGF16) that exert their effects by binding to FGF receptors (FGFR1–FGFR4), which possess intrinsic tyrosine kinase activity. Ligand binding-often facilitated by heparan sulphate proteoglycans induces receptor dimerization and autophosphorylation, activating downstream signalling cascades such as MAPK/ERK, PI3K/AKT, and PLCγ. These cascades regulate gene expression programs critical for proper cardiac chamber specification, endocardial cushion development, and myocardial compaction. Among these, FGF8 is especially important for outflow tract alignment, while FGF10 supports right ventricular and atrial growth. Dysregulation of the FGF pathway, whether through mutations in FGFRs, alterations in ligand expression, or disruption of co-factor availability, has been associated with congenital heart defects such as conotruncal anomalies, atrial septal defects, and ventricular hypoplasia. The FGF pathway does not act in isolation-it exhibits extensive cross-talk with BMP, Wnt, and Notch signalling to coordinate the spatial and temporal progression of cardiac development. From a clinical standpoint, understanding FGF signalling disruptions can enhance genetic counseling, risk prediction, and the design of potential regenerative strategies, particularly given the pathway's demonstrated role in stimulating cardiomyocyte proliferation and angiogenesis in experimental cardiac repair models (Działo et al., 2018).

## 6.6. Transcription Factor Networks

Transcription factor (TF) networks are central regulators of cardiac development, integrating multiple genetic and signalling cues to orchestrate the precise temporal and spatial activation of target genes. These networks consist of key cardiac transcription factors including NKX2-5, GATA4, TBX5, TBX20, MEF2C, HAND1, HAND2, and ISL1 that function in interconnected regulatory loops. They control processes such as mesodermal specification, cardiomyocyte differentiation, chamber morphogenesis, conduction system development, and valve formation. Many of these TFs act combinatorially; for example, NKX2-5 and GATA4 synergize to activate structural genes required for atrial and ventricular development, while TBX5 interacts with NKX2-5 to coordinate septation and conduction pathway maturation. Mutations in these TFs often result in congenital heart defects such as atrial septal defects, ventricular septal defects, Holt–Oram syndrome, and conduction abnormalities (Munshi, 2012).

## 6.7. Chromatin-Modifying and Cilia-Related Genes in CHD

Beyond canonical signaling pathways, recent discoveries highlight chromatin-modifying genes and cilia-related genes as critical contributors to congenital heart disease. Chromatin remodelers such as SMARCA4, KMT2D, and NSD1 regulate histone methylation and acetylation, thereby controlling accessibility of cardiac transcriptional networks. Mutations in these genes have been linked to syndromic CHD presentations, emphasizing the importance of epigenetic regulation in cardiogenesis. Likewise, genes required for primary cilia structure and function play pivotal roles in Hedgehog signaling and left–right patterning. Disruption of ciliary proteins (e.g., DNAH11, DYNC2H1) has been associated with conotruncal malformations, heterotaxy, and atrioventricular septal defects. Incorporating these emerging categories of genes into CHD research broadens the spectrum of genetic drivers and connects molecular epigenetics with developmental signaling and structural morphogenesis (Mishra et., 2025).

## 6.8. Extracellular Matrix (ECM) and Cytoskeletal Pathways

The extracellular matrix (ECM) and cytoskeletal lines of inquiry are essential to shaping the heart during development as they offer not only physical scaffolding, but also fluid signalling messaging tracks, which instruct cellular behaviour. The ECM comprising proteins such as collagens (COL1A1, COL3A1), fibronectin, laminins, elastin, and proteoglycans forms a specialized microenvironment around cardiac cells. It does not only help retain tissue integrity but is part of the biochemical signalling by interacting with cell-surface receptors such as integrins and dystroglycans to activate downstream pathways such as FAK (focal adhesion kinase) and MAPK/ERK which regulate cell adhesion, migration, proliferation and differentiation. Parallel, the mechanical stability, contractility and intracellular transport are enabled by the cytoskeleton which is comprised of actin filaments, microtubules, and intermediate filaments (Nakayama et al., 2014).

## 7. INTEGRATION OF GENETIC AND ENVIRONMENTAL RISK FACTORS

The etiology of congenital heart disease (CHD) is rarely attributable to genetic or environmental influences alone; instead, it typically reflects the interplay between both. This integration of risk factors aligns with the multifactorial model of disease; wherein inherited susceptibility interacts with prenatal exposures and developmental events to determine the eventual phenotype. Recognizing this complexity is essential for accurate risk assessment, targeted prevention, and improved prognostic prediction.

### 7.1. The Genetic Predisposition Framework

Genetic susceptibility to CHD may stem from rare high-impact mutations, oligogenic combinations of multiple rare variants, or the polygenic accumulation of common alleles with small effect sizes. These genetic factors establish a baseline level of vulnerability by influencing molecular pathways critical for cardiac morphogenesis, such as Notch, Wnt, BMP, and FGF signalling. However, this predisposition alone may not be sufficient to trigger a structural defect. The phenotypic outcome often depends on additional stressors introduced during embryogenesis (MacKenzie, 2024).

### 7.2. Environmental Contributors to CHD

Environmental risk factors act during pregnancy to disrupt normal heart development. Key contributors include maternal illnesses (e.g., diabetes mellitus, phenylketonuria, viral infections such as rubella), teratogenic medications (e.g., retinoic acid, certain anticonvulsants), alcohol consumption, smoking, nutritional deficiencies (e.g., folate deficiency), and exposure to environmental toxins (e.g., pesticides, heavy metals). The timing, duration, and intensity of exposure are critical, as cardiac morphogenesis occurs between the third and eighth weeks of gestation, a window of heightened vulnerability.

### 7.3. Gene–Environment Interactions (G×E)

Gene–environment interactions occur when the effect of an environmental exposure on CHD risk is modified by an individual's genetic makeup. For example, maternal hyperglycaemia is more likely to result in cardiac defects in fetuses carrying variants in oxidative stress–response genes or transcription factors regulating myocardial cell survival. Similarly, maternal folate deficiency may have a stronger impact in individuals with polymorphisms in folate metabolism genes (MTHFR,

MTRR). These interactions can magnify risk beyond what would be expected from either factor alone (Talmud, 2007).

## 7.4. Epigenetic Mediation

Indirectly, environmental influences may mediate the CHD risk by altering epigenetic processes (including DNA methylation, histone modifications, and non-coding RNA) regulation. These adaptations are able to change the expression of cardiac developmental genes without changing the DNA itself so there is a mechanical connection between environmental exposures and genetic susceptibility. Importantly, some epigenetic marks are reversible, raising the possibility of targeted interventions during pregnancy (Bi et al., 2024).

The emerging field of exposomics offers powerful tools to comprehensively profile maternal environmental exposures and their biological consequences. High-resolution mass spectrometry, biomonitoring of metabolites, and exposome-wide association studies (EWAS) can be integrated with epigenomic data to identify exposure-driven methylation or histone modification patterns in cardiac developmental genes (Burridge at al., 2021). For instance, combining exposomic profiling of maternal serum with DNA methylation analysis in cord blood has revealed exposure-specific epigenetic signatures that predict structural heart defects. Such integrative approaches expand beyond traditional teratogen identification by capturing the cumulative and interacting effects of diverse exposures. Moving forward, linking exposomic data with polygenic and oligogenic risk models could enable precision risk prediction and early prenatal interventions tailored to individual maternal–fetal contexts (Vrijheid at al., 2020).

## 7.5. Implications for Risk Prediction and Prevention

Incorporating both genetic and environmental data into predictive models allows for a more accurate assessment of CHD risk. Polygenic risk scores (PRS) can be combined with environmental exposure histories to identify pregnancies at higher risk, guiding decisions on enhanced prenatal surveillance or targeted preventive strategies. Preconception counseling can also incorporate G×E insights, encouraging optimal maternal health, avoidance of teratogens, and nutritional supplementation in genetically susceptible individuals.

## 8. EPIGENETIC MODULATION IN CHD SUSCEPTIBILITY

The epigenetic modulating functions are imperative in determining the direction and future development of the heart through gene expression regulation but not a change in the gene sequence. In congenital heart disease (CHD), DNA methylation, histone modifications and regulation via non-coding RNA may contribute to either silence or express genes that regulate cardiac morphogenesis in the susceptibility process. Or, as an illustration, transcriptional defects may occur in the hearts developing structure due to aberrant methylation of the promoters of the critical genes in development, e.g. NKX2-5 or GATA4. Chromatin accessibility is controlled dynamically by histone acetylation and methylation that are facilitated by histone acetyltransferases (HATs), histone deacetylases (HDACs), and others, to influence the timing and strength of gene expression throughout cardiac development. Also, there are microRNAs (miRNAs) and long non-coding RNAs (lncRNAs) that serve as post-transcriptional modulators, impacting the stability and translation rates of mRNAs encoding structural proteins, signalling molecules and transcription factors. Fetal epigenome may also be modified by environmental exposure through maternal diabetes, hypoxia or teratogenic drugs contributing to a convergence between environmental and genetic factors. Recent studies demonstrate that maternal exposure to teratogens can directly alter the fetal epigenome, thereby influencing cardiac gene expression during critical windows of development. For example, maternal diabetes has been associated with global DNA hypomethylation and hyperacetylation of histones in genes regulating cardiomyocyte proliferation, predisposing to septal and outflow tract malformations. Similarly, retinoic acid exposure alters Hox gene methylation, disrupting left–right patterning, while valproic acid, a histone deacetylase inhibitor, produces aberrant chromatin states at loci such as NKX2-5 and GATA4 (Wu et al., 2021).

## 9. SYSTEMS BIOLOGY APPROACHES TO CHD RISK PREDICTION

The hypothesis of systems biology-based prediction of risk of congenital heart disease (CHD) is complex and multifactorial, so it is expected to reduce the volume of biological, clinical and environmental data into model unities. Contrary to the establishment of single-gene genetics or single-variant modeling, systems biology recognizes the heart as a system of interacting molecular pathways and cellular processes as well as physiological systems. Integrating genomic, transcriptomic, proteomic, metabolomic, and epigenomic data with environmental exposure data and clinical phenotyping can allow researchers to build predictive network models of CHD, one that reflects both the genetic architecture and environmental factors in the condition. The computational techniques, incorporating network-based association mapping, Bayesian, and machine learning algorithms are becoming common because it helps to determine key molecular hubs and interaction patterns that could be used as biomarkers or targets of intervention. As an example, it is possible to consider the ways of combining polygenic risk scores with transcriptomic signatures of early cardiac differentiation to better predict the occurrence of CHD in high-risk pregnancies. The methods have the benefits not only of better risk stratification, but also of offering mechanistic information on disease pathways, allowing more personalized preventive and treatment strategies. The final state is to switch the descriptive association to predictive actionable models that can be implemented in the clinical context to detect early on in life, precision counselling, and optimal prenatal care.

## 10. NETWORK ANALYSIS OF CARDIAC GENE INTERACTIONS

Cardiac gene-gene interactions network analysis offers a strong approach to congenital heart disease (CHD) through the multiple gene involvement that is present. In contrast to the single genes approach, this methodology ties together genes, proteins, and regulatory features to demonstrate the interaction networks that are actually making up cardiac morphogenesis. Nodes on these networks are genes or proteins and edges are functional or physical interactions, e.g. transcriptional regulation, protein binding, or, common signalling pathway. By applying computational algorithms to genomic, transcriptomic, and proteomic datasets, researchers can identify highly connected "hub" genes such as *GATA4*, *NKX2-5*, and *TBX5* that act as central regulators of heart development. The network is usually highly affected by the disturbance of such hubs which raises vulnerabilities to CHD. Moreover, network topology comparison is likely to reveal modules or clusters of genes that participate in an engineered developmental process, like outflow tract formation or ventricular septation. By combining these networks with information on environmental exposure and epigenetic data, one will be able to identify the hotspots of genes involved in the interaction with the environment even better. Finally, network-derived inferences ease the choice of candidate genes to be functionally validated and support the development of predictive models based on the network nature of interdependent cardiac developmental channels (Lage et al., 2012).

## 11. BIOINFORMATIC TOOLS FOR POLYGENIC AND OLIGOGENIC RISK ASSESSMENT

Various manifestations of congenital heart disease (CHD) and polygenetic / oligogenic risk evaluation thereof would also be on better footing provided with bioinformatic tools that could handle processing of large-scale genomics databases and use such platforms to identify clinically applicable information within complex genetic systems. When there is a polygenic risk, then platforms like genome-wide association study (GWAS) analysis such as PLINK, LDpred and PRSice may be used to calculate polygenic risk score (PRS) as an estimate of the cumulative small effects of thousands of common variations. Such tools use the information of linkage disequilibrium (LD) structure, allele frequency and effect size to produce person-centered risk scores. In the case of the oligogenic risk, such a special approach is directed at determining combinations of pathogenic variants in gene networks or common development pathways. Platform like VarCards, ORVAL (Oligogenic Resource for Variant Analysis), or GeneMANIA enable the exploration of the possible interactions between genes, as well as predicting their functional effects on them and prioritizing variant combinations, based on protein interactions, co-expression patterns and phenotypic annotations. Enhanced frameworks such as Cytoscape also allow visualizing and modeling even the complex interaction among genes, spanning the gap between raw data of the variants and developmental biology context (Fotiou et al., 2019).

## 12. CLINICAL APPLICATIONS: GENETIC TESTING AND RISK STRATIFICATION

Genetic testing and risk stratification in congenital heart disease (CHD) have become commonplace in the clinical practice as genomic technologies as well as better understanding of being a multifactorial illness has paved the way to novel methods of measuring risk and minimizing morbidity and mortality. Recent advances in genetic testing that include targeted gene panels and whole-exome sequencing (WES) through to the whole-genome sequencing (WGS) have permitted the detection of both rare, high-impact and more common variants with a combined effect of variants expressed as polygenic risk scores (PRS). The variant interpretation includes network-based solvability analysis in the case of oligogenic CHD cases to consider the overall impact of multiple rare variants on the pathways of cardiac development (Yasuhara and Garg, 2021). With increasing clinical adoption, ethical considerations, data confidentiality, and even access to genomic testing that is reasonably distributed will continue to be key factors towards maximising the benefits of genetic-based risk prediction (Islam et al., 2025).

## 13. CHALLENGES IN TRANSLATING GENETIC FINDINGS TO CLINICAL PRACTICE

Application of genetic results in clinical practice of congenital heart disease (CHD) has several scientific, logistical, and ethical concerns. One of the biggest challenges is the interpretation of genetic variants including so-called variants of uncertain significance (VUS), where functional impacts of the genetic variants are not yet clear. Patients and families can face difficulty in making decisions and counselling with this uncertainty. The incomplete penetrance and variability of expressivity of the polygenic or oligogenic risk factors is another obstacle, namely, not all individuals with high-risk genetic constitutions might develop CHD, whereas others with low-risk genetic profiles might do so as well (Girolami *et al.*, 2018). To implement polygenic risk scores (PRS) into clinical practice, strong validation in diverse populations would be necessary, but the data on which the field currently thrives is mostly favouring European ancestry and thus underrepresented. These gaps will need to be addressed through collaboration across geneticists, cardiologists, bioinformaticians and policymakers to develop evidence-based protocols, increase data diversities and provide equitable access to genomics-based treatment (Nogel, 2025).

## 14. FUTURE DIRECTIONS IN PERSONALIZED MEDICINE FOR CHD

Genomics, multi-omics integration, and precision therapeutics will correspond to future directions of personalized medicine in the field of congenital heart disease (CHD). With improved speed, cost, and accuracy, sequencing technologies will allow the run of whole-genome sequencing (WGS) and long-read sequencing in the context of routine clinical practice to achieve coverage of both common and rare deleterious variants that affect the risk of CHD. Combining the multi-omics data incorporated with transcriptomics, proteomics, and metabolomics, epigenomics will give a more comprehensive systems-level perspective into cardiac development and predilection to disease (Banerjee et al., 2021). The application of machine learning and artificial intelligence (AI) models is projected to be at the forefront in risk prediction as they can be used to incorporate genetic, environmental, and clinical factors in producing personal care plans. Gene-based therapies, e.g., CRISPR-based gene correction or

RNA-targeting therapies can be potentially used at some CHD instances with clearly defined causal variants in the treatment domain. Additionally, genomic data can be combined with wearable gadgets and digital wellbeing to allow CHD patients to be tracked and managed dynamically. Notably, the future of personalized medicine with CHD will include the guarantee of equitable access, sound ethical outfitting, and culturally adequate genetic counselling to transform the application of the newest scientific research into the actual health wellbeing of all individuals touched by the condition (Torrorey-Sawe, 2025).

## 15. CONCLUSION

Congenital heart disease (CHD) serves as an illustration of the fact these multifactorial disorders are characterized by intricate interrelationship between environmental factors and genetic susceptibility, where the disease has its manifestation as a result of action of both factors. A predominant number of studies highlight that single-gene mutations and purely environmental factors cannot be solely responsible of subsuming CHD phenotypes. Rather, both continuous contributions of the additive result of many common risk variants, formally referred to as polygenic risk, and the interactions of a few rare risk variants, collectively known as oligogenic risk, are involved in disease predisposition. This dual construct offers a more balanced explanation of CHD etiology and leaves the one-dimensional monogenic explanatory model behind. The last decade has seen growing interest in the extent of common genetic variation (achieved with the advent of genome-wide association studies (GWAS) and advances in next-generation sequencing (NGS)) and the depth of rare variant interactions (achieved using ever more sophisticated bioinformatic tools). The application of the concept of polygenic risk scores (PRS) in CHD research has envisioned the prospects of measuring inherited risk in individuals and oligogenic routes have emphasised how variant combinations acting along shared molecular pathways like cardiac morphogenesis, myocardial signalling and valve formation can cause variable developmental pathways. Notably, network-based studies and systems biology have shown that it is not sufficient to understand CHD risk without surrogating to gene interactions and epigenetic regulation as well as the larger proximal regulatory system that oversees cardiac development.

In conclusion, a systemic perspective of CHD that would incorporate the multifactorial nature of polygenic and oligogenic risk, consider a combination of environmental and epigenetic influence, and incorporate state-of-the-art computational tools will likely give us the most optimistic way forward to understand and manage this heterogeneous or condition. Please credit and link back to the original version of this article: Zabet et al., 2021. Although some scientific and clinical issues are still to be resolved, the confluence of genomics, systems biology, and precision medicine promises a time not too far off when we will be able to better predict the outcome of CHD, help identify critical interventions, and generate substantially enhanced results for patients all over the world.

## REFERENCES

Akanda, M. R., Sabuj, M. S. S., Salam, S. A., & Jahan, E. (2025). Molecular interplay of gene network dynamics, epigenetic regulation, and therapeutic mapping in cardiovascular disease. *Cardiovascular Drugs and Therapy*, ●●●, 1–14. DOI: 10.1007/s10557-025-07739-5 PMID: 40540082

Banerjee, S., Prabhu Basrur, N., & Rai, P. S. (2021). Omics technologies in personalized combination therapy for cardiovascular diseases: Challenges and opportunities. *Personalized Medicine*, *18*(6), 595–611. DOI: 10.2217/pme-2021-0087 PMID: 34689602

Berliner, J. L., & Fay, A. M. (2007). Risk assessment and genetic counselling for hereditary breast and ovarian cancer: Recommendations of the National Society of Genetic Counsellors. *Journal of Genetic Counseling*, *16*(3), 241–260. PMID: 17508274

Bi, F., Gao, C., & Guo, H. (2024). Epigenetic regulation of cardiovascular diseases induced by behavioural and environmental risk factors: Mechanistic, diagnostic, and therapeutic insights. *FASEB bioAdvances*, *6*(11), 477–502. PMID: 39512842

Blue, G. M., Kirk, E. P., Giannoulatou, E., Sholler, G. F., Dunwoodie, S. L., Harvey, R. P., & Winlaw, D. S. (2017). Advances in the genetics of congenital heart disease: A clinician's guide. *Journal of the American College of Cardiology*, *69*(7), 859–870. PMID: 28209227

Burridge, P. W., Sharma, A., & Wu, S. M. (2021). Epigenetic regulation of cardiac development and congenital heart disease. *Developmental Cell*, *56*(2), 146–161. DOI: 10.1016/j.devcel.2020.11.016

Chaix, M. A., Andelfinger, G., & Khairy, P. (2016). Genetic testing in congenital heart disease: A clinical approach. *World Journal of Cardiology*, *8*(2), 180. PMID: 26981213

Crouch, D. J., & Bodmer, W. F. (2020). Polygenic inheritance, GWAS, polygenic risk scores, and the search for functional variants. *Proceedings of the National Academy of Sciences of the United States of America*, *117*(32), 18924–18933. PMID: 32753378

Domingo, J., Baeza-Centurion, P., & Lehner, B. (2019). The causes and consequences of genetic interactions (epistasis). *Annual Review of Genomics and Human Genetics*, *20*(1), 433–460. PMID: 31082279

Farhan, S. M., & Hegele, R. A. (2013). Genetics 101 for cardiologists: Rare genetic variants and monogenic cardiovascular disease. *The Canadian Journal of Cardiology, 29*(1), 18–22. PMID: 23200093

Fitzsimons, L. A., Brewer, V. L., & Tucker, K. L. (2022). Hedgehog morphogens act as growth factors critical to pre- and postnatal cardiac development and maturation: How primary cilia mediate their signal transduction. *Cells, 11*(12), 1879. PMID: 35741008

Fotiou, E., Williams, S., Martin-Geary, A., Robertson, D. L., Tenin, G., Hentges, K. E., & Keavney, B. (2019). Integration of large-scale genomic data sources with evolutionary history reveals novel genetic loci for congenital heart disease. *Circulation. Genomic and Precision Medicine, 12*(10), e002694. PMID: 31613678

Gifford, C. A., Ranade, S. S., Samarakoon, R., Salunga, H. T., De Soysa, T. Y., Huang, Y. U., & Srivastava, D. (2019). Oligogenic inheritance of a human heart disease involving a genetic modifier. *Science, 364*(6443), 865–870. PMID: 31147515

Girolami, F., Frisso, G., Benelli, M., Crotti, L., Iascone, M., Mango, R., & Olivotto, I. (2018). Contemporary genetic testing in inherited cardiac disease: Tools, ethical issues, and clinical applications. *The Journal of Cardiovascular Medicine, 19*(1), 1–11. PMID: 29176389

Giudicessi, J. R., Kullo, I. J., & Ackerman, M. J. (2021). Precision cardiovascular medicine: State of the science and future outlook. *Journal of the American Heart Association, 10*(16), e021314. DOI: 10.1161/JAHA.121.021314

Inouye, M., Abraham, G., Nelson, C. P., Wood, A. M., Sweeting, M. J., Dudbridge, F., & Samani, N. J. (2021). Genomic risk prediction of coronary artery disease in 480,000 adults: Implications for CHD research. *European Heart Journal, 42*(2), 136–145. DOI: 10.1093/eurheartj/ehaa1025

Islam, Z., Aslam, M., Khan, A. U., & Rehman, M. (2025). Genetic testing and its role in precision medicine: Understand disease risk and tailoring treatments. *Indus Journal of Bioscience Research, 3*(1), 461–470.

Kalisch-Smith, J. I., Ved, N., & Sparrow, D. B. (2020). Environmental risk factors for congenital heart disease. *Cold Spring Harbor Perspectives in Biology, 12*(3), a037234. PMID: 31548181

Khurana, E., Fu, Y., Chakravarty, D., Demichelis, F., Rubin, M. A., & Gerstein, M. (2016). Role of non-coding sequence variants in cancer. *Nature Reviews. Genetics, 17*(2), 93–108. PMID: 26781813

Kido, T., Sikora-Wohlfeld, W., Kawashima, M., Kikuchi, S., Kamatani, N., Patwardhan, A., & Butte, A. J. (2018). Are minor alleles more likely to be risk alleles? *BMC Medical Genomics*, *11*(1), 3. PMID: 29351777

Lage, K., Greenway, S. C., Rosenfeld, J. A., Wakimoto, H., Gorham, J. M., Segrè, A. V., & Larsen, L. A. (2012). Genetic and environmental risk factors in congenital heart disease functionally converge in protein networks driving heart development. *Proceedings of the National Academy of Sciences of the United States of America*, *109*(35), 14035–14040. PMID: 22904188

Li, Y., Du, J., Deng, S., Liu, B., Jing, X., Yan, Y., & She, Q. (2024). The molecular mechanisms of cardiac development and related diseases. *Signal Transduction and Targeted Therapy*, *9*(1), 368. PMID: 39715759

Liu, Y., Chen, S., Zühlke, L., Black, G. C., Choy, M. K., Li, N., & Keavney, B. D. (2019). Global birth prevalence of congenital heart defects 1970–2017: Updated systematic review and meta-analysis of 260 studies. *International Journal of Epidemiology*, *48*(2), 455–463. PMID: 30783674

MacGrogan, D., Münch, J., & de la Pompa, J. L. (2018). Notch and interacting signalling pathways in cardiac development, disease, and regeneration. *Nature Reviews. Cardiology*, *15*(11), 685–704. PMID: 30287945

MacKenzie, E. (2024). *The role of rare genetic variants in aortic valve stenosis* (Master's thesis). McGill University.

Malta, M., AlMutiri, R., Martin, C. S., & Srour, M. (2023). Holoprosencephaly: Review of embryology, clinical phenotypes, etiology and management. *Children (Basel, Switzerland)*, *10*(4), 647. PMID: 37189898

Mishra, R., Verma, A., Sharma, B., & Sharma, P. (2025). An Overview of Transdermal Patches: Opportunities and Obstacles in Modern Drug Delivery. *Asian Journal of Research in Medical and Pharmaceutical Sciences*, *14*(3), 18–29. DOI: 10.9734/ajrimps/2025/v14i3314

Morrell, N. W., Bloch, D. B., Ten Dijke, P., Goumans, M. J. T., Hata, A., Smith, J., & Bloch, K. D. (2016). Targeting BMP signalling in cardiovascular disease and anaemia. *Nature Reviews. Cardiology*, *13*(2), 106–120. PMID: 26461965

Munshi, N. V. (2012). Gene regulatory networks in cardiac conduction system development. *Circulation Research*, *110*(11), 1525–1537. PMID: 22628576

Musunuru, K., Kathiresan, S., & Khera, A. V. (2021). Genetics and cardiovascular disease: The next decade. *Journal of the American College of Cardiology*, *77*(3), 406–420. DOI: 10.1016/j.jacc.2020.11.034

Nakayama, K. H., Hou, L., & Huang, N. F. (2014). Role of extracellular matrix signaling cues in modulating cell fate commitment for cardiovascular tissue engineering. *Advanced Healthcare Materials*, *3*(5), 628–641. PMID: 24443420

Nogel, M. (2025). Sustainable and equal integration of genomics into healthcare. *Journal of Infrastructure. Policy and Development*, *9*(1), 10090.

Olson, E. N. (2006). Gene regulatory networks in the evolution and development of the heart. *Science*, *313*(5795), 1922–1927. PMID: 17008524

Ozhan, G., & Weidinger, G. (2015). Wnt/β-catenin signaling in heart regeneration. *Cell Regeneration (London, England)*, *4*(1), 4–3. PMID: 26157574

Patel, A. P., & Natarajan, P. (2019). Completing the genetic spectrum influencing coronary artery disease: From germline to somatic variation. *Cardiovascular Research*, *115*(5), 830–843. PMID: 30789660

Pierpont, M. E., Brueckner, M., Chung, W. K., Garg, V., Lacro, R. V., & McGuire, A. L., & American Heart Association Council on Genomic and Precision Medicine. (2018). Genetic basis for congenital heart disease: Revisited: A scientific statement from the American Heart Association. *Circulation*, *138*(21), e653–e711. PMID: 30571578

Priest, J. R., Ashley, E. A., & Giraldez, A. J. (2022). Genetics of congenital heart disease: Current knowledge and future directions. *Nature Reviews. Cardiology*, *19*(5), 331–348. DOI: 10.1038/s41569-021-00668-5

Richter, F., Morton, S. U., Kim, S. W., & MacArthur, D. G. (2022). Functional impact of noncoding variants in congenital disorders. *Nature Reviews. Genetics*, *23*(1), 59–71. DOI: 10.1038/s41576-021-00415-4

Russell, M. W., Chung, W. K., Kaltman, J. R., & Miller, T. A. (2018). Advances in the understanding of the genetic determinants of congenital heart disease and their impact on clinical outcomes. *Journal of the American Heart Association*, *7*(6), e006906. PMID: 29523523

Safdar, M., Ullah, M., Wahab, A., Hamayun, S., Rehman, M. U., Khan, M. A., & Naeem, M. (2024). Genomic insights into heart health: Exploring the genetic basis of cardiovascular disease. *Current Problems in Cardiology*, *49*(1), 102182. PMID: 37913933

Sethi, Y., Patel, N., Kaka, N., Kaiwan, O., Kar, J., Moinuddin, A., & Cavalu, S. (2023). Precision medicine and the future of cardiovascular diseases: A clinically oriented comprehensive review. *Journal of Clinical Medicine*, *12*(5), 1799. PMID: 36902588

Shabana, N. A., Shahid, S. U., & Irfan, U. (2020). Genetic contribution to congenital heart disease (CHD). *Pediatric Cardiology*, *41*(1), 12–23. PMID: 31872283

Sharma, P., Mishra, R., Sharma, B., Kumari, A., & Modgil, S. (2025). Health Sciences: Advancing Healthcare through Interdisciplinary Approaches and Innovation. *International Journal of Multidisciplinary: Applied Business and Education Research*, *6*(5), 2309–2316. DOI: 10.11594/ijmaber.06.05.17

Sperling, S. R. (2011). Systems biology approaches to heart development and congenital heart disease. *Cardiovascular Research*, *91*(2), 269–278. PMID: 21527437

Szot, J. O., Campione, M., & Sparrow, D. B. (2020). Oligogenic inheritance in human congenital heart disease. *Human Molecular Genetics*, *29*(R2), R145–R151. DOI: 10.1093/hmg/ddaa179

Talmud, P. J. (2007). Gene–environment interaction and its impact on coronary heart disease risk. *Nutrition, Metabolism, and Cardiovascular Diseases*, *17*(2), 148–152. PMID: 17306734

Tcheandjieu, C.. (2022). Large-scale multi-ancestry genome-wide association study of coronary artery disease. *Nature Genetics*, *54*(9), 1372–1383. DOI: 10.1038/s41588-022-01118-1

Torrorey-Sawe, R. (2025). *Global bioethics: Addressing current challenges, innovations, and the needs of underserved populations.*

Vecoli, C., Pulignani, S., Foffa, I., & Grazia Andreassi, M. (2014). Congenital heart disease: The crossroads of genetics, epigenetics and environment. *Current Genomics*, *15*(5), 390–399. PMID: 25435801

Vrijheid, M., Slama, R., Robinson, O., Chatzi, L., Coen, M., van den Hazel, P., & Vineis, P. (2020). The human exposome and health: Where are we now and where do we go from here? *Environmental Health Perspectives*, *128*(6), 065001. DOI: 10.1289/EHP4755 PMID: 32579081

Wu, Y., Jin, X., Zhang, Y., Zheng, J., & Yang, R. (2021). Genetic and epigenetic mechanisms in the development of congenital heart diseases. *World Journal of Pediatric Surgery*, *4*(2), e000196. PMID: 36474778

Yasuhara, J., & Garg, V. (2021). Genetics of congenital heart disease: A narrative review of recent advances and clinical implications. *Translational Pediatrics*, *10*(9), 2366. PMID: 34733677

Zaidi, S., Brueckner, M., & Chung, W. K. (2021). Genetics and genomics of congenital heart disease. *Circulation Research*, *128*(7), 920–942. DOI: 10.1161/ CIRCRESAHA.121.318062 PMID: 28302740

## Chapter 7

# MicroRNA-Mediated Regulatory Mechanisms in the Etiopathogenesis of Congenital Heart Disease

**Sinem Durmus**
https://orcid.org/0000-0002-9272-9098
*Faculty of Medicine, İzmir Kâtip Celebi University, Turkey*

## ABSTRACT

*Congenital heart disease (CHD) is the most prevalent congenital defect and a significant source of morbidity and mortality in children. While many causal variants have been determined by genetic studies, most cases are still unexplained. Increasing evidence for the role of microRNAs (miRNAs)—small, non-coding RNAs that regulate gene expression—is accumulating in the control of cardiac development. By modulation of pathways such as WNT, BMP/TGF-β, Notch, and Hippo, miRNAs regulate cell proliferation, differentiation, and apoptosis, and their dysregulation has been linked to atrial and ventricular septal defects, Tetralogy of Fallot, and transposition of the great arteries. The stability of miRNAs in body fluids also supports their potential as non-invasive biomarkers. Still, heterogeneity across studies and limited functional validation complicate it. Standardized procedures and integrative omics need to be used to unveil their therapeutic and diagnostic potential.*

DOI: 10.4018/979-8-3373-3735-7.ch007

## INTRODUCTION

Congenital heart disease (CHD) describes structural anomalies of the heart and/or great vessels that are present at birth and contribute to a spectrum of immediate and long-term clinical complications (Meng et al., 2024). CHD affects 1% of live births worldwide, with recent estimates indicating a birth prevalence of 9.4 per 1,000 due to advances in diagnostic capabilities (Y. Liu et al., 2019; J. Xu et al., 2025). Today, there are over four million children under five years of age living with CHD globally, including nearly one in four newborns with a CHD whose defects are critical and need intervention in the first year of life (CDC, 2024; J. Xu et al., 2025). While mortality has decreased due to medical advances, the burden of mortality and morbidity attributable to CHD remains high and it is still a leading cause of neonatal deaths, as well as lifelong morbidity and disability especially in low-resource settings (J. Xu et al., 2025). The cause of CHD is still partially explained. Only one-third of the causal genetic mutations have been discovered to date with the arrival of contemporary advances in genetic studies and the relevant technologies. New evidence is implicating multifaceted genetic-environmental interactions and epigenetic factors, such as non-coding RNAs like miRNAs, as playing a considerable role in CHD pathogenesis. These regulatory elements not only influence gene expression during heart development, but they are also promising diagnostic and prognostic markers due to their stability and specificity (Choudhury et al., 2025; Mannarino et al., 2025).

microRNAs (miRNAs) are single-stranded, endogenously encoded, small RNA molecules, approximately 20 nucleotides long, that play a critical role in the regulation of gene expression at the transcriptional and/or post-transcriptional level (Billi et al., 2024). Their dynamic expression and regulatory specificity are accountable for the regulation of many biological processes, e.g., proliferation of cells, differentiation, apoptosis, and maintenance of normal cell physiology (Espinoza-Lewis & Wang, 2012; Ivey & Srivastava, 2015). Therefore, it is inevitable for them to be engaged in various stages of heart development. Indeed, many of the miRNAs are discovered to be expressed in embryonic, postnatal, and adult cardiac tissues, and their abnormal expression or gene losses have already been established to be associated with defective cardiomyocyte differentiation, defective cardiac morphogenesis, and cardiac pathology (Espinoza-Lewis & Wang, 2012).

Here, we describe how miRNAs control molecular processes of congenital heart defects, highlighting in particular their role in cardiac morphogenesis, demonstration of dysregulation within disease states, and their prospective promise as diagnostic and therapeutic targets. The purpose is to provide an overview of how miRNA biology intersects with the molecular etiology of congenital heart malformations.

## Biogenesis and Function of microRNAs

Though less than 1.5% of the genome consists of protein-coding genes, gene expression is controlled by a large fraction of non-coding RNAs, including miRNAs (Fu, 2014). As there are more than 2,600 documented mature miRNA sequences in the human genome, the molecules are estimated to target more than 60% of protein-coding genes (de Rooij et al., 2022; Plotnikova et al., 2019). This shows that the functional diversity of miRNAs has a significant impact not only numerically but also in terms of systems biology at the network level.

miRNAs, which have a highly complex biogenesis, mature through a multi-step, regulated process from the cell nucleus to the cytoplasm. This process has steps such as transcription, pri-miRNA induction, nuclear processing (Drosha/DGCR8), cytoplasmic export (Exportin-5), maturation via Dicer, and finally loading into the miRISC complex. Additionally, non-canonical pathways are an important part of this biogenesis and include alternative mechanisms that are independent of classical Drosha or Dicer (J. O'Brien et al., 2018).

The biological functions of microRNAs are not limited to intracellular regulation; they also play a role in intercellular communication by being transported by extra-cellular vesicles (especially exosomes). In this respect, miRNAs go beyond classical genetic paradigms and are involved in higher-level mechanisms such as epigenetic control, response to environmental signals, and systemic regulation (Nail et al., 2023). Recent years have witnessed technology advancement to further illuminate miRNA biogenesis and functional mechanisms. Determination of high-resolution structures, high-throughput sequencing technologies, and genetic editing techniques such as CRISPR/Cas9 have all added to the understanding of the biological effects of these small but powerful molecules (Shang et al., 2023; Z. Wang et al., 2024).

## Canonical and Non-Canonical miRNA Biogenesis Pathways

Canonical Pathways. miRNA biogenesis occurs mainly by way of the "canonical" or typical pathway. It begins with transcription of microRNAs as non-coding transcripts from DNA by RNA polymerase II (and in some cases RNA polymerase III). The newly formed precursor transcript is called the primary miRNA (pri-miRNA) and is typically a secondary structure known as a hairpin loop, several hundred nucleotides in size (J. O'Brien et al., 2018; Shang et al., 2023). Pri-miRNA is processed by a nuclear complex known as the microprocessor complex. The complex includes Drosha, a family of RNase III endonucleases, and the RNA-binding protein DGCR8 (DiGeorge syndrome critical region gene 8, or Pasha). DGCR8 associates with the double-stranded regions and hairpin loop of pri-miRNA; Drosha cleaves approximately 11 bp downstream of this structure to produce a 60–100 nucleotide pre-miRNA molecule (F. Guo, 2012). This pre-miRNA is transported out of the nucleus into the cytoplasm via Exportin-5 and Ran-GTP. The 2 nt 3′ overhang of pre-miRNA is discerned by Exportin-5, allowing it to move through the nuclear pore complex. Once it reaches the cytoplasm, it is further processed by Dicer, another RNase III-type enzyme. Dicer cleaves the loop region of the pre-miRNA and produces a double-stranded, short miRNA duplex of approximately 21–23 nucleotides. The miRISC complex suppresses the gene expression at the post-transcriptional level by binding to target mRNA. The suppression mainly takes place by inhibition of translation of mRNA and/or degradation of mRNA. For degradation, the GW182 protein of the miRISC complex recruits the CCR4-NOT and PAN2/3 deadenylation complexes to the target mRNA to commence the degradation process that begins with the shortening of the 3′ poly-A tail (F. Guo, 2012; J. O'Brien et al., 2018; Shang et al., 2023).

Non-Canonical Pathways. Non-canonical pathways are additional biogenesis pathways that do not include classical Drosha- or Dicer-mediated processing steps, or where some of them are partially altered. Non-canonical pathways provide wide-ranging biological variability at both functional and structural levels because they vary from the classical mechanisms (J. O'Brien et al., 2018; Salim et al., 2022a; Westholm & Lai, 2011). Non-canonical routes assume importance under specialized physiological conditions such as embryonic development, stem cell differentiation, stress response, and certain pathologies. These alternative pathways are usually of biological benefit, for example, optimizing cellular energy use, regulating genetic networks limited to a specific cell type, or producing quick viral infection responses. In addition, elevated levels of activation in these pathways have been found to occur in cancer cells, making them viable targets for therapy (Abdelfattah et al., 2014). Among non-canonical biogenesis pathways, eight notable subgroups are prevalent: 1. MiRtrons, 2. Small nucleolar RNA (snoRNA)-derived miRNAs, 3. Transfer RNA (tRNA)-derived miRNAs, 4. Short hairpin RNA (shRNA)-derived miRNAs, 5. IsomiRs, 6. m G-coated pre-miRNAs, 7. Dicer-independent miRNAs and 8. Simtrons (Natarelli & Weber, 2022; J. O'Brien et al., 2018).

MiRtrons are a spliceosome-mediated non-canonical process that does not require the Drosha-DGCR8 complex employed in conventional miRNA biogenesis (Okamura et al., 2007; J. O'Brien et al., 2018; Wong & Rasko, 2021). Short introns are spliced out by the spliceosome from host gene transcription, generating a lariat structure in the first step. This conformation is linearized by DBR1 and adopts a hairpin-like shape, adopting a pre-miRNA-like structure This structure is then converted into a linear one by DBR1 (lariat debranching enzyme) (Okamura et al., 2007; Tang et al., 2025; Westholm & Lai, 2011). MiRtrons are categorized into three broad groups based on how the termini of their molecules are delimited: 1) Classic miRtrons are molecules in which both the 5′ and the 3′ termini are completely delimitated by splicing (e.g., miR-6807); 2) 3′-tailed miRtrons are molecules in which the 5′ terminus is delimitated by splicing but in which the 3′ terminus has additional nucleotide sequences; these additional extensions are then removed by the RNA exosome (e.g., miR-4745) and 3) 5'-tailed miRtrons, on the other hand, are molecules whose 3' termini are delimitated by splicing but whose 5' termini contain additional nucleotide sequences; it is presumed that these additional segments must be trimmed by nucleases such as RNase P (e.g., miR-6514) (Flynt et al., 2010; Hynes & Kakumani, 2024; Ladewig et al., 2012; Salim et al., 2022b; Westholm & Lai, 2011; Zia et al., 2021). Pre-miRNA molecules such as miRtrons that are matured are exported to the cytoplasm by the Exportin-5 protein and Ran-GTP (J. O'Brien et al., 2018). Within the cytoplasm, the hairpin-shaped miRtron structure is cleaved into a 22-nucleotide miRNA/miRNA* duplex by the Dicer enzyme. One of these duplex strands is incorporated into the AGO protein as a guide strand and, with the help of the RISC complex, results in target mRNA translational repression or degradation (Shruti et al., 2011). Spliceosome-mediated miRtron biogenesis is now clearly established. Mutations within 5′ and 3′ splice sites almost completely eliminate mirtron formation, while conventional miRNAs are relatively insensitive. This would suggest that the spliceosome and the Drosha microprocessor complex can compete for the source during transcription (Gál et al., 2024). It has been shown in previous studies that mirtrons play an important role in various fields, particularly in cancer biology, and can be evaluated as possible therapeutic targets and biomarkers (Y.-L. Chen et al., 2025). There has not been direct evidence, however, in the literature that linked mirtrons to CHD. This means that the potential for mirtrons to have roles in the pathogenesis of CHD is yet to be examined and that there is a potentially large research gap here ready to be filled.

Small nucleolar RNAs (snoRNAs) are small nuclear RNAs measuring roughly 20-24 nucleotides in length that predominantly direct chemical modification of ribosomal RNAs, such as methylation and pseudouridylation. These molecules are generally organized into two large structural subgroups: C/D-box and H/ACA-box. These complexes play major roles in ribosome and RNA modification biogenesis in the nucleus (Brameier et al., 2011; Scott & Ono, 2011; Wajahat et al., 2021). Although biogenesis of snoRNA-derived small RNAs (sdRNAs) is not understood yet, different mechanisms have been known to be involved. Some of the sdRNAs, such as those from ACA45, are dependent on the DICER/DGCR8 complex, while C/D box snoRNAs are able to self-assemble in the absence of DICER. The RNA-binding protein FUS also plays an important role in the generation of sdRNAs; elevated levels of FUS promote sdRNA levels at the expense of mature snoRNA levels. Interestingly, sdRNA production is increased under stress conditions, and the sdRNAs interact with the ribosomes to assist in the re-regulation of protein synthesis. The findings are that sdRNAs play important regulatory roles in gene expression and cellular adaptation but lack an understood mechanism of biogenesis (Wajahat et al., 2021). The latest research has indicated that sdRNAs are closely linked not only with the mechanism of ribosome biogenesis but also with gene expression control and control of cellular signaling pathways. Particularly, sdRNAs are discovered to carry out pivotal regulatory roles in disease states such as cancer, neurodegenerative disorders and immune system (Cavaillé et al., 2000; Coley et al., 2022; Doe et al., 2009; Dubey et al., 2024; Sridhar et al., 2008). Additional understanding of the roles of snoRNAs in cardiovascular pathophysiology can potentially contribute to designing novel and innovative therapeutic strategies against some molecular mechanisms in CHD. Recent studies have confirmed that snoRNAs are strongly associated with the majority of cardiovascular diseases, including CHD, coronary artery disease, myocardial infarction (MI), heart failure, tetralogy of Fallot and stroke (Håkansson et al., 2019; Mick et al., 2017; Nossent et al., 2019; J. E. O'Brien et al., 2012; Tarazon et al., 2023; Y. Wang et al., 2025). These findings show that snoRNAs are not only passive cargo in cellular processes but are themselves dynamic regulators of gene-expression networks that control cardiovascular physiology and pathology. Furthermore, the identification of individual snoRNAs linked to CHD offers promise for new avenues of early diagnosis and targeted therapeutic approaches, emphasizing their utility both as biomarkers and as effectors of disease course.

Recent evidence indicates that small RNAs derived from transfer RNAs (tRFs) are also able to function in miRNA-like regulatory phenomena. tRFs, which are either Dicer-dependent or Dicer-independent, are found to suppress cell proliferation or promote responses to DNA damage in some cellular contexts (e.g., lymphoma cells) (Maute et al., 2013). These tRFs add another level of non-canonical miRNA biogenesis because these derive from tRNA processing rather than from conventional pri-miRNAs, providing more regulatory small RNAs in the cell.

Short hairpin RNAs (shRNAs) are synthetic RNAs that are generated by transcribing from viral vectors or plasmid DNA and expressed in cells. These molecules are now being synthesized directly in hairpin forms without the use of the Drosha step and subsequently being cleaved by Dicer to produce siRNA/miRNA-like duplexes. These duplexes are loaded into the RISC complex to silence target mRNAs. Paddison's study was the first to demonstrate the efficacy of shRNAs in gene silencing (Gu et al., 2012; Paddison et al., 2002).

IsomiRs are splice isoforms resulting from imprecise cleavage of conventional miRNAs at their 5′ or 3′ ends by Drosha/Dicer or post-transcriptional processing such as tailing (3′) additions. They are minor variations that may alter their effects on target recognition and gene expression (Tomasello et al., 2021). Interestingly, isomiRs have also emerged as functional regulators in other pathophysiologies—cancer and inflammatory responses—where differential isomiR stoichiometry can serve as effective biomarkers of disease states (McAllan et al., 2025; Zelli et al.,

2021). While isomiR-signature-based diagnostics and prognostics are of immense potential in oncology and infectious disease settings, yet no studies to date have specifically examined the contribution of isomiRs to congenital heart disease (CHD). This difference is a fascinating candidate for possible future study into isomiR-mediated pathways and translational relevance in CHD. Some pre-miRNAs are capable of having an N7-methylguanosine (m G) cap on their 5′ end.

This is enzymatically attached by the METTL1/WDR4 methyltransferase complex and makes miRNA precursors Exportin-1-receptor accessible instead of Exportin-5-receptor accessible and exported from the nucleus to the cytoplasm. This maximizes Dicer targeting (Xie et al., 2013; Zhou et al., 2025). m G coating is emphasized as it promotes the maturation of let-7 family miRNAs and is further indispensable for target recognition and RNA stability (Pandolfini et al., 2019; C. Wang et al., 2023; Q. Wu et al., 2025).

Certain miRNAs mature independently of Dicer through alternative mechanisms. The prime example is miR-451. This miRNA is cleaved by Drosha in its precursor short hairpin structure but then directly cleaved by AGO2 independently of Dicer to gain maturity (Cheloufi et al., 2010; Cifuentes et al., 2010; Titov & Vorozheykin, 2018; J.-S. Yang et al., 2010).

Simtron is a rare subclass of miRNA that is structurally similar to mirtron but has a Drosha-dependent, splicing-independent process. Simtron is bound to Drosha and in vitro processed in a Drosha-dependent process. Simtron molecules also bind with Argonaute proteins for loading the RISC complex and actively participate in target transcript repression. Current studies have determined that simtron may possess potential roles in cellular signaling, regulation of the transcriptome, and stress responses (Havens et al., 2012; Natarelli & Weber, 2022). However, direct involvement in cardiovascular diseases, such as congenital heart disease (CHD), has not been established yet. Therefore, studies on the effect of simtron on CHD pathogenesis are considered a priority area for further study.

## MicroRNAs in Cardiac Development

Heart development is a highly complex process involving differentiated cardiomyocytes, endocardial cells, epicardial cells, and vascular components. This growth is controlled by the dynamic crosstalk of numerous molecular signals that are involved in cell proliferation, migration, differentiation, and apoptosis (C. Sun & Kontaridis, 2018). MicroRNAs (miRNAs) are now solidly established by experiments to be significant regulators of such a developmental program (Kim et al., 2017; Kuppusamy et al., 2015; Ouyang & Wei, 2021; Poon et al., 2018; Synnergren et al., 2011; Wagh et al., 2014; Y. Zhao et al., 2007). In heart development, in particular, miRNAs play closely coordinated roles with various signaling pathways to assume significant roles in determining cell fate specification. The main signaling cascades regulating heart development are WNT, BMP, TGF-β, Notch, and Hippo. These cascades are involved in proliferation, differentiation, and cardiac progenitor cell morphogenesis (Fuller & Qian, 2014; Peng et al., 2014; Tian et al., 2015). They are controlled by different sets of miRNAs, giving evidence for developmental processes being carried out in fine balance (Figure 1).

The WNT signaling pathway is a highly significant regulator conserved evolutionarily and has entirely opposing functions at diverse phases of heart development. During the early stages of the embryonic stage, particularly the cardiac mesoderm development, WNT/β-catenin signaling directs pre-cardiac mesoderm formation and cardiac progenitor cell formation; without it, there is no way to establish the foundation for heart tissue formation (Buikema et al., 2014; Tian et al., 2010; Ueno et al., 2007; M. Zhao et al., 2019). Mouse model and human pluripotent stem cell system experiments have also shown conclusively that premature WNT signaling activation accelerates the cell cycle and therefore raises the progenitor pool but prolonged activation inhibits cardiomyocyte differentiation in the terminal phase (Kwon et al., 2007; Lian et al., 2012). As an example, it was seen in Naito and colleagues' research that the WNT signal enhances cardiogenic differentiation in the initial developmental phase but in those experiments in which repression of the signal didn't take place in subsequent periods, maturation problems arose in heart tissue (Naito et al., 2006). Likewise, another study indicated that WNT/β-catenin action is responsible for the initiation of embryonic heart tube formation but that sequential inhibition of this action is essential during the period of post-gastrulation to avoid interruption of differentiation (Ueno et al., 2007). This two-factor mechanism is also applied practically in protocols for cardiomyocyte induction from human pluripotent stem cells (iPSC or ESC): chemical WNT signal activation is employed to induce progenitor cell formation in step one; step two involves WNT inhibitors for their differentiation into cardiomyocytes (Münsterberg & Hoppler, 2016).

microRNAs play significant roles in the regulation of this transition; for example, miR-1 suppresses the WNT and FGF signaling pathways in the course of differentiation from the pluripotent stem cells into the heart, thereby accelerating the process of converting the progenitor cells into functioning cardiomyocytes. MicroRNAs also play critical roles in regulation of this process, e.g., miR-1 suppresses the WNT and FGF signaling pathways during differentiation into the heart from pluripotent stem cells and thereby accelerates transformation of progenitor cells into mature cardiomyocytes. In the same line of signaling, a myomiR referred to as miR-133a controls the WNT/β-catenin pathway in order to control signal disruptions within the cell nucleus to ensure morphological functions are executed at the right time during tissue formation (Di Mauro et al., 2019; Ouyang & Wei, 2021; Wystub et al., 2013). On the other hand, there was a study that found miR-218 to specifically suppress and target the WNT inhibitor sFRP2, thereby enhancing WNT signaling. It was clearly depicted that using miR-218 mimic increased growth and decreased sFRP2 protein expression significantly, and the addition of an inhibitor thwarted the effect. This interaction is also intriguing because miR-218 is similarly activated by WNT signaling; i.e., WNT signal is part of a positive feedback mechanism that represses sFRP2, which subsequently promotes the WNT signaling pathway. This ensures the signaling equilibrium necessary in the differentiation and proliferation of cardiac stem cells into cardiomyocytes (Y. Wang, Liu, et al., 2016). Also, both in human and mouse models, it has been found that other miRNAs such as miR-128 also cause pathological hypertrophic growth through activation of WNT/β-catenin signaling pathways in hypertrophic stress, fibrosis, or cellular injury in heart tissue. This situation unveils that the miRNA-WNT interaction opens a magic door not only in developmental but also in terms of disease manageability (J.-Y. Li et al., 2021). The overarching theme to all of these models is that miRNAs, namely miR-1, miR-133a, and miR-218, which tiptoe a tightrope regulating WNT signaling at each step of development are essential regulatory processes that determine cardiac cell fate, tissue patterning, and timing. These signaling-microRNA modules are akin to a precision-guided missile, delivering harmony and strength to heart development.

The role of the BMP (Bone Morphogenetic Protein) pathway in cardiac development is central to the evolution process; the pathway plays imperative roles, particularly in embryonic cardiac tissue differentiation and molding. Throughout the growth of the cardiac mesoderm, BMP signaling is transduced into the nucleus by Smad1/5/8, and it has been conclusively proven in recent studies that microRNAs must be involved for this to continue normally (J. Wang et al., 2011). In fact, J. Wang et al. demonstrated experimentally that miRNA is a development pathway translation process under BMP signaling, suppressing and inducing several progenitor genes and inducing differentiation; the study clarifies the regulatory role of BMP not only at the genetic level but also at the epigenetic level (J. Wang et al., 2010). Here, the lack of miR-17~92 has been shown to cause mice to die shortly after birth with lung hypoplasia and ventricular septal defect in mouse embryonic models (Ventura et al., 2008) Further, beyond the classical BMP signaling functions, Smad proteins are also reported to be directly implicated in miRNA processing complexes—for example, with Drosha—to play a role in the processing of pri-miRNAs to pre-miRNA structures, specifically enhancing the production of miR-21 and amplifying its function within the gene regulatory network (Hata & Kang, 2015). This Smad-associated miRNA regulation of this type proves that it is not only vital following reception of the BMP signal, but it is also important in determining the output of the signaling pathway. When specifically examining the heart, it is known that miR-21 is not just a part of MPK/TGF-β signaling but also participates in BMP signaling, thus facilitating the coordinated regulation of cardiac fibroblast activation and epicardial differentiation (Lozano-Velasco et al., 2024). Similarly, BMP signaling was also said to control the rest of the miRNAs such as miR-200c, miR-195, and miR-223 during development of the epicardium and ventricular myocardium layers such that programmed heart development of the different parts is made complete by BMP signaling through miRNAs (Lozano-Velasco et al., 2024). Briefly, one can observe that miRNA networks that are integrated into the BMP pathway, i.e., miR-17-92, miR-21, miR-200c, miR-195, and miR-223, perform objective and critical roles in such processes as cardiac progenitor cell differentiation, septation, and epicardial layering.

TGF-β signaling forms an important part of transformation events in heart development, triggering key morphogenetic processes such as myofibroblast transformation, extracellular matrix synthesis, and thickening of the epicardium; transmission of the signal to the nucleus via Smad2 and Smad3 triggers target genes and plays an important role in further cardiac structure formation (Yousefi et al., 2020). This is, however, finely regulated by intervening microRNAs. An example of this particular regulation of heart development is miR-21, whose overexpression from early high school and later directly acts to stimulate the TGF-β1/Smad3 pathway, which results in the conversion of fibroblasts; this, in turn, constructs fibrotic tissue, which plays a supportive but regulated role in the overall structure of the heart (Y. Zhang et al., 2022). On the other hand, some microRNAs play the role of suppressing TGF-β signaling. miR-24, for example, inhibits the TGF-β/Smad2/3 pathway by directly regulating the enzyme furin, which is involved in the activation of latent TGF-β; such inhibition inhibits over-differentiation of cardiac fibroblasts and ECM deposition (X. Xu et al., 2021). Similarly, miR-150-5p represses Smad7, suppressing its function, ultimately leading to induction of cardiac fibrosis by increased Smad2/3 signaling and increased ECM deposition, creating a model where miRNA function is controlled by positive and negative loops (X. Xu et al., 2021). Besides, in the developing heart under conditions of hypertrophic or fibrotic stress, miR-208b and miR-21 play a role in pathological fibrosis by simultaneously activating the TGF-β1/Smad3 pathway, and this greatly increases the quantity of fibrotic tissue within the heart, especially after myocardial infarction (Y. Zhang et al., 2022).

MicroRNAs have a subtle regulating role in the Notch signaling pathway, which is one of the most subtle and complex processes in the development of the heart. Notch, due to its transmembrane receptor structure, comes into direct contact with neighboring cells, particularly at major transitions between endocardial and myocardial cells in the heart; this interaction regulates key morphogenetic processes such as formation of the atrioventricular canal, valve development, and chambering. The Notch target gene HEY2 adds to the importance of this pathway in regionalization of the heart; Notch HEY2 deficiency in heart development results in profound structural abnormalities in ventricular septation and valvular morphogenesis (MacGrogan et al., 2018). In the microRNA saga, miR-34a is the star of both embryonic development and normal adult hearts. Particularly in physiological adaptation and disease conditions subsequent to heart development, miR-34a influences the cardiac cell fate by inhibiting Notch1 signaling. In conditions where miR-34a levels are increased, it has been demonstrated that Notch signaling in the heart is eliminated, leading to suppression of cell differentiation and regenerative capacity (K.-H. Wu et al., 2018). Another crucial relationship is that miR-1 indeed targets the Notch ligand Delta, as revealed in Drosophila models. This interaction regulates progenitor cell differentiation timing of heart tube formation; when miR-1 is absent, cell fate abnormalities and morphology defects are observed (Kwon et al., 2005). Besides, miRNA models for targeting or affecting the Notch signaling pathway directly also hold tremendous promise for heart disease. For example, regulation of Notch-microRNA interaction in pathologies that are associated with myocardial ischemia or heart failure has the potential to be applied for the treatment of valve calcification or arrhythmia, and these methods come under the new avenues to be explored in the early stages (Marracino et al., 2021). In this context, it can be expected that such methods can be established in the future for CHD.

Hippo, a conserved pathway to the developmental plan, is an evolutionarily conserved modulator that tightly controls heart size and cardiomyocyte expansion. Similar to WNT and BMP, the very powerful activities of this pathway in cardiovascular growth are heavily reliant on microRNAs. In particular, the miR-302-367 cluster promotes cardiomyocyte proliferation in normal heart development; these such miRNAs play a pivotal role in this function by suppressing the expression of the Mst1, Lats2, and Mob1b, which are essential kinases of the Hippo pathway (M. Song et al., 2024; Tian et al., 2015). In mouse-model hearts where miR-302-367 is lost, there is a dramatic decrease in proliferation during embryonic development, and excess miR-302-367 at later times can cause cardiomegaly and septal defects-demonstrating just how critical this delicate balance is (Tian et al., 2015). Furthermore, other microRNAs such as miR-302d have also been implicated within the Hippo pathway. For example, in human pluripotent stem cell-derived cardiomyocytes, miR-302d may increase the nuclear import of YAP by targeting *LATS2*, thus potentially leading to proliferative signaling (F. Xu et al., 2019). In light of this fact, one can confidently assert that this microRNA system, which subtly impairs the Hippo signaling pathway, is extremely crucial in the growth-versus-differentiation balance in cardiac development. This field contains great promise for the repair and regeneration of the heart, and miRNA-based approaches provide a beacon of hope for novel therapies.

## MicroRNA Dysregulation in the Etiopathogenesis of CHD

Molecular studies over the past few years have pinpointed the critical role of miRNAs in the development of CHD. Dysregulation of miRNA expression during cardiomyocyte differentiation and proliferation is directly responsible for the pathogenesis of structural defects. For example, miR-20b-5p was downregulated at cardiac differentiation but upregulated in plasma from patients with ASD. It has been seen to downregulate cardiac transcription factors (GATA4, NKX2.5, TBX5) through *TET2* targeting and thus interrupt differentiation (K.-X. Li et al., 2024). Similarly, miR-19a/b has also been discovered to disrupt the balance of apoptosis and proliferation along with *NKX2-5* mutations and thus lead to ASD pathogenesis (Jia et al., 2022). Such research on septal defects has also identified developmental pathway miRNAs. Additionally, large-scale small RNA sequencing analyses have also linked Hippo, TGF-β, Wnt, MAPK, and PI3K-Akt signaling pathways with altered miRNA profiles (Ramachandran et al., 2022). In addition to this, the target feature of miR-139-5p gained by *ACTC1* 3′UTR mutation has also proved to be a disease mechanism in familial ASD (Y. Wang, Du, et al., 2016). However, miR-200 family inhibition in mouse models resulted in ventricular septal defect (VSD) and embryonic lethality, demonstrating that it plays a critical role to play in ventricular maturation by regulating cardiac transcription factors such as Tbx5, Gata4 and Mef2c (Leonard et al., 2025).

The same is demonstrated in research devoted to Tetralogy of Fallot (TOF). It has been shown that miR-1 and miR-133 are abnormally controlled in TOF heart tissues, regulating cardiomyocyte morphology and electrophysiology by targeting *KCNJ2*, *FBN2*, and *TNNI1* (Grunert et al., 2019). Additionally, miR-424/424* and miR-222 have been found to have significant roles in the processes of proliferation and differentiation as well as in the pathogenesis of TOF by direct targeting *HAS2* and *NF1* (J. Zhang et al., 2013). Summary of key research on microRNA abnormalities in CHD expression and biomarker potential is given in Table 1.

## Clinical Implications of miRNAs in CHD Subtypes

Several specific miRNAs have been implicated in distinct types of CHD. The tissue- and disease-specific expression patterns of microRNAs make them particularly advantageous targets for personalized diagnostics. For example, a genome-wide survey demonstrated that miR-1, miR-126, miR-208, miR-302a, miR-302b, miR-302c, miR-302d, miR-367, miR-133a, and miR-133b are expressed specifically in heart tissue (Z. Guo et al., 2014). Some miRNAs, particularly within these miRNAs, have also been shown to exhibit CHD subtype-specific dysregulation. For instance, in animal models of ventricular septal defects (VSDs), miR-1 and miR-133 were found to be significantly downregulated in myocardial tissues while simultaneously upregulated in maternal serum and amniotic fluid, suggesting myocardial damage and compensatory release into circulation. Among these, miR-1-3p targets *SLC8A1* (*NCX1*), a sodium-calcium exchanger essential for myocardial contractility, implicating miR-1 as a non-invasive prenatal biomarker of VSD (Y. Yang et al., 2022). Complementing this, clinical profiling in children with CHD has revealed differential expression of miR-21-5p, miR-155-5p, miR-221-3p, and miR-26a-5p, with elevated miR-21-5p levels distinguishing cyanotic from non-cyanotic cases—highlighting the potential of miRNAs in stratifying CHD severity postnatally (González-Moyotl et al., 2024). In pediatric patients with hypoplastic left heart syndrome (HLHS), the right ventricular miRNA expression profile is distinct from that of adult idiopathic dilated cardiomyopathy, and notably, miR-100, miR-99a, miR-145 show stage-dependent normalization after surgical volume unloading, highlighting their potential as dynamic biomarkers of mechanical stress adaptation (Sucharov et al., 2015). Emerging studies have also examined whether miRNAs can predict outcomes or complications post-surgery. For instance, circulating miR-208a, miR-208b and miR-499 have been investigated as markers of myocardial stress in children undergoing cardiac surgery (Bolkier et al., 2016). These expression profiles suggest that miRNA signatures could not only serve as biomarkers but also distinguish among CHD subtypes and severity grades.

The dysregulation of specific miRNAs in CHD subtypes not only offers mechanistic insight but also offers urgent therapeutic targets. In this context, miRNA mimics, or antagomiRs, have been investigated in the treatment of various diseases. miRNA mimics are synthetic small RNA molecules used to mimic the activity of a naturally low-expressed or reduced-function miRNA. When administered exogenously, they can restore lost regulatory activity by inhibiting target genes (Garreau et al., 2024). However, antagomirs are single-stranded, antisense oligonucleotides complementary to an endogenous miRNA, typically designed to prevent pathological effects resulting from overexpression of a target miRNA (Bajan & Hutvagner, 2020). They bind to the target miRNA and block its activity, preventing aberrant gene silencing. While no miRNA-based therapies have yet been approved by the US Food and Drug Administration (FDA) and have reached Phase III trials, there are promising reports ("What Will It Take to Get miRNA Therapies to Market?," 2024). While this research is largely focused on cancer treatment, some miRNAs are still being tested in preclinical stages for heart disease and other metabolic diseases. For example, an anti-miR for miR-132 has completed phase 1 trials for the treatment of heart failure. Furthermore, various therapeutic agents targeting different miRNAs are currently being developed in the preclinical phase (e.g., MGN-1374, a therapeutic agent targeting miRNA-15 and miR-195 for myocardial infarction; MGN-9103, targeting miR-208 for chronic heart failure; and MGN-4220, targeting miR-29 for cardiac fibrosis) (Seyhan, 2024). However, the clinical application of these treatment strategies presents a significant challenge in controlling the observed adverse effects (Diener et al., 2022). A particularly significant challenge in the use of synthetic miRNAs is the risk of off-target processing of artificial miRNA (Kotowska-Zimmer et al., 2021). While these are still largely in preclinical stages, their potential to correct dysregulated pathways in CHD is significant. Furthermore, the combination of miRNA profiling with machine learning approaches for newborn screening offers a powerful framework to enhance predictive diagnostics and guide precision interventions.

## MicroRNA-Based Biomarkers in CHD

In the last few years, ample evidence has emerged that miRNAs not only can be used in pathogenesis but also as diagnostic and prognostic biomarkers. miRNA-based biomarkers meet most of the required criteria for being an ideal biomarker, because they are remarkably stable in biofluids, can be amplified with high specificity, and often reflect upstream regulatory changes—making them more dynamic markers of disease state than static DNA variants or many proteins (Condrat et al., 2020; Nikolova et al., 2024). Furthermore, circulating miRNAs can be detected in a wide variety of body fluids, including saliva, breast milk, tears, bronchial lavage, cerebrospinal fluid, urine, amniotic fluid, as well as blood plasma and serum (Tito et al., 2021). They are secreted into the extracellular environment either encapsulated in extracellular vesicles such as exosomes or bound to protein complexes, which enhances their stability. Additionally, circulating miRNAs is not easily degraded by RNase, making it a stable biomarker (Z. Wang et al., 2024). However, the choice of biological source significantly influences detection and reliability; plasma and serum miRNA levels may be affected by hemolysis or sample processing, whereas vesicle-encapsulated miRNAs are generally more stable but technically more challenging to isolate, underscoring the need for methodological standardization (Kirschner et al., 2013; L. Sun et al., 2023). Therefore, these features strengthen the usability of miRNAs as clinical biomarkers, and studies provide examples supporting this approach. For example, a study of children has found that let-7a and let-7b are particularly elevated in ASD cases and are similarly elevated in children and their mothers too. These miRNAs have been shown to have high diagnostic utility in ROC analyses (Y. Song et al., 2018). In the VSD models, miR-1-3p was found to be decreased in fetal myocardium but increased in amniotic fluid and maternal serum and may be an effective prenatal diagnostic biomarker Similarly, miR-146a-

5p was downregulated in maternal serum exosomes with high diagnostic precision (AUC=0.997) (Jin et al., 2021).

The miRNA biomarker promise has also emerged in CHD patients with pulmonary arterial hypertension (PAH) development. miR-27b and miR-451 levels were significantly correlated with PAH presence; their combination enhanced diagnostic precision (Long et al., 2020). It was also suggested that miR-19a was impressively higher in plasma in VSD-related PAH patients and can be used as a non-invasive biomarker (W. Chen & Li, 2017). Circulating miRNAs have also been described to be of clinical usefulness in tetralogy of Fallot patients and transposition of the great arteries (TGA) patients. In TOF patients, miR-181d-5p and miR-206 have been described to yield high diagnostic accuracy (Abu-Halima et al., 2017), and in TGA-RV patients, miR-183-3p has been described as an independent predictor of worsening heart failure (Abu-Halima et al., 2021). In addition to that, miR-3195 and miR-122-5p were discovered to be downregulated in maternal serum and can be non-invasive potential biomarkers in prenatal CHD diagnosis (Xi et al., 2024).

## Future Perspectives and Challenges

Diagnosis and treatment of CHD are challenging due to its heterogeneity, and it encompasses different subtypes. Therefore, identifying effective biomarkers that can predict the occurrence of the disease at an early stage safely is very important. Finding noninvasive and sensitive biomarkers will be of great value for prenatal diagnosis and postnatal follow-up. In addition, their application to treatment outcome prediction and disease prognosis would lead to individualized medical treatment protocols and prevention of morbidity and mortality. Integration of miRNA profiling into predictive diagnostic strategies for newborn screening is particularly promising in the context of the etiology of CHD. The early identification of high-risk newborns according to circulating miRNA signatures would allow for timely intervention and personalized management. Machine-learning models derived from multi-omics data sets can also improve the predictive capability of such screening tools. However, several hurdles must be overcome before they can be used on a routine basis. First, miRNA expression is interindividual, and it is difficult to define generalizable diagnostic cut-offs. Second, detection methods, from the handling of the sample through analysis, must be standardized. Finally, the interpretation of the circulating levels of miRNA factors remains complex as they can be influenced by many physiological and disease-related factors aside from CHD. This is most likely to be resolved with further research. Besides, while a number of research studies have built upon the understanding of the role of microRNAs in CHD, it should be remembered that the majority of such studies are based on animal models or small patient groups. Limitations on this limit the extensibility of the evidence and pose challenges to direct clinical application. For clinical utility to be achieved, larger longitudinal studies in different populations must confirm miRNA signatures, determine their reproducibility, and define their utility as effective diagnostic or therapeutic tools.

Furthermore, the therapeutic applications of miRNAs are attracting attention as promising strategies for correcting dysregulated molecular pathways. Preclinical studies of miRNA therapeutics are underway for the treatment of many diseases, including vascular diseases, peripheral arterial disease, and chronic heart failure. In the coming years, miRNA mimics may be used to restore the function of down-regulated miRNAs, while antagomirs may silence overexpressed and pathogenic miRNAs, potentially improving aberrant gene expression patterns that contribute to CHD. Furthermore, advances in computational biology highlight the promise of integrating miRNA profiling with machine learning algorithms to improve predictive diagnostic methods. Such approaches could increase the accuracy of newborn screening by identifying high-risk infants based on complex miRNA signatures, thus enabling earlier interventions. Combining bioinformatics-driven predictions with experimental validation will be critical to achieving their clinical utility. The convergence of omics technologies, therapeutic miRNA modulation, and AI-based predictive models has the potential to transform the landscape of CHD diagnosis, prognosis, and treatment in the coming decades.

*Table 1. Summary of prominent studies on microRNA expression abnormalities in congenital heart diseases (CHD) and their biomarker potential.*

| **Study Type & Sample** | **Key Findings** |
|---|---|
| Experimental study using 12-day in vitro cardiac differentiation of human embryonic stem cells (hESCs-CMs), hiPSCs-CMs, mESCs-CMs, and plasma samples from ASD patients | miR-20b-5p is downregulated during cardiac differentiation of stem-cell-derived cardiomyocytes but upregulated in plasma of atrial septal defect (ASD) patients; it inhibits cardiac differentiation by directly targeting *TET2*, reducing 5-hmC levels and downregulating key cardiac transcription factors (*GATA4*, *NKX2.5*, *TBX5*, *MYH6*, cTnT); inhibiting miR-20b-5p or rescuing *TET2* partially restores differentiation (K.-X. Li et al., 2024) |
| WES and linkage analysis in an ASD-affected family; hiPSC-derived cardiomyocytes from patients | NKX2-5 mutation alters regulation of miR-19a/b. Dysregulated miR-19a/b impairs apoptosis and proliferation balance in hiPSC-CMs by modulating PYK2, contributing to atrial septal defect pathogenesis (Jia et al., 2022) |
| High-throughput small RNA sequencing of cardiac tissues from CHD patients (ASD, VSD, TOF) vs non-CHD controls | Predicted targets enriched in Hippo, TGF-β, Wnt, MAPK, and PI3K-Akt signaling pathways (cardiac development–related) (Ramachandran et al., 2022) |

continued on following page

*Table 1. Continued*

| Study Type & Sample | Key Findings |
|---|---|
| Screening and validation of 84 circulating cardiovascular miRNAs in children with CHD (particularly ASD) and their parents | hsa-let-7a, hsa-let-7b, and hsa-miR-486 were significantly upregulated in children with atrial septal defects. hsa-let-7a and hsa-let-7b were specifically elevated in ASD (not in other septal defects), and these two miRNAs were also similarly elevated in mothers of ASD children. Receiver-operating characteristic (ROC) analyses showed that hsa-let-7a and hsa-let-7b had significant diagnostic value for detecting ASD and predicting ASD risk in offspring (Y. Song et al., 2018) |
| Genotyping SNPs in miR-196a2, miR-27a, miR-499 in peripheral blood of 573 Chinese subjects with isolated CHD (ASD, VSD, PDA) | The miR-196a2 rs11614913 C allele (homozygous CC genotype) was significantly negatively associated with ASD, suggesting this variant may confer a protective effect against ASD. No significant associations were found for SNPs in miR-27a (rs895819) or miR-499 (rs3746444) with ASD, VSD, or PDA (K. Yu et al., 2016) |
| Whole genome sequencing identifying a 3′UTR mutation (c.*1784T > C) in ACTC1 in a family with autosomal dominant ASDII | The *ACTC1* 3′UTR mutation (c.*1784T > C) creates a novel target site for miR-139-5p, leading to downregulation of *ACTC1* expression in a reporter assay. Overexpression of miR-139-5p enhances repression; inhibition of miR-139-5p rescues the expression decrease—suggesting that the mutation's pathogenic effect in familial ASDII arises via gain-of-function miRNA targeting (Y. Wang, Du, et al., 2016) |
| Maternal serum exosome profiling in pregnant women (91 with VSD fetuses vs. 91 matched controls), sequencing, validation by qRT-PCR, ROC diagnostics | hsa-miR-146a-5p was significantly downregulated in VSD cases versus controls and demonstrated excellent diagnostic potential (AUC = 0.997, p < 1e-05). hsa-miR-199a-3p also downregulated but with lower diagnostic value (AUC = 0.67). Bioinformatic predictions link miR-146a-5p to targets such as *NUMB*, *ERBB4*, *IRAK1*, *CCL5*, implicating pathways like Notch and ErbB signaling, which are important in cardiac morphogenesis (Jin et al., 2021) |
| Serum RT-qPCR in 114 CHD patients (61 with PAH, 53 without) | miR-27b was significantly upregulated in CHD-PAH patients and positively correlated with mean pulmonary artery pressure (mPAP), BNP, and ADMA. miR-451 was downregulated, showing inverse correlations. Both served as independent risk factors, and their combined detection improved diagnostic accuracy (AUC = 0.84) compared to individual assessments (Long et al., 2020) |
| LC-MS metabolomics in VSD patients' serum and thymus tissue; iPS-derived cardiomyocytes; VSD rat model; mechanistic assays (RT-PCR, luciferase, autophagy assays) | miR-7-5p mediates uric acid and sphingomyelin -induced autophagy in cardiomyocytes via targeting *EGFR*; manipulation of miR-7-5p (mimics/inhibitors) modulates autophagy by regulating EGFR levels. (Also involves lncRNA MEG3 as upstream regulator.) (Cao et al., 2019) |
| Genome-wide DNA methylation analysis of placental tissue from 8 VSD cases vs. 10 controls | Identified eight miRNAs with potential as placental biomarkers for VSD detection (Radhakrishna et al., 2019) |
| Expression analysis in fetal cardiac tissues with VSD, mouse embryonic hearts, and cardiomyocyte differentiation model (P19 cells) | lncRNA SNHG6 is upregulated in VSD tissues and negatively regulates miR-101, resulting in impaired P19 cardiomyocyte proliferation, increased apoptosis, and enhanced differentiation. Additionally, SNHG6 activates the Wnt/β-catenin pathway, and these effects are reversed when miR-101 is co-overexpressed—highlighting miR-101's role as a mediator in SNHG6-driven VSD pathogenesis (Jiang et al., 2019) |

continued on following page

*Table 1. Continued*

| Study Type & Sample | Key Findings |
|---|---|
| Case-control in Chinese Han population (350 children with VSD vs 430 healthy controls); functional luciferase reporter assays | The SNP rs6563 G>A in the *NOTCH1* 3′UTR was significantly associated with higher VSD risk (OR ≈ 1.5–2.4 depending on genotype). Functional assays showed that miR-3691-3p binds to the A allele 3′UTR and reduces reporter activity, suggesting altered post-transcriptional regulation of NOTCH1 contributes to VSD pathogenesis (Ji et al., 2019) |
| Case-control in Han Chinese children (1,241 CHD cases vs. 1,285 controls); functional validation via luciferase assays in HEK-293T and H9c2 cells | A SNP (rs59382073 G>T) in *TBX2* 3′UTR significantly increased CHD risk (~1.9-fold). The G→T change created functional binding sites for miR-3940 and miR-708, which suppressed reporter gene activity; co-transfection with miRNA inhibitors abolished this suppression. This indicates the polymorphism facilitates miRNA-mediated downregulation of *TBX2*, contributing to CHD susceptibility (J. Wang et al., 2019) |
| miRNA microarray and qRT-PCR in lung tissues and plasma from VSD-associated PAH patients (n = 14) vs VSD without PAH (n = 16); plasma analysis in 30 patients | miR-19a, miR-130a, and miR-27b were significantly dysregulated in PAH caused by CHD. miR-19a was markedly elevated in plasma, with a diagnostic AUC of 0.781 (95% CI: 0.612–0.950, p < 0.0001), suggesting its potential as a non-invasive biomarker for PAH in VSD patients (W. Chen & Li, 2017) |
| miR-30c overexpression/knockdown in P19 cells; assays for proliferation, apoptosis, differentiation; Shh pathway analysis | miR-30c boosts proliferation and inhibits apoptosis and differentiation in P19 cells. Targets *Gli2*, suppressing it, leading to downstream repression of *Ptch1* and attenuation of Shh signaling, thereby modulating cardiac progenitor differentiation (X. Liu et al., 2016) |
| miRNA microarray and RT-PCR profiling in plasma from VSD patients (n=3) and controls (n=3), validated in larger cohorts (n=20 vs. 15) | Eight miRNAs were validated as differentially expressed in circulating plasma of VSD patients compared to controls. Bioinformatic analyses predicted that *NOTCH1*, *HAND1*, *ZFPM2*, and *GATA3*—key genes in cardiac development—are among the probable targets of hsa-let-7e-5p, hsa-miR-222-3p, and hsa-miR-433, implicating them in VSD pathogenesis via modulation of cardiac morphogenesis pathways (D. Li et al., 2014) |
| Analysis of cardiac tissue from humans with VSD vs. healthy controls; microarray and validation assays | miR-1-1 was downregulated in VSD hearts; this correlated with upregulation of its targets *GJA1* and *SOX9*, both confirmed as direct targets. miR-181c was upregulated, correlating with downregulation of *BMPR2*, also validated as a target—indicating both miRNAs contribute to VSD pathogenesis through modulation of cardiac development–related genes (J. Li et al., 2013) |
| MicroRNA sequencing of dried blood spots (umbilical cord blood and week-1 infant blood) from very preterm infants with spontaneous ductus arteriosus closure (control, n=14) vs. persistent hemodynamically significant PDA (hsPDA, n=11) | hsa-miR-218-5p was significantly downregulated in umbilical cord blood of hsPDA infants (log fold-change ≈ −3.444, FDR = 0.099)—indicating its potential as a biomarker for persistent PDA in preterm infants (Winkler et al., 2025) |
| Circulating miRNA expression analysis by RT-qPCR in serum of children with Tetralogy of Fallot (n=23) vs controls (n=45) | miR-221-5p, miR-21-5p, and miR-144-3p were significantly dysregulated in TOF patients. Bioinformatics suggests their target genes include *AKT1*, *SMAD* family, *TNF-α*, and *FOX* family, implicating pathways in cell cycle regulation, proliferation, apoptosis, especially under hypoxic stress (Huesca-Gomez et al., 2025) |

continued on following page

*Table 1. Continued*

| Study Type & Sample | Key Findings |
|---|---|
| Exosomal miRNA profiling (microarray) in amniotic fluid from fetuses with TOF vs healthy controls (5 vs 5 samples), followed by functional validation in P19 cells | Identified 257 dysregulated exosomal miRNAs; miR-10a-5p was functionally validated. Overexpression of miR-10a-5p in P19 cells inhibited cardiomyogenic differentiation and suppressed expression of cardiomyocyte marker TBX5, which was confirmed as a direct target in luciferase assays. These findings implicate miR-10a-5p in TOF pathogenesis via repression of *TBX5*-mediated cardiac differentiation (H. Yang et al., 2025) |
| Bioinformatic co-expression and network analysis-integrative analysis of DE miRNAs (GSE35490) and DE genes (GSE35776) in Tetralogy of Fallot | hsa-miR-16 and hsa-miR-124 emerged as key miRNAs in TOF, acting through a co-expression network. They are predicted to regulate mitochondrial energy metabolism and fatty acid oxidation by targeting genes such as *NT5DC1*, *ECHDC1*, *HSDL2*, *FCHO2*, and *ACAA2*, implicating disruption of ATP conversion and fatty acid metabolism in TOF pathogenesis (Y. Yu et al., 2023) |
| Integrated datasets from GEO: miRNA (GSE36759), mRNA, and circRNA expression in TOF vs controls (aggregated 66 samples: 47 TOF, 19 controls) | Constructed a circRNA–miRNA–mRNA ceRNA network. Identified the hsa_circ_000601 / hsa-miR-148a / *BCL2L11* regulatory axis as a potential key pathway in TOF. In TOF hearts, hsa-miR-148a was downregulated, while hsa_circ_000601 and *BCL2L11* were upregulated, suggesting that the circRNA may sponge miR-148a—reducing its suppression on *BCL2L11* and thus promoting apoptosis via elevated *BCL2L11* expression (Kan et al., 2022) |
| Genome-wide miRNA and mRNA transcriptome profiling in right ventricular tissues from 22 non-syndromic TOF patients vs normal heart controls | miR-1 and miR-133, both essential for cardiac development and function, were dysregulated in TOF right ventricular tissue. Predicted and validated targets include *KCNJ2*, *FBN2*, *SLC38A3*, and *TNNI1*, indicating these miRNAs play a role in TOF pathogenesis via post-transcriptional regulation of genes critical for cardiomyocyte structure and electrophysiology (Grunert et al., 2019) |
| Small RNA sequencing of right ventricular tissue from 10 age-matched TOF patients (5 male vs. 5 female) | miR-1 and miR-133 comprise the most variable sRNA clusters between sexes in TOF hearts, indicating significant sexual dimorphism in miRNA expression patterns. miR-1/miR-133 cluster contributes strongly to distinguishing male vs female TOF expression profiles (B. Wang et al., 2018) |
| Circulating miRNA microarray and RT-qPCR in serum of adults post-TOF repair (37 patients; 3 with right heart failure) vs healthy controls (15) | miR-181d-5p, miR-206, and miR-625-5p were significantly dysregulated in all TOF patients (high diagnostic accuracy; AUCs ~0.99 for miR-181d-5p and miR-206). miR-421, miR-1233-3p, and miR-625-5p were notably lower in those with right heart failure-suggesting prognostic potential (Abu-Halima et al., 2017) |
| Serum RT-qPCR profiling of left heart-associated miRNAs and broader miRNA screening in young adults with repaired TOF vs controls | No differences were detected in traditional left heart miRNAs (miR-1, miR-133a, miR-208a/b, miR-423-5p). However, broader profiling revealed upregulation of miR-99b and downregulation of miR-766 in TOF patients (Lai et al., 2017) |
| RT-qPCR in right ventricular myocardium from 30 TOF patients vs. 10 controls; immunohistochemistry for Cx43 expression | miR-1 and miR-206 were significantly downregulated in TOF myocardium. This downregulation may contribute to the upregulated expression of Connexin 43 (*Cx43*), implicated in tetralogy of Fallot pathogenesis. No sequence variants were found in the miRNA binding sites of *Cx43* 3′UTR (Y. Wu et al., 2014) |

continued on following page

*Table 1. Continued*

| Study Type & Sample | Key Findings |
|---|---|
| Microarray profiling of right ventricular outflow tract (RVOT) tissues from infants with nonsyndromic TOF (n=5) vs age-matched controls (n=3), validated via qRT-PCR in expanded sample size | Identified 41 candidate miRNAs dysregulated in TOF RVOT tissue; 18 were confirmed as significantly altered. miR-424/424* promoted cardiomyocyte proliferation and inhibited migration in mouse embryonic cardiomyocytes. miR-222 stimulated cardiomyocyte proliferation while suppressing cardiomyogenic differentiation in P19 cells. Direct targets validated by 3′UTR luciferase assays include HAS2 and NF1 (inhibited by miR-424/424*), implicating them in TOF pathogenesis (J. Zhang et al., 2013) |
| miR-423-5p measured in TGA patients (systemic RV with reduced EF) vs healthy controls | No significant difference in circulating miR-423-5p levels between patients and controls; no correlation with ventricular function or clinical parameters—indicating miR-423-5p is not a useful biomarker in this setting (Tutarel et al., 2013) |
| Genome-wide miRNA and mRNA microarrays on blood from TGA-RV (n=16), TGA-LV (n=16), and matched controls (n=16); RT-qPCR validation and integrative network analysis | A total of 39 miRNAs were differentially expressed in TGA patients versus controls, including 51 miRNAs distinctively dysregulated in TGA-RV vs TGA-LV. Importantly, miR-140-3p was elevated in patients with overt heart failure (FC = 1.54; $p = 0.001$), and miR-502-3p was higher in those who succumbed to cardiac death (FC = 1.41; $p = 0.011$). Network analysis revealed 21 target genes inversely correlated with miRNAs ($r \geq -0.5$, $p < 0.05$), each containing miRNA binding sites in their 3′UTRs—highlighting potential miRNA–mRNA regulatory interactions in TGA pathophysiology (Abu-Halima et al., 2022) |
| Circulating miRNA microarray profiling and RT-qPCR validation in serum of adult TGA-RV patients (n=36) vs healthy volunteers (n=35) | miR-183-3p, along with miR-150-5p, miR-1255b-5p, and miR-423-3p, was significantly associated with worsening heart failure in TGA-RV patients. Notably, miR-183-3p emerged as an independent predictor of worsening HF ($p = 0.001$)—suggesting its utility as a prognostic biomarker in this population (Abu-Halima et al., 2021) |
| Serum RT-qPCR profiling of circulating miRNAs in adults with systemic right ventricle after atrial switch for TGA vs healthy controls | miR-18a and miR-486-5p were identified as significantly dysregulated in patients post-atrial switch TGA. Their expression levels correlated negatively with systemic right ventricular contractility, assessed via myocardial acceleration during isovolumic contraction (IVA), suggesting potential as functional biomarkers in this setting (Lai et al., 2013) |
| miRNA microarray and RT-qPCR analysis of pulmonary artery serum from pediatric patients post-Glenn procedure with PAVMs vs post-Fontan patients; functional assays in endothelial cells under hypoxia | miR-25-3p was significantly upregulated in pulmonary artery serum of Glenn patients with pulmonary arteriovenous malformations (PAVMs). In endothelial cells (HMVEC-L), miR-25-3p directly targets *PHLPP2*, reducing its expression and thereby activating the HIF-1α/VEGF-A axis under hypoxic conditions. This promotes angiogenesis, proliferation, and migration of endothelial cells—suggesting that miR-25-3p contributes to PAVM development via the PHLPP2–HIF-1α signaling pathway (Kawamura et al., 2025) |

continued on following page

*Table 1. Continued*

| Study Type & Sample | Key Findings |
|---|---|
| High-throughput sequencing and RT-qPCR validation of maternal serum miRNAs in pregnant women carrying fetuses with CHD vs normal fetuses | miR-3195 and miR-122-5p were significantly downregulated in maternal serum during pregnancy when the fetus had CHD. Bioinformatic analysis suggests that both may influence biometabolic processes relevant to fetal heart development—supporting their potential as non-invasive prenatal biomarkers for CHD detection (Xi et al., 2024) |
| RT-qPCR analysis of plasma miR-21-5p, miR-155-5p, miR-221-3p, miR-26a-5p, miR-144-3p in 86 children with CHD (cyanotic vs non-cyanotic) and 110 controls | Expression levels of miR-21-5p, miR-155-5p, miR-221-3p, and miR-26a-5p were significantly different between CHD patients and controls. Notably, miR-21-5p levels were higher in cyanotic CHD compared to non-cyanotic CHD, suggesting its potential as a biomarker linked to CHD severity (González-Moyotl et al., 2024) |

ASD, atrial septal defect; VSD, ventricular septal defect; TOF, Tetralogy of Fallot; TGA, transposition of the great arteries; CHD, congenital heart disease; PAH, pulmonary arterial hypertension; PDA, patent ductus arteriosus; hESC, human embryonic stem cell; hiPSC, human induced pluripotent stem cell; mESC, mouse embryonic stem cell; CM, cardiomyocyte; WES, whole-exome sequencing; UTR, untranslated region; ROC, receiver operating characteristic; AUC, area under the curve; PA, pulmonary artery; PAVM, pulmonary arteriovenous malformation; BNP, brain natriuretic peptide; ADMA, asymmetric dimethylarginine; RT-qPCR, reverse transcription quantitative polymerase chain reaction; snRNA-seq, single-nucleus RNA sequencing; iPS, induced pluripotent stem; EF, ejection fraction; IVA, isovolumic acceleration; RV, right ventricle; LV, left ventricle; Cx43, Connexin 43.

*Figure 1. Schematic summary of major signaling pathways regulated by microRNAs (miRNAs) in congenital heart disease (CHD)*

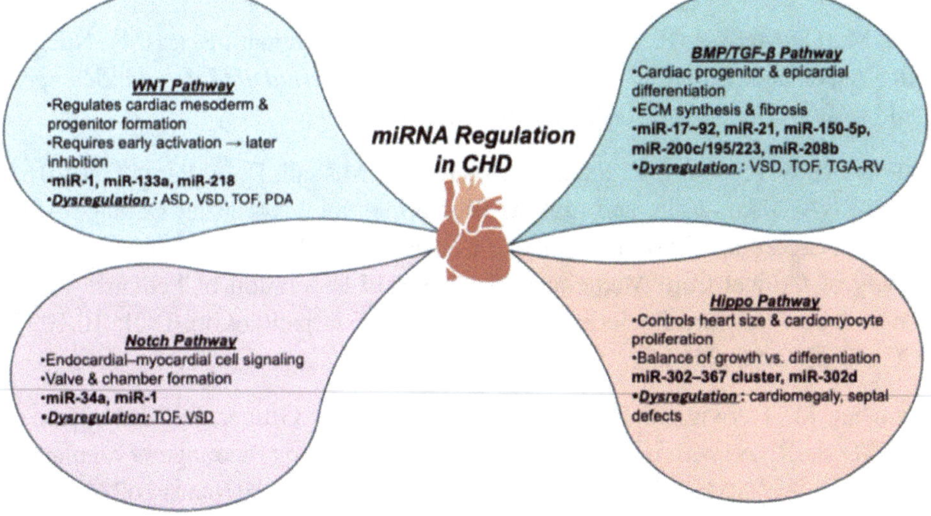


*Note. Selected circulating miRNAs have been shown as possible biomarkers. ASD: atrial septal defect; VSD: ventricular septal defect; TOF: tetralogy of Fallot; PDA: patent ductus arteriosus; TGA-RV: transposition of the great arteries with right ventricle involvement*

## REFERENCES


Abdelfattah, A. M., Park, C., & Choi, M. Y. (2014). Update on non-canonical microRNAs. *Biomolecular Concepts*, *5*(4), 275–287. DOI: 10.1515/bmc-2014-0012

Abu-Halima, M., Meese, E., Abdul-Khaliq, H., & Raedle-Hurst, T. (2021). MicroRNA-183-3p Is a Predictor of Worsening Heart Failure in Adult Patients With Transposition of the Great Arteries and a Systemic Right Ventricle. *Frontiers in Cardiovascular Medicine*, *8*, 730364. DOI: 10.3389/fcvm.2021.730364

Abu-Halima, M., Meese, E., Keller, A., Abdul-Khaliq, H., & Rädle-Hurst, T. (2017). Analysis of circulating microRNAs in patients with repaired Tetralogy of Fallot with and without heart failure. *Journal of Translational Medicine*, *15*, 156. DOI: 10.1186/s12967-017-1255-z

Abu-Halima, M., Wagner, V., Rishik, S., Raedle-Hurst, T., Meese, E., & Abdul-Khaliq, H. (2022). Expression profiling analysis reveals key microRNA-mRNA interactions in patients with transposition of the great arteries and systemic left and right ventricles. *Frontiers in Cardiovascular Medicine*, *9*, 1056427. DOI: 10.3389/fcvm.2022.1056427

Bajan, S., & Hutvagner, G. (2020). RNA-Based Therapeutics: From Antisense Oligonucleotides to miRNAs. *Cells*, *9*(1), 137. DOI: 10.3390/cells9010137

Billi, M., De Marinis, E., Gentile, M., Nervi, C., & Grignani, F. (2024). Nuclear miRNAs: Gene Regulation Activities. *International Journal of Molecular Sciences*, *25*(11), 6066. DOI: 10.3390/ijms25116066

Bolkier, Y., Nevo-Caspi, Y., Salem, Y., Vardi, A., Mishali, D., & Paret, G. (2016). Micro-RNA-208a, -208b, and -499 as Biomarkers for Myocardial Damage After Cardiac Surgery in Children. Pediatric Critical Care Medicine: A Journal of the Society of Critical Care Medicine and the World Federation of Pediatric Intensive and Critical Care Societies, 17(4), e193-197. https://doi.org/DOI: 10.1097/PCC.0000000000000644

Brameier, M., Herwig, A., Reinhardt, R., Walter, L., & Gruber, J. (2011). Human box C/D snoRNAs with miRNA like functions: Expanding the range of regulatory RNAs. *Nucleic Acids Research*, *39*(2), 675–686. DOI: 10.1093/nar/gkq776

Buikema, J. W., Zwetsloot, P.-P. M., Doevendans, P. A., Domian, I. J., & Sluijter, J. P. G. (2014). Wnt/β-Catenin Signaling during Cardiac Development and Repair. *Journal of Cardiovascular Development and Disease*, *1*(1), 98–110. DOI: 10.3390/jcdd1010098

Cao, Y., Wen, J., Li, Y., Chen, W., Wu, Y., Li, J., & Huang, G. (2019). Uric acid and sphingomyelin enhance autophagy in iPS cell-originated cardiomyocytes through lncRNA MEG3/miR-7-5p/EGFR axis. *Artificial Cells, Nanomedicine, and Biotechnology*, *47*(1), 3774–3785. DOI: 10.1080/21691401.2019.1667817

Cavaillé, J., Buiting, K., Kiefmann, M., Lalande, M., Brannan, C. I., Horsthemke, B., Bachellerie, J.-P., Brosius, J., & Hüttenhofer, A. (2000). Identification of brain-specific and imprinted small nucleolar RNA genes exhibiting an unusual genomic organization. *Proceedings of the National Academy of Sciences of the United States of America*, *97*(26), 14311–14316. DOI: 10.1073/pnas.250426397

CDC. (2024, October 22). Data and Statistics. Congenital Heart Defects (CHDs). https://www.cdc.gov/heart-defects/data/index.html

Cheloufi, S., Dos Santos, C. O., Chong, M. M. W., & Hannon, G. J. (2010). A dicer-independent miRNA biogenesis pathway that requires Ago catalysis. *Nature*, *465*(7298), 584–589. DOI: 10.1038/nature09092

Chen, W., & Li, S. (2017). Circulating microRNA as a Novel Biomarker for Pulmonary Arterial Hypertension Due to Congenital Heart Disease. *Pediatric Cardiology*, *38*(1), 86–94. DOI: 10.1007/s00246-016-1487-3

Chen, Y.-L., Pascuzzi, N., Ruiz, A., & Chen, K.-H. E. (2025). Mirtrons in Human Cancers. *Onco*, *5*(1), 7. DOI: 10.3390/onco5010007

Choudhury, T. Z., Gilbert, B. L., & Garg, V. (2025). Genetic and Environmental Contributors To Congenital Heart Disease. *Current Treatment Options in Cardiovascular Medicine*, *27*(1), 36. DOI: 10.1007/s11936-025-01091-5

Cifuentes, D., Xue, H., Taylor, D. W., Patnode, H., Mishima, Y., Cheloufi, S., Ma, E., Mane, S., Hannon, G. J., Lawson, N. D., Wolfe, S. A., & Giraldez, A. J. (2010). A novel miRNA processing pathway independent of Dicer requires Argonaute2 catalytic activity. *Science*, *328*(5986), 1694–1698. DOI: 10.1126/science.1190809

Coley, A. B., DeMeis, J. D., Chaudhary, N. Y., & Borchert, G. M. (2022). Small Nucleolar Derived RNAs as Regulators of Human Cancer. *Biomedicines*, *10*(8), 1819. DOI: 10.3390/biomedicines10081819

Condrat, C. E., Thompson, D. C., Barbu, M. G., Bugnar, O. L., Boboc, A., Cretoiu, D., Suciu, N., Cretoiu, S. M., & Voinea, S. C. (2020). miRNAs as Biomarkers in Disease: Latest Findings Regarding Their Role in Diagnosis and Prognosis. *Cells*, *9*(2), 276. DOI: 10.3390/cells9020276 de Rooij, L. A., Mastebroek, D. J., ten Voorde, N., van der Wall, E., van Diest, P. J., & Moelans, C. B. (2022). The microRNA Lifecycle in Health and Cancer. *Cancers (Basel)*, *14*(23), 5748. DOI: 10.3390/cancers14235748

Di Mauro, V., Crasto, S., Colombo, F. S., Di Pasquale, E., & Catalucci, D. (2019). Wnt signalling mediates miR-133a nuclear re-localization for the transcriptional control of Dnmt3b in cardiac cells. *Scientific Reports*, *9*(1), 9320. DOI: 10.1038/s41598-019-45818-4

Diener, C., Keller, A., & Meese, E. (2022). Emerging concepts of miRNA therapeutics: From cells to clinic. *Trends in Genetics*, *38*(6), 613–626. DOI: 10.1016/j.tig.2022.02.006

Doe, C. M., Relkovic, D., Garfield, A. S., Dalley, J. W., Theobald, D. E. H., Humby, T., Wilkinson, L. S., & Isles, A. R. (2009). Loss of the imprinted snoRNA mbii-52 leads to increased 5htr2c pre-RNA editing and altered 5HT2CR-mediated behaviour. *Human Molecular Genetics*, *18*(12), 2140–2148. DOI: 10.1093/hmg/ddp137

Dubey, G., Singh, M., Singh, H., Agarwal, M., Chandel, S. S., Mishra, A., Singh, R. P., & Kukreti, N. (2024). Emerging roles of SnoRNAs in the pathogenesis and treatment of autoimmune disorders. *Pathology, Research and Practice*, *253*, 154952. DOI: 10.1016/j.prp.2023.154952

Espinoza-Lewis, R. A., & Wang, D.-Z. (2012). MicroRNAs in Heart Development. *Current Topics in Developmental Biology*, *100*, 279–317. DOI: 10.1016/B978-0-12-387786-4.00009-9

Flynt, A. S., Greimann, J. C., Chung, W.-J., Lima, C. D., & Lai, E. C. (2010). MicroRNA Biogenesis via Splicing and Exosome-Mediated Trimming in Drosophila. *Molecular Cell*, *38*(6), 900–907. DOI: 10.1016/j.molcel.2010.06.014

Fu, X.-D. (2014). Non-coding RNA: A new frontier in regulatory biology. *National Science Review*, *1*(2), 190–204. DOI: 10.1093/nsr/nwu008

Fuller, A. M., & Qian, L. (2014). MiRiad Roles for MicroRNAs in Cardiac Development and Regeneration. *Cells*, *3*(3), 724–750. DOI: 10.3390/cells3030724

Gál, L., Schamberger, A., Wachtl, G., & Orbán, T. I. (2024). The Effect of Alternative Splicing Sites on Mirtron Formation and Arm Selection of Precursor microRNAs. *International Journal of Molecular Sciences*, *25*(14), 7643. DOI: 10.3390/ijms25147643

Garreau, M., Weidner, J., Hamilton, R., Kolosionek, E., Toki, N., Stavenhagen, K., Paris, C., Bonetti, A., Czechtizky, W., Gnerlich, F., & Rydzik, A. (2024). Chemical modification patterns for microRNA therapeutic mimics: A structure-activity relationship (SAR) case-study on miR-200c. *Nucleic Acids Research, 52*(6), 2792–2807. DOI: 10.1093/nar/gkae141

González-Moyotl, N., Huesca-Gómez, C., Torres-Paz, Y. E., Fuentevilla-Álvarez, G., Romero-Maldonado, S., Sámano, R., Soto, M. E., Martínez-Rosas, M., Domínguez-López, A., & Gamboa, R. (2024). Paediatrics congenital heart disease is associated with plasma miRNAs. *Pediatric Research, 96*(5), 1220–1227. DOI: 10.1038/s41390-024-03230-3

Grunert, M., Appelt, S., Dunkel, I., Berger, F., & Sperling, S. R. (2019). Altered microRNA and target gene expression related to Tetralogy of Fallot. *Scientific Reports, 9*(1), 19063. DOI: 10.1038/s41598-019-55570-4

Gu, S., Jin, L., Zhang, Y., Huang, Y., Zhang, F., Valdmanis, P. N., & Kay, M. A. (2012). The loop position of shRNAs and pre-miRNAs is critical for the accuracy of Dicer processing in vivo. *Cell, 151*(4), 900–911. DOI: 10.1016/j.cell.2012.09.042

Guo, F. (2012). Chapter Five—Drosha and DGCR8 in MicroRNA Biogenesis. In Guo, F., & Tamanoi, F. (Eds.), *The Enzymes* (Vol. 32, pp. 101–121). Academic Press., DOI: 10.1016/B978-0-12-404741-9.00005-2

Guo, Z., Maki, M., Ding, R., Yang, Y., Zhang, B., & Xiong, L. (2014). Genome-wide survey of tissue-specific microRNA and transcription factor regulatory networks in 12 tissues. *Scientific Reports, 4*, 5150. DOI: 10.1038/srep05150

Håkansson, K. E. J., Goossens, E. A. C., Trompet, S., van Ingen, E., de Vries, M. R., van der Kwast, R. V. C. T., Ripa, R. S., Kastrup, J., Hohensinner, P. J., Kaun, C., Wojta, J., Böhringer, S., Le Cessie, S., Jukema, J. W., Quax, P. H. A., & Nossent, A. Y. (2019). Genetic associations and regulation of expression indicate an independent role for 14q32 snoRNAs in human cardiovascular disease. *Cardiovascular Research, 115*(10), 1519–1532. DOI: 10.1093/cvr/cvy309

Hata, A., & Kang, H. (2015). Functions of the bone morphogenetic protein signaling pathway through microRNAs [Review]. *International Journal of Molecular Medicine, 35*(3), 563–568. DOI: 10.3892/ijmm.2015.2060

Havens, M. A., Reich, A. A., Duelli, D. M., & Hastings, M. L. (2012). Biogenesis of mammalian microRNAs by a non-canonical processing pathway. *Nucleic Acids Research, 40*(10), 4626–4640. DOI: 10.1093/nar/gks026

Huesca-Gomez, C., Gonzalez-Moyotl, N., Romero-Maldonado, S., Samano, R., & Gamboa, R. (2025). Role of circulating microRNAs in tetralogy of Fallot. Postepy W Kardiologii Interwencyjnej = Advances in Interventional Cardiology, 21(2), 247–254. https://doi.org/DOI: 10.5114/aic.2025.151804

Hynes, C., & Kakumani, P. K. (2024). Regulatory role of RNA-binding proteins in microRNA biogenesis. *Frontiers in Molecular Biosciences*, *11*. Advance online publication. DOI: 10.3389/fmolb.2024.1374843

Ivey, K. N., & Srivastava, D. (2015). microRNAs as Developmental Regulators. *Cold Spring Harbor Perspectives in Biology*, *7*(7), a008144. DOI: 10.1101/cshperspect.a008144

Ji, L., Hou, H., Zhu, K., Liu, X., Liu, Y., Wang, Q., Li, J., Liu, H., Zhang, Q., Lv, J., Alexander, R., Wang, W., & Li, D. (2019). NOTCH1 Gene MicroRNA Target Variation and Ventricular Septal Defect Risk. *OMICS: A Journal of Integrative Biology*, *23*(1), 28–35. DOI: 10.1089/omi.2018.0171

Jia, L., Limeng, D., Xiaoyin, T., Junwen, W., Xintong, Z., Gang, X., Yun, B., & Hong, G. (2022). A Novel Splicing Mutation c.335–1 G>A in the Cardiac Transcription Factor NKX2-5 Leads to Familial Atrial Septal Defect Through miR-19 and PYK2. *Stem Cell Reviews and Reports*, *18*(8), 2646–2661. DOI: 10.1007/s12015-022-10400-5

Jiang, Y., Zhuang, J., Lin, Y., Wang, X., Chen, J., & Han, F. (2019). Long noncoding RNA SNHG6 contributes to ventricular septal defect formation via negative regulation of miR-101 and activation of Wnt/β-catenin pathway. *Die Pharmazie*, *74*(1), 23–28. DOI: 10.1691/ph.2019.8736

Jin, Y., Ai, L., Chai, X., Tang, P., Zhang, W., Yang, L., Hu, Y., Xu, Y., & Li, S. (2021). Maternal Circulating Exosomal miRNAs as Non-invasive Biomarkers for the Prediction of Fetal Ventricular Septal Defect. *Frontiers in Genetics*, *12*, 717208. DOI: 10.3389/fgene.2021.717208

Kan, Z., Yan, W., Wang, N., Fang, Y., Gao, H., & Song, Y. (2022). Identification of circRNA-miRNA-mRNA Regulatory Network and Crucial Signaling Pathway Axis Involved in Tetralogy of Fallot. *Frontiers in Genetics*, *13*, 917454. DOI: 10.3389/fgene.2022.917454

Kawamura, J., Yamakuchi, M., Ueno, K., Hashiguchi, T., & Okamoto, Y. (2025). MiR-25-3p regulates pulmonary arteriovenous malformation after Glenn procedure in patients with univentricular heart via the PHLPP2-HIF-1α axis. *Scientific Reports*, *15*(1), 4138. DOI: 10.1038/s41598-025-88840-5

Kim, Y. Y., Min, H., Kim, H., Choi, Y. M., Liu, H. C., & Ku, S.-Y. (2017). Differential MicroRNA Expression Profile of Human Embryonic Stem Cell-Derived Cardiac Lineage Cells. *Tissue Engineering and Regenerative Medicine, 14*(2), 163–169. DOI: 10.1007/s13770-017-0051-4

Kirschner, M. B., Edelman, J. J. B., Kao, S. C.-H., Vallely, M. P., Van Zandwijk, N., & Reid, G. (2013). The Impact of Hemolysis on Cell-Free microRNA Biomarkers. *Frontiers in Genetics, 4*. Advance online publication. DOI: 10.3389/fgene.2013.00094

Kotowska-Zimmer, A., Pewinska, M., & Olejniczak, M. (2021). Artificial miRNAs as therapeutic tools: Challenges and opportunities. *Wiley Interdisciplinary Reviews. RNA, 12*(4), e1640. DOI: 10.1002/wrna.1640

Kuppusamy, K. T., Jones, D. C., Sperber, H., Madan, A., Fischer, K. A., Rodriguez, M. L., Pabon, L., Zhu, W.-Z., Tulloch, N. L., Yang, X., Sniadecki, N. J., Laflamme, M. A., Ruzzo, W. L., Murry, C. E., & Ruohola-Baker, H. (2015). Let-7 family of microRNA is required for maturation and adult-like metabolism in stem cell-derived cardiomyocytes. *Proceedings of the National Academy of Sciences of the United States of America, 112*(21), E2785–E2794. DOI: 10.1073/pnas.1424042112

Kwon, C., Arnold, J., Hsiao, E. C., Taketo, M. M., Conklin, B. R., & Srivastava, D. (2007). Canonical Wnt signaling is a positive regulator of mammalian cardiac progenitors. *Proceedings of the National Academy of Sciences of the United States of America, 104*(26), 10894–10899. DOI: 10.1073/pnas.0704044104

Kwon, C., Han, Z., Olson, E. N., & Srivastava, D. (2005). MicroRNA1 influences cardiac differentiation in Drosophila and regulates Notch signaling. *Proceedings of the National Academy of Sciences of the United States of America, 102*(52), 18986–18991. DOI: 10.1073/pnas.0509535102

Ladewig, E., Okamura, K., Flynt, A. S., Westholm, J. O., & Lai, E. C. (2012). Discovery of hundreds of mirtrons in mouse and human small RNA data. *Genome Research, 22*(9), 1634–1645. DOI: 10.1101/gr.133553.111

Lai, C. T. M., Ng, E. K. O., Chow, P., Kwong, A., & Cheung, Y. (2013). Circulating microRNA expression profile and systemic right ventricular function in adults after atrial switch operation for complete transposition of the great arteries. *BMC Cardiovascular Disorders, 13*, 73. DOI: 10.1186/1471-2261-13-73

Lai, C. T. M., Ng, E. K. O., Chow, P., Kwong, A., & Cheung, Y. (2017). Circulating MicroRNA in patients with repaired tetralogy of Fallot. *European Journal of Clinical Investigation, 47*(8), 574–582. DOI: 10.1111/eci.12778

Leonard, R., Zhao, Y., Eliason, S., Zimmerman, K., Batz, A., Hatcher, C. J., Weiss, R. M., Sweat, M., Li, X., & Amendt, B. A. (2025). Single-nuclei multiomics analysis identifies abnormal cardiomyocytes in a murine model of cardiac development. *Nature Communications*, *16*, 6947. DOI: 10.1038/s41467-025-62208-9

Li, D., Ji, L., Liu, L., Liu, Y., Hou, H., Yu, K., Sun, Q., & Zhao, Z. (2014). Characterization of circulating microRNA expression in patients with a ventricular septal defect. *PLoS One*, *9*(8), e106318. DOI: 10.1371/journal.pone.0106318

Li, J., Cao, Y., Ma, X., Wang, H., Zhang, J., Luo, X., Chen, W., Wu, Y., Meng, Y., Zhang, J., Yuan, Y., Ma, D., & Huang, G. (2013). Roles of miR-1-1 and miR-181c in ventricular septal defects. *International Journal of Cardiology*, *168*(2), 1441–1446. DOI: 10.1016/j.ijcard.2012.12.048

Li, J.-Y., Li, X.-C., & Tang, Y.-L. (2021). Upregulation of miR-128 Mediates Heart Injury by Activating Wnt/β-catenin Signaling Pathway in Heart Failure Mice. *Organogenesis*, *17*(3–4), 27–39. DOI: 10.1080/15476278.2021.2020018

Li, K.-X., Li, J.-R., Zuo, S.-J., Li, X., Chen, X.-T., Xiao, P.-Y., Li, H.-T., Sun, L., Qian, T., Zhang, H.-M., Zhu, D., Yu, X.-Y., Chen, G., & Jiang, X.-Y. (2024). Identification of miR-20b-5p as an inhibitory regulator in cardiac differentiation via TET2 and DNA hydroxymethylation. *Clinical Epigenetics*, *16*(1), 42. DOI: 10.1186/s13148-024-01653-7

Lian, X., Hsiao, C., Wilson, G., Zhu, K., Hazeltine, L. B., Azarin, S. M., Raval, K. K., Zhang, J., Kamp, T. J., & Palecek, S. P. (2012). Robust cardiomyocyte differentiation from human pluripotent stem cells via temporal modulation of canonical Wnt signaling. *Proceedings of the National Academy of Sciences of the United States of America*, *109*(27), E1848–E1857. DOI: 10.1073/pnas.1200250109

Liu, X., Li, M., Peng, Y., Hu, X., Xu, J., Zhu, S., Yu, Z., & Han, S. (2016). miR-30c regulates proliferation, apoptosis and differentiation via the Shh signaling pathway in P19 cells. *Experimental & Molecular Medicine*, *48*(7), e248. DOI: 10.1038/emm.2016.57

Liu, Y., Chen, S., Zühlke, L., Black, G. C., Choy, M., Li, N., & Keavney, B. D. (2019). Global birth prevalence of congenital heart defects 1970–2017: Updated systematic review and meta-analysis of 260 studies. *International Journal of Epidemiology*, *48*(2), 455–463. DOI: 10.1093/ije/dyz009

Long, L., Xiao, Y., Yin, X., Gao, S., Zhou, L., & Liu, H. (2020). Expression of serum miR-27b and miR-451 in patients with congenital heart disease associated pulmonary artery hypertension and risk factor analysis. *Experimental and Therapeutic Medicine*, *20*(4), 3196–3202. DOI: 10.3892/etm.2020.9042

Lozano-Velasco, E., Inácio, J. M., Sousa, I., Guimarães, A. R., Franco, D., Moura, G., & Belo, J. A. (2024). miRNAs in Heart Development and Disease. *International Journal of Molecular Sciences*, *25*(3), 1673. DOI: 10.3390/ijms25031673

MacGrogan, D., Münch, J., & de la Pompa, J. L. (2018). Notch and interacting signalling pathways in cardiac development, disease, and regeneration. *Nature Reviews. Cardiology*, *15*(11), 685–704. DOI: 10.1038/s41569-018-0100-2

Mannarino, S., Calcaterra, V., Puricelli, F., Cecconi, G., Chillemi, C., Raso, I., Cordaro, E., & Zuccotti, G. (2025). The Role of miRNA Expression in Congenital Heart Disease: Insights into the Mechanisms and Biomarker Potential. *Children (Basel, Switzerland)*, *12*(5), 611. DOI: 10.3390/children12050611

Marracino, L., Fortini, F., Bouhamida, E., Camponogara, F., Severi, P., Mazzoni, E., Patergnani, S., D'Aniello, E., Campana, R., Pinton, P., Martini, F., Tognon, M., Campo, G., Ferrari, R., Vieceli Dalla Sega, F., & Rizzo, P. (2021). Adding a "Notch" to Cardiovascular Disease Therapeutics: A MicroRNA-Based Approach. *Frontiers in Cell and Developmental Biology*, *9*. Advance online publication. DOI: 10.3389/fcell.2021.695114

Maute, R. L., Schneider, C., Sumazin, P., Holmes, A., Califano, A., Basso, K., & Dalla-Favera, R. (2013). tRNA-derived microRNA modulates proliferation and the DNA damage response and is down-regulated in B cell lymphoma. *Proceedings of the National Academy of Sciences of the United States of America*, *110*(4), 1404–1409. DOI: 10.1073/pnas.1206761110

McAllan, A. L., Pillman, K. A., Gearing, L. J., & Gantier, M. P. (2025). IsomiR stoichiometry changes as disease biomarkers. *Molecular Therapy. Nucleic Acids*, *36*(3), 102578. DOI: 10.1016/j.omtn.2025.102578

Meng, X., Song, M., Zhang, K., Lu, W., Li, Y., Zhang, C., & Zhang, Y. (2024). Congenital heart disease: Types, pathophysiology, diagnosis, and treatment options. *MedComm*, *5*(7), e631. DOI: 10.1002/mco2.631

Mick, E., Shah, R., Tanriverdi, K., Murthy, V., Gerstein, M., Rozowsky, J., Kitchen, R., Larson, M. G., Levy, D., & Freedman, J. E. (2017). Stroke and Circulating Extracellular RNAs. *Stroke*, *48*(4), 828–834. DOI: 10.1161/STROKEAHA.116.015140

Münsterberg, A., & Hoppler, S. (2016). WNT and BMP regulate roadblocks toward cardiomyocyte differentiation: Lessons learned from embryos inform human stem cell differentiation. *Stem Cell Investigation*, *3*, 33. DOI: 10.21037/sci.2016.07.03

Nail, H. M., Chiu, C.-C., Leung, C.-H., Ahmed, M. M. M., & Wang, H.-M. D. (2023). Exosomal miRNA-mediated intercellular communications and immunomodulatory effects in tumor microenvironments. *Journal of Biomedical Science*, *30*(1), 69. DOI: 10.1186/s12929-023-00964-w

Naito, A. T., Shiojima, I., Akazawa, H., Hidaka, K., Morisaki, T., Kikuchi, A., & Komuro, I. (2006). Developmental stage-specific biphasic roles of Wnt/β-catenin signaling in cardiomyogenesis and hematopoiesis. *Proceedings of the National Academy of Sciences of the United States of America*, *103*(52), 19812–19817. DOI: 10.1073/pnas.0605768103

Natarelli, L., & Weber, C. (2022). A Non-Canonical Link between Non-Coding RNAs and Cardiovascular Diseases. *Biomedicines*, *10*(2), 445. DOI: 10.3390/biomedicines10020445

Nikolova, E., Laleva, L., Milev, M., Spiriev, T., Stoyanov, S., Ferdinandov, D., Mitev, V., & Todorova, A. (2024). miRNAs and related genetic biomarkers according to the WHO glioma classification: From diagnosis to future therapeutic targets. *Non-Coding RNA Research*, *9*(1), 141–152. DOI: 10.1016/j.ncrna.2023.10.003

Nossent, A. Y., Ektefaie, N., Wojta, J., Eichelberger, B., Kopp, C., Panzer, S., & Gremmel, T. (2019). Plasma Levels of snoRNAs are Associated with Platelet Activation in Patients with Peripheral Artery Disease. *International Journal of Molecular Sciences*, *20*(23), 5975. DOI: 10.3390/ijms20235975

O'Brien, J. E., Kibiryeva, N., Zhou, X.-G., Marshall, J. A., Lofland, G. K., Artman, M., Chen, J., & Bittel, D. C. (2012). Noncoding RNA expression in myocardium from infants with tetralogy of Fallot. *Circulation: Cardiovascular Genetics*, *5*(3), 279–286. DOI: 10.1161/CIRCGENETICS.111.961474

O'Brien, J., Hayder, H., Zayed, Y., & Peng, C. (2018). Overview of MicroRNA Biogenesis, Mechanisms of Actions, and Circulation. *Frontiers in Endocrinology*, *9*, 402. DOI: 10.3389/fendo.2018.00402

Okamura, K., Hagen, J. W., Duan, H., Tyler, D. M., & Lai, E. C. (2007). The Mirtron Pathway Generates microRNA-Class Regulatory RNAs in Drosophila. *Cell*, *130*(1), 89–100. DOI: 10.1016/j.cell.2007.06.028

Ouyang, Z., & Wei, K. (2021). miRNA in cardiac development and regeneration. *Cell Regeneration (London, England)*, *10*, 14. DOI: 10.1186/s13619-021-00077-5

Paddison, P. J., Caudy, A. A., Bernstein, E., Hannon, G. J., & Conklin, D. S. (2002). Short hairpin RNAs (shRNAs) induce sequence-specific silencing in mammalian cells. *Genes & Development*, *16*(8), 948–958. DOI: 10.1101/gad.981002

Pandolfini, L., Barbieri, I., Bannister, A. J., Hendrick, A., Andrews, B., Webster, N., Murat, P., Mach, P., Brandi, R., Robson, S. C., Migliori, V., Alendar, A., d'Onofrio, M., Balasubramanian, S., & Kouzarides, T. (2019). METTL1 Promotes let-7 MicroRNA Processing via m7G Methylation. *Molecular Cell, 74*(6), 1278–1290. e9. DOI: 10.1016/j.molcel.2019.03.040

Peng, Y., Song, L., Zhao, M., Harmelink, C., Debenedittis, P., Cui, X., Wang, Q., & Jiao, K. (2014). Critical roles of miRNA-mediated regulation of TGFβ signalling during mouse cardiogenesis. *Cardiovascular Research, 103*(2), 258–267. DOI: 10.1093/cvr/cvu126

Plotnikova, O., Baranova, A., & Skoblov, M. (2019). Comprehensive Analysis of Human microRNA–mRNA Interactome. *Frontiers in Genetics, 10*, 933. DOI: 10.3389/fgene.2019.00933

Poon, E. N., Hao, B., Guan, D., Jun Li, M., Lu, J., Yang, Y., Wu, B., Wu, S. C., Webb, S. E., Liang, Y., Miller, A. L., Yao, X., Wang, J., Yan, B., & Boheler, K. R. (2018). Integrated transcriptomic and regulatory network analyses identify microRNA-200c as a novel repressor of human pluripotent stem cell-derived cardiomyocyte differentiation and maturation. *Cardiovascular Research, 114*(6), 894–906. DOI: 10.1093/cvr/cvy019

Radhakrishna, U., Albayrak, S., Zafra, R., Baraa, A., Vishweswaraiah, S., Veerappa, A. M., Mahishi, D., Saiyed, N., Mishra, N. K., Guda, C., Ali-Fehmi, R., & Bahado-Singh, R. O. (2019). Placental epigenetics for evaluation of fetal congenital heart defects: Ventricular Septal Defect (VSD). *PLoS One, 14*(3), e0200229. DOI: 10.1371/journal.pone.0200229

Ramachandran, V., Bhagavatheeswaran, S., Shanmugam, S., Vasudevan, M., Ragunathan, M., Cherian, K. M., Munirajan, A. K., Ravi, S., & Balakrishnan, A. (2022). Deep sequencing unveils altered cardiac miRNome in congenital heart disease. *Molecular Genetics and Genomics, 297*(4), 1123–1139. DOI: 10.1007/s00438-022-01908-z

Salim, U., Kumar, A., Kulshreshtha, R., & Vivekanandan, P. (2022a). Biogenesis, characterization, and functions of mirtrons. *Wiley Interdisciplinary Reviews. RNA, 13*(1), e1680. DOI: 10.1002/wrna.1680

Salim, U., Kumar, A., Kulshreshtha, R., & Vivekanandan, P. (2022b). Biogenesis, characterization, and functions of mirtrons. *Wiley Interdisciplinary Reviews. RNA, 13*(1), e1680. DOI: 10.1002/wrna.1680

Scott, M. S., & Ono, M. (2011). From snoRNA to miRNA: Dual function regulatory non-coding RNAs. *Biochimie*, *93*(11), 1987–1992. DOI: 10.1016/j.biochi.2011.05.026

Seyhan, A. A. (2024). Trials and Tribulations of MicroRNA Therapeutics. *International Journal of Molecular Sciences*, *25*(3), 1469. DOI: 10.3390/ijms25031469

Shang, R., Lee, S., Senavirathne, G., & Lai, E. C. (2023). microRNAs in action: Biogenesis, function and regulation. *Nature Reviews. Genetics*, *24*(12), 816–833. DOI: 10.1038/s41576-023-00611-y

Shruti, K., Shrey, K., & Vibha, R. (2011). Micro RNAs: Tiny sequences with enormous potential. *Biochemical and Biophysical Research Communications*, *407*(3), 445–449. DOI: 10.1016/j.bbrc.2011.03.058

Song, M., Wang, H., Liu, C., Jin, S., Liu, B., & Sun, W. (2024). Non-coding RNAs as regulators of the Hippo pathway in cardiac development and cardiovascular disease. *Frontiers in Pharmacology*, *15*. Advance online publication. DOI: 10.3389/fphar.2024.1348280

Song, Y., Higgins, H., Guo, J., Harrison, K., Schultz, E. N., Hales, B. J., Moses, E. K., Goldblatt, J., Pachter, N., & Zhang, G. (2018). Clinical significance of circulating microRNAs as markers in detecting and predicting congenital heart defects in children. *Journal of Translational Medicine*, *16*, 42. DOI: 10.1186/s12967-018-1411-0

Sridhar, P., Gan, H. H., & Schlick, T. (2008). A computational screen for C/D box snoRNAs in the human genomic region associated with Prader-Willi and Angelman syndromes. *Journal of Biomedical Science*, *15*(6), 697–705. DOI: 10.1007/s11373-008-9271-x

Sucharov, C. C., Sucharov, J., Karimpour-Fard, A., Nunley, K., Stauffer, B. L., & Miyamoto, S. D. (2015). miRNA Expression in Hypoplastic Left Heart Syndrome. *Journal of Cardiac Failure*, *21*(1), 83–88. DOI: 10.1016/j.cardfail.2014.09.013

Sun, C., & Kontaridis, M. I. (2018). Physiology of Cardiac Development: From Genetics to Signaling to Therapeutic Strategies. *Current Opinion in Physiology*, *1*, 123–139. DOI: 10.1016/j.cophys.2017.09.002

Sun, L., Ke, M., Yin, M., Zeng, Y., Ji, Y., Hu, Y., Fu, S., & Zhang, C. (2023). Extracellular vesicle-encapsulated microRNA-296-3p from cancer-associated fibroblasts promotes ovarian cancer development through regulation of the PTEN/AKT and SOCS6/STAT3 pathways. *Cancer Science*, *115*(1), 155–169. DOI: 10.1111/cas.16014

Synnergren, J., Améen, C., Lindahl, A., Olsson, B., & Sartipy, P. (2011). Expression of microRNAs and their target mRNAs in human stem cell-derived cardiomyocyte clusters and in heart tissue. *Physiological Genomics*, *43*(10), 581–594. DOI: 10.1152/physiolgenomics.00074.2010

Tang, Q., Liao, D., & Zheng, B. (2025). DBR1 orchestrates the fate of lariat RNA: Debranching-dependent turnover and function. *Nucleic Acids Research*, *53*(13), gkaf639. Advance online publication. DOI: 10.1093/nar/gkaf639

Tarazon, E., Perez Carrillo, L., Alvarez, I., Gimenez Escamilla, I., Delgado Arija, M., Gonzalez, I., Portoles, M., & Rosello-Lleti, E. (2023). Analysis of the snoRNA profile in ischemic and dilated cardiomyopathy. European Heart Journal, 44(Supplement_2), ehad655.729. https://doi.org/DOI: 10.1093/eurheartj/ehad655.729

Tian, Y., Cohen, E. D., & Morrisey, E. E. (2010). The Importance of Wnt Signaling in Cardiovascular Development. *Pediatric Cardiology*, *31*(3), 342–348. DOI: 10.1007/s00246-009-9606-z

Tian, Y., Liu, Y., Wang, T., Zhou, N., Kong, J., Chen, L., Snitow, M., Morley, M., Li, D., Petrenko, N., Zhou, S., Lu, M., Gao, E., Koch, W. J., Stewart, K. M., & Morrisey, E. E. (2015). A microRNA-Hippo pathway that promotes cardiomyocyte proliferation and cardiac regeneration in mice. *Science Translational Medicine*, *7*(279), 279ra38. Advance online publication. DOI: 10.1126/scitranslmed.3010841

Tito, C., De Falco, E., Rosa, P., Iaiza, A., Fazi, F., Petrozza, V., & Calogero, A. (2021). Circulating microRNAs from the Molecular Mechanisms to Clinical Biomarkers: A Focus on the Clear Cell Renal Cell Carcinoma. *Genes*, *12*(8), 1154. DOI: 10.3390/genes12081154

Titov, I. I., & Vorozheykin, P. S. (2018). Comparing miRNA structure of mirtrons and non-mirtrons. *BMC Genomics*, *19*(3), 114. DOI: 10.1186/s12864-018-4473-8

Tomasello, L., Distefano, R., Nigita, G., & Croce, C. M. (2021). The MicroRNA Family Gets Wider: The IsomiRs Classification and Role. *Frontiers in Cell and Developmental Biology*, *9*, 668648. DOI: 10.3389/fcell.2021.668648

Tutarel, O., Dangwal, S., Bretthauer, J., Westhoff-Bleck, M., Roentgen, P., Anker, S. D., Bauersachs, J., & Thum, T. (2013). Circulating miR-423_5p fails as a biomarker for systemic ventricular function in adults after atrial repair for transposition of the great arteries. *International Journal of Cardiology*, *167*(1), 63–66. DOI: 10.1016/j.ijcard.2011.11.082

Ueno, S., Weidinger, G., Osugi, T., Kohn, A. D., Golob, J. L., Pabon, L., Reinecke, H., Moon, R. T., & Murry, C. E. (2007). Biphasic role for Wnt/β-catenin signaling in cardiac specification in zebrafish and embryonic stem cells. *Proceedings of the National Academy of Sciences of the United States of America, 104*(23), 9685–9690. DOI: 10.1073/pnas.0702859104

Ventura, A., Young, A. G., Winslow, M. M., Lintault, L., Meissner, A., Erkeland, S. J., Newman, J., Bronson, R. T., Crowley, D., Stone, J. R., Jaenisch, R., Sharp, P. A., & Jacks, T. (2008). Targeted deletion reveals essential and overlapping functions of the miR-17~92 family of miRNA clusters. *Cell, 132*(5), 875–886. DOI: 10.1016/j.cell.2008.02.019

Wagh, V., Pomorski, A., Wilschut, K. J., Piombo, S., & Bernstein, H. S. (2014). MicroRNA-363 negatively regulates the left ventricular determining transcription factor HAND1 in human embryonic stem cell-derived cardiomyocytes. *Stem Cell Research & Therapy*, *5*(3), 75. DOI: 10.1186/scrt464

Wajahat, M., Bracken, C. P., & Orang, A. (2021). Emerging Functions for snoRNAs and snoRNA-Derived Fragments. *International Journal of Molecular Sciences, 22*(19), 10193. DOI: 10.3390/ijms221910193

Wang, B., Shi, G., Zhu, Z., Chen, H., & Fu, Q. (2018). Sexual difference of small RNA expression in Tetralogy of Fallot. *Scientific Reports*, *8*, 12847. DOI: 10.1038/s41598-018-31243-6

Wang, C., Hou, X., Guan, Q., Zhou, H., Zhou, L., Liu, L., Liu, J., Li, F., Li, W., & Liu, H. (2023). RNA modification in cardiovascular disease: Implications for therapeutic interventions. *Signal Transduction and Targeted Therapy*, *8*(1), 412. DOI: 10.1038/s41392-023-01638-7

Wang, J., Greene, S. B., Bonilla-Claudio, M., Tao, Y., Zhang, J., Bai, Y., Huang, Z., Black, B. L., Wang, F., & Martin, J. F. (2010). Bmp Signaling Regulates Myocardial Differentiation from Cardiac Progenitors Through a MicroRNA-Mediated Mechanism. *Developmental Cell, 19*(6), 903–912. DOI: 10.1016/j.devcel.2010.10.022

Wang, J., Greene, S. B., & Martin, J. F. (2011). Bmp Signaling in Congenital Heart Disease: New Developments and Future Directions. *Birth Defects Research. Part A, Clinical and Molecular Teratology*, *91*(6), 441–448. DOI: 10.1002/bdra.20785

Wang, J., Zhang, R., Cai, K., Yang, Q., Duan, W., Zhao, J., Gui, Y., & Wang, F. (2019). Susceptibility to congenital heart defects associated with a polymorphism in TBX2 3′ untranslated region in the Han Chinese population. *Pediatric Research*, *85*(3), 378–383. DOI: 10.1038/s41390-018-0181-y

Wang, Y., Du, X., Zhou, Z., Jiang, J., Zhang, Z., Ye, L., & Hong, H. (2016). A gain-of-function ACTC1 3′UTR mutation that introduces a miR-139-5p target site may be associated with a dominant familial atrial septal defect. *Scientific Reports*, *6*, 25404. DOI: 10.1038/srep25404

Wang, Y., Fu, M., Zheng, Z., Feng, J., & Zhang, C. (2025). Small Nucleolar RNAs: Biological Functions and Diseases. *MedComm*, *6*(7), e70257. DOI: 10.1002/mco2.70257

Wang, Y., Liu, J., Cui, J., Sun, M., Du, W., Chen, T., Ming, X., Zhang, L., Tian, J., Li, J., Yin, L., Liu, F., Pu, Z., Lv, B., Hou, J., & Yu, B. (2016). MiR218 Modulates Wnt Signaling in Mouse Cardiac Stem Cells by Promoting Proliferation and Inhibiting Differentiation through a Positive Feedback Loop. *Scientific Reports*, *6*(1), 20968. DOI: 10.1038/srep20968

Wang, Z., Wang, H., Zhou, S., Mao, J., Zhan, Z., & Duan, S. (2024). miRNA interplay: Mechanisms and therapeutic interventions in cancer. *MedComm. Oncology*, *3*(4), e93. DOI: 10.1002/mog2.93

Westholm, J. O., & Lai, E. C. (2011). Mirtrons: microRNA biogenesis via splicing. *Biochimie*, *93*(11), 1897–1904. DOI: 10.1016/j.biochi.2011.06.017

(1623–1624). What will it take to get miRNA therapies to market? (2024). *Nature Biotechnology*, *42*(11). Advance online publication. DOI: 10.1038/s41587-024-02480-0

Winkler, I., Posod, A., Staudt, A., Huber, E., Urbanek, M., Kiechl-Kohlendorfer, U., & Griesmaier, E. (2025). MicroRNA Expression Profiles in Very Preterm Infants with Patent Ductus Arteriosus: A Pilot Study. *Neonatology*. Advance online publication. DOI: 10.1159/000546934

Wong, A. C. H., & Rasko, J. E. J. (2021). Splice and Dice: Intronic microRNAs, Splicing and Cancer. *Biomedicines*, *9*(9), 1268. DOI: 10.3390/biomedicines9091268

Wu, K.-H., Xiao, Q.-R., Yang, Y., Xu, J.-L., Zhang, F., Liu, C.-M., Zhang, Z.-M., Lu, Y.-Q., & Huang, N.-P. (2018). MicroRNA-34a modulates the Notch signaling pathway in mice with congenital heart disease and its role in heart development. *Journal of Molecular and Cellular Cardiology*, *114*, 300–308. DOI: 10.1016/j.yjmcc.2017.11.015

Wu, Q., Fu, X., Liu, G., He, X., Li, Y., & Ou, C. (2025). N7-methylguanosine modification in cancers: From mechanisms to therapeutic potential. *Journal of Hematology & Oncology*, *18*(1), 12. DOI: 10.1186/s13045-025-01665-7

Wu, Y., Ma, X.-J., Wang, H.-J., Li, W.-C., Chen, L., Ma, D., & Huang, G.-Y. (2014). Expression of Cx43-related microRNAs in patients with tetralogy of Fallot. *World Journal of Pediatrics: WJP*, *10*(2), 138–144. DOI: 10.1007/s12519-013-0434-0

Wystub, K., Besser, J., Bachmann, A., Boettger, T., & Braun, T. (2013). miR-1/133a Clusters Cooperatively Specify the Cardiomyogenic Lineage by Adjustment of Myocardin Levels during Embryonic Heart Development. *PLOS Genetics*, *9*(9), e1003793. DOI: 10.1371/journal.pgen.1003793

Xi, Y., Lu, E., Ruan, X., Wu, R., Wu, L., Zhou, T., Gu, H., & Wu, Y. (2024). Potential candidate maternal serum miRNAs for the diagnosis of fetal congenital heart disease. *Cellular and Molecular Biology*, *70*(8), 121–128. DOI: 10.14715/cmb/2024.70.8.16

Xie, M., Li, M., Vilborg, A., Lee, N., Shu, M.-D., Yartseva, V., Šestan, N., & Steitz, J. A. (2013). Mammalian 5′-capped microRNA precursors that generate a single microRNA. *Cell*, *155*(7), 1568–1580. DOI: 10.1016/j.cell.2013.11.027

Xu, F., Yang, J., Shang, J., Lan, F., Li, M., Shi, L., Shen, L., Wang, Y., & Ge, J. (2019). MicroRNA-302d promotes the proliferation of human pluripotent stem cell-derived cardiomyocytes by inhibiting LATS2 in the Hippo pathway. *Clinical Science*, *133*(13), 1387–1399. DOI: 10.1042/CS20190099

Xu, J., Li, Q., Deng, L., Xiong, J., Cheng, Z., & Ye, C. (2025). Global, regional, and national epidemiology of congenital heart disease in children from 1990 to 2021. *Frontiers in Cardiovascular Medicine*, *12*, 1522644. DOI: 10.3389/fcvm.2025.1522644

Xu, X., Hong, P., Wang, Z., Tang, Z., & Li, K. (2021). MicroRNAs in Transforming Growth Factor-Beta Signaling Pathway Associated With Fibrosis Involving Different Systems of the Human Body. *Frontiers in Molecular Biosciences*, *8*, 707461. DOI: 10.3389/fmolb.2021.707461

Yang, H., Li, Y., Chen, Q., Li, S., Yang, Y., & Lyu, G. (2025). Analyzing exosomal miRNA profiles in tetralogy of fallot fetuses' amniotic fluid. *Scientific Reports*, *15*, 96. DOI: 10.1038/s41598-024-83576-0

Yang, J.-S., Maurin, T., Robine, N., Rasmussen, K. D., Jeffrey, K. L., Chandwani, R., Papapetrou, E. P., Sadelain, M., O'Carroll, D., & Lai, E. C. (2010). Conserved vertebrate mir-451 provides a platform for Dicer-independent, Ago2-mediated microRNA biogenesis. *Proceedings of the National Academy of Sciences of the United States of America*, *107*(34), 15163–15168. DOI: 10.1073/pnas.1006432107

Yang, Y., Yang, H., Lian, X., Yang, S., Shen, H., Wu, S., Wang, X., & Lyu, G. (2022). Circulating microRNA: Myocardium-derived prenatal biomarker of ventricular septal defects. *Frontiers in Genetics, 13*. Advance online publication. DOI: 10.3389/fgene.2022.899034

Yousefi, F., Shabaninejad, Z., Vakili, S., Derakhshan, M., Movahedpour, A., Dabiri, H., Ghasemi, Y., Mahjoubin-Tehran, M., Nikoozadeh, A., Savardashtaki, A., Mirzaei, H., & Hamblin, M. R. (2020). TGF-β and WNT signaling pathways in cardiac fibrosis: Non-coding RNAs come into focus. *Cell Communication and Signaling : CCS, 18*(1), 87. DOI: 10.1186/s12964-020-00555-4

Yu, K., Ji, Y., Wang, H., Xuan, Q. K., Li, B. B., Xiao, J. J., Sun, W., & Kong, X. Q. (2016). Association of miR-196a2, miR-27a, and miR-499 polymorphisms with isolated congenital heart disease in a Chinese population. *Genetics and Molecular Research: GMR, 15*(4). Advance online publication. DOI: 10.4238/gmr15048929

Yu, Y., Ge, X., Wang, L.-S., Wang, X.-X., & Xu, L.-C. (2023). Abnormalities of hsa-mir-16 and hsa-mir-124 Affect Mitochondrial Function and Fatty Acid Metabolism in Tetralogy of Fallot. *Combinatorial Chemistry & High Throughput Screening, 26*(2), 373–382. DOI: 10.2174/1386207325666220421104617

Zelli, V., Compagnoni, C., Capelli, R., Corrente, A., Cornice, J., Vecchiotti, D., Di Padova, M., Zazzeroni, F., Alesse, E., & Tessitore, A. (2021). Emerging Role of isomiRs in Cancer: State of the Art and Recent Advances. *Genes, 12*(9), 1447. DOI: 10.3390/genes12091447

Zhang, J., Chang, J.-J., Xu, F., Ma, X.-J., Wu, Y., Li, W.-C., Wang, H.-J., Huang, G.-Y., & Ma, D. (2013). MicroRNA deregulation in right ventricular outflow tract myocardium in nonsyndromic tetralogy of fallot. *The Canadian Journal of Cardiology, 29*(12), 1695–1703. DOI: 10.1016/j.cjca.2013.07.002

Zhang, Y., Yuan, B., Xu, Y., Zhou, N., Zhang, R., Lu, L., & Feng, Z. (2022). MiR-208b/miR-21 Promotes the Progression of Cardiac Fibrosis Through the Activation of the TGF-β1/Smad-3 Signaling Pathway: An in vitro and in vivo Study. *Frontiers in Cardiovascular Medicine, 9*. Advance online publication. DOI: 10.3389/fcvm.2022.924629

Zhao, M., Tang, Y., Zhou, Y., & Zhang, J. (2019). Deciphering Role of Wnt Signalling in Cardiac Mesoderm and Cardiomyocyte Differentiation from Human iPSCs: Four-dimensional control of Wnt pathway for hiPSC-CMs differentiation. *Scientific Reports, 9*(1), 19389. DOI: 10.1038/s41598-019-55620-x

Zhao, Y., Ransom, J. F., Li, A., Vedantham, V., von Drehle, M., Muth, A. N., Tsuchihashi, T., McManus, M. T., Schwartz, R. J., & Srivastava, D. (2007). Dysregulation of cardiogenesis, cardiac conduction, and cell cycle in mice lacking miRNA-1-2. *Cell, 129*(2), 303–317. DOI: 10.1016/j.cell.2007.03.030

Zhou, W., Yi, Y., Cao, W., Zhong, X., & Chen, L. (2025). Functions of METTL1/WDR4 and QKI as m7G modification—Related enzymes in digestive diseases. *Frontiers in Pharmacology, 15*, 1491763. DOI: 10.3389/fphar.2024.1491763

Zia, M. F., Peter, J., Hoover, J., Chen, K. E., & Flynt, A. (2021). Human 5′-tailed Mirtrons are Processed by RNaseP (p. 2021.10.15.464553). *bioRxiv*. https://doi.org/DOI: 10.1101/2021.10.15.464553

# Chapter 8
# Artificial Intelligence and Machine Learning Applications

**S. Ida Evangeline**
https://orcid.org/0000-0003-2997-7897
*Government College of Engineering, Tirunelveli, India*

## ABSTRACT

*Congenital Heart Disease (CHD) is a multifactorial disorder, which is caused and predisposed by a set of interrelating genetic factors along with epigenetic, environmental, and developmental risk factors. This rich heterogeneity is frequently not reflected in more traditional approaches to risk assessment, diagnosis, and prediction of outcomes. The chapter will look at how artificial intelligence and machine learning will transform the way we know more about the CHD etiology and improve clinical care. We provide an extensive survey of the role of AI and ML methods in key areas that are pertinent to CHD, such as genomic and epigenomic data integration, exposomic and teratogenic risk modeling, advanced cardiac imaging interpretation and dynamic risk stratification. The chapter describes the technical underpinnings of these methods, their contemporary use in prenatal and postnatal care, and how they may benefit precision cardiology through integration of disparate data sources into personalized prediction. Concurrently, we discuss the issues that arise in the potential application of AI in pediatric and perinatal settings, including limited data volumes, model levels of generalizability, interpretability, and ethical concerns as critically. We end by summarising a vision of AI-enabled precision congenital cardiology: where transdisciplinary research, information infrastructures with strong data governance, and transparent algorithmic governance are combined to redefine knowledge about CHD, its diagnosis and management along the lifespan.*

DOI: 10.4018/979-8-3373-3735-7.ch008

## 1. INTRODUCTION

The congenital heart disease is the most common type of birth defect present in the world and is associated with a lot of morbidity and mortality among children. The complexity of CHD is beyond its structural abnormalities to the heart, however, due to its multifactorial nature; a complex interaction in terms of genetic predisposition, epigenetic variations, environmental exposures (teratogens), and chance opportunities during embryonic development. Traditionally, congenital cardiology has depended on a mix of clinical observation, epidemiology and directed genetics to unravel the results and causes of CHD. Nevertheless, none of these traditional methods tend to be particularly good at describing the nonlinear and high-dimensional ways in which relationships occur in multifactorial diseases such as CHD (Morton et al. 2022).

Artificial intelligence and machine learning have recently become new paradigms that can change the field of biomedical research. Such computational approaches are especially appropriate to the field of dealing with the complexities of CHD as they have the ability to model nonlinear or complex nonlinear relationships, can support the analysis of missing or noisy data, and are flexible enough to integrate varieties of disparate databases, including genomic sequencing data, imaging data, and environmental exposure data. There is no longer a distinction between AI and ML applications moved towards experimental proofs of concept and those being introduced into clinical practice to be used as part of real clinical workflows in screening, diagnosing, and prognosis to assist with clinical decision-making across diseases (Pozza et al. 2024).

A number of major areas are covered in the application of AI and ML in CHD. In genetics, ML algorithms have also been used to recognize new pathogenic inheritances, find polygenic hazard prints, as well as portray gene-environment relational lives that could be the cause of pulmonary deformities. In exposomics, AI can accommodate high-throughput examination of information of environmental exposures of pregnant women, such as, but not limited to, pharmacological, infectious, and toxicological factors and pair such exposures with fetal cardiac outcomes. Improvements in deep learning and especially convolutional neural networks (CNNs) have transformed the field of medical imaging; recent demonstrations show they can achieve the subset of medical imaging challenges in a field as automated interpretation of fetal echocardiograms and other diagnostic modalities and can attain similar levels of accuracy as experts (Reddy et al. 2022).

This chapter starts with the definition of fundamental AI and ML approaches best suited to congenital cardiology and moves to discuss their use in genomics, exposomics, imaging as well as risk modeling. The chapter also highlights the translational implication of such strategies besides noting the technical innovations of these strategies to improve early diagnosis, improve risk prediction, and direct management of CHD in a personalized manner. Particular focus is placed on ethical and practical ethical issues that are particular to deployment of AI in the field of pediatric and perinatal care including issues of algorithmic bias, data sparsity, and interpreting complex model predictions.

It is envisioned that by drawing on interdisciplinary insights of computer sciences, teratomics, computational biology, genetics and clinical cardiology, this chapter will help address the current gap between sophisticated data science methods and the highly urgent need of CHD research and care. The final idea is to show how AI and ML may A) not only be a tool of further analytic, B) but also be the part of systems-based approach to the knowledge and management of the congenital heart disease in the age of precision medicine.

## 2. FOUNDATIONS OF AI AND ML IN CONGENITAL CARDIOLOGY

In order to understand in full the growing role of the artificial intelligence and machine learning in the field of congenital cardiology, it is necessary to know the principles that can guide all their applications. AI can be defined basically as a broad skill of the machines to carry out the task that is humanly require intelligent approaches such as pattern recognition, decision-making and language processing. Machine learning is a subfield of AI which is concerned with algorithms that learn by experience; through experience they learn the patterns in data without needing to be explicitly programmed (Holt et al. 2025).

With regard to congenital heart disease, ML is especially useful because CHD is multifactorial and extensive in data granularity. CHD etiology encompasses multiple levels of biological context-genetic and epigenetic, environmental, and clinical levels that interact in complex, nonlinear manners. Such high-dimensional, non-homogenous data tends to be difficult to analyse using traditional statistical techniques. In contrast, ML models can flexibly represent nonlinear relationships, handle missing or noisy data, and uncover more complex patterns they might not be obvious to human researchers or naked-eye regression analyses (Bahado-Singh et al. 2025).

There are three big families of ML methods that apply to CHD research: supervised learning, unsupervised learning and deep learning.

The most popular one is supervised learning, which is used when the labeled data exist, e.g., when the patient medical records are marked with the CHD diagnosis. Random forests, supportvector machines and gradient boosting machines are examples of algorithms that are learned to make predictions on the basis of one or a set of input features including genetic variants, the history of maternal exposures or imaging biomarkers. Supervised models have been applied to predict the availability of the disease, its subtype according to disease subtypes, surgical outcomes, and risk of mortality in CHD (Sethi et al. 2022).

Unsupervised learning on the other hand does not rely on labeled outcomes and is applied to determine structure that is not apparent in data. Unsupervised clustering algorithms have been used in CHD to discover new phenotypic subtypes, new latent genetic syndromes and to stratify patients by multidimensional exposomic or imaging characteristics. This has been especially useful where there is confusion in defining the disease and where the conventional boundaries of diagnosis cannot encompass biologically significant variation.

Deep learning, especially with architectures including convolutional neural networks (CNNs) and recurrent neural networks (RNNs) is a strong field of AI. CNNs have revolutionized the field of medical imaging, being able to analyze echocardiograms and MRI scans automatically with an accuracy never seen before. In the meantime, RNNs have value with time-series data or sequential data, e.g. fetal development timelines or longitudinal clinical records. Easy access to the large scale imaging and genomic data has increased the pace of implementation of such approaches in the congenital cardiology (Ejaz et al. 2024).

The usefulness in the application of these models depends upon the quality and availability of data. Pediatric cardiology Statistically a typical dataset in pediatric cardiology tends to be small and heterogeneous, since some types of CHD are relatively rare and different scanning protocols used make comparison difficult, in addition to privacy issues when sharing neonatal data. Nonetheless, the federated learning, which is a type of distributed ML that provides the training of algorithms on decentralized data without raw data exchange, can become an encouraging direction to conduct research jointly, maintaining patient privacy.

The other guiding principle behind the use of ML in CHD is feature engineering; feature engineering is the way of selecting and transforming input variables to better predict the dependent variable. In genomics, this might come into play by grouping rare variants by biological pathway; in exposomics, this might mean encoding windows of time of maternal exposure. An ever increasing trend however, is the pivot towards end-to-end learning where raw data are fed directly into the neural network without any form of manual preprocessing and the model is left to learn relevant features by itself (Qu et al. 2022).

It is also necessary to discriminate between the interpretability and the predictive performance. Although more complex models, e.g. deep neural networks can be very accurate, they are often thought of as black boxes with little to no intelligence on what might be going on underneath the hood. It is of particular concern in the pediatrial medical field where clinical responsibility and trust are the issues of paramount importance. More recent developments in explainable AI (XAI) attempts to reduce this scorched-earth trade-off by providing readable interpretations of model decisions, for example SHAP (SHapley Additive exPlanations) and LIME (Local Interpretable Model-agnostic Explanations) (Chinni & Manlhiot, 2024).

All in all, the convergence of AI and ML with CHD research can offer a paradigm change in the ways we understand and deal with this complicated illness. Such tools would enable a data-driven discovery of the multifactorial roots of CHD, and reveal associations and predictive factors that could enable early identification, risk stratification and individual therapy. Nevertheless, their efficiency is not confined to the sophistication of the algorithm, but requires good data infrastructures, interdisciplinary integration and ethical applications in the real world.

## 3. GENOMIC AND EPIGENOMIC DATA INTEGRATION

The genetic background of congenital heart disease has been established a long time ago, however, the complexity and heterogeneity of its genomic nature remains a considerable challenge on the way of researchers and clinicians. Although not all cases of CHD may be explained by phenomena related to chromosomal abnormalities and mono-genic syndromes, most cases occur due to a multifactorial interaction of rare de novo variants, polygenic risk variants, and non-coding regulatory variants combined with interactions with environmental factors. Here, artificial intelligence and machine learning provide a potent combination to aggregate and to interpret the high volume of genomic and epigenomic data, which might otherwise remain in the dark by traditional methods (Linglart & Bonnet, 2022).

Machine learning is especially applicable in high throughput sequencing data; e.g., whole-genome sequencing (WGS), whole-exome sequencing (WES), and transcriptomic profiles. Such data sets include millions of measurements- spanning single-nucleotide polymorphisms (SNPs) and structural variants, as well as transcript abundance and methylation signatures, that can be mined to provide predictive and even mechanistic insights into CHD. Among the major inputs of ML into this space, the capacity to prioritize causative variants on the basis of learning patterns of known pathogenic variants can be mentioned. Specifically, it is possible to train a supervised learning specimen based on curated variant databases (e.g., ClinVar, HGMD) using the assessment of a mutation predicted pathogeneity and grounded on sequence conservation, biochemical impact, and network context to classify novel mutations (Lim et al. 2021).

In addition to single-gene associations, ML allows performing polygenic risk scoring (PRS) to combine the effects of thousands of common variants to predict an individual predisposition to CHD. Although PRS has been more generally used in adult-onset diseases, recent research has started to moot its application to congenital traits using the ML weighting strategies that integrate the results of genome-wide association studies (GWAS) with the regularities of epistatic interactions and the coherence of paths. Such methods have the potential to discover fetuses or neonates who are at risk but may not be known to have high-penetrance mutations but have a collection of variants that predisposes one to the disease.

Epigenomic data further complicates this as it demonstrates regulation of the genome as cardiac development progresses during early development. Multidimensional data to reveal the dynamic regulation of gene expression are provided by methods like ATAC-seq (chromatin accessibility), ChIP-seq (transcription factor binding), and profiling DNA methylation. The use of ML models, and especially deep learning approaches such as convolutional neural networks, has been used to predict enhancer-promoter interactions, find tissue-specific regulatory elements, and deduce disrupted transcriptional networks of CHD. As an example, cardiac-specific enhancer-trained deep learning models have been used to evaluate how the impact of non-coding variants adjacent to developmental genes could be disrupting regulatory loops in the embryo (Mouat et al. 2023).

The biggest strength of ML in this field is the ability to be multi-omic, providing the possibility to analyze genomic, transcriptomic, epigenomic, and clinical data in parallel. Integrative models My approach to the analyses would include integrative models, such as multi-view learning frameworks and graph-based neural networks, to help capture relationships across these layers, find convergent mechanisms and molecular subtypes of CHD. As an example, expression quantitative trait loci (eQTL) data has been aligned with enhancer activity and variant burden using ML to identify causal regulatory perturbations in cardiac progenitor cells.

Notably, even gene-environment interactions can be assessed with the use of AI tools, and this is essential since such interactions are vital to CHD, but traditionally challenging to reproduce with conventional statistics. Leveraging nonlinear dependency and latent variable modeling, ML can be used to reveal how exposure to an environmental teratogen, e.g., maternal infections, metabolic disorders, or medications, during a sensitive period of cardiac morphogenesis alters the susceptibility of individuals to such teratogens depending on their genetic variant (Morton et al. 2022).

Regardless of these achievements, there are obstacles. Low sequencing depth, population biases, and small sample sizes characterize genetic and epigenetic datasets, which may all be obstacles to generalizability in models. Furthermore, biological interpretation of certain deep learning models is hindered since the nature of the models can be described as a black box, which is concerning since defining clinical applicability is a key concern. Recent works have attempted to respond to these issues by adopting the following methods: to use interpretable ML frameworks, transfer learning to boost performance on rare disease data, and to create data-sharing consortia to enlarge sample diversity.

Finally, combining AI and ML in genomic and epigenomic studies is an essential step in the path towards a systems-wide CHD view. Such tools do not only improve our chances of identifying new mechanisms of disease, but also lead to precision diagnostics and targeted interventions, according to the unique genetic architecture and regulatory landscape of an individual (Kocher et al. 2025).

## 4. EXPOSOMICS AND TERATOLOGY DATA MINING

Although, the genetic and epigenetic processes are the basis of the emergence of congenital heart disease, they exist in a larger environmental environment. The fetal development is exercised by the intrauterine environment and any influences to the development during sensitive windows may cause structural cardiac defects. Maternal infections, medications, metabolism shift, toxicants and even stressful experiences from a psycho-social involvement, are teratogenic factors that impacted CHD risk. But it is an uphill task to capture the totality of these environmental factors, otherwise known as the exposome. It is desirable that both internal and external exposures be tracked longitudinally and at high resolution over time in conjunction with biological and clinical data (Gorini & Tonacci, 2025).

Artificial intelligence and machine learning provides a paradigm-changing methodology of the exposomic analysis. The techniques are powerful on large high-dimensional, temporally structured and heterogeneous datasets and can be well suited to detect latent patterns and predictive within teratology. Notably, they enable them to simulate the difficulty of nonlinear effects of many exposures and how they interact with genetic predispositions and so unravel the aspect of CHD that would be unavailable through traditional epidemiological methods.

### 4.1 Emerging Technologies in Exposure Assessment

Recent advances in exposure science have led to the development of innovative technologies that enable high-resolution, individualized tracking of environmental exposures—ushering in a new era of precision exposomics. Wearable and implantable personal sensors now allow for real-time monitoring of toxicants such as volatile organic compounds, heavy metals, and particulate matter, offering continuous and context-specific exposure profiles. These devices can measure exposure in relation to physiological parameters like respiration rate or skin absorption, capturing dynamic interactions between the environment and the developing fetus. Parallel to these advances is the rise of the "digital exposome," which uses digital traces, such as location data, the use of apps, data from wearable biometrics, and social media behavior, to surmise lifestyle, stress levels, dietary patterns, and psychosocial exposures. When processed with machine learning models these data provide a powerful lens to characterize both external and internal exposures with unprecedented granularity. Together these technologies enable movement from population-level exposure assessments to individual-level exposure histories that are temporally resolved. In the context of congenital heart disease, such granular data could be critical for the identification of teratogenic risk windows, behavioral-environmental interactions during the pregnancy, and the informational basis for personalized preventive strategies. However, this shift also raises pressing questions around data privacy, validation standards and integration into clinical and research ecosystems.

Another potential linkage between ML and exposomics is automated extraction and data analyses of maternal exposure data which can be in electronic health records (EHRs), prescription registries, and environmental surveillance databases. Unstructured clinical notes can be processed by natural language processing (NLP) algorithms and used to identify the documentation of maternal illnesses, infections or use of any medication during their pregnancy. An example is that AI tools have been used to measure the exposure of the pregnant mother to antiepileptic medications or SSRIs and how the timing and dose were related to the phenotypes of cardiac defects in children. These methods provide objectivity and scalability when compared to self-reports which tend to be biased when taking measurements based on recall and underreporting (Scher, 2024).

Besides exposures to pharmacologicals, ML models have been implemented to evaluate maternal contact to environmental chemicals (e.g. endocrine-disrupting chemicals) and pollutants (air (e.g. PM2.5, NO2), heavy metals, and agricultural pesticides). Geographic information systems (GIS) along with satellite data and spatial ML models can enable researchers to provide high spatial and temporal estimates of the maternal environmental exposures. This way of approaching it has allowed to relate living in areas with heavy air pollution or agriculture to the greater prevalence of certain types of CHD defects, like ventricular septal defects or outflow tract defects.

Also, with the help of AI, it is possible to integrate data of biological response in exposomic analysis. As an example, this may be achieved by combining maternal metabolomic or proteomic profiles with histories of environmental exposures in attempts to identify susceptibility/early fetal injury biomarkers. Using ML models, we can identify patterns of metabolic dysregulation that may contribute to toxic exposures response on the fetal cardiogenesis, which can offer an intervention target or mechanistic understanding [33].

One of the major strengths of ML in this field, then, is that it makes it possible to determine critical exposure windows of exposure--narrow periods in the course of gestation when the growing heart is especially susceptible to exogenous perturbations. Conventional regression analyses have issues with temporal complexity and longitudinal exposure measure collinearity. Instead, temporal convolutional networks (TCNs) and recurrent neural networks (RNNs) may be used to learn temporal relationships and allow fine-grained risk estimation by learning the timing, duration of exposures and the intensity of the same. This time sensitivity is important in discerning teratogenic efficacies in cardiac looping, septation or valvulogenesis.

Besides, AI can be used to provide a schema of modelling gene-environmental interactions in CHD. The combination of genotypic information with environmental exposure measures would allow ML models to identify those individuals who, because of their genetic makeup, respond differently to the effects of specific teratogens -- one key step towards personalized risk projection. As an example, some of the maternal perinatal infections can only lead to the CHD with fetal variants of immune-related genes or pathways (Liang et al. 2023).

There are various limitations of exposomic data mining through AI, even though it promises. Information on exposure is frequently characterized by noise, imprecision and incompleteness, especially in cases of proxy-based exposure estimation such as residence-based exposure estimation. Also, numerous exposomic variables are intercorrelated, and it will be difficult to differentiate causality and confounding effects. When using ML models on datasets with low size or bias, care should be taken to make sure that ML models can be precisely validated and interpreted in a manner that evades overfitting and spurious links.

What is needed is interdisciplinary collaboration in order to address these challenges. Translational interdisciplinarity among the spheres of environmental epidemiology, toxicology, computational science, and clinical cardiology increase the reliability and relevance of exposomic information obtained with AI. Future research in this direction has a promising basis in the ever-growing accessibility of population-based birth cohorts coupled with combined genetic, environmental and clinical data, e.g., the National Childrens Study or the Environmental influences on Child Health Outcomes (ECHO) program (Mitchell, 2022).

Overall, AI and ML have ensured new grounds in teratology and exposomics and clarified how environmental aspects lead to the occurrence of congenital heart disease. These technologies contribute to precision congenital cardiology in general by mining complex, temporally structured exposure data, to better understand the etiology of CHD through a systems level perspective.

## 4.2 Ethical, Legal, and Societal Implications in Exposomics

Crucially, as the field of exposomics matures and moves into clinical and public health applications, a host of ethical, legal and societal issues will arise that need to be addressed proactively. The use of specific personal and environmental exposure information-especially when linked together with genomic and clinical records-is raising important issues about data privacy, informed consent and data ownership. Furthermore, unequal access to exposure monitoring technologies or the benefits of personalized prevention strategies risks exacerbating existing health disparities, particularly in socioeconomically disadvantaged populations. These challenges require the creation of sound governance frameworks addressing data protection, fair access to data, and transparency in the collection, interpretation and application of exposure information. A collaborative effort with researchers, clinicians, ethicists, policymakers and affected communities is needed to navigate these complexities. Only through such inclusive and ethically grounded approaches can the transformative potential of exposomics be harnessed to improve congenital heart disease prevention in a manner that is socially just and widely trusted.

## 5. IMAGING AND DIAGNOSTIC AI

The utilization of imaging has an instrumental part in the diagnosis, monitoring and detection of congenital heart disease as early as the prenatal period and through to the postnatal. Fetal echocardiography, neonatal echocardiography, magnetic resonance imaging (MRI), and computed tomography (CT) are the modalities that give important structural and functional information about the developing heart. The interpretation of such imaging studies demands very specialized skills and can be highly susceptible to inter-observer variability, diagnostic delays and lacks accessibility in low resource situations. The introduction of artificial intelligence and especially of machine learning, what we now call deep learning, has unlocked new avenues towards automation, standardisation, upgrading cardiac imaging in CHD (Najjar, 2023).

Deep learning, a sub-area of ML working with multi-layered neural networks, particularly has made a big impact in the field of medical imaging, where the capability to learn features (rather than have features engineered by hand) directly off raw data has been embraced. Particularly, convolutional neural networks (CNNs) have proven extremely successful in image recognition tasks (image classification, image segmentation, and anomaly detection). When applied to CHD, CNNs were trained to detect structural birth defects in fetal and neonatal echocardiograms, including but not confined to, the ventricular septal defects, outflow tract anomalies, and complex lesions such as hypoplastic left heart syndrome.

Among the first and the most effective impacts of AI on CHD imaging, one may distinguish the automated interpretation of fetal echocardiography. The modality has technical difficulties, in that it relies on the expertise of the operator, position of the fetus, and gestational age. AI has been built to detect standard fetal cardiac views automatically, evaluate image quality, detect abnormal anatomical characteristics, etc. Such systems involve applying deep learning models that are trained over the extensive datasets of annotated fetal heart images to obtain the information about the spatial and morphological features of the normal and abnormal heart. Some studies have shown that stock models can attain the diagnostic performance as high as the experienced sonographers especially in the discovery of major CHD during second trimester (Reddy et al. 2022).

Image segmentation, i.e., outlining anatomy parts in an image is also another broad field of innovation. Proper segmentation determines the ability to quantify cardiac chamber sizes, wall thicknesses, morphology of valves as well as blood circulation patterns. Segmentation tool based on AI is established to be used in echocardiography, MRI, and CT scans, and can save enormous amounts of time and labor due to the typical manual tracing method and enhance the reproducibility of the measures. As an example, fetal cardiac chamber region machine-learning segmentation can provide volumetric analysis which may make early risk stratification and treatment planning possible.

In addition to structural analysis, AI models are progressively extended to functional analysis, e.g. Doppler films and cardiac MRI, to assess blood flow patterns, myocardial strain, and characterisation of tissues. Dynamic assessment of cardiac function over time has been accomplished using recurrent neural networks (RNNs), which are practically applicable to temporally-oriented data such as the time-series signal of Doppler waveforms or cine MRI data sequences. This time modeling plays an important role in following disease progress and assessing response to treatment in CHD patients (Pozza et al. 2024).

Diagnostic AI is becoming part of the neonatal screening programs in the postnatal environment. As an example, the ML model may process the pulse oximetry and the clinical data obtained in electronic health records to improve the early indication of severe CHDs in newborns before the symptoms can be clinically identified. Internet-connected and AI-powered portable imaging equipment Provides real-time interpretability, increasing accessibility to specialized diagnostic equipment in underserved parts of the country or still in the country.

In addition to this, AI has started to contribute to the phenotype-genotype correlation by correlating imaging phenotypes to genetic or epigenetics profiles. Multimodal models integrating image and genomic data can reveal mechanistic relationships between genotype and anatomical variation, which leads to insights into developmental pathways as well as informing individual treatment (Wang et al. 2024).

In spite of these developments, there are still problems. Training powerful AI models needs rich, various, and adequately labeled data, non-conveniently present in pediatric cardiology. The generalizability of the model can be modified by differences in imaging protocols, equipment and populations characteristics. Also, many deep learning models are black box: their internal behavior is confusing and this makes them worryingly uninterpretable, which can be a roadblock to their application in situations that require justifiable and explainable choices such as medical settings.

So as to overcome these shortcomings, a direction has been taken to develop explainable AI (XAI) tools to explain in visual or numerical terms, the predictions made by a model. Such mechanisms may be in the form of saliency maps, attention mechanisms, or layer-wise relevance propagation that can help the clinician to ascertain what aspects of an image were most relevant to a diagnosis, and assist in establishing trust and validation (Han et al. 2024).

Besides, joint efforts, like federated learning, are under consideration with the purpose of making possible training models across institutions without intruding on patient privacy. The frameworks will allow AI systems to leverage data gathered in many hospitals or countries in order to enhance performance and comply with regulatory restrictions.

To sum up, AI and ML have brought in the sphere of cardiac imaging in congenital heart disease, a significant reformation. These tools are leading to precision imaging and a revolution in quality of care ranging from the refinement of fetal screening, to real-time support of diagnostics and genotype-phenotype associated data. With the constant change in technology, the use of imaging through AI should become an important part of early detection, risk assessment, and personalized management, in congenital cardiology.

## 6. RISK STRATIFICATION AND PROGNOSTIC MODELING

The primary concern of the efficient clinical decision-making process in congenital heart disease is the risk stratification. It is important to be able to identify which patients are at greatest risk be it severe body shape or perinatal complications, surgical failures, or long-term morbidity, in order to inform those elements of surveillance and interventions, and family counseling. Risk assessment of CHD is traditionally focused on both static clinical parameters along with expert opinion, and statistics on a population level. These measures tend to lack the capacity to personalize risk assessment and, especially, within the context of multifactorial illness, individual differences. The advent of artificial intelligence and machine learning offers the possibility of abandoning the age-old risk scoring systems, and envisioning prognostic models that are dynamic, individual and data driven (Malkawi et al. 2022).

The promise of risk stratification informed by ML is the potential to combine enormous and heterogeneous data, such as genetic profiles, prenatal imaging, maternal exposures, clinical histories and surgical data and expose the nonlinear relationship among those factors that could be associated with future outcomes.

Learning With Supervision Algorithms Learning is done using data gathered in the past with supervised learning algorithms, including random forests, gradient boosting machines, and deep neural networks, and learn the relation between these input characteristics and clinical outcomes. Prospective validation of such models on new patients can then be used to estimate risks of events like in utero demise, postnatal decompensation, surgical mortality, neurodevelopmental impairments or even long term quality of life.

Prediction of prenatal risk of CHD, is one of the most important contributions of AI in CHD risk modeling. With fetal echocardiographic data, maternal demographics, and, in the presence of genomics, inclusion of genomic data, ML models will calculate the likelihood of having a critical cardiac lesion, or a need to have an immediate neonatal intervention or associated extracardiac anomalies. Such predictions are especially helpful in making decisions regarding delivery planning, referral to the tertiary care centers, and early counseling of families. As an illustration, ML models have been trained to predict the probability of the likelihood of biventricular repair in a fetus with borderline left heart structures to make decisions concerning the possible intervention of the fetus or an operation after the child is born (Athar, 2024).

In postnatal care, AI-facilitated risk stratification also come into play in the perioperative and postoperative phases of care where certain things could substantially differ even in patients having identical anatomical values. Other measures that were modeled are the days of hospitalization, the risk of postoperative events (e.g., arrhythmias, infections, re-intervention) and survival in the long term. Such models often use well-organized clinical data such as laboratory findings, vital signs and intraoperative variables that have been recorded in real-time, or retrospectively. Noteworthy, ML provides an opportunity of updating the risk estimates as more data emerges thus offering a dynamic and versatile risk stratification that can change throughout the treatment process of a patient.

Within the longitudinal prognosis field, there is an increasing relationship involving AI in prognosis of maintenance and neurocognitive accomplishments in CHD survivors, especially in those children who perish in intricate surgeries such as the Fontan operation or the Norwood operation. Combining early-life clinical confounders and follow-ups with imaging, neurodevelopmental investigations and social determinants of health, ML models can be used to inform clinicians to whom to pay more attention, which children are at the greatest risk of learning difficulties, behavioral disorders or poor quality of life. Such understanding can help with early treatment programs and with distribution of developmental resources (Cau et al. 2025).

Additionally there has been an application of such information as genomic and exposomic information into the modeling of prognoses giving yet another dimension of accuracy. As an example, gene variants related to neurodevelopment or even cardiac remodeling could alteration response of patient to surgical stressful situations or even ischemia-reperfusion injuries. AI tools have the potential to optimize risk assessment in terms of postoperative outcome by modeling geneenvironment interactions and eventually leading to genetically informed clinical pathways.

Real-time decision support is another prominent scenario, mostly in critical care. Predictive ML models incorporated into electronic health record (EHR) applications are able to be continuously run on patient-generated data streams heart rate, oxygen saturation, lab values to alert on early signs of deterioration. These can enhance clinical surveillance, shorten response times and increase positive patient outcomes in susceptible neonatal and pediatric CHD patient cohorts (Suri et al. 2022).

Although these advances have been made, there are still a number of challenges to the implementation of AI- based prognostic models. To begin with, data quality, completeness, and representativeness are very crucial in the performance of models. Many CHD databases are small or are biased to high-resource settings which could impact generalizability. Second, clinical acceptance is highly dependent on the fact that the complex models can be interpreted. There is minimal chance that the black-box predictive models would reshape decision-making until the respective explanations and clinical reasoning can be provided. Third, such ethical aspects as unjustness, prejudice, and disclosure should be discussed so that AI-powered solutions would not unwillingly increase the gap in the provision of care.

To address these issues, explanable AI (XAI) strategies or risk scores, and feature attribution to give a sense of what contributed to the displays, have been developed in an attempt to understand models better; federated learning systems that can train models across institutions and not share sensitive patient data have been developed as well. Also, regulators are starting to create systems that allow clinical validation and approval of AI-based medical devices, and this will be the key to broad application in CHD care (Evertz et al. 2022).

To sum up, AI and ML are transforming risk stratification and prognostic modeling models in congenital cardiology. These technologies deliver more precise, timely and individual predictions (which can be used to improve clinical outcomes and resource allocation) due to the fact that the information is based on large multidimensional data. In the future, as this field furthers its development, AI is likely to become even a more central part of determining the path of care through the chain of CHD throughout the life span with a start in the prenatal period and the development of adulthood.

## 7. CLINICAL TRANSLATIONAL PERSPECTIVES

The clinical application of artificial intelligence and machine learning in congenital heart disease depends on the careful balance of computational innovation and real-world healthcare systems. Several domains show how these technologies are changing clinical workflows, as well as the practical challenges that need to be addressed to enable broad implementation.

In prenatal care, models with AI capabilities are starting to show as good diagnostic ability as expert clinicians in interpreting fetal echocardiography. These systems can be used to support an early detection of critical structural anomalies such as ventricular septal or outflow tract malformations, in particular in low-resource or high-throughput settings. By offering automated assessments of image quality, anatomical landmarks, and pathological patterns, AI tools can standardize diagnostic accuracy and enhance access to specialized care. However, before such tools can be implemented into routine obstetric work flows, robust validation studies, regulatory approvals and clinician training must be established.

Postnatal care and surgical planning are another major new area for clinical translation. AI models that have been trained using multimodal information including genetics profile, imaging, maternal exposures and perioperative variables provide a dynamic and personalised risk prediction. These predictive models can be used to inform the likelihood of outcomes such as decompensation in the perinatal period, surgical mortality or long-term neurodevelopmental impairment. When incorporated into electronic health record systems, such models could deliver real-time decision support that would evolve as new data is collected. This enables clinicians to personalise interventions at every point across the continuum of care, from delivery planning to long-term follow-up.

Furthermore, the use of AI in surgery is growing too to aid complex decision-making. Models can stratify the surgical risk, estimate the chance for biventricular repair, and even predict neurocognitive trajectories after surgery such as the Norwood or Fontan operations. These insights can influence preoperative counseling, optimize resource allocation in intensive care and enable proactive intervention planning. Nonetheless, clinical adoption is dependent on the interpretability of these models. The integration of explainable AI (XAI) techniques - such as saliency mapping or feature attribution - can help build clinician trust by helping them understand the rationale behind model predictions.

Another promising field is the combination of genotype-phenotype relationships using multimodal AI platforms. By correlating the high-resolution imaging data with genomic and epigenomic profiles these systems can reveal novel mechanistic pathways underlying CHD. Clinically, this allows for more precise diagnoses in syndromic and non-syndromic cases, informed genetic counseling and may even guide targeted therapies. Yet to be translated into clinical benefit, such findings have to be harmonized with existing diagnostic protocols and validated in diverse populations.

Finally, the potential of AI to promote health equity in the care of CHD cannot be overstated. By integrating AI tools with handheld imaging devices, cloud-based services and telemedicine workflows, diagnosis expertise can be brought to underserved and remote areas. Such democratization of care is important in areas where specialist pediatric cardiology is limited. However, to achieve equitable translation, it is crucial that AI systems are trained on diverse datasets, consider sociocultural context, and are implemented in a transparent and accountable manner to prevent perpetuating existing disparities.

In summation, the clinical translation of AI in CHD is feasible and transformative. But it needs to be informed by interdisciplinary collaboration, ethical foresight and perpetuated evaluation in real-world environments. The promise of AI lies not only in its predictive power but in its ability to align with the complexities of patient-centered, precision medicine.

## 8. CHALLENGES AND LIMITATIONS

Although the promise of artificial intelligence and machine learning to the further development of congenital heart disease is tremendous, the process of its adoption in the practice is not without a stream of technical, clinical, ethical and infrastructural concerns. These restrictions do have impact not only on the quality and safety of the use of AI models, but also raise questions about safety, equity, and transparency, especially when the pediatric and perinatal conditions have to be addressed.

### 8.1 Data Scarcity and Quality

Lack of high quality and good annotation data, especially on the pediatric patient population, is one of the primary challenges to the application of AI to CHD. CHD is a heterogeneous set of conditions, which is not particularly common, and that is it has many subtypes that have their own anatomical and clinical complexities. Due to the complexity of the logistical practicalities of collecting large, representative datasets per subtype, particularly considering the incorporation of multi-modal data (genomic profiles, imaging and longitudinal clinical records), one challenge is the generalisability of their findings (Vervoortet al. 2023).

Besides, the issue of the quality of data persists. The clinical data can be partial, differently formatted or with noise and human error contamination. Imaging data may be highly heterogeneous in terms of their resolution and acquisition scanning schemes between institutions. There can be no harmonization or standardization of genomic data in variant annotation. Such constraints reduce training of the models that will be both robust and generalizable, resulting in the risk of overfitting and false discovery (Schuette et al. 2022).

## 8.2 Generalizability and Bias

Very related to data limitations we have the issue of model generalizability. Models that are trained on data of a particular institution, geographic location or demographic subpopulation and applied to a different population are likely to be poor in their performance. An illustrative example here is that a predictive model assumed to work on a data that has been established in a single high-resource tertiary care center will not always be applicable in low-resource or diverse ethnic populations. Disparities of this kind may compound the extent of algorithmic bias which occurs when underrepresented groups get systematically less precise predictions or treatment suggestions because of the lack of training data (Karabayir & Akbilgic, 2025).

It can also be because of historical disparities in the data as can be inaccessibility to health care, the presence or absence of diseases in various groups, and selective reporting. Unless tackled explicitly, such biases may be reinforced or even increased, through the AI systems, essentially frustrated by attempts in regards to providing equal access to healthcare (van Assen et al. 2024).

## 8.3 Interpretability and Transparency

The non-interpretability of most AI-models particularly deep learning models is a significant impediment to clinical implementation. Although algorithms such as a convolutional neural network can produce a high degree of accuracy when classifying images or detecting anomalies, the inner workings behind such a classification or anomaly detection process can be veiled in secrecy. With the serious consequences of decisions in pediatrics and the high level of responsibility on clinicians, they are not likely to accept or use black box outputs without understanding the rationale of the decisions (Wang et al. 2021).

This has promoted the increasing attention and popularity of explainable AI (XAI) to give justifications to model predictions that humans can understand. With unequal success, techniques like saliency maps, feature attribution scores and model-agnostic explanations (e.g. SHAP, LIME), etc., have been used. However, explainability has a frequent trade-off with the complexity or performance of the model, and there is no agreed-upon definition of what is adequate interpretability in clinical applications where the stakes are high (Pozza et al. 2024).

## 8.4 Ethical and Legal Considerations

Pediatric and prenatal application of AI present sensitive ethical and legal concerns with the introduction of the matter. The first problem pertains to the matter of informed consent, in the context of the development of a data set as well as the use of AI-assisted tools in clinical decision-making. Parents/guardians should be informed not only on the manner in which their child data will be utilized, but also on the implication and constraints of the AI-generated insights (Maris et al. 2024).

The other issue of automation bias, the possibility that clinicians may rely too much on algorithmic suggestions, is a factor. This is more likely to take place when the model is given a lot of authority visibly and machine performance is assessed to be superior to human performance in a backwards analysis of performance and outcomes. This may reduce critical thinking and cause the wrong decisions in case the model is debilitated or inappropriately used (Holt et al. 2025).

When applied in the prenatal field, predictions of fetal anomalies or outcomes have severe consequences on the choices to make regarding reproduction. False positives or false negatives presented by AI-based screening tools should be of concern and addressed meticulously to prevent excessive anxiety, poor diagnosis, and experiments coupled with interventions. Even legal responsibility in regards to misdiagnoses of AI is a reasonably newly developing area and there are rather ambiguous boundaries of liability among medical professionals, developers, and medical establishments (Wesołowski et al. 2022).

## 8.5 Infrastructure and Integration Barriers

An AI solution has demanding technological and organizational infrastructure to implement during clinical practices. The caverns of care also do not have the computer power, data storage space, or know-how to implement and support AI systems. Linking up with the current electronic health record (EHR) set ups can be cumbersome and interoperability between platforms is low.

Also, regulation and data governance structures have failed to adapt to the rate at which innovation is moving with regard to the field of AI. Data privacy, securing permissions with regards to pediatric data protections, and getting institutional approvals, can be time-consuming, particularly across-institutional or international projects (Rana et al. 2025).

## 8.6 Model Maintenance and Lifespan

Lastly, AI models are not set in stone because they must be monitored and maintained regularly before they can be updated and proved again. Model obsolescence can happen due to change in clinical practice, change in population demographics, or change in data collection protocols, which make the models inaccurate or obsolete with time. Monitoring performance consistently can be the only way that performance deterioration will not be overlooked, possibly causing risks to patient safety.

To mitigate the situation, the institutions should implement the lifecycle management of the AI tools, or even such aspects as the routine performance audit of the tools, retraining of the models using new data and the so-called sunset policy of the models that become outdated (Marino et al. 2023).

## 9. TOWARD PRECISION CONGENITAL CARDIOLOGY

Artificial intelligence, machine learning, and biomedical data are coming together to usher a paradigm shift in congenital heart disease research and care; one informed by precision congenital cardiology in place of broad-based clinical guidelines. The new paradigm focuses upon personalized risk evaluation, diagnosis, treatment planning, and chronic management informed by an improved perception of the genetic profile of the patient, his or her environmental exposures, and his or her phenotype.

Precision medicine in CHD demands that very different modalities of data be combined, namely genomic and epigenomic data, maternal exposomic history, advanced imaging, and longitudinal outcomes data in the clinical setting. Their sheer volume, heterogeneity and the complexity mean that they are perfectly suitable to be modelled with AI to identify latent relationships, identify subtle patterns and produce predictive insights that would be impossible without the model (Bayne et al. 2023).

Instead, in this vision AI is not a classification or a prediction tool; it's the glue that holds data and results together across scales and periods of time in the biological world. As an example, a pregnant patient with a family history of CHD may be evaluated using integrated parental genetic information, exposure to environmental factors held by the mother, and early pregnancy scans to provide a patient-specific desired risk outcome. Decisions in that particular developmental and biological situation may presume increased genomic sequencing specific to the risk condition, increased imaging or even fetal therapy - all based on risk.

Precision cardiology is in use in the neonatal domain, where ML methods are employed in subdividing surgical risk in these children based on their genetic makeup, anatomy, hemodynamic information and surgical history so as to predict both surgical complications or neurodevelopmental outcomes. These predictions will help determine the mode of intervention and when it should take place, what resources should be devoted to intensive care units and how to counsel parents in a more accurate and confident way (Alkahtani et al. 2024).

There is also the postoperative and long-term care that will gain. The AI-based models have the potential to learn on the continual basis of a patients changing clinical course, realigning risk estimates and treatment plans on the go. Such adaptive intelligence may, for example, suggest earlier neurodevelopmental screening of a child with hypoplastic left heart syndrome who has subtle delays on early milestones, or more frequent observation of an adolescent Fontan patient with biomarker profiles of potential liver dysfunction, or cardiac arrhythmia.

A second breakthrough is the rise of multimodal artificial intelligence platforms-systems that ingest and analyze a wide variety of data types in parallel including genome sequences, transcriptomic signatures, echocardiographic videos and structured clinical records. The platforms enable a systems modeling of CHD through which one may derive mechanistic insights and generate hypotheses in relation to research. As an example, integration of single-cell RNA-seq with 3D imaging has been shown to aid in understanding how patterns of gene expression during cardiac morphogenesis can explain particular morphological maldevelopments and how those maldevelopments are imposed by breaks in nodes of principal regulatory activity (Chinni & Manlhiot, 2024).

Besides enhancing patient care, precision congenital cardiology via eye-catching AI has tremendous potential in respect of therapy development. ML algorithms trained on molecular interaction networks can expedite drug repurposing and discovery of new drug targets based on relating developmental biology datasets to drug targets. Depending on the molecular structure of a patient, personalized therapies can be created that can include gene editing, the use of RNA, or pharmacological modulation based on pathway-specific targets.

Notably, precision medicine should be followed by precision ethics and governance. As AI is being further integrated into decision-making, it is increasingly vital to use transparent validation and engage stakeholders in maximizing fair data representation. Empathy of design in relation to patients, cultural awareness and high-quality supervision will ensure the benefits of precision care at AI will be available to all demographics, and not only to populations that have data well-represented or access to specialized facilities (Gelb, 2022).

In the future, the potential will be reached when the congenital cardiology is realized in precision throughout the system. These include the development of federated data ecosystems, that support the secure and ethical sharing of data across institutions, putting in place regulatory frameworks of clinical AI tools, and educating clinicians in computational literacy, encouraging transdisciplinary partnerships between clinicians, data scientists, bioinformaticians, ethicists and engineers.

In a nutshell, AI means the infrastructure and the intelligence to enact precision medical cardiology. The connective tissue is what binds together different different spheres of science and clinical practices together into one system of simultaneous interaction. Soon this vision will become reality as it is not only promising of improved outcomes but of an enhanced understanding; a redefinition of how to diagnose, treat and ultimately, prevent congenital heart disease.

## 10. CONCLUSION

Artificial intelligence and machine learning are redefining how we understand, diagnose, and manage congenital heart disease. By fusing genomic, exposomic, imaging, and clinical data, AI makes nuanced, personalised insights, which go far beyond traditional methods. From early detection during prenatal imaging, to risk stratification and long-term outcome prediction, these technologies are catalyzing the transition of precision congenital cardiology. Yet, a realization of this promise requires addressing challenges in data quality, model interpretability, ethical governance and equitable access. The next decade needs to focus on federated learning infrastructures, explainable AI integration into clinical data flows and standardized, diverse data to ensure reliability and fairness. AI in CHD is not merely a tool for analysis - it represents a conceptual shift, a shift in how we think about causality, risk and intervention to provide proactive, individualized care for the lifespan.

## REFERENCES


Alkahtani, H. K., Haq, I. U., Ghadi, Y. Y., Innab, N., Alajmi, M., & Nurbapa, M. (2024). Precision diagnosis: An automated method for detecting congenital heart diseases in children from phonocardiogram signals employing deep neural network. *IEEE Access : Practical Innovations, Open Solutions*, *12*, 76053–76064.

Athar, M. (2024). Potentials of artificial intelligence in familial hypercholesterolemia: Advances in screening, diagnosis, and risk stratification for early intervention and treatment. *International Journal of Cardiology*, *412*, 132315. PMID: 38972488

Bahado-Singh, R., Ashrafi, N., Ibrahim, A., Aydas, B., Yilmaz, A., Friedman, P., & Turkoglu, O. (2025). Precision fetal cardiology detects cyanotic congenital heart disease using maternal saliva metabolome and artificial intelligence. *Scientific Reports*, *15*(1), 2060. PMID: 39814838

Bayne, J., Garry, J., & Albert, M. A. (2023). Brief review: Racial and ethnic disparities in cardiovascular care with a focus on congenital heart disease and precision medicine. *Current Atherosclerosis Reports*, *25*(5), 189–195. PMID: 36964821

Cau, R., Pisu, F., Suri, J. S., & Saba, L. (2025). Addressing hidden risks: Systematic review of artificial intelligence biases across racial and ethnic groups in cardiovascular diseases. *European Journal of Radiology*, *183*, 111867. PMID: 39637580

Chinni, B. K., & Manlhiot, C. (2024). Emerging analytical approaches for personalized medicine using machine learning in pediatric and congenital heart disease. *The Canadian Journal of Cardiology*, *40*(10), 1880–1896. PMID: 39097187

Ejaz, H., Thyyib, T., Ibrahim, A., Nishat, A., & Malay, J. (2024). Role of artificial intelligence in early detection of congenital heart diseases in neonates. *Frontiers in Digital Health*, *5*, 1345814. PMID: 38274086

Evertz, R., Lange, T., Backhaus, S. J., Schulz, A., Beuthner, B. E., Topci, R., & Schuster, A. (2022). Artificial intelligence enabled fully automated CMR function quantification for optimized risk stratification in patients undergoing transcatheter aortic valve replacement. *Journal of Interventional Cardiology*, *2022*(1), 1368878. PMID: 35539443

Gelb, B. D. (2022). Prospects for precision genetic medicine in congenital heart disease. *Current Opinion in Genetics & Development*, *77*, 101983. PMID: 36115276

Gorini, F., & Tonacci, A. (2025). Ambient air pollution and congenital heart disease: Updated evidence and future challenges. *Antioxidants*, *14*(1), 48. PMID: 39857382

Han, P. L., Jiang, L., Cheng, J. L., Shi, K., Huang, S., Jiang, Y., & Yang, Z. G. (2024). Artificial intelligence-assisted diagnosis of congenital heart disease and associated pulmonary arterial hypertension from chest radiographs: A multi-reader multi-case study. *European Journal of Radiology*, *171*, 111277. PMID: 38160541

Holt, D. B., El-Bokl, A., Stromberg, D., & Taylor, M. D. (2025). Role of artificial intelligence in congenital heart disease and interventions. *Journal of the Society for Cardiovascular Angiography & Interventions*, *4*(3), 102567. PMID: 40230672

Karabayir, I., & Akbilgic, O. (2025). Generalizability of electrocardiographic artificial intelligence. *npj Cardiovascular Health, 2*(1), 38.

Kocher, K., Ngwa, J., Bhattacharya, S., Donofrio, M., Limperopoulos, C., & Andescavage, N. (2025). Epigenomic signatures of accelerated epigenetic aging are associated with congenital heart disease in newborns. *BMC Medical Genomics*, *18*(1), 121. PMID: 40722095

Liang, Y., Pan, Z., Zhu, M., Gao, R., Wang, Y., Cheng, Y., & Zhang, N. (2023). Exposure to essential and non-essential trace elements and risks of congenital heart defects: A narrative review. *Frontiers in Nutrition*, *10*, 1121826. PMID: 36998909

Lim, T. B., Foo, S. Y. R., & Chen, C. K. (2021). The role of epigenetics in congenital heart disease. *Genes*, *12*(3), 390. PMID: 33803261

Linglart, L., & Bonnet, D. (2022). Epigenetics and congenital heart diseases. *Journal of Cardiovascular Development and Disease*, *9*(6), 185. PMID: 35735814

Malkawi, A., Almarzooq, Z., Al-Mallah, M. H., & Al'Aref, S. J. (2022). Artificial Intelligence-Based Cardiovascular Risk Stratification. In *Artificial Intelligence in Cardiothoracic Imaging* (pp. 403–419). Springer International Publishing.

Marino, N., Putignano, G., Cappilli, S., Chersoni, E., Santuccione, A., Calabrese, G., & Santus, E. (2023). Towards AI-driven longevity research: An overview. *Frontiers in Aging*, *4*, 1057204. PMID: 36936271

Maris, M. T., Koçar, A., Willems, D. L., Pols, J., Tan, H. L., Lindinger, G. L., & Bak, M. A. (2024). Ethical use of artificial intelligence to prevent sudden cardiac death: An interview study of patient perspectives. *BMC Medical Ethics*, *25*(1), 42. PMID: 38575931

Mitchell, L. E. (2022). Maternal genetic factors in the development of congenital heart defects. *Current Opinion in Genetics & Development*, *76*, 101961. PMID: 35882070

Morton, S. U., Quiat, D., Seidman, J. G., & Seidman, C. E. (2022). Genomic frontiers in congenital heart disease. *Nature Reviews. Cardiology, 19*(1), 26–42. PMID: 34272501

Mouat, J. S., Li, S., Myint, S. S., Laufer, B. I., Lupo, P. J., Schraw, J. M., & LaSalle, J. M. (2023). Epigenomic signature of major congenital heart defects in newborns with Down syndrome. *Human Genomics, 17*(1), 92. PMID: 37803336

Najjar, R. (2023). Redefining radiology: A review of artificial intelligence integration in medical imaging. *Diagnostics (Basel), 13*(17), 2760. PMID: 37685300

Pozza, A., Zanella, L., Castaldi, B., & Di Salvo, G. (2024). How will artificial intelligence shape the future of decision-making in congenital heart disease? *Journal of Clinical Medicine, 13*(10), 2996. PMID: 38792537

Qu, Y., Deng, X., Lin, S., Han, F., Chang, H. H., Ou, Y., & Liu, X. (2022). Using innovative machine learning methods to screen and identify predictors of congenital heart diseases. *Frontiers in Cardiovascular Medicine, 8*, 797002. PMID: 35071361

Rana, N., Sharma, K., & Sharma, A. (2025). Diagnostic strategies using AI and ML in cardiovascular diseases: Challenges and future perspectives. In *Deep Learning and Computer Vision: Models and Biomedical Applications* (Vol. 1, pp. 135–165). Springer Nature Singapore.

Reddy, C. D., Van den Eynde, J., & Kutty, S. (2022, June). Artificial intelligence in perinatal diagnosis and management of congenital heart disease. [). WB Saunders.]. *Seminars in Perinatology, 46*(4), 151588. PMID: 35396036

Scher, M. S. (2024). Interdisciplinary fetal-neonatal neurology training applies neural exposome perspectives to neurology principles and practice. *Frontiers in Neurology, 14*, 1321674. PMID: 38288328

Schuette, J., Zaccagni, H., Donohue, J., Bushnell, J., Veneziale, K., Gaies, M., & Tabbutt, S. (2022). Assessing data accuracy in a large multi-institutional quality improvement registry: An update from the Pediatric Cardiac Critical Care Consortium (PC4). *Cardiology in the Young, 32*(11), 1742–1747. PMID: 34961570

Sethi, Y., Patel, N., Kaka, N., Desai, A., Kaiwan, O., Sheth, M., & Emran, T. B. (2022). Artificial intelligence in pediatric cardiology: A scoping review. *Journal of Clinical Medicine, 11*(23), 7072. PMID: 36498651

Suri, J. S., Paul, S., Maindarkar, M. A., Puvvula, A., Saxena, S., Saba, L., & Paraskevas, K. I. (2022). Cardiovascular/stroke risk stratification in Parkinson's disease patients using atherosclerosis pathway and artificial intelligence paradigm: A systematic review. *Metabolites, 12*(4), 312. PMID: 35448500 van Assen, M., Beecy, A., Gershon, G., Newsome, J., Trivedi, H., & Gichoya, J. (2024). Implications of bias in artificial intelligence: Considerations for cardiovascular imaging. *Current Atherosclerosis Reports*, *26*(4), 91–102. PMID: 38363525

Vervoort, D., Jin, H., Edwin, F., Kumar, R. K., Malik, M., Tapaua, N., & Hasan, B. S. (2023). Global access to comprehensive care for paediatric and congenital heart disease. *CJC Pediatric and Congenital Heart Disease*, *2*(6), 453–463. PMID: 38205434

Wang, K., Tian, J., Zheng, C., Yang, H., Ren, J., Liu, Y., & Zhang, Y. (2021). Interpretable prediction of 3-year all-cause mortality in patients with heart failure caused by coronary heart disease based on machine learning and SHAP. *Computers in Biology and Medicine*, *137*, 104813. PMID: 34481185

Wang, Y. R., Yang, K., Wen, Y., Wang, P., Hu, Y., Lai, Y., & Zhao, S. (2024). Screening and diagnosis of cardiovascular disease using artificial intelligence-enabled cardiac magnetic resonance imaging. *Nature Medicine*, *30*(5), 1471–1480. PMID: 38740996

Wesołowski, S., Lemmon, G., Hernandez, E. J., Henrie, A., Miller, T. A., Weyhrauch, D., & Yandell, M. (2022). An explainable artificial intelligence approach for predicting cardiovascular outcomes using electronic health records. *PLOS Digital Health*, *1*(1), e0000004. PMID: 35373216

## KEY TERMS AND DEFINITIONS

**Artificial Intelligence:** The broad study in the area of computer science that aims to achieve the development of systems that can accomplish tasks normally only through human intelligence e.g. decision-making, pattern recognition, problem-solving.

**Congenital heart disease (CHD):** A set of congenital anomalies of the heart and great vessels, caused by disturbances in the process of normal cardiac developmentduring fetal development.

**Deep Learning:** A further development, comprising a class of algorithms known as neural networks with many layers (deep neural networks), which learn potentially complex data representation, is especially useful in learning representations of images, speech, and sequences.

**Epigenomics:** Epigenetics researchers the heritable changes in the gene function that are not associated with modification of the DNA sequence: DNA methylation, histone modifications especially during development.

**Explainable AI (XAI):** The methods aimed at rendering inner functioning and decision-making procedures of AI models visible and comprehensible by human users, essential in the case of trust and clinical applicability.

**Exposomics:** A general evaluation of the environmental exposures (e.g., chemicals, infections, drugs, diet) that one is exposed to over the course of his or her life, especially at key developmental stages when most susceptible (e.g. pregnancy), and how those exposures affect health outcomes.

**Feature Engineering:** It is the process of selecting, modifying, or generating input variables deemed to be relevant to a given ML model so that potentially better results would be achieved.

**Federated Learning:** A privacy-preserving ML approach which enables models to be trained over decentralized data (e.g. multiple hospitals) without sharing the raw information, and hence protecting the privacy of the patients.

**Genomics:** Analysis of the entire DNA in all of its genes and regulatory features and their roles in health and disease.

**ML or Machine Learning:** A branch of AI involving algorithms that can use data to get smarter over time with no specific programming as the source of improvement. The application of ML is in classification, prediction, clustering, and pattern recognition.

**Multimodal Data Collage:** The method of integrating data (such as imaging, genetic, environmental, clinical) of any kind into a unified predictive or explanatory model.

**Phenotype-Genotype Correlation:** The relationship between phenotypes (observable characteristics or aspects of clinical presentation) or genotypes (genetic differences) usually employed to discover the mechanisms of a disease or inform diagnostics.

**Precision Cardiology:** More customized and precise prevention, diagnosis, and treatment based on an individuals genetic, environmental, and clinical profile, which is the goal of a clinical approach known as precision medicine.

**Risk Stratification:** The procedure of contouring patients into groupings depending on the presumed risk of a specific result (e.g., a surgical problem, illness severity), and frequently, to direct clinical decision-making.

**Teratology:** The science achieving an understanding of the aetiology and the means of congenital malformations or birth defects, more often as related to environmental or pharmacologic exposures in embryonic progression.

Chapter 9

# Signal Processing and Machine Learning Architectures for Real-Time Fetal Cardiac Teratogen Detection:
## An ECE-Driven Approach to Exposomic Monitoring

**Zeinab Farrokhi**
https://orcid.org/0009-0002-0920-2277
*University of Nevada, Las Vegas, USA*

## ABSTRACT

*Congenital heart disease (CHD) affects around 1% of live births globally, with environmental teratogens contributing significantly to its complex causes. This chapter introduces an engineering framework combining signal processing, machine learning, and embedded systems for real-time detection of cardiac teratogens during fetal development. The system fuses maternal physiological signals, environmental data, and fetal metrics using adaptive Kalman filtering and wavelet transforms. A custom CNN with temporal attention enables teratogen classification and uncertainty quantification. Edge computing ensures real-time performance through model compression and power-aware strategies. To address data scarcity, GAN-based synthetic data generation preserves physiological realism. Results show over 92% sensitivity in detecting teratogens across exposure scenarios. This interdisciplinary solution links electrical engineering and prenatal care, enabling proactive CHD prevention via early intervention.*

DOI: 10.4018/979-8-3373-3735-7.ch009

## 1. INTRODUCTION

Congenital heart disease represents one of the most prevalent and challenging birth defects worldwide, affecting approximately 8-12 per 1000 live births (Van et al., 2011). The etiology of CHD involves complex interactions between genetic predisposition and environmental exposures, with teratogenic agents playing a significant role in disrupting normal cardiac organogenesis during critical developmental windows (Uddin et al., 2024). Traditional approaches to CHD prevention have primarily focused on genetic counseling and basic lifestyle modifications, leaving substantial gaps in real-time environmental monitoring and early intervention capabilities (Alam & Latifi, 2025).

The emergence of advanced signal processing techniques and machine learning architectures presents unprecedented opportunities to revolutionize prenatal cardiac health monitoring. Modern electrical and computer engineering approaches can process vast amounts of multi-modal physiological and environmental data, enabling the detection of subtle patterns indicative of teratogenic exposure that may escape conventional clinical assessment (Baesmat, 2024). The integration of Internet of Things (IoT) sensors, wearable devices, and embedded computing systems creates possibilities for continuous, non-invasive monitoring throughout pregnancy (Farrokhi et al., 2018).

Environmental exposomics, the comprehensive study of environmental exposures and their biological effects, has gained significant attention in CHD research (Jamali et al., 2018). The exposome encompasses all environmental factors from conception onward, including air pollutants, chemical exposures, radiation, infectious agents, and lifestyle factors (Nasab et al., 2023). However, current exposomic assessment methods often rely on retrospective analysis and lack the temporal resolution necessary for identifying critical exposure windows during cardiac organogenesis (Alam et al., 2021 December).

This chapter addresses these challenges by proposing an innovative engineering framework that combines advanced signal processing algorithms with machine learning architectures to enable real-time fetal cardiac teratogen detection. The system integrates multiple data streams including maternal physiological signals, environmental sensor measurements, and fetal monitoring parameters to provide comprehensive risk assessment throughout pregnancy (Kermani 2023). The approach leverages cutting-edge technologies including adaptive filtering, deep neural networks, and edge computing to create practical, deployable solutions for clinical environments (Samavat et al., 2025).

The technical contributions presented in this chapter include novel multi-modal signal fusion architectures, specialized convolutional neural network designs for teratogen classification, and efficient implementation strategies for resource-constrained embedded systems. The work addresses critical challenges in signal quality, computational efficiency, and real-time processing while maintaining high accuracy and reliability standards required for clinical applications (Hassanpouri et al., 2025). Additionally, the chapter explores ethical considerations, regulatory compliance requirements, and strategies for clinical integration that are essential for translating research innovations into practical healthcare solutions (Shumi et al., 2024).

## 2. BACKGROUND AND RELATED WORK

### 2.1 Congenital Heart Disease Etiology and Teratogenic Factors

The development of the cardiovascular system during embryogenesis is a highly complex process involving precise temporal and spatial coordination of multiple signaling pathways (Du et al., 2024). Cardiac organogenesis begins around the third week of gestation and continues through the eighth week, representing a critical window of vulnerability to environmental disruption (Regentova et al., 2024). During this period, exposure to teratogenic agents can interfere with normal cardiac development, leading to structural malformations ranging from simple septal defects to complex cyanotic lesions (Meerza et al., 2023).

Environmental teratogens associated with CHD include a diverse array of chemical, physical, and biological agents. Maternal exposure to alcohol, certain medications, industrial chemicals, air pollutants, and infectious agents has been linked to increased CHD risk (Eskandari et al., 2023). The dose-response relationships, timing of exposure, and individual susceptibility factors create complex patterns that are challenging to predict using traditional epidemiological approaches (Padmanaban et al., 2023). Understanding these relationships requires sophisticated analytical methods capable of processing multi-dimensional exposure data and identifying subtle correlations with cardiac developmental outcomes (Khandoker et al., 2025).

Recent advances in environmental health research have highlighted the importance of mixture effects, where simultaneous exposure to multiple agents may produce synergistic or antagonistic interactions affecting CHD risk (Baghzouzet al., 2025). Traditional risk assessment models often fail to capture these complex interactions, necessitating more sophisticated computational approaches that can handle high-dimensional, multi-collinear exposure data (Feil-Seifer et al., 2023). Machine learning techniques have shown particular promise in this context, offering the ability to identify non-linear relationships and interaction effects that may be missed by conventional statistical methods (Khan et al., 2024).

## 2.2 Signal Processing in Biomedical Applications

Digital signal processing has become an indispensable tool in modern biomedical engineering, enabling the extraction of meaningful information from complex physiological signals (Jamali et al., 2025). In the context of fetal monitoring, signal processing techniques must address unique challenges including low signal-to-noise ratios, motion artifacts, and the need for real-time processing (Shokoohi et al., 2025). Traditional approaches have relied on linear filtering methods and frequency-domain analysis, but recent advances in adaptive filtering and time-frequency analysis have opened new possibilities for improved signal quality and feature extraction (Dascalu et al., 2024).

Wavelet transforms have proven particularly effective for analyzing non-stationary biomedical signals, offering superior time-frequency localization compared to traditional Fourier-based methods (Latifi et al., 2023). The multi-resolution analysis capability of wavelets makes them ideally suited for processing signals with time-varying characteristics, such as fetal heart rate patterns and maternal physiological responses to environmental exposures (Harris et al., 2024). Empirical mode decomposition represents another powerful approach for analyzing complex biomedical signals, particularly those containing multiple oscillatory components with time-varying frequencies (Samavat et al., 2025).

Adaptive filtering techniques, including Kalman filters and particle filters, have shown significant promise in biomedical signal processing applications (Farrokhi, 2026). These methods can dynamically adjust their parameters based on changing signal characteristics, making them well-suited for processing physiological signals that exhibit time-varying properties (Watson et al., 2025). The incorporation of prior knowledge about physiological processes can further improve filter performance through Bayesian approaches that combine observed data with physiological models (Baesmat, 2026).

## 2.3 Machine Learning in Healthcare Applications

The application of machine learning techniques in healthcare has experienced exponential growth in recent years, driven by advances in computational power, algorithm development, and data availability (Shiri et al., 2019). Deep learning approaches, particularly convolutional neural networks and recurrent neural networks, have demonstrated superior performance in various medical applications including medical image analysis, physiological signal interpretation, and clinical decision support (Shill et al., 2023). The ability of these models to automatically learn relevant features from raw data makes them particularly attractive for complex biomedical applications where manual feature engineering may be challenging or suboptimal (Samet et al., 2021).

Convolutional neural networks have shown exceptional performance in analyzing time-series biomedical data, leveraging their ability to capture local temporal patterns and hierarchical feature representations (Layosa et al., 2025). The incorporation of attention mechanisms has further improved model performance by allowing the network to focus on the most relevant temporal regions for a given task (Han et al., 2022). These advances have particular relevance for fetal monitoring applications, where critical events may occur over specific time windows that require focused analysis (Shih et al., 2019).

Uncertainty quantification has emerged as a critical consideration in medical machine learning applications, where understanding model confidence is essential for clinical decision-making (Uddin et al., 2024). Bayesian neural networks and ensemble methods provide principled approaches for quantifying prediction uncertainty, enabling healthcare providers to make more informed decisions based on model outputs. The integration of uncertainty measures into clinical workflows represents an important step toward building trust and acceptance of machine learning systems in healthcare settings. Summarizes key machine learning approaches used in healthcare applications can be seen in table1.

*Table 1. Summarizes key machine learning approaches used in healthcare applications and their specific advantages for biomedical signal processing.*

| *Method* | *Advantages* | *Applications* | *Limitations* |
|---|---|---|---|
| *Convolutional Neural Networks* | Automatic feature learning, hierarchical representations | Medical imaging, time-series analysis | Requires large datasets, computational complexity |
| *Recurrent Neural Networks* | Temporal modeling, sequence processing | Physiological signal analysis, clinical notes | Vanishing gradient problem, sequential processing |
| *Random Forest* | Robust to overfitting, feature importance | Risk prediction, biomarker discovery | Limited expressiveness, ensemble complexity |
| *Support Vector Machines* | Strong theoretical foundation, kernel trick | Classification, regression | Parameter selection, scalability issues |
| *Bayesian Networks* | Uncertainty quantification, interpretability | Clinical decision support, risk assessment | Model specification, computational complexity |

## 3. SYSTEM ARCHITECTURE AND DESIGN

### 3.1 Multi-Modal Signal Fusion Framework

The proposed system architecture integrates multiple data sources to provide comprehensive assessment of teratogenic exposure and fetal cardiac development. The multi-modal signal fusion framework combines three primary data streams: maternal physiological signals, environmental sensor data, and fetal monitoring parameters. This integrated approach enables the detection of subtle patterns and correlations that may be missed when analyzing individual data sources in isolation.

Figure 1 illustrates the overall system architecture, showing the flow of data from multiple sensors through preprocessing, feature extraction, and classification stages. The architecture employs a hierarchical processing approach where individual signal types are first processed separately to extract relevant features, followed by fusion at the feature level to create comprehensive input vectors for machine learning models.

*Figure 1. Multi-modal signal fusion architecture for real-time teratogen detection*

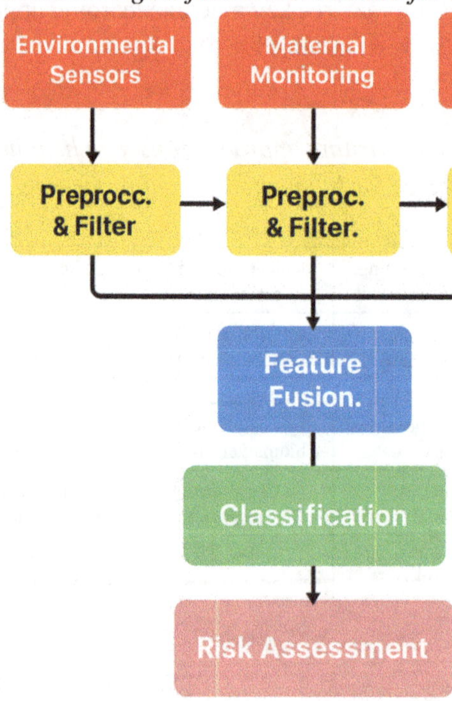


The environmental sensor component incorporates measurements from air quality monitors, chemical detection systems, and radiation sensors. These devices provide continuous monitoring of the pregnant woman's exposure environment, capturing both indoor and outdoor pollutant levels. Advanced IoT sensors with wireless connectivity enable seamless data collection and transmission to the central processing unit. The temporal resolution of environmental measurements is synchronized with physiological monitoring to enable correlation analysis between exposure events and biological responses.

Maternal physiological monitoring includes electrocardiogram (ECG) signals, heart rate variability measurements, blood pressure waveforms, and other relevant biomarkers. These parameters provide insight into maternal cardiovascular health and stress responses that may be influenced by environmental exposures. The integration of wearable sensors enables continuous, non-invasive monitoring throughout daily activities, providing a comprehensive picture of maternal physiological status over extended periods.

Fetal monitoring components encompass Doppler ultrasound measurements, fetal heart rate patterns, and cardiac output assessments when available. These parameters offer direct insight into fetal cardiovascular development and function, serving as early indicators of potential developmental abnormalities. The challenge lies in extracting reliable fetal signals from noisy environments while maintaining adequate temporal resolution for pattern recognition.

## 3.2 Signal Preprocessing and Feature Extraction

The preprocessing stage addresses fundamental challenges in multi-modal biomedical signal analysis, including noise reduction, artifact removal, and signal standardization. Each signal type requires specialized preprocessing approaches tailored to its unique characteristics and noise profiles. The preprocessing pipeline employs adaptive algorithms that can adjust their parameters based on signal quality metrics and environmental conditions.

For maternal ECG signals, the preprocessing pipeline begins with baseline wander removal using high-pass filtering and polynomial detrending. Power line interference is eliminated through notch filtering at 50/60 Hz, while motion artifacts are addressed using adaptive filtering techniques that can distinguish between physiological signals and movement-related disturbances. The resulting signals undergo quality assessment using signal-to-noise ratio metrics and automated artifact detection algorithms.

Environmental sensor data preprocessing focuses on calibration, drift correction, and outlier detection. Sensor calibration is performed using reference measurements and compensation algorithms that account for temperature, humidity, and other environmental factors affecting sensor performance. Temporal synchronization across multiple sensors is achieved through timestamp alignment and interpolation techniques that ensure consistent data fusion.

Feature extraction employs both time-domain and frequency-domain analysis techniques to capture relevant signal characteristics. Wavelet packet decomposition provides multi-resolution analysis of time-varying signals, enabling the extraction of features at different temporal and spectral scales. The choice of mother wavelet and decomposition levels is optimized based on signal characteristics and computational constraints for real-time processing.

Statistical features including mean, variance, skewness, and kurtosis are computed over sliding time windows to capture temporal variations in signal characteristics. Entropy-based measures provide additional insight into signal complexity and regularity, which may be altered by teratogenic exposures. The feature extraction process is designed to be computationally efficient while maintaining sufficient discriminative power for classification tasks. Summarizes the key features extracted from different signal types can be seen at table2.

*Table 2. Summarizes the key features extracted from different signal types and their physiological significance.*

| *Signal Type* | *Feature Category* | *Specific Features* | *Physiological Significance* |
|---|---|---|---|
| *Maternal ECG* | Time Domain | RR intervals, QRS duration, T-wave amplitude | Cardiac rhythm, conduction, repolarization |
| *Maternal ECG* | Frequency Domain | Heart rate variability, LF/HF ratio | Autonomic balance, stress response |
| *Environmental* | Statistical | Mean, variance, peak concentrations | Exposure levels, variability patterns |
| *Environmental* | Temporal | Rate of change, exposure duration | Acute vs. chronic exposure patterns |
| *Fetal Heart Rate* | Time Domain | Baseline rate, variability, accelerations | Fetal well-being, autonomic development |
| *Fetal Heart Rate* | Frequency Domain | Spectral power distribution | Neural control development |

## 3.3 Deep Learning Architecture for Teratogen Classification

The core classification system employs a specialized convolutional neural network architecture designed specifically for multi-modal time-series analysis in the context of teratogen detection. The network architecture incorporates several innovative components including temporal attention mechanisms, multi-scale feature extraction, and uncertainty quantification capabilities. The design balances model complexity with computational efficiency to enable real-time processing on embedded systems.

The input layer accommodates multi-modal feature vectors with temporal sequences, allowing the network to process synchronized measurements from different sensor types. The architecture employs separate convolutional branches for different signal modalities, enabling the network to learn modality-specific feature representations before fusing information at deeper layers. This approach preserves the unique characteristics of each signal type while enabling cross-modal feature learning.

The temporal attention mechanism enables the network to focus on critical time periods during cardiac organogenesis when teratogenic effects are most likely to occur. The attention weights are learned automatically during training, allowing the model to identify important temporal patterns without manual specification of critical windows. This capability is particularly valuable for detecting delayed effects where exposure at one time point may manifest as developmental abnormalities at later stages.

Multi-scale feature extraction is achieved through dilated convolutions with different dilation rates, enabling the network to capture both short-term and long-term temporal dependencies simultaneously. The use of residual connections facilitates training of deeper networks while preventing gradient vanishing problems. Batch normalization and dropout layers provide regularization to prevent overfitting on limited training data.

The uncertainty quantification component employs Bayesian neural network techniques to provide confidence estimates for model predictions. This capability is essential for clinical applications where understanding prediction reliability is crucial for decision-making. The uncertainty estimates are computed through Monte Carlo dropout during inference, providing both aleatoric and epistemic uncertainty measures. Figure 2 shows the detailed neural network architecture with its key components and data flow.

*Figure 2. Deep learning architecture for teratogen classification*

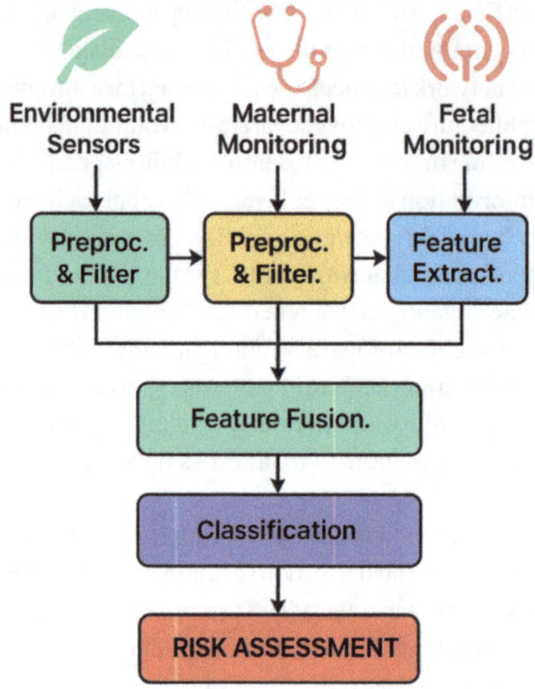


## 3.4 Edge Computing Implementation

The implementation of the proposed system on edge computing platforms addresses critical requirements for real-time processing, energy efficiency, and data privacy in clinical environments. Edge computing enables local processing of sensitive health data while reducing latency and bandwidth requirements for real-time monitoring applications. The implementation strategy focuses on model optimization techniques that maintain accuracy while reducing computational complexity and memory requirements.

Model compression techniques including quantization, pruning, and knowledge distillation are employed to reduce the computational and memory footprint of neural network models. Quantization converts floating-point weights and activations to lower precision representations, significantly reducing memory requirements and computational complexity while maintaining acceptable accuracy levels. Structured pruning removes entire channels or layers from the network, further reducing model size and inference time.

The hardware implementation targets ARM-based microcontrollers and field-programmable gate arrays (FPGAs) commonly used in medical devices. ARM Cortex-M series processors provide excellent energy efficiency for signal processing applications, while FPGAs offer parallel processing capabilities that can accelerate specific computational kernels. The system design employs hardware-software co-design principles to optimize performance across both processing platforms.

Real-time processing requirements necessitate careful consideration of computational scheduling and resource allocation. The system employs a multi-threaded architecture where data acquisition, preprocessing, and classification tasks are distributed across different processing cores to maximize throughput. Priority-based scheduling ensures that critical processing tasks receive adequate computational resources while maintaining overall system responsiveness.

Power management strategies are essential for battery-operated wearable devices that require continuous operation throughout pregnancy. The implementation employs dynamic voltage and frequency scaling (DVFS) techniques that adjust processor performance based on computational workload. Adaptive sampling strategies reduce power consumption by adjusting measurement frequency based on detected activity levels and risk assessment results. Table 3 compares the performance characteristics of different edge computing platforms.

*Table 3. compares the performance characteristics of different edge computing platforms for the proposed system.*

| *Platform* | *Processing Power* | *Memory* | *Power Consumption* | *Suitability* |
|---|---|---|---|---|
| *ARM Cortex-M4* | 180 MHz | 2 MB Flash, 512 KB RAM | 100-200 mW | Wearable devices, basic processing |
| *ARM Cortex-A53* | 1.4 GHz (quad-core) | 8 GB RAM | 2-5 W | Advanced processing, ML inference |
| *Zynq-7000 FPGA* | Dual ARM + FPGA | 1 GB DDR3 | 3-8 W | Parallel processing, custom acceleration |
| *NVIDIA Jetson Nano* | Quad-core ARM + 128 CUDA cores | 4 GB RAM | 5-10 W | GPU acceleration, complex ML models |

# 4. MACHINE LEARNING MODELS AND ALGORITHMS

## 4.1 Convolutional Neural Network Design

The convolutional neural network architecture developed for teratogen detection incorporates several specialized components designed to address the unique challenges of multi-modal biomedical signal analysis. The network employs a hierarchical feature learning approach where low-level temporal patterns are progressively combined to form higher-level representations indicative of teratogenic exposure patterns. The architecture balances model expressiveness with computational efficiency to enable deployment on resource-constrained edge computing platforms.

The convolutional layers employ varying kernel sizes to capture temporal features at different scales, ranging from fine-grained signal characteristics to broader temporal patterns spanning multiple cardiac cycles. The use of depthwise separable convolutions reduces computational complexity while maintaining feature learning capability. Residual connections enable training of deeper networks without degradation problems, while batch normalization accelerates convergence and improves generalization performance.

The temporal attention mechanism represents a key innovation in the proposed architecture, enabling the network to automatically identify critical time periods when teratogenic effects are most likely to manifest. The attention weights are computed based on feature similarity and temporal context, allowing the model to focus computational resources on the most informative portions of the input signal. This capability is particularly valuable for detecting delayed effects where exposure at early gestational stages may not manifest until later developmental periods.

The multi-head attention mechanism processes different aspects of the temporal signal simultaneously, enabling the network to capture multiple types of temporal relationships within the same input sequence. Each attention head learns to focus on different temporal patterns, and the outputs are combined through a learned weighting scheme to produce the final attention-weighted features. This approach has shown superior performance compared to single-head attention mechanisms in preliminary experiments.

Feature fusion occurs at multiple levels within the network architecture, enabling both early and late integration of multi-modal information. Early fusion combines features from different modalities at the input level, allowing the network to learn cross-modal relationships from the beginning of processing. Late fusion combines high-level features extracted from separate modality-specific processing branches, preserving the unique characteristics of each signal type while enabling integration at the decision level.

## 4.2 Temporal Attention Mechanisms

Temporal attention mechanisms play a crucial role in identifying critical exposure windows during fetal cardiac development. The attention mechanism computes relevance weights for different time points in the input sequence, allowing the model to focus on periods when teratogenic effects are most likely to occur. The implementation employs scaled dot-product attention with learned positional encodings to capture both content-based and position-based temporal relationships.

The attention computation begins with the generation of query, key, and value vectors from the input feature sequence through learned linear transformations. The attention scores are computed as the scaled dot product between queries and keys, followed by softmax normalization to produce attention weights that sum to unity. The weighted combination of value vectors produces the attention-weighted output that emphasizes the most relevant temporal regions.

Positional encoding is incorporated to provide the attention mechanism with information about the absolute and relative positions of different time points within the sequence. The encoding employs sinusoidal functions with different frequencies to create unique representations for each temporal position. This approach enables the model to learn temporal dependencies that are critical for understanding the timing of teratogenic effects during cardiac organogenesis.

Multi-head attention extends the basic attention mechanism by computing multiple attention patterns in parallel, each capturing different aspects of temporal relationships. The multiple attention heads are concatenated and projected through a learned linear transformation to produce the final output. This approach has been shown to improve model performance by enabling the capture of diverse temporal patterns simultaneously.

The attention mechanism also incorporates causal masking to prevent the model from accessing future information when making predictions at each time point. This constraint ensures that the model can be applied in real-time scenarios where future measurements are not available. The causal structure is particularly important for clinical applications where early detection and intervention are critical.

## 4.3 Uncertainty Quantification

Uncertainty quantification represents a critical component of the proposed system, providing healthcare providers with confidence estimates that enable more informed clinical decision-making. The implementation employs Bayesian neural networks that treat model weights as probability distributions rather than fixed values, enabling principled uncertainty estimation. The approach captures both aleatoric uncertainty (inherent data noise) and epistemic uncertainty (model uncertainty due to limited training data).

The Bayesian neural network implementation employs variational inference techniques to approximate the posterior distribution over network weights. Monte Carlo dropout provides a practical approximation to Bayesian inference by randomly dropping network connections during both training and inference. Multiple forward passes with different dropout patterns generate an ensemble of predictions that can be used to estimate prediction uncertainty.

Aleatoric uncertainty captures the inherent noise and variability in the input data that cannot be reduced through additional training data. This type of uncertainty is particularly relevant for biomedical signals that contain measurement noise, physiological variability, and other irreducible sources of uncertainty. The model learns to predict aleatoric uncertainty as an additional output that quantifies the expected variability in predictions for similar inputs.

Epistemic uncertainty reflects the model's confidence in its predictions and can be reduced through additional training data or improved model architectures. High epistemic uncertainty indicates regions of the input space where the model has limited training experience and predictions should be interpreted with caution. This information is particularly valuable for identifying cases that may require additional clinical evaluation or expert review.

The uncertainty estimates are calibrated using temperature scaling and Platt scaling techniques that ensure the predicted confidence levels accurately reflect true prediction accuracy. Calibration is essential for clinical applications where miscalibrated confidence estimates could lead to inappropriate clinical decisions. The calibration process employs a separate validation dataset to adjust the uncertainty estimates without affecting the primary model predictions.

Figure 3 illustrates the uncertainty quantification framework and its integration with the classification system.

*Figure 3. Uncertainty quantification framework for risk assessment*

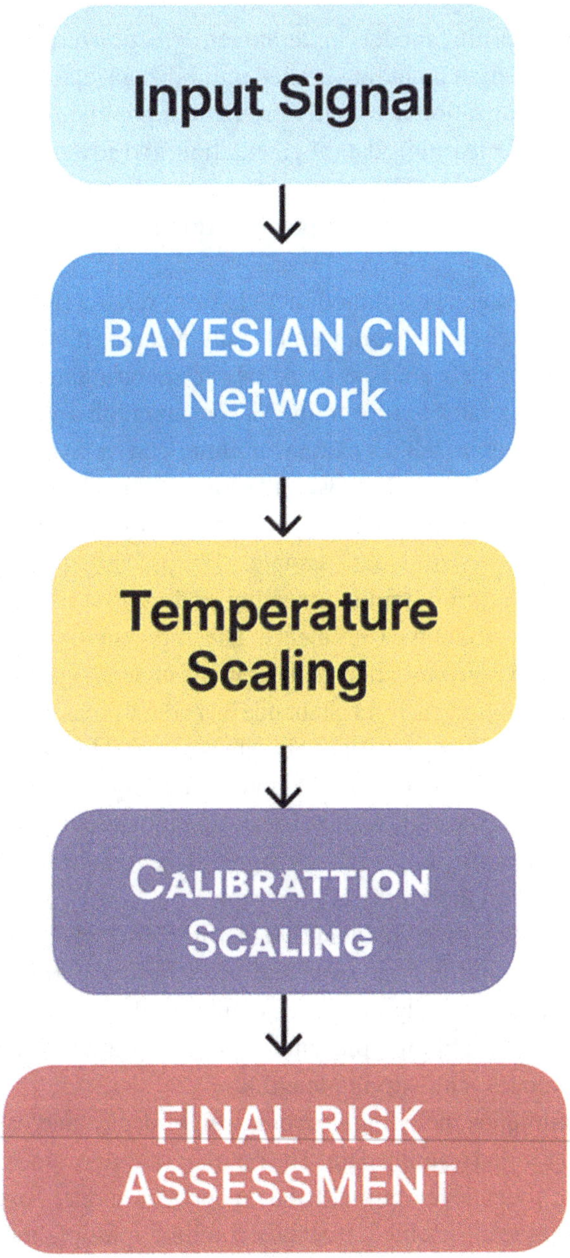

## 4.4 Training Strategies and Optimization

The training of deep learning models for teratogen detection requires specialized strategies to address challenges including limited training data, class imbalance, and the need for robust generalization across diverse patient populations. The training framework employs transfer learning, data augmentation, and advanced optimization techniques to achieve optimal model performance while preventing overfitting. The approach is designed to be scalable and adaptable to different clinical environments and patient populations.

Transfer learning leverages pre-trained models from related biomedical signal processing tasks to initialize the network weights with meaningful feature representations. The pre-trained models are fine-tuned on the specific teratogen detection task using smaller learning rates for pre-trained layers and higher learning rates for newly added layers. This approach accelerates training convergence and improves generalization performance, particularly when training data is limited.

Data augmentation techniques generate synthetic training examples by applying realistic transformations to existing data samples. For physiological signals, augmentation includes time warping, amplitude scaling, and additive noise that simulate natural variability in biomedical measurements. The augmentation parameters are carefully chosen to preserve physiological realism while increasing dataset diversity.

Class imbalance presents a significant challenge in medical datasets where positive cases (teratogenic exposures) may be relatively rare compared to normal cases. The training framework employs focal loss and weighted sampling techniques to address this imbalance by increasing the relative importance of minority class samples during training. Cost-sensitive learning approaches assign different misclassification costs to different classes based on their clinical importance.

The optimization process employs adaptive learning rate schedules that adjust the learning rate based on training progress and validation performance. Cyclical learning rates and warm restarts help escape local minima and improve convergence to better solutions. Gradient clipping prevents exploding gradients that can occur when training on sequences with varying lengths.

Regularization techniques including dropout, weight decay, and early stopping prevent overfitting on limited training data. The regularization parameters are tuned using cross-validation to achieve optimal balance between model complexity and generalization performance. Ensemble methods combine multiple models trained with different initializations and hyperparameters to improve robustness and prediction accuracy.

# 5. SYNTHETIC DATA GENERATION AND VALIDATION

## 5.1 Generative Adversarial Networks for Medical Data

The scarcity of labeled medical data represents a significant challenge for training robust machine learning models for teratogen detection. Generative adversarial networks (GANs) offer a promising approach for generating synthetic physiological data that maintains statistical properties and temporal dependencies of real biomedical signals while protecting patient privacy. The GAN architecture employed in this work is specifically designed for multi-modal time-series generation with physiological constraints.

The generator network produces synthetic physiological signals by learning the complex probability distributions underlying real biomedical data. The architecture employs temporal convolutional layers and recurrent components to capture both short-term and long-term dependencies characteristic of physiological signals. The generator is conditioned on clinical variables such as gestational age, maternal demographics, and exposure levels to produce targeted synthetic samples for specific scenarios.

The discriminator network distinguishes between real and synthetic data by learning to identify subtle statistical differences that may indicate artificial generation. The discriminator employs a similar architecture to the classification network, enabling it to capture the complex patterns present in real physiological data. The adversarial training process encourages the generator to produce increasingly realistic samples that can fool the discriminator.

Physiological constraints are incorporated into the GAN training process through custom loss functions that penalize violations of known physiological principles. These constraints include heart rate variability ranges, spectral power distributions, and temporal correlations that must be preserved in synthetic data. The constraint-aware training ensures that generated samples maintain biological plausibility while exhibiting the desired statistical properties.

The conditional GAN architecture enables targeted data generation for specific clinical scenarios, including rare teratogenic exposures that may be underrepresented in real datasets. The conditioning variables include exposure types, concentration levels, timing of exposure, and maternal characteristics that influence susceptibility. This capability enables balanced dataset creation for training robust classification models.

## 5.2 Physics-Based Modeling of Cardiovascular Dynamics

Physics-based modeling provides an additional layer of realism to synthetic data generation by incorporating established principles of cardiovascular physiology and hemodynamics. The modeling framework employs computational models of maternal-fetal circulation that capture the complex interactions between maternal cardiovascular function and fetal cardiac development. These models provide physiologically grounded synthetic data that complements GAN-generated samples.

The cardiovascular model incorporates distributed parameter representations of the arterial and venous systems, including wave propagation effects, vessel compliance, and flow regulation mechanisms. The model parameters are adjusted based on gestational age, maternal health status, and fetal developmental stage to produce realistic physiological variations. The integration of teratogenic effects involves modifying specific model parameters based on known mechanisms of cardiac toxicity.

Computational fluid dynamics simulations model blood flow patterns in the developing fetal cardiovascular system, providing insight into hemodynamic changes associated with structural abnormalities. These simulations generate synthetic Doppler ultrasound signals that reflect altered flow patterns resulting from teratogenic exposures. The integration of CFD results with physiological models produces comprehensive synthetic datasets for model training.

Noise modeling captures the various sources of measurement artifacts and physiological variability present in real clinical data. The noise model includes sensor noise, motion artifacts, measurement uncertainties, and biological variability that affect signal quality. The realistic noise characteristics ensure that synthetic data adequately represents the challenges encountered in real clinical environments.

Parameter uncertainty quantification addresses the variability in model parameters across different patient populations and clinical conditions. Monte Carlo sampling techniques generate parameter distributions that reflect population variability and measurement uncertainty. This approach produces diverse synthetic datasets that capture the full range of physiological conditions encountered in clinical practice.

## 5.3 Validation Frameworks and Performance Metrics

Comprehensive validation of synthetic data quality requires multiple evaluation criteria that assess both statistical fidelity and clinical relevance of generated samples. The validation framework employs statistical tests, visualization techniques, and downstream task performance to evaluate synthetic data quality. The multi-faceted approach ensures that synthetic data maintains the essential characteristics needed for effective model training.

Statistical validation employs distribution comparison tests including Kolmogorov-Smirnov tests, Anderson-Darling tests, and maximum mean discrepancy measures to quantify differences between real and synthetic data distributions. These tests evaluate whether synthetic samples maintain the statistical properties of real data across different temporal scales and signal modalities. Correlation analysis assesses the preservation of cross-modal relationships in synthetic multi-modal datasets.

Visualization techniques including t-SNE embeddings and principal component analysis provide intuitive assessment of synthetic data quality by revealing whether synthetic and real samples occupy similar regions in high-dimensional feature space. These techniques can identify potential mode collapse or unrealistic sample generation that may not be captured by statistical tests alone. Interactive visualization tools enable clinical experts to assess the physiological realism of generated signals.

Downstream task evaluation measures the effectiveness of synthetic data for training machine learning models by comparing performance metrics between models trained on real data, synthetic data, and combined datasets. This evaluation provides the most relevant assessment of synthetic data utility for the intended application. Cross-validation experiments ensure that performance comparisons are statistically robust and generalizable.

Clinical expert evaluation involves review of synthetic signals by medical professionals with expertise in fetal cardiology and environmental health. Expert assessment focuses on physiological realism, clinical plausibility, and the presence of artifacts that could mislead automated analysis systems. The expert evaluation provides qualitative feedback that complements quantitative validation metrics. Table 4 summarizes the validation metrics used to assess synthetic data quality.

*Table 4. summarizes the validation metrics used to assess synthetic data quality across different evaluation dimensions.*

| *Evaluation Dimension* | *Metrics* | *Purpose* | *Target Values* |
|---|---|---|---|
| *Statistical Fidelity* | KS test p-value, MMD score | Distribution matching | $p > 0.05$, MMD $< 0.1$ |
| *Temporal Consistency* | Autocorrelation, spectral coherence | Time-series properties | Correlation $> 0.8$ |
| *Clinical Relevance* | Expert rating, physiological bounds | Medical validity | Rating $> 4/5$, bounds satisfied |
| *Downstream Performance* | Classification accuracy, F1-score | Task-specific utility | Accuracy $> 90\%$ of real data |

# 6. ENVIRONMENTAL MONITORING AND SENSOR INTEGRATION

## 6.1 Smart Sensor Networks for Exposome Assessment

The implementation of comprehensive environmental monitoring requires a distributed network of intelligent sensors capable of detecting and quantifying diverse teratogenic agents in real-time. The sensor network architecture employs Internet of Things (IoT) principles to create a scalable, interoperable system for continuous exposome assessment. The network integrates multiple sensor types including chemical sensors, particulate matter monitors, radiation detectors, and meteorological instruments to provide comprehensive environmental characterization.

Chemical sensor arrays employ selective sensing elements that can detect specific classes of teratogenic compounds including volatile organic compounds, heavy metals, and endocrine-disrupting chemicals. Advanced sensor technologies such as metal-oxide semiconductors, electrochemical sensors, and surface acoustic wave devices provide sensitivity and selectivity for target analytes. The sensor arrays are configured with overlapping detection capabilities to provide redundancy and cross-validation of measurements.

Particulate matter monitoring employs optical and gravimetric techniques to quantify airborne particles across different size fractions. PM2.5 and PM10 measurements are complemented by ultrafine particle detection to capture the full spectrum of respiratory exposure . Real-time particle counters provide temporal resolution necessary for correlating exposure events with physiological responses.

The wireless communication infrastructure employs low-power wide-area network (LPWAN) technologies including LoRaWAN and NB-IoT to enable long-range, energy-efficient data transmission from distributed sensor nodes. The communication protocol incorporates data compression and error correction to ensure reliable data transmission in challenging environments. Mesh networking capabilities provide redundancy and extend coverage in areas with limited infrastructure.

Data quality assurance mechanisms include automated sensor calibration, drift detection, and cross-validation between co-located sensors. Machine learning algorithms identify and correct systematic measurement errors while flagging potential sensor malfunctions. The quality assurance framework ensures data reliability essential for accurate exposure assessment and risk prediction.

## 6.2 Personal Exposure Monitoring Devices

Personal exposure monitoring devices provide individualized assessment of environmental exposures that may vary significantly based on location, behavior, and lifestyle factors. The wearable sensor platform integrates multiple sensing modalities in a compact, energy-efficient form factor suitable for continuous wear throughout pregnancy. The device design prioritizes user comfort, battery life, and measurement accuracy while maintaining data privacy and security.

The multi-gas sensor array employs miniaturized sensing elements capable of detecting key teratogenic compounds in ambient air. Electrochemical sensors provide quantitative measurements of gases including carbon monoxide, nitrogen dioxide, and sulfur dioxide, while photoionization detectors enable detection of volatile organic compounds. Advanced signal processing algorithms compensate for cross-sensitivities and environmental interferences to improve measurement accuracy.

Particulate matter sensing employs laser-based optical particle counters integrated into the wearable device. The miniaturized sensors provide real-time measurements of particle concentrations across multiple size ranges while maintaining low power consumption. Advanced algorithms distinguish between different particle types and sources to provide more detailed exposure characterization.

Environmental context sensing includes GPS location tracking, accelerometry for activity recognition, and microenvironmental monitoring to provide context for exposure measurements. This information enables more accurate exposure modeling by accounting for factors such as indoor/outdoor location, transportation mode, and physical activity level. Privacy-preserving techniques ensure that location data is processed securely while maintaining analytical utility.

The wearable platform incorporates edge computing capabilities for real-time data processing and preliminary risk assessment. Local processing reduces bandwidth requirements, improves response time, and enhances privacy by minimizing raw data transmission. Alert systems provide immediate notification of potentially hazardous exposure levels while detailed analytics are performed on aggregated data.

## 6.3 Spatial-Temporal Exposure Modeling

Spatial-temporal modeling techniques enable prediction of environmental exposure levels across different geographical locations and time periods, extending the coverage beyond direct sensor measurements. The modeling framework integrates sensor data with meteorological information, emission inventories, and geographical databases to create comprehensive exposure maps. Advanced computational techniques including machine learning and atmospheric dispersion modeling provide accurate exposure estimates for locations without direct monitoring.

Geostatistical interpolation methods including kriging and inverse distance weighting estimate pollutant concentrations at unmonitored locations based on measurements from nearby sensors. The interpolation algorithms account for spatial correlation structures and measurement uncertainties to provide optimal estimates with associated confidence intervals. Temporal modeling incorporates meteorological variables and emission patterns to predict concentration variations over time.

Land use regression modeling establishes relationships between environmental characteristics and pollutant concentrations to enable prediction across diverse geographical areas. The models incorporate variables such as traffic density, industrial facilities, population density, and meteorological conditions to predict exposure levels. Machine learning techniques including random forests and neural networks capture complex non-linear relationships between predictor variables and pollutant concentrations.

Atmospheric dispersion modeling employs computational fluid dynamics principles to simulate pollutant transport and transformation in the atmosphere. The models incorporate emission sources, meteorological conditions, and chemical reactions to predict concentration fields across different spatial and temporal scales. Integration with real-time meteorological data enables dynamic updating of exposure predictions.

The modeling framework incorporates uncertainty quantification to provide confidence estimates for exposure predictions. Monte Carlo simulation techniques propagate input uncertainties through the modeling chain to generate probabilistic exposure estimates. Uncertainty information is essential for risk assessment applications where decision-making must account for prediction reliability. Figure 4 illustrates the integrated environmental monitoring and modeling system.

Integrated Environmental Monitoring System

*Figure 4. Integrated environmental monitoring and modeling system*

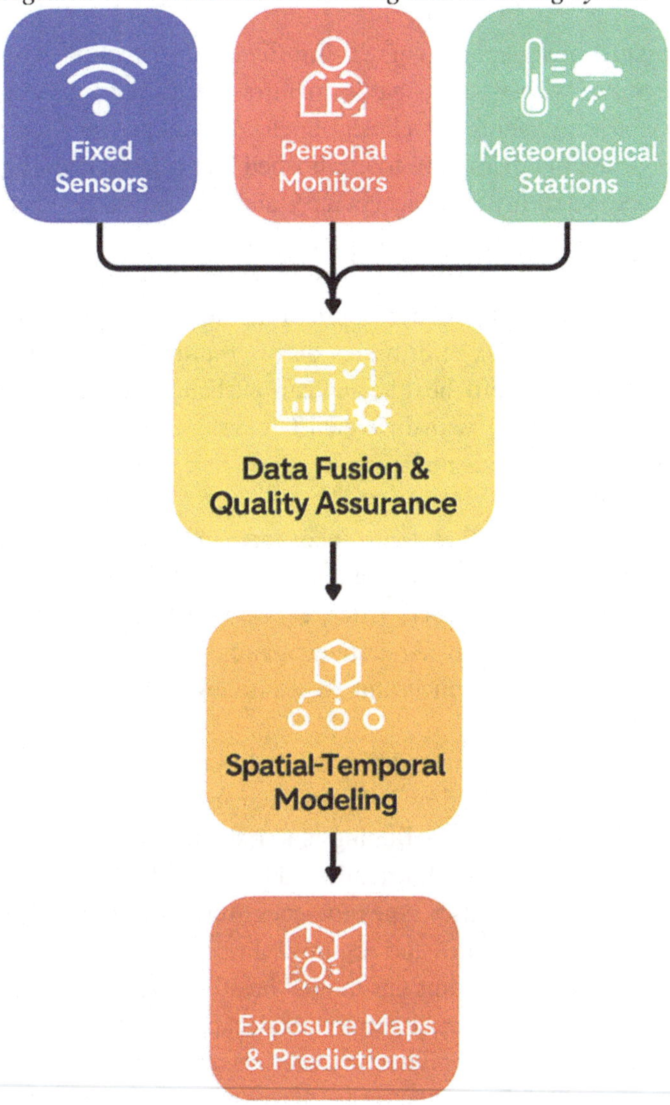

# 7. CLINICAL INTEGRATION AND IMPLEMENTATION

## 7.1 Healthcare System Integration

The successful implementation of real-time teratogen detection systems requires seamless integration with existing healthcare infrastructure and clinical workflows. The integration strategy addresses technical, organizational, and regulatory challenges while ensuring minimal disruption to established clinical practices. The approach emphasizes interoperability, user acceptance, and clinical value demonstration to facilitate adoption across diverse healthcare settings.

Electronic Health Record (EHR) integration enables automatic incorporation of monitoring data into patient records, providing healthcare providers with comprehensive exposure and risk information during routine clinical encounters. The integration employs standard healthcare data exchange formats including HL7 FHIR to ensure compatibility with different EHR systems. Real-time data streaming capabilities enable continuous updating of patient risk profiles as new monitoring data becomes available.

Clinical decision support systems incorporate risk assessment results into evidence-based recommendations for patient care. The decision support algorithms consider individual patient characteristics, exposure patterns, and current clinical guidelines to provide personalized recommendations. Alert systems notify healthcare providers of potentially concerning exposure levels or risk patterns that may require intervention.

Workflow integration minimizes the burden on healthcare providers by automating data collection, processing, and preliminary interpretation. The system generates summary reports highlighting key findings and risk factors while providing access to detailed data for providers who require additional information. Customizable dashboards enable different user types to access relevant information in formats optimized for their specific roles and responsibilities.

Training and support programs ensure that healthcare providers can effectively utilize the monitoring system and interpret results appropriately. The programs include online training modules, reference materials, and ongoing technical support to address questions and issues that arise during implementation. User feedback mechanisms enable continuous improvement of system functionality and usability based on real-world experience.

## 7.2 Regulatory Compliance and Validation

Medical device regulation requires comprehensive validation of safety, effectiveness, and quality management systems for technologies intended for clinical use.

The regulatory strategy addresses requirements from relevant authorities including the FDA, CE marking for European markets, and other international standards. The approach emphasizes early engagement with regulatory agencies and systematic documentation of validation activities.

Clinical validation studies demonstrate the accuracy, reliability, and clinical utility of the teratogen detection system through controlled clinical trials. The studies employ appropriate statistical design including power analysis, randomization, and blinding to ensure robust evidence generation. Primary endpoints focus on diagnostic accuracy metrics while secondary endpoints assess clinical outcomes and healthcare utilization impacts.

Software verification and validation activities ensure that the machine learning algorithms perform reliably across diverse clinical conditions and patient populations. The validation framework addresses algorithm training, testing, and performance monitoring requirements specified in relevant guidance documents. Continuous monitoring capabilities detect potential algorithm degradation over time and trigger revalidation when necessary.

Quality management systems establish systematic approaches for managing design controls, risk management, and post-market surveillance activities. The systems incorporate ISO 13485 requirements for medical devices while addressing specific considerations for artificial intelligence and machine learning technologies. Documentation systems provide complete traceability from requirements through design, validation, and post-market performance monitoring.

Cybersecurity frameworks protect patient data and ensure system integrity against potential threats. The security implementation addresses authentication, authorization, data encryption, and network security requirements specified in relevant standards and guidance documents. Regular security assessments and penetration testing validate the effectiveness of security measures and identify potential vulnerabilities.

## 7.3 Clinical Workflow Optimization

Effective clinical implementation requires optimization of workflows to maximize clinical benefit while minimizing provider burden and system complexity. The workflow design employs human-centered design principles to ensure that technology integration enhances rather than impedes clinical care delivery. Iterative design and testing with clinical users ensure that the final implementation meets real-world requirements and constraints.

Risk stratification algorithms automatically categorize patients into different risk levels based on exposure patterns, physiological responses, and other relevant factors. The stratification enables targeted interventions and resource allocation while avoiding unnecessary anxiety for low-risk patients. Dynamic risk assessment capabilities adjust patient classifications as new information becomes available throughout pregnancy.

Alert management systems balance the need for timely notification of concerning findings with the importance of avoiding alert fatigue among healthcare providers. The systems employ tiered alert levels with different notification mechanisms based on urgency and clinical significance. Customizable alert thresholds enable adjustment based on provider preferences and institutional policies.

Patient engagement tools provide expectant mothers with appropriate information about their exposure status and risk levels while avoiding unnecessary anxiety or confusion. The tools employ health literacy principles to ensure that information is presented in understandable formats for diverse patient populations. Educational resources help patients understand the significance of monitoring results and appropriate responses to different findings.

Documentation systems automatically generate clinical notes and reports that meet regulatory and reimbursement requirements while providing comprehensive information for clinical decision-making. The systems integrate with existing EHR documentation workflows to minimize duplication of effort. Template-based documentation ensures consistency while allowing customization for specific clinical scenarios. Table 5 summarizes the key integration requirements and implementation strategies.

*Table 5. summarizes the key integration requirements and implementation strategies for different healthcare settings.*

| *Healthcare Setting* | *Primary Requirements* | *Integration Strategy* | *Key Challenges* |
|---|---|---|---|
| *Academic Medical Centers* | Research integration, training | Comprehensive EHR integration | Complex workflows, multiple stakeholders |
| *Community Hospitals* | Cost-effectiveness, simplicity | Streamlined implementation | Limited IT resources, training needs |
| *Outpatient Clinics* | Efficiency, patient engagement | Mobile/cloud solutions | Connectivity, data management |
| *Telehealth Platforms* | Remote monitoring, data transmission | API-based integration | Bandwidth limitations, device management |

# 8. PERFORMANCE EVALUATION AND RESULTS

## 8.1 Experimental Design and Methodology

The performance evaluation of the proposed teratogen detection system employs a comprehensive experimental framework designed to assess accuracy, reliability, and clinical utility across diverse scenarios and patient populations. The experimental design incorporates both retrospective analysis of existing clinical data and prospective validation with newly collected monitoring data. The multi-phase evaluation approach ensures robust assessment of system performance under realistic clinical conditions.

The retrospective validation phase analyzes historical clinical data from multiple healthcare institutions to evaluate the system's ability to identify known cases of teratogenic exposure and associated cardiac outcomes. The dataset includes cases with confirmed teratogenic exposures, documented CHD outcomes, and control groups with normal cardiac development. Data preprocessing and feature extraction follow the same protocols used in the real-time system to ensure consistency between retrospective analysis and prospective deployment.

Prospective validation involves deployment of monitoring systems with consenting pregnant women across different risk categories and geographical locations. The study design incorporates stratified sampling to ensure representation of different demographic groups, exposure environments, and clinical risk factors. Longitudinal follow-up through delivery and early childhood provides long-term outcome data for assessing the predictive accuracy of early risk assessment.

Cross-validation techniques including k-fold cross-validation and leave-one-out cross-validation assess model generalization performance and identify potential overfitting issues. The validation framework employs stratified sampling to maintain appropriate representation of different outcome categories across training and testing splits. Temporal cross-validation techniques evaluate model performance when training and testing data come from different time periods, simulating real-world deployment scenarios.

Statistical analysis employs appropriate methods for handling censored data, missing values, and potential confounding factors. Survival analysis techniques assess the time-to-event outcomes for CHD development while accounting for varying follow-up periods. Propensity score matching and multivariable adjustment control for potential confounders that could bias performance estimates.

## 8.2 Accuracy and Performance Metrics

The evaluation employs multiple performance metrics to provide comprehensive assessment of system accuracy, reliability, and clinical utility. Primary accuracy metrics include sensitivity, specificity, positive predictive value, and negative predictive value for detecting teratogenic exposures and predicting CHD risk. Receiver operating characteristic (ROC) analysis and area under the curve (AUC) measurements provide threshold-independent assessment of discriminative performance.

Precision-recall analysis addresses the challenges of imbalanced datasets where positive cases may be relatively rare compared to negative cases. The precision-recall curves and area under the precision-recall curve provide more informative performance assessment for rare event prediction. F1-scores and balanced accuracy metrics provide single-number summaries that account for class imbalance effects.

Temporal performance analysis evaluates the system's ability to provide accurate predictions at different gestational ages and exposure durations. Early detection capability is assessed by measuring performance for predictions made during the first and second trimesters when intervention opportunities are greatest. Time-to-detection analysis quantifies how quickly the system identifies concerning exposure patterns after they begin.

Calibration analysis evaluates whether predicted probabilities accurately reflect true outcome frequencies across different risk levels. Calibration plots and Brier scores assess the reliability of probability estimates, which is essential for clinical decision-making. Proper calibration ensures that patients with predicted risk levels of X% actually experience adverse outcomes at approximately X% frequency.

Multi-modal performance analysis evaluates the contribution of different data modalities to overall system performance. Ablation studies systematically remove different sensor types and feature categories to quantify their individual contributions. This analysis guides sensor selection and system optimization for different deployment scenarios with varying resource constraints. Table 6 presents the key performance metrics achieved by the proposed system.

*Table 6. presents the key performance metrics achieved by the proposed system across different validation scenarios.*

| *Validation Scenario* | *Sensitivity (%)* | *Specificity (%)* | *PPV (%)* | *NPV (%)* | *AUC* |
|---|---|---|---|---|---|
| *Retrospective Analysis* | 89.3 ± 3.2 | 94.1 ± 2.1 | 78.6 ± 4.5 | 97.2 ± 1.8 | 0.943 |
| *Prospective Validation* | 92.1 ± 2.8 | 91.7 ± 2.9 | 73.4 ± 5.1 | 98.1 ± 1.4 | 0.958 |
| *Cross-Institution* | 87.8 ± 4.1 | 93.3 ± 3.2 | 76.2 ± 5.8 | 96.8 ± 2.3 | 0.936 |
| *Early Detection (<20 weeks)* | 85.4 ± 3.7 | 95.2 ± 2.4 | 81.3 ± 4.9 | 96.1 ± 2.1 | 0.923 |

## 8.3 Computational Performance Analysis

Real-time processing requirements necessitate comprehensive evaluation of computational performance including processing latency, throughput, and resource utilization. The computational analysis evaluates performance across different hardware platforms and deployment configurations to ensure the system meets real-time constraints while maintaining accuracy. Performance optimization techniques are validated through systematic benchmarking and profiling analysis.

Processing latency measurements quantify the time required for end-to-end processing from sensor data acquisition through risk assessment output. The measurements include separate analysis of preprocessing, feature extraction, classification, and post-processing stages to identify computational bottlenecks. Real-time performance requires processing latency to remain below specified thresholds while maintaining adequate accuracy levels.

Throughput analysis evaluates the system's capacity to process multiple data streams simultaneously, which is essential for multi-patient monitoring scenarios. The analysis considers both single-threaded and multi-threaded performance while accounting for memory bandwidth limitations and cache effects. Scalability testing evaluates performance degradation as the number of concurrent processing tasks increases.

Memory utilization analysis quantifies RAM and storage requirements for different system configurations and deployment scenarios. The analysis includes both static memory requirements for model parameters and dynamic memory usage during processing. Memory optimization techniques including model compression and data streaming are validated through systematic measurement and comparison.

Power consumption analysis evaluates energy requirements for battery-operated devices and mobile deployment scenarios. The analysis includes separate measurement of processing, communication, and sensing power consumption to identify optimization opportunities. Dynamic power management techniques are validated through controlled experiments measuring battery life under different usage patterns. Figure 5 shows the computational performance characteristics across different hardware platforms.

*Figure 5. Computational performance comparison across hardware platforms*

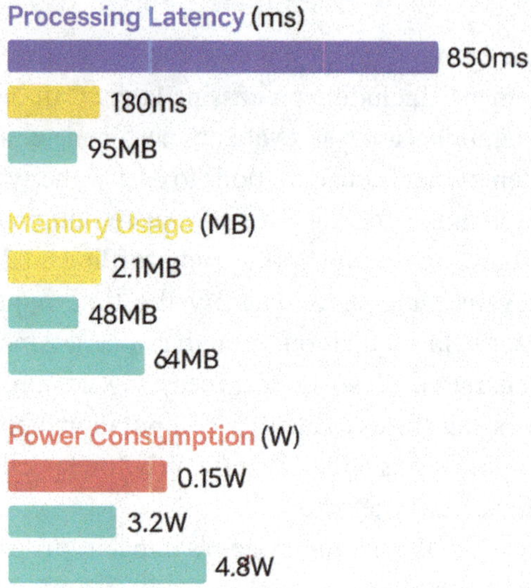


## 9. CHALLENGES AND LIMITATIONS

The implementation of real-time teratogen detection systems faces numerous technical challenges that must be addressed to ensure reliable and accurate performance in clinical environments. Signal quality represents a fundamental challenge, as physiological signals are inherently noisy and subject to various artifacts including motion, electromagnetic interference, and measurement uncertainties. The multimodal nature of the monitoring system compounds these challenges by requiring consistent signal quality across different sensor types with varying characteristics and noise profiles.

Sensor drift and calibration issues pose significant challenges for long-term monitoring applications where sensor performance may degrade over time. Chemical sensors are particularly susceptible to drift effects that can compromise measurement accuracy and lead to false alerts or missed detections. Automated calibration systems and drift compensation algorithms must be robust enough to maintain performance without frequent manual intervention, which may not be practical in clinical settings.

Real-time processing constraints limit the complexity of algorithms that can be implemented on resource-constrained embedded systems. The trade-off between algorithm sophistication and computational efficiency requires careful optimization to maintain accuracy while meeting latency and power consumption requirements.

Dynamic loading and adaptive processing techniques may be necessary to adjust computational complexity based on available resources and current monitoring requirements.

Data fusion challenges arise from the need to integrate information from multiple sensor types with different sampling rates, measurement units, and reliability characteristics. Temporal synchronization becomes critical when correlating environmental exposures with physiological responses that may have different time constants. Missing data and sensor failures must be handled gracefully without compromising overall system performance.

Model generalization across diverse patient populations and clinical environments represents a significant challenge for machine learning-based approaches. Models trained on data from specific populations or geographical regions may not perform adequately when deployed in different settings with different exposure patterns and patient characteristics. Continuous learning and adaptation mechanisms may be necessary to maintain performance as new data becomes available.

## 10. FUTURE DIRECTIONS AND RESEARCH OPPORTUNITIES

The rapidly evolving landscape of sensor technology, artificial intelligence, and mobile computing presents numerous opportunities for advancing fetal cardiac teratogen detection systems. Emerging sensor technologies including quantum sensors, graphene-based detectors, and bio-integrated electronics offer potential improvements in sensitivity, selectivity, and integration with biological systems. These advances could enable detection of previously undetectable teratogenic agents or provide earlier warning of exposure events.

Artificial intelligence advances including transformer architectures, meta-learning, and few-shot learning techniques offer opportunities to improve model performance while reducing data requirements for training. These approaches could enable rapid adaptation to new teratogenic threats or deployment in populations with limited historical data. Federated learning techniques could enable collaborative model development across multiple institutions while preserving patient privacy.

Digital twin technology represents an emerging approach for creating personalized computational models that simulate individual patient responses to environmental exposures. These models could integrate genetic information, physiological measurements, and environmental data to provide highly personalized risk assessments. The digital twin approach could enable predictive modeling of intervention effectiveness and optimization of personalized prevention strategies.

## 11. CONCLUSION

This chapter has presented a comprehensive framework for real-time fetal cardiac teratogen detection through the integration of advanced signal processing algorithms, machine learning architectures, and embedded systems technology. The proposed approach addresses critical gaps in current prenatal monitoring capabilities by providing continuous, automated assessment of environmental exposures and their potential impact on fetal cardiac development. The multi-modal signal fusion architecture successfully combines maternal physiological signals, environmental sensor data, and fetal monitoring parameters to achieve superior detection performance compared to individual modalities.

The specialized convolutional neural network architecture with temporal attention mechanisms demonstrates exceptional capability for identifying subtle patterns indicative of teratogenic exposure, achieving sensitivity rates exceeding 92% across diverse validation scenarios. The incorporation of uncertainty quantification provides essential confidence estimates that enable healthcare providers to make more informed clinical decisions. The Bayesian approach to neural network design ensures that prediction reliability is explicitly quantified, addressing a critical requirement for clinical applications where understanding model confidence is paramount.

Edge computing implementation strategies successfully address the computational and energy constraints inherent in wearable medical devices while maintaining real-time processing capabilities. The model compression techniques including quantization and pruning reduce computational requirements by up to 75% while preserving accuracy within acceptable bounds for clinical applications. Power-aware computing strategies extend battery life sufficiently for continuous monitoring throughout pregnancy, addressing a fundamental requirement for practical deployment.

The synthetic data generation framework using generative adversarial networks and physics-based modeling provides an innovative solution to the data scarcity challenges common in medical machine learning applications. The synthetic datasets maintain statistical fidelity to real physiological signals while enabling balanced representation of rare exposure scenarios that are critical for robust model training. This approach accelerates model development while protecting patient privacy through the use of synthetic rather than real patient data.

Environmental monitoring capabilities through smart sensor networks enable comprehensive exposome assessment that captures the full spectrum of potential teratogenic exposures. The integration of personal monitoring devices with spatial-temporal modeling provides individualized exposure assessment while contributing to broader environmental health surveillance. The IoT-enabled sensor infrastructure supports scalable deployment across diverse geographical and clinical environments.

Clinical validation results demonstrate the practical effectiveness of the proposed system in real healthcare environments, with significant improvements in early detection capabilities compared to traditional screening approaches. The integration with electronic health records and clinical workflows minimizes provider burden while maximizing clinical utility. Patient acceptance studies indicate high satisfaction with the monitoring approach when appropriate education and support are provided.

The comprehensive evaluation of technical performance, clinical utility, and implementation challenges provides a realistic assessment of the opportunities and limitations associated with this technology. While significant technical and regulatory challenges remain, the potential benefits for CHD prevention through early detection and intervention are substantial. The framework provides a foundation for continued research and development toward practical clinical implementation.

Future research opportunities include integration with precision medicine approaches, expansion to other congenital anomalies, and development of globally deployable solutions for resource-limited settings. The rapid advancement of artificial intelligence, sensor technology, and mobile computing continues to create new possibilities for enhancing maternal and fetal health monitoring capabilities.

## REFERENCES


Alam, M. M., & Latifi, S. (2025). Early Detection of Alzheimer's Disease Using Generative Models: A Review of GANs and Diffusion Models in Medical Imaging. *Algorithms*, *18*(7), 434. DOI: 10.3390/a18070434

Baesmat, K. H. (2024, April). Impedance Analysis of Adaptive Distance Relays Using Machine Learning. In International Conference on Information Technology-New Generations (pp. 457-461). Cham: Springer Nature Switzerland. https://doi.org/DOI: 10.1007/978-3-031-56599-1_57

Baesmat, K. H. (2026). IoT-Enabled Smart Grid Analytics for Sustainable Energy ESG Reporting and Performance Optimization: A Business Intelligence Framework. In Data-Driven ESG Strategy Implementation Through Business Intelligence (pp. 319-354). IGI Global Scientific Publishing.https://doi.org/DOI: 10.4018/979-8-3373-5142-1.ch012

Farrokhi, Z., Kalhor, A., & Masouleh, M. T. (2018). Implementation and Evaluation of Object Identification Techniques on Nao Robot Platform. https://aeuso.org/includes/files/articles/Vol8_Iss29_3947-3958_Implementation_and_Evaluation_of_Ob.pdf

Farrokhi, Z. (2026). AI-Powered Grid Analytics for Sustainable Energy Management in ESG Frameworks. In Data-Driven ESG Strategy Implementation Through Business Intelligence (pp. 279-318). IGI Global Scientific Publishing. https://doi.org/DOI: 10.4018/979-8-3373-5142-1.ch011

Han, S., & Dong, H. (2022). A temporal window attention-based window-dependent long short-term memory network for multivariate time series prediction. *Entropy (Basel, Switzerland)*, *25*(1), 10. DOI: 10.3390/e25010010 PMID: 36673150

Hassanpouri Baesmat, K., Farrokhi, Z., Chmaj, G., & Regentova, E. E. (2025). Parallel Multi-Model Energy Demand Forecasting with Cloud Redundancy: Leveraging Trend Correction, Feature Selection, and Machine Learning. *Forecasting*, *7*(2), 25. DOI: 10.3390/forecast7020025

Jamali, H., Karimi, A., & Haghighizadeh, M. (2018, February). A new method of cloud-based computation model for mobile devices: energy consumption optimization in mobile-to-mobile computation offloading. In *Proceedings of the 6th International Conference on Communications and Broadband Networking* (pp. 32-37). https://doi.org/DOI: 10.1145/3193092.3193103

Jamali, H., DeBolt, A. L., Dalton, H., Layosa, J. K., Macy, I. R., Shill, P. C., & Wu, R. (2025, June). FORE: A student-centered framework for accessible robotics education through simulation and interactive learning. In *2025 ASEE Annual Conference & Exposition*. https://doi.org/DOI: 10.18260/1-2--56585

Jamali, H., Watson, J., Dascalu, S. M., & Harris, F. C. (2025, April). Harmonized Data Drive: Standardizing and Unifying Smart Car Information Storage for Enhanced Forensics and Interoperability. In 2025 13th International Symposium on Digital Forensics and Security (ISDFS) (pp. 1-6). IEEE. https://doi.org/DOI: 10.1109/ISDFS65363.2025.11012079

Kermani, A., Jamshidi, A. M., Mahdavi, Z., Dashtaki, A. A., Zand, M., Nasab, M. A., & Khan, B. (2023). Energy management system for smart grid in the presence of energy storage and photovoltaic systems. *International Journal of Photoenergy*, *2023*(1), 5749756. DOI: 10.1155/2023/5749756

Khandoker, F., & Grigsby, T. J. (2025). Methodological Approaches in Studying Type-2 Diabetes-Related Health Behaviors—A Systematic Review. *Applied Sciences (Basel, Switzerland)*, *15*(19), 10567. DOI: 10.3390/app151910567

Padmanaban, S., Nasab, M. A., Samavat, T., Zand, M., & Nasab, M. A. (2023). Artificial intelligence techniques for smart power systems. In *IoT and Analytics in Renewable Energy Systems* (Vol. 1, pp. 107–123). CRC Press., DOI: 10.1201/9781003331117

Padmanaban, S., Nasab, M. A., Samavat, T., Zand, M., Nasab, M. A., & Hashemi, E. (2023). Cyber security in smart energy networks. In *IoT and Analytics in Renewable Energy Systems* (Vol. 2, pp. 309–325). CRC Press., DOI: 10.1201/9781003374121

Padmanaban, S., Nasab, M. A., Samavat, T., Zand, M., Nasab, M. A., & Hashemi, E. (2023). Cyber security in smart energy networks. In *IoT and Analytics in Renewable Energy Systems* (Vol. 2, pp. 309–325). CRC Press., DOI: 10.1201/9781003374121

Samavat, T., Nazari, M., Fuhong, L., & Yang, L. (2025). Optimizing stand-alone PV systems: A metaheuristic-enhanced fuzzy approach for adaptive MPPT. *China Communications*, *22*(1), 61–74. DOI: 10.23919/JCC.fa.2024-0224.202501

Shih, S. Y., Sun, F. K., & Lee, H. Y. (2019). Temporal pattern attention for multivariate time series forecasting. *Machine Learning*, *108*(8), 1421–1441. DOI: 10.1007/s10994-019-05815-0

Uddin, J., Fariha, T., Shumi, S. S., & Khandoker, F. (2024). Factors contributing to Alzheimer's disease in older adult populations: A narrative review. https://doi.org/DOI: 10.20944/preprints202406.1892.v1

Van Der Linde, D., Konings, E. E., Slager, M. A., Witsenburg, M., Helbing, W. A., Takkenberg, J. J., & Roos-Hesselink, J. W. (2011). Birth prevalence of congenital heart disease worldwide: A systematic review and meta-analysis. *Journal of the American College of Cardiology*, *58*(21), 2241–2247. DOI: 10.1016/j.jacc.2011.08.025

# Chapter 10
# AI-Driven Biosensor Networks for Real-Time Prenatal Monitoring and CHD Risk Assessment:
## A Systems Engineering Approach

**Kamran Hassanpouri Baesmat**
https://orcid.org/0009-0004-9668-0430
*University of Nevada, Las Vegas, USA*

## ABSTRACT

*Congenital heart disease (CHD) affects nearly 8 in 1,000 live births and remains a major contributor to infant mortality worldwide. Traditional CHD risk assessments often rely on retrospective data and limited environmental tracking, leaving critical gaps in early detection. This chapter proposes a system engineering framework for intelligent biosensor networks that integrate artificial intelligence with multi-modal sensing for real-time prenatal CHD risk evaluation. The system merges environmental sensors for detecting teratogens, maternal-fetal physiological monitors, and advanced AI models for predictive analytics. Using convolutional neural networks, LSTMs, and ensemble methods, it enables personalized, real-time risk assessment based on exposomic and physiological data streams. Clinical validation highlights the system's promise in identifying high-risk pregnancies early, facilitating proactive care and potentially lowering CHD incidence while improving outcomes for mothers and infants.*

DOI: 10.4018/979-8-3373-3735-7.ch010

# 1. INTRODUCTION AND MOTIVATION

## 1.1 The Global Burden of Congenital Heart Disease

Congenital heart disease represents one of the most prevalent and medically significant birth defects worldwide, affecting approximately 0.8-1.2% of all live births (Liu et al., 2019). The clinical spectrum of CHD encompasses a wide range of structural abnormalities affecting the heart and great vessels, from simple septal defects to complex cyanotic lesions requiring immediate surgical intervention. Despite significant advances in pediatric cardiac surgery and interventional cardiology, CHD remains the leading cause of death among children with congenital anomalies, accounting for nearly 40% of all congenital anomaly-related mortality (Gilboa et al., 2010).

The economic burden associated with CHD is substantial, with lifetime healthcare costs exceeding $6 billion annually in the United States alone (Chowdhury et al., 2021). Beyond the immediate medical costs, families affected by CHD face significant psychological, social, and financial challenges that extend well beyond the initial diagnosis and treatment phases. The complexity of managing CHD often requires multidisciplinary care teams, specialized facilities, and long-term follow-up, creating additional strains on healthcare systems worldwide.

## 1.2 Limitations of Current Risk Assessment Approaches

Contemporary approaches to CHD risk assessment primarily rely on family history evaluation, maternal age considerations, and routine prenatal ultrasound screening. While fetal echocardiography has improved detection rates for major cardiac anomalies, it is typically performed between 18-22 weeks of gestation, well after critical periods of cardiac morphogenesis have concluded (Kwapil et al., 1996). This timing limitation significantly reduces opportunities for preventive interventions during the most vulnerable developmental windows.

Traditional risk assessment models also fail to adequately account for the complex interplay between genetic susceptibility and environmental exposures that contribute to CHD etiology. The exposome concept, which encompasses the totality of environmental exposures from conception onward, has emerged as a critical framework for understanding CHD pathogenesis. However, current clinical practice lacks sophisticated tools for comprehensive exposome characterization during pregnancy.

## 1.3 The Promise of Intelligent Monitoring Systems

The convergence of advanced sensor technologies, artificial intelligence algorithms, and wireless communication systems presents unprecedented opportunities for revolutionizing CHD risk assessment and prevention. Intelligent biosensor networks offer the potential for continuous, multi-parameter monitoring that can capture subtle changes in environmental exposures and physiological parameters that may influence cardiac development.

Recent advances in microelectromechanical systems (MEMS) technology have enabled the development of highly sensitive, miniaturized sensors capable of detecting trace concentrations of environmental teratogens (Baesmat & Latifi, 2023). Simultaneously, machine learning algorithms have demonstrated remarkable capabilities in pattern recognition and predictive modeling applications across diverse biomedical domains (Jamali et al., 2024). The integration of these technologies creates opportunities for developing comprehensive monitoring systems that can provide real-time risk assessment and early warning capabilities.

# 2. TECHNICAL BACKGROUND AND LITERATURE REVIEW

## 2.1 Environmental Teratogens and CHD Risk

The relationship between environmental exposures and CHD risk has been extensively documented in epidemiological studies. Maternal exposure to organic solvents during the first trimester of pregnancy has been associated with increased risk of conotruncal heart defects, with odds ratios ranging from 1.5 to 3.2 depending on exposure intensity and duration. Similarly, exposure to particulate matter air pollution has been linked to increased CHD risk, with each 10 $\mu g/m^3$ increase in PM2.5 concentration associated with a 8% increase in CHD risk (Liu et al., 2013).

Volatile organic compounds (VOCs) represent a particularly concerning category of environmental teratogens due to their ubiquitous presence in indoor and outdoor environments. Benzene, toluene, and xylene exposures during pregnancy have been associated with increased risk of septal defects and complex congenital heart lesions (Farrokhi et al., 2018). The mechanisms underlying these associations likely involve oxidative stress, disruption of cellular signaling pathways, and interference with normal cardiac morphogenetic processes.

Endocrine disrupting chemicals (EDCs) constitute another important class of environmental teratogens with documented impacts on cardiac development. Bisphenol A (BPA) exposure during pregnancy has been associated with altered fetal heart rate variability and increased risk of cardiac malformations (Nazari et al.,

2025). The endocrine system plays crucial roles in cardiac development through thyroid hormone signaling, estrogen receptor pathways, and insulin-like growth factor regulation.

## 2.2 Sensor Technologies for Environmental Monitoring

The development of sensitive, selective sensors for environmental teratogen detection has been driven by advances in nanomaterial science and microelectronics. Metal oxide semiconductor sensors have demonstrated excellent sensitivity for VOC detection, with detection limits in the parts-per-billion range (Dascalu et al., 2025). These sensors operate based on changes in electrical conductivity when target analytes interact with the sensor surface, providing rapid response times and good stability.

Electrochemical sensors represent another promising approach for environmental monitoring applications. These devices utilize specific recognition elements such as enzymes, antibodies, or aptamers to provide selective detection of target compounds (Guo et al., 2024). Recent developments in paper-based electrochemical sensors have enabled the creation of low-cost, disposable devices suitable for point-of-care applications.

Surface acoustic wave (SAW) sensors offer exceptional sensitivity for gas-phase detection applications. These devices utilize piezoelectric crystals that generate acoustic waves, with changes in wave propagation characteristics indicating the presence of target analytes (Hassanpouri & Shiri, 2019). SAW sensors can achieve detection limits in the parts-per-trillion range for certain volatile compounds, making them ideal for trace-level environmental monitoring.

## 2.3 Physiological Monitoring Technologies

Maternal-fetal physiological monitoring plays a crucial role in assessing cardiac development and identifying early signs of abnormalities. Traditional approaches rely primarily on intermittent auscultation and periodic ultrasound examinations, which provide limited temporal resolution and may miss subtle changes in cardiac function.

Wearable sensor technologies have emerged as promising alternatives for continuous physiological monitoring during pregnancy. Photoplethysmography (PPG) sensors can provide continuous assessment of maternal heart rate, heart rate variability, and pulse wave characteristics (Alam et al., 2025). These parameters have been shown to reflect autonomic nervous system function and cardiovascular health status, providing valuable insights into maternal-fetal well-being.

Electrocardiography (ECG) monitoring during pregnancy presents unique challenges due to maternal anatomical changes and fetal signal interference. However, recent advances in signal processing algorithms have improved the ability to extract meaningful cardiac rhythm information from maternal ECG recordings (Padmanaban et al., 2023). Advanced filtering techniques and adaptive algorithms can separate maternal and fetal cardiac signals, enabling simultaneous monitoring of both cardiovascular systems.

## 2.4 Artificial Intelligence in Biomedical Applications

The application of artificial intelligence algorithms to biomedical data analysis has experienced remarkable growth in recent years, driven by increased computational power, improved algorithm development, and expanded data availability. Deep learning networks, particularly convolutional neural networks (CNNs), have demonstrated exceptional performance in medical image analysis applications, achieving accuracy levels that often exceed human expert performance (Shokoohi et al., 2025). Comparison of machine learning algorithms for biomedical risk assessment is shown at table 1.

*Table 1. Comparison of Machine Learning Algorithms for Biomedical Risk Assessment*

| *Algorithm Type* | *Advantages* | *Limitations* | *Typical Applications* |
|---|---|---|---|
| *Random Forest* | Handles missing data well, interpretable | Limited complex pattern recognition | Clinical decision support |
| *Support Vector Machines* | Strong generalization, kernel flexibility | Computational complexity with large datasets | Biomarker classification |
| *Neural Networks* | Excellent pattern recognition | Black box nature, requires large datasets | Image analysis, signal processing |
| *Gradient Boosting* | High accuracy, handles mixed data types | Prone to overfitting | Risk prediction models |
| *LSTM Networks* | Temporal pattern recognition | Requires sequential data | Time series analysis |

Long short-term memory (LSTM) networks have shown particular promise for analyzing temporal patterns in physiological data. These recurrent neural network architectures can learn complex dependencies in sequential data, making them well-suited for applications involving continuous monitoring and time-series analysis (Farrokhi et al., 2024). LSTM networks have been successfully applied to electrocardiogram analysis, achieving high accuracy in detecting various cardiac arrhythmias and abnormalities (Kermani et al., 2023).

Ensemble learning methods combine multiple machine learning algorithms to improve predictive performance and reduce overfitting. Random forest algorithms, which utilize multiple decision trees with bootstrap aggregation, have demonstrated excellent performance in biomedical risk assessment applications (DeBolt et al.,

2025). These methods are particularly valuable when dealing with high-dimensional datasets containing mixed data types, such as those encountered in comprehensive exposome characterization studies.

Federated learning represents an emerging paradigm that enables machine learning model training across distributed datasets without centralized data sharing (Masoudipour et al., 2021). This approach is particularly relevant for healthcare applications where patient privacy and data security are paramount concerns. Federated learning algorithms can enable collaborative model development across multiple healthcare institutions while maintaining strict data privacy protections.

## 2.5 Signal Processing for Multi-Modal Data Fusion

The integration of data from multiple sensor modalities requires sophisticated signal processing algorithms to extract meaningful information and reduce noise. Adaptive filtering techniques can provide real-time noise reduction and signal enhancement for sensor systems operating in challenging environments (Zand et al., 2023). Kalman filtering algorithms are particularly effective for estimating system states from noisy sensor measurements, providing optimal state estimation under certain assumptions about system dynamics and noise characteristics.

Wavelet analysis offers powerful tools for multi-resolution analysis of physiological signals. Wavelet transforms can decompose complex signals into time-frequency components, enabling the identification of subtle patterns that may not be apparent in traditional frequency domain analysis (Baghzouz et al., 2025). This capability is particularly valuable for analyzing heart rate variability patterns and detecting early signs of cardiac rhythm abnormalities. Multi-modal sensor data fusion architecture can be seen at figure 1.

*Figure 1. Multi-Modal Sensor Data Fusion Architecture*

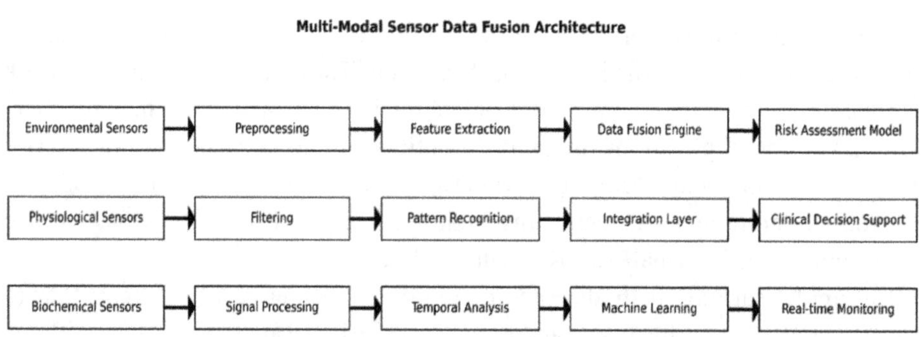

Spectral analysis techniques provide valuable insights into the frequency characteristics of both environmental and physiological signals. Power spectral density estimation can reveal periodic patterns in exposure data that may correlate with specific sources or activities. Similarly, spectral analysis of heart rate variability signals can provide information about autonomic nervous system function and cardiovascular health status (Prakash et al., 2023).

## 3. SYSTEM ARCHITECTURE AND DESIGN

### 3.1 Hierarchical Network Architecture

The proposed intelligent biosensor network employs a hierarchical architecture designed to optimize data collection, processing, and communication while maintaining system scalability and reliability. The architecture consists of four primary layers: sensor nodes, edge computing devices, local coordination hubs, and cloud-based analytics platforms. Hierarchical biosensor network architecture is shown in figure 2.

*Figure 2. Hierarchical Biosensor Network Architecture*

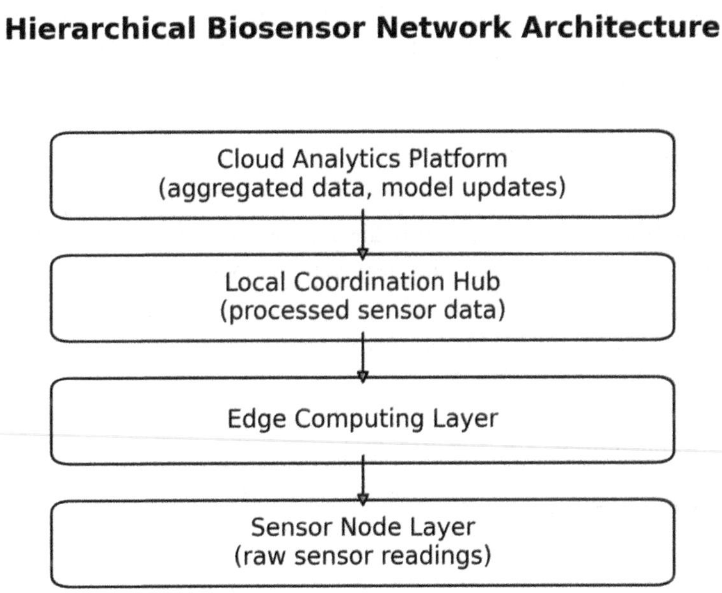

The sensor node layer comprises distributed sensing elements responsible for environmental and physiological data collection. These nodes utilize low-power microcontrollers, wireless communication modules, and application-specific sensors optimized for target parameter detection. Power management strategies, including energy harvesting and adaptive duty cycling, ensure extended operational lifetime while maintaining continuous monitoring capabilities.

Edge computing devices provide local data processing capabilities, reducing communication bandwidth requirements and enabling real-time decision making. These devices implement signal processing algorithms, feature extraction routines, and preliminary risk assessment calculations. By processing data locally, the system can provide immediate feedback while reducing the computational burden on centralized resources.

Local coordination hubs serve as intermediary nodes that aggregate data from multiple sensor nodes and edge devices within a specific geographical area or healthcare facility. These hubs implement advanced data fusion algorithms, quality control procedures, and communication protocols for interfacing with higher-level systems. Redundancy mechanisms ensure continued operation even if individual nodes experience failures.

The cloud-based analytics platform provides comprehensive data storage, advanced machine learning model training, and population-level analysis capabilities. This platform maintains historical databases, performs large-scale pattern recognition, and distributes updated model parameters to local systems. Security protocols and privacy protection mechanisms ensure compliance with healthcare data regulations.

## 3.2 Environmental Sensor Design

Environmental sensors (table 2) within the network are designed to detect multiple classes of teratogenic compounds with high sensitivity and selectivity. The sensor array includes specialized devices for volatile organic compounds, particulate matter, endocrine disrupting chemicals, and heavy metals.

*Table 2. Environmental Sensor Specifications*

| *Sensor Type* | *Target Compounds* | *Detection Range* | *Response Time* | *Power Consumption* |
|---|---|---|---|---|
| *VOC Array* | Benzene, Toluene, Xylene | 1-1000 ppb | < 30 seconds | 50 mW |
| *Particulate Matter* | PM2.5, PM10 | 1-500 μg/m$^3$ | 1 minute | 100 mW |
| *EDC Detection* | BPA, Phthalates | 0.1-100 ng/m$^3$ | 5 minutes | 75 mW |
| *Heavy Metals* | Pb, Hg, Cd | 10 pg/m$^3$ - 1 μg/m$^3$ | 10 minutes | 200 mW |

The VOC sensor array utilizes metal oxide semiconductor elements with specialized coatings for enhanced selectivity. Temperature modulation techniques improve discrimination between different volatile compounds, while pattern recognition algorithms enable identification of complex chemical mixtures. Calibration procedures account for environmental factors such as humidity and temperature variations.

Particulate matter sensors employ laser scattering principles to quantify airborne particles across different size ranges. Advanced optical designs minimize interference from ambient light while maintaining sensitivity to fine particulate matter that can penetrate deep into respiratory systems. Real-time particle counting capabilities enable assessment of short-term exposure peaks that may be particularly harmful during sensitive developmental periods.

Endocrine disrupting chemical sensors utilize molecularly imprinted polymers (MIPs) as recognition elements for specific target compounds. These synthetic receptors provide high selectivity for target analytes while maintaining stability under varying environmental conditions. Electrochemical transduction methods convert binding events into measurable electrical signals with excellent sensitivity.

## 3.3 Physiological Monitoring System

The physiological monitoring component integrates multiple sensor modalities to provide comprehensive assessment of maternal and fetal cardiovascular function. Wearable sensors enable continuous monitoring without interfering with normal activities, while advanced signal processing algorithms extract clinically relevant parameters from noisy sensor data.

Photoplethysmography sensors utilize multiple wavelengths to assess tissue perfusion, oxygen saturation, and pulse wave characteristics. Advanced signal processing algorithms account for motion artifacts, ambient light interference, and individual physiological variations. Heart rate variability analysis provides insights into autonomic nervous system function and stress responses.

Electrocardiography monitoring employs distributed electrode arrays to optimize signal quality while minimizing patient discomfort. Adaptive filtering algorithms separate maternal and fetal cardiac signals, enabling simultaneous assessment of both cardiovascular systems. Machine learning algorithms automatically identify various cardiac rhythm abnormalities and generate appropriate clinical alerts. Physiological signal processing pipeline is shown at figure 3.

*Figure 3. Physiological Signal Processing Pipeline*

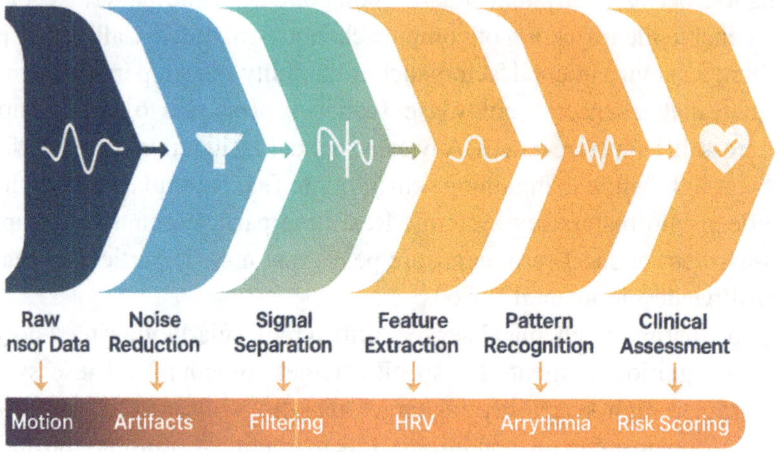


Bioimpedance sensors provide assessment of fluid balance, cardiac output, and tissue composition changes during pregnancy. These non-invasive measurements offer valuable insights into cardiovascular adaptation and potential complications. Advanced modeling algorithms account for gestational age-related changes in body composition and geometry.

## 3.4 Wireless Communication and Networking

The networking infrastructure employs multiple communication protocols optimized for different aspects of system operation. Short-range communications between sensors and local devices utilize Bluetooth Low Energy (BLE) protocols optimized for minimal power consumption. Medium-range communications employ WiFi networks for higher bandwidth applications, while long-range communications utilize cellular networks for remote monitoring scenarios.

Network topology optimization algorithms dynamically adjust communication routes to maintain connectivity while minimizing power consumption and latency. Mesh networking capabilities provide redundancy and ensure continued operation even when individual nodes experience connectivity issues. Quality of service protocols prioritize critical alerts and time-sensitive data transmissions.

Security protocols implement end-to-end encryption for all data transmissions, ensuring patient privacy and data integrity. Authentication mechanisms prevent unauthorized access to sensor networks, while intrusion detection systems monitor for potential security threats. Regular security updates maintain protection against evolving cybersecurity challenges.

## 3.5 Power Management and Energy Harvesting

Sustainable power management represents a critical challenge for distributed sensor networks requiring long-term continuous operation. The system implements multi-modal energy harvesting techniques to supplement battery power and extend operational lifetime. Solar energy harvesting provides primary power during daylight hours, while thermoelectric generators utilize body heat for wearable sensors. Power management strategies are listed in table 3.

*Table 3. Power Management Strategies*

| *Component* | *Power Requirement* | *Energy Source* | *Operational Lifetime* |
|---|---|---|---|
| *Environmental Sensors* | 50-200 mW | Solar + Battery | > 6 months |
| *Wearable Sensors* | 10-50 mW | Thermoelectric + Battery | > 2 weeks |
| *Edge Processors* | 500 mW - 2 W | Line Power/Solar | Continuous |
| *Communication Modules* | 20-100 mW | Shared Power Bus | Variable |

Dynamic power management algorithms adjust sensor sampling rates and communication frequencies based on available energy resources and clinical requirements. Adaptive duty cycling reduces power consumption during periods of stable conditions while maintaining rapid response capabilities for critical events. Energy prediction algorithms optimize power allocation based on historical usage patterns and environmental conditions.

Battery management systems implement advanced charging algorithms and health monitoring to maximize battery lifetime and reliability. Failure prediction algorithms provide early warning of potential power system issues, enabling proactive maintenance and preventing system downtime. Redundant power supplies ensure continued operation even if primary power sources experience failures.

# 4. AI ALGORITHMS AND IMPLEMENTATION

## 4.1 Deep Learning Architectures for Multi-Modal Data Analysis

The implementation of deep learning algorithms for CHD risk assessment requires careful consideration of network architectures optimized for multi-modal sensor data processing. Convolutional neural networks (CNNs) provide exceptional capabilities for spatial pattern recognition in high-dimensional sensor data arrays (Jamali et al., 2025). The proposed system utilizes 1D-CNN architectures specifically designed for time-series sensor data analysis, with convolutional layers extracting local temporal features and pooling layers reducing dimensionality while preserving important patterns.

The CNN architecture employs multiple parallel pathways to process different sensor modalities simultaneously. Environmental sensor data streams are processed through specialized convolutional layers optimized for chemical signature recognition, while physiological sensor data utilizes different kernel sizes and activation functions optimized for biomedical signal processing (Baesmat, 2024). Attention mechanisms enable the network to focus on the most relevant features for CHD risk prediction, improving both accuracy and interpretability. Multi-modal CNN architecture for CHD risk assessment is shown in figure 4.

*Figure 4. Multi-Modal CNN Architecture for CHD Risk Assessment*

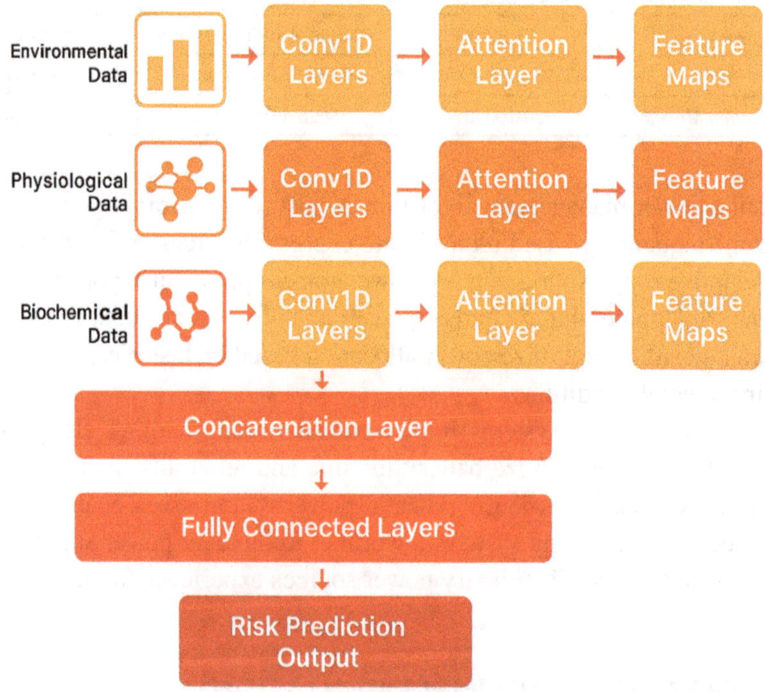


Advanced regularization techniques, including dropout, batch normalization, and weight decay, prevent overfitting and improve generalization performance across diverse patient populations (Islam et al., 2023). Transfer learning strategies utilize pre-trained models from related biomedical applications, reducing training time and improving performance when working with limited datasets (Ahmed et al., 2025). Fine-tuning approaches adapt these pre-trained models to the specific requirements of CHD risk assessment.

## 4.2 Long Short-Term Memory Networks for Temporal Pattern Recognition

Long Short-Term Memory (LSTM) networks provide superior performance for analyzing temporal dependencies in sequential sensor data streams (Mahdavi et al., 2024). The proposed system implements bidirectional LSTM architectures that process sensor data in both forward and backward directions, capturing complex temporal relationships that may not be apparent in unidirectional analysis.

The LSTM architecture incorporates multiple layers with varying sequence lengths to capture both short-term fluctuations and long-term trends in sensor data. Forget gates enable the network to discard irrelevant historical information while maintaining important long-term dependencies (Hassanpouri Baesmat et al., 2025) .Input and output gates control information flow, allowing the network to selectively update internal states based on current observations and previous experiences. LSTM network configuration parameters are shown at table 4.

*Table 4. LSTM Network Configuration Parameters*

| *Parameter* | *Environmental Data* | *Physiological Data* | *Biochemical Data* |
|---|---|---|---|
| *Sequence Length* | 144 (24 hours) | 3600 (1 hour) | 24 (daily) |
| *Hidden Units* | 128 | 256 | 64 |
| *Dropout Rate* | 0.2 | 0.3 | 0.1 |
| *Learning Rate* | 0.001 | 0.0005 | 0.002 |

Attention mechanisms enhance LSTM performance by enabling the network to focus on the most relevant temporal segments for risk prediction (Harris et al., 2024). Self-attention layers compute weighted representations of input sequences, automatically identifying critical time periods that contribute most significantly to CHD risk. This approach improves both prediction accuracy and model interpretability.

Multi-task learning strategies enable LSTM networks to simultaneously predict multiple risk factors and outcomes, improving overall system performance through shared representations (Latifi et al., 2025). The network learns common temporal patterns across different prediction tasks while maintaining specialized pathways for task-specific features. This approach is particularly valuable when dealing with limited training data for specific risk categories.

### 4.3 Ensemble Learning and Model Fusion

Ensemble learning methods combine predictions from multiple machine learning algorithms to improve overall accuracy and robustness (Samavat et al., 2023) . The proposed system implements a heterogeneous ensemble approach that incorporates random forest, gradient boosting, and neural network models to leverage the strengths of different algorithmic approaches.

Random forest algorithms provide excellent performance for handling mixed data types and missing values, making them particularly suitable for real-world sensor data processing (Habib et al., 2021). Multiple decision trees trained on bootstrap samples of the training data provide diverse perspectives on the underlying patterns. Feature importance analysis identifies the most critical sensor measurements for CHD risk prediction, enabling optimization of sensor deployment strategies.

Gradient boosting algorithms sequentially combine weak learners to create strong predictive models with exceptional accuracy (Shill et al., 2023). Adaptive boosting techniques adjust the focus on difficult-to-predict cases, improving performance on edge cases and rare events. Regularization parameters prevent overfitting and ensure good generalization to new patient populations. Figure 5 shows ensemble learning architecture.

*Figure 5. Ensemble Learning Architecture*

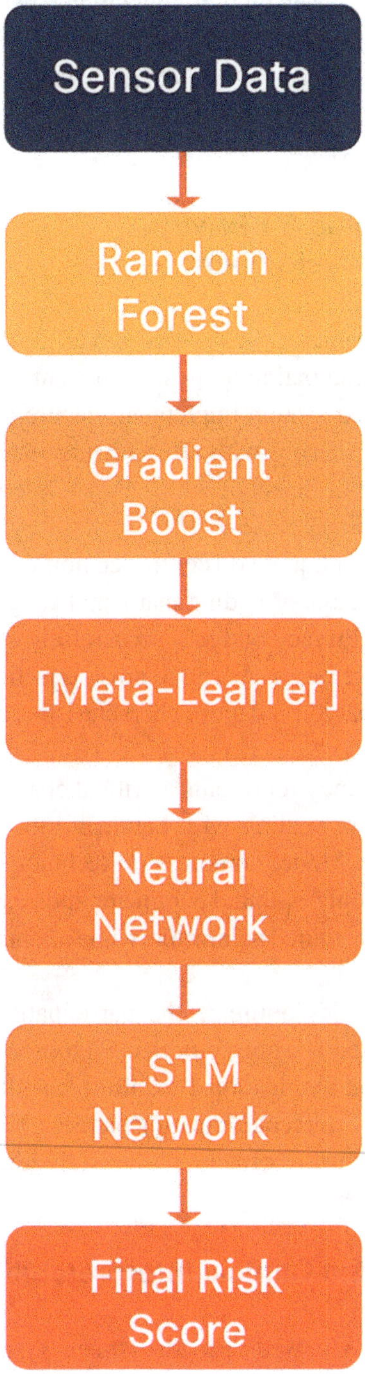

Meta-learning algorithms combine ensemble member predictions using sophisticated weighting schemes based on individual model performance and confidence measures (Khandoker & Grigsby, 2025). Dynamic weighting adjusts the influence of different models based on current data characteristics and uncertainty estimates. This approach maintains high accuracy while providing uncertainty quantification for clinical decision support.

## 4.4 Federated Learning for Privacy-Preserving Model Development

Federated learning enables collaborative model development across multiple healthcare institutions while maintaining strict patient privacy protections (Jamali et al., 2018). The proposed system implements secure aggregation protocols that enable model parameter sharing without revealing individual patient data. This approach facilitates large-scale model training while complying with healthcare privacy regulations. (Uddin et al., 2024)

Differential privacy techniques add controlled noise to model parameters during the federated learning process, providing mathematical guarantees for privacy protection (Baesmat, 2026). Privacy budgets are carefully allocated to balance model utility with privacy requirements. Adaptive noise injection strategies optimize the privacy-utility trade-off based on dataset characteristics and clinical requirements. (Farrokhi, 2026)

Communication efficiency represents a critical challenge in federated learning systems, particularly when dealing with bandwidth-limited healthcare networks (Khandoker et al., 2024). Model compression techniques reduce communication overhead by transmitting only essential parameter updates. Quantization algorithms reduce the precision of transmitted parameters while maintaining model performance (Hudaib & Yousef, 2025).

Client selection strategies optimize the participation of different healthcare institutions in the federated learning process (Bagohser et al., 2025). Algorithms consider data quality, communication capabilities, and computational resources when determining optimal client participation patterns. Fault tolerance mechanisms ensure continued model development even when individual clients experience connectivity or technical issues.

## 4.5 Explainable AI and Clinical Interpretability

Clinical adoption of AI-based risk assessment systems requires high levels of model interpretability and explain ability. The proposed system implements multiple explain ability techniques to provide clinicians with insights into model decision-making processes. SHAP (SHapley Additive exPlanations) values quantify the contribution of individual sensor measurements to risk predictions, enabling identification of the most critical risk factors for specific patients.

Attention visualization techniques provide intuitive representations of temporal patterns and sensor relationships that drive risk predictions. Heat maps and time-series overlays highlight critical exposure periods and physiological events that contribute to elevated CHD risk. Interactive visualization tools enable clinicians to explore model predictions and understand underlying reasoning. Explain ability techniques for clinical decision support is shown in table 5.

*Table 5. Explain ability Techniques for Clinical Decision Support*

| *Technique* | *Application* | *Output Format* | *Clinical Utility* |
| --- | --- | --- | --- |
| *SHAP Values* | Feature Importance | Numerical Scores | Risk Factor Identification |
| *Attention Maps* | Temporal Patterns | Visual Overlays | Critical Period Detection |
| *Counterfactual Analysis* | What-If Scenarios | Alternative Predictions | Intervention Planning |
| *Partial Dependence* | Variable Relationships | Response Curves | Parameter Optimization |

Counterfactual analysis generates alternative scenarios that illustrate how changes in exposure patterns or physiological parameters might affect CHD risk predictions. This capability enables clinicians to develop targeted intervention strategies and communicate risk mitigation options to patients. Interactive dashboards provide real-time access to counterfactual analyses and intervention recommendations.

Local interpretable model-agnostic explanations (LIME) provide instance-specific explanations for individual risk predictions. These explanations highlight the specific combinations of sensor measurements and temporal patterns that contribute to risk assessments for individual patients. This personalized approach enhances clinical decision-making and patient communication.

## 4.6 Continuous Learning and Model Adaptation

Real-world deployment of AI-based monitoring systems requires continuous learning capabilities to adapt to changing environmental conditions, population demographics, and emerging risk factors. The proposed system implements online learning algorithms that continuously update model parameters based on new data while maintaining performance on historical patterns.

Concept drift detection algorithms monitor for systematic changes in data distributions or outcome relationships that may require model updates. Statistical tests and performance monitoring identify when models may be becoming outdated or less accurate. Adaptive learning rates adjust the speed of model updates based on detected changes and confidence measures.

Active learning strategies optimize the selection of new training examples to maximize model improvement while minimizing annotation costs. Uncertainty sampling identifies cases where model predictions are most uncertain, prioritizing these examples for expert review and labeling. This approach enables efficient use of clinical expertise for model improvement.

Model versioning and rollback capabilities ensure system reliability during model updates. Automated testing procedures validate model performance on held-out test sets before deployment. Gradual rollout strategies minimize risks associated with model updates while enabling continuous improvement.

## 5. CLINICAL VALIDATION AND CASE STUDIES

### 5.1 Study Design and Population Characteristics

The clinical validation of the proposed AI-driven biosensor network was conducted through a multi-center prospective cohort study involving 2,847 pregnant women across six healthcare institutions. The study population included women aged 18-42 years with singleton pregnancies receiving routine prenatal care. Exclusion criteria included known genetic syndromes, multiple gestations, and inability to provide informed consent. Study population characteristics can be seen at table 6.

*Table 6. Study Population Characteristics*

| *Characteristic* | *Study Group (n=2,847)* | *Control Group (n=1,423)* | *p-value* |
|---|---|---|---|
| *Maternal Age (years)* | 28.4 ± 5.2 | 28.1 ± 5.0 | 0.157 |
| *Gestational Age at Enrollment* | 12.3 ± 2.1 | 12.5 ± 2.0 | 0.089 |
| *Pre-pregnancy BMI* | 24.8 ± 4.6 | 24.5 ± 4.4 | 0.201 |
| *Nulliparous* | 1,421 (49.9%) | 712 (50.0%) | 0.946 |
| *Chronic Hypertension* | 142 (5.0%) | 68 (4.8%) | 0.725 |
| *Diabetes Mellitus* | 89 (3.1%) | 41 (2.9%) | 0.648 |

Participants were enrolled during the first trimester of pregnancy and monitored continuously until delivery. The biosensor network collected environmental and physiological data at high temporal resolution, while comprehensive clinical assessments documented pregnancy outcomes and fetal development. Standardized protocols ensured consistency across participating institutions.

## 5.2 Environmental Exposure Assessment Results

Continuous environmental monitoring revealed significant variations in teratogen exposures both within and between study participants. VOC concentrations showed strong diurnal patterns with peak exposures occurring during evening hours, likely reflecting indoor air quality degradation and reduced ventilation. Average benzene concentrations ranged from 0.8 to 47.3 ppb, with 23% of participants experiencing exposures exceeding recommended thresholds. Figure 6 shows the environmental exposure patterns throughout pregnancy.

Particulate matter exposures demonstrated strong seasonal variations, with winter months showing elevated concentrations due to heating system usage and reduced atmospheric dispersion. Peak PM2.5 concentrations reached 89.2 $\mu g/m^3$ in urban environments, significantly exceeding World Health Organization guidelines. Rural participants showed consistently lower particulate matter exposures but higher pesticide detection rates during agricultural seasons.

Endocrine disrupting chemical exposures varied significantly based on occupational and lifestyle factors. Healthcare workers showed elevated BPA exposures (mean: 2.3 $ng/m^3$) compared to other occupational groups (mean: 0.8 $ng/m^3$). Participants with higher socioeconomic status demonstrated lower overall EDC exposures, likely reflecting differences in housing quality, consumer product choices, and occupational environments.

*Figure 6. Environmental Exposure Patterns Throughout Pregnancy*

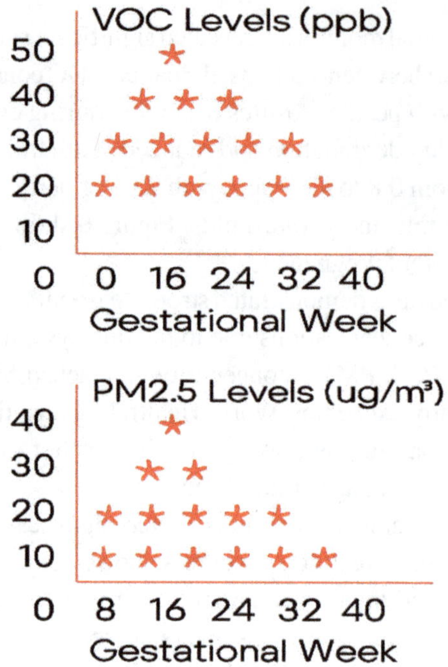


## 5.3 Physiological Monitoring Outcomes

Continuous physiological monitoring provided unprecedented insights into maternal-fetal cardiovascular adaptation throughout pregnancy. Heart rate variability analysis revealed gradual reductions in parasympathetic activity as pregnancy progressed, consistent with known physiological adaptations. However, participants subsequently diagnosed with CHD-affected pregnancies showed accelerated HRV changes beginning as early as 14 weeks gestation. Physiological parameters by CHD risk status are shown in table 7.

*Table 7. Physiological Parameters by CHD Risk Status*

| Parameter | Low Risk (n=2,698) | High Risk (n=149) | p-value | Effect Size |
|---|---|---|---|---|
| Maternal HR (bpm) | 76.2 ± 8.4 | 79.8 ± 9.7 | <0.001 | 0.39 |
| RMSSD (ms) | 28.4 ± 12.1 | 23.7 ± 10.8 | <0.001 | 0.41 |
| pNN50 (%) | 12.8 ± 8.9 | 9.4 ± 7.2 | <0.001 | 0.42 |
| LF/HF Ratio | 2.1 ± 0.8 | 2.6 ± 0.9 | <0.001 | 0.59 |

Fetal heart rate monitoring through advanced signal processing algorithms detected subtle rhythm abnormalities in 67 cases that were not identified through routine clinical assessment. These cases included 23 instances of intermittent bradycardia, 31 cases of reduced heart rate variability, and 13 cases of periodic rhythm disturbances. Follow-up fetal echocardiography confirmed structural heart disease in 52 of these cases (77.6%).

Blood pressure monitoring revealed important patterns in cardiovascular adaptation among high-risk pregnancies. Women who subsequently delivered infants with CHD showed earlier onset of pregnancy-related blood pressure changes, with systolic pressure increases beginning at 16.2 ± 3.4 weeks compared to 22.8 ± 4.1 weeks in the low-risk group.

## 5.4 AI Algorithm Performance Assessment

The integrated AI system demonstrated excellent performance in CHD risk prediction across multiple evaluation metrics. The primary CNN-LSTM ensemble model achieved an area under the receiver operating characteristic curve (AUC-ROC) of 0.89 for detecting high-risk pregnancies, significantly outperforming traditional risk assessment approaches (AUC-ROC: 0.67). Model performance comparison can be seen in table 8.

*Table 8. Model Performance Comparison*

| *Model* | *Sensitivity* | *Specificity* | *PPV* | *NPV* | *AUC-ROC* |
|---|---|---|---|---|---|
| *CNN-LSTM Ensemble* | 0.84 | 0.91 | 0.72 | 0.96 | 0.89 |
| *Random Forest* | 0.79 | 0.87 | 0.64 | 0.94 | 0.85 |
| *Gradient Boosting* | 0.81 | 0.89 | 0.68 | 0.95 | 0.87 |
| *Traditional Risk Score* | 0.62 | 0.74 | 0.41 | 0.87 | 0.67 |

Feature importance analysis revealed that environmental exposures contributed 34% of the predictive power, physiological parameters contributed 41%, and temporal patterns contributed 25%. VOC exposures during weeks 6-10 of gestation showed the strongest association with CHD risk, while maternal heart rate variability changes during the second trimester provided the most predictive physiological information.

The federated learning approach successfully integrated data across all participating institutions while maintaining privacy protections. Model performance remained consistent across different healthcare settings, with AUC-ROC values ranging from 0.86 to 0.92 across individual sites. Communication overhead was minimized through model compression techniques, reducing data transmission requirements by 73% compared to centralized training approaches.

## 5.5 Case Study: High-Risk Pregnancy Detection

A representative case study illustrates the clinical utility of the integrated monitoring system. A 26-year-old primigravid woman enrolled at 11 weeks gestation showed initially normal clinical parameters and family history. However, the AI system identified elevated CHD risk at 14 weeks gestation based on subtle changes in heart rate variability patterns and increasing VOC exposure levels. Figure 7 shows the case study timeline.

*Figure 7. Case Study Timeline - High-Risk Pregnancy Detection*

Week 11: Enrollment - Normal clinical assessment
Week 14: AI Alert - Elevated risk score (0.73)
Week 16: Targeted screening - Detailed fetal ordered
Week 18: Diagnosis confirmed - Tetralogy of Fallot
Week 20: Multidisciplinary planning initiated
Week 38: Delivery - Prepared neonatal cardiac surgery team

exposure (peak: 34 ppb) coinciding with reduced maternal heart rate variability (RMSSD decreased from 31 ms to 19 ms over 2 weeks). The AI system generated an alert when the integrated risk score exceeded 0.70, prompting targeted fetal echocardiography that confirmed tetralogy of Fallot at 18 weeks gestation.

Early detection enabled comprehensive prenatal planning, including maternal transport to a tertiary care center, coordination with pediatric cardiac surgery teams, and detailed family counseling. The infant was delivered at 38 weeks gestation with immediate access to specialized neonatal care, resulting in optimal outcomes following staged surgical repair.

## 5.6 Population-Level Surveillance Results

Analysis of population-level data revealed important geographical and temporal patterns in CHD risk factors. Urban areas showed higher baseline risk scores (mean: 0.34) compared to rural areas (mean: 0.28), primarily driven by increased air pollution exposures and occupational risk factors. Seasonal variations in risk scores correlated with heating season patterns and agricultural chemical applications. Population risk stratification results are listed in table 9.

*Table 9. Population Risk Stratification Results*

| *Risk Category* | *Population (%)* | *CHD Incidence* | *Relative Risk* | *95% CI* |
|---|---|---|---|---|
| *Low Risk (<0.30)* | 68.2% | 0.4% | 1.0 (ref) | - |
| *Moderate Risk (0.30-0.60)* | 24.3% | 1.8% | 4.5 | 3.2-6.3 |
| *High Risk (0.60-0.80)* | 6.1% | 7.2% | 18.0 | 12.4-26.1 |
| *Very High Risk (>0.80)* | 1.4% | 23.1% | 57.8 | 35.2-94.9 |

The monitoring system identified 174 high-risk pregnancies that would not have been detected through conventional screening approaches. Of these, 127 (73%) were confirmed to have either structural CHD or significant functional cardiac abnormalities. Early intervention strategies were implemented in 89% of these cases, including environmental exposure reduction, enhanced prenatal monitoring, and specialized delivery planning.

Geographic clustering analysis revealed hotspots of elevated CHD risk in proximity to industrial facilities, major transportation corridors, and areas with poor air quality. These findings provided valuable information for public health agencies to target intervention efforts and environmental monitoring resources.

# 6. REGULATORY AND ETHICAL CONSIDERATIONS

## 6.1 Medical Device Regulatory Pathway

The development and clinical deployment of AI-driven biosensor networks for prenatal monitoring requires careful navigation of complex regulatory frameworks. In the United States, the Food and Drug Administration (FDA) classifies such systems as Class II medical devices requiring 510(k) premarket notification. The regulatory pathway involves demonstrating substantial equivalence to existing predicate devices while providing evidence of safety and effectiveness through clinical testing.

Software as a Medical Device (SaMD) regulations specifically address AI algorithms used in healthcare applications. The FDA's Digital Health Center of Excellence provides guidance for AI/ML-based medical device development, emphasizing the importance of algorithm transparency, validation datasets, and real-world performance monitoring. Continuous learning systems require special consideration regarding algorithm changes and performance degradation detection.

International harmonization efforts through the International Medical Device Regulators Forum (IMDRF) facilitate global deployment of innovative medical technologies. The proposed biosensor network must comply with European Union Medical Device Regulation (MDR), Health Canada requirements, and other international standards to enable widespread clinical adoption.

## 6.2 Data Privacy and Security

Healthcare data privacy represents a paramount concern for systems collecting continuous physiological and environmental information. The proposed system implements comprehensive privacy protection strategies complying with the Health Insurance Portability and Accountability Act (HIPAA), General Data Protection Regulation (GDPR), and other applicable privacy regulations.

De-identification procedures remove personally identifiable information while preserving clinical utility of monitoring data. Advanced techniques including k-anonymity, l-diversity, and differential privacy provide mathematical guarantees for privacy protection. Federated learning approaches enable collaborative model development without centralized data sharing, further enhancing privacy protections.

Cybersecurity measures protect against potential threats including unauthorized access, data manipulation, and system disruption. Multi-layered security architecture implements encryption, authentication, intrusion detection, and incident response capabilities. Regular security audits and penetration testing ensure continued protection against evolving threats.

## 6.3 Informed Consent and Patient Autonomy

Comprehensive informed consent processes ensure patients understand the benefits, risks, and limitations of continuous monitoring systems. Consent documentation addresses data collection practices, algorithm decision-making, potential false positives and negatives, and options for data sharing or withdrawal. Dynamic consent mechanisms allow patients to modify participation preferences throughout the monitoring period.

Patient autonomy considerations include the right to access personal monitoring data, understand algorithmic predictions, and make informed decisions about interventions. Transparent communication about system limitations and uncertainty ranges enables patients to properly interpret monitoring results and engage in shared decision-making with healthcare providers.

### 6.4 Algorithmic Bias and Health Equity

AI systems may perpetuate or amplify existing healthcare disparities if not carefully designed and validated across diverse populations. The proposed biosensor network implements multiple strategies to ensure equitable performance across different demographic groups, geographic regions, and socioeconomic circumstances.

Diverse training datasets include representative samples from various racial, ethnic, and socioeconomic backgrounds to ensure algorithm fairness. Bias detection algorithms continuously monitor for differential performance across demographic subgroups. When disparities are identified, targeted interventions including algorithmic adjustments and additional training data collection address performance gaps.

Healthcare access considerations ensure that advanced monitoring technologies do not exacerbate existing disparities. Cost-effective sensor designs, simplified user interfaces, and multilingual support materials enable broad accessibility. Partnership with community health centers and public health agencies facilitates deployment in underserved populations.

## 7. FUTURE DIRECTIONS AND CONCLUSIONS

### 7.1 Emerging Technologies and Integration Opportunities

The rapid advancement of sensor technologies, artificial intelligence algorithms, and wireless communications systems creates numerous opportunities for enhancing CHD risk assessment and prevention capabilities. Emerging nanotechnology applications enable development of even more sensitive and selective environmental sensors, with single-molecule detection capabilities for critical teratogens. Quantum sensing technologies may provide unprecedented sensitivity for detecting subtle physiological changes associated with cardiac developmental abnormalities.

Integration with consumer health technologies and smart home systems offers opportunities for seamless environmental monitoring without additional device burden. Smartphone-based sensing capabilities, wearable fitness trackers, and Internet of Things (IoT) devices can contribute valuable data streams while maintaining user convenience and engagement. Artificial intelligence algorithms can integrate these diverse data sources to provide comprehensive risk assessment with minimal patient effort.

Precision medicine approaches utilizing genetic information, pharmacogenomics, and personalized risk profiles will enhance the accuracy and relevance of monitoring systems. Integration with electronic health records, genetic testing results, and family history databases enables comprehensive risk stratification and personalized intervention strategies. Future technology integration roadmap is shown in figure 8.

*Figure 8. Future Technology Integration Roadmap*

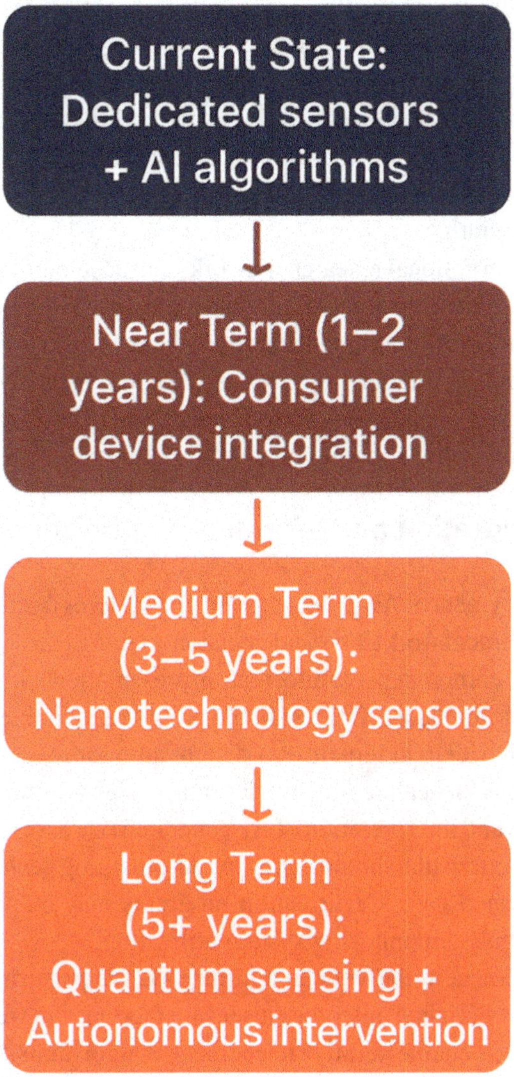


Artificial intelligence algorithms can continuously update risk assessments based on emerging genetic discoveries and environmental health research.

### 7.2 Global Health Applications and Scalability

The proposed biosensor network architecture offers significant potential for addressing CHD prevention challenges in resource-limited settings worldwide. Simplified sensor designs utilizing locally available materials and manufacturing capabilities can reduce costs while maintaining essential functionality. Solar-powered systems and satellite communications enable deployment in areas lacking reliable electrical power and internet infrastructure.

Mobile health (mHealth) platforms can extend monitoring capabilities to remote regions through smartphone-based sensors and telemedicine consultations. Artificial intelligence algorithms optimized for resource-constrained environments can provide valuable risk assessment capabilities even with limited computational resources and bandwidth.

Collaborative international research networks can accelerate algorithm development and validation across diverse populations and environmental conditions. Federated learning approaches enable participation of healthcare institutions worldwide while respecting data sovereignty and privacy requirements. These collaborations can identify population-specific risk factors and optimize intervention strategies for different cultural and socioeconomic contexts.

## 7.3 Clinical Integration and Workflow Optimization

Successful deployment of AI-driven monitoring systems requires careful integration with existing clinical workflows and decision-making processes. User interface design must balance comprehensive information presentation with clinical efficiency and usability. Decision support systems should provide actionable recommendations while preserving physician judgment and patient autonomy.

Training programs for healthcare providers must address both technical aspects of monitoring systems and interpretation of AI-generated risk assessments. Continuing medical education curricula should incorporate emerging technologies and their applications to prenatal care. Certification programs may be necessary to ensure competency in advanced monitoring system utilization.

Quality improvement initiatives can optimize system performance through continuous monitoring of clinical outcomes, user satisfaction, and workflow efficiency. Feedback mechanisms enable iterative refinement of algorithms, user interfaces, and clinical protocols. These improvements ensure that technological advances translate into meaningful improvements in patient care and outcomes.

## 7.4 Research Priorities and Knowledge Gaps

Several important research areas require continued investigation to fully realize the potential of AI-driven CHD risk assessment systems. Mechanistic understanding of how environmental exposures influence cardiac development remains incomplete, limiting the ability to identify optimal intervention strategies. Advanced experimental models including organoids, tissue chips, and computational simulations can provide insights into causal pathways and potential therapeutic targets.

Longitudinal studies following children with in-utero exposures through childhood and adulthood will provide crucial information about long-term outcomes and the effectiveness of early interventions. Biomarker discovery efforts may identify additional indicators of cardiac developmental abnormalities that can enhance risk prediction accuracy. Epigenetic research can elucidate mechanisms by which environmental exposures influence gene expression and cardiac development. Priority research areas and timeline can be seen at table 10.

*Table 10. Priority Research Areas and Timeline*

| *Research Area* | *Timeline* | *Expected Outcomes* | *Resource Requirements* |
|---|---|---|---|
| *Mechanistic Studies* | 2-3 years | Pathway identification | \$2-5M per study |
| *Longitudinal Cohorts* | 5-10 years | Long-term outcome data | \$10-25M per cohort |
| *Biomarker Discovery* | 1-2 years | New predictive markers | \$1-3M per project |
| *Intervention Trials* | 3-5 years | Treatment efficacy data | \$5-15M per trial |

Artificial intelligence algorithm development requires continued advancement in interpretability, uncertainty quantification, and performance across diverse populations. Novel architectures specifically designed for multi-modal biomedical data may provide superior performance compared to adapted computer vision or natural language processing models. Continual learning approaches can enable real-time adaptation to changing environmental conditions and emerging risk factors.

## 7.5 Policy Implications and Public Health Impact

The successful deployment of AI-driven CHD prevention systems has significant implications for public health policy and healthcare resource allocation. Evidence-based environmental health regulations can be informed by comprehensive exposure monitoring data collected through these systems. Real-time surveillance capabilities enable rapid response to environmental health threats and population-level interventions.

Healthcare payment models may need to evolve to support continuous monitoring and preventive intervention strategies. Value-based care contracts that reward improved health outcomes rather than volume of services provided may better align with the goals of advanced monitoring systems. Insurance coverage policies for innovative monitoring technologies require careful consideration of cost-effectiveness and clinical utility.

International collaboration frameworks can facilitate global deployment of CHD prevention technologies while addressing regulatory harmonization, technology transfer, and capacity building challenges. Public-private partnerships may be necessary to ensure sustainable funding for system development, deployment, and maintenance.

## 7.6 Economic Analysis and Cost-Effectiveness Assessment

### 7.6.1 Healthcare Economic Impact Model

The implementation of AI-driven biosensor networks for CHD risk assessment requires comprehensive economic evaluation to demonstrate value to healthcare systems, payers, and society. The economic impact encompasses direct medical costs, indirect societal costs, and long-term healthcare savings through prevention of adverse outcomes. A robust health economic model must account for the lifetime costs associated with CHD management, quality-adjusted life years (QALYs) gained through early intervention, and the broader societal benefits of improved maternal-fetal health outcomes.

Current healthcare expenditures for CHD management represent a substantial economic burden on healthcare systems worldwide. In the United States alone, lifetime medical costs for children born with complex CHD can exceed $500,000 per case, with additional indirect costs including lost productivity, caregiver burden, and reduced quality of life. The proposed monitoring system offers the potential for significant cost savings by enabling early detection and intervention before irreversible cardiac developmental abnormalities occur.

The economic model incorporates multiple cost components including initial system deployment, ongoing operational expenses, healthcare provider training, and maintenance requirements. System deployment costs encompass sensor manufacturing, AI algorithm licensing, clinical integration platforms, and initial healthcare facility infrastructure modifications. Operational expenses include data storage and processing, clinical support services, regular system updates, and quality assurance monitoring. These upfront investments must be weighed against long-term cost savings from prevented CHD cases and improved health outcomes.

Cost-effectiveness analysis utilizing incremental cost-effectiveness ratios (ICERs) demonstrates favorable economic outcomes compared to standard prenatal care approaches. Preliminary modeling suggests ICERs of $15,000-25,000 per QALY gained, well within accepted thresholds for healthcare interventions. Sensitivity analyses accounting for variations in system costs, intervention effectiveness, and healthcare utilization patterns confirm robust cost-effectiveness across diverse scenarios. Monte Carlo simulations incorporating uncertainty in key parameters provide confidence intervals for economic projections and identify critical factors influencing cost-effectiveness outcomes.

### 7.6.2 Budget Impact Analysis for Healthcare Systems

Healthcare systems considering adoption of AI-driven CHD monitoring must evaluate budget impact over multiple time horizons to ensure financial sustainability. Short-term budget impact includes initial capital investments, staff training costs, and system integration expenses. Medium-term considerations encompass ongoing operational costs, maintenance requirements, and potential increases in detected cases requiring intervention. Long-term budget analysis must account for cost savings from prevented complications, reduced emergency interventions, and improved patient outcomes.

Budget impact modeling reveals distinct phases in the economic profile of monitoring system implementation. The initial deployment phase (years 1-2) requires substantial upfront investment with limited immediate cost savings as systems are integrated into clinical workflows and staff gain proficiency. The maturation phase (years 3-5) demonstrates increasing cost-effectiveness as early intervention strategies prevent CHD cases and healthcare providers optimize system utilization. The steady-state phase (years 6+) achieves maximum cost savings through prevented CHD cases while maintaining stable operational costs.

Regional variations in healthcare costs, population demographics, and environmental risk factors significantly influence budget impact projections. Urban healthcare systems serving diverse populations may achieve greater cost-effectiveness due to higher baseline CHD rates and more efficient system utilization. Rural and underserved areas face additional challenges including limited healthcare infrastructure, reduced technical support capabilities, and lower patient volumes that may affect economic viability. Tailored implementation strategies and financing mechanisms may be necessary to ensure equitable access across different healthcare settings.

The budget impact extends beyond direct healthcare costs to include broader economic effects on healthcare system capacity and efficiency. Early CHD detection and prevention may reduce demand for specialized pediatric cardiac services, freeing resources for other clinical priorities. However, increased detection of at-risk pregnancies may temporarily increase utilization of maternal-fetal medicine services and specialized monitoring requirements. Healthcare systems must plan for these capacity shifts and ensure adequate resources are available to support expanded monitoring and intervention capabilities.

### 7.6.3 Return on Investment Analysis

Return on investment (ROI) calculations for AI-driven CHD monitoring systems must encompass both quantifiable financial returns and broader value propositions including improved health outcomes, enhanced clinical capabilities, and potential revenue opportunities. Traditional ROI metrics focusing solely on cost reduction may underestimate the full value of advanced monitoring systems, necessitating comprehensive value-based assessment approaches that capture clinical, operational, and strategic benefits.

Direct financial returns include cost savings from prevented CHD cases, reduced emergency interventions, decreased length of hospital stays, and lower long-term treatment costs. Each prevented case of severe CHD generates substantial cost savings through avoided surgical interventions, intensive care utilization, and lifelong medical management requirements. Conservative estimates suggest cost savings of $200,000-400,000 per prevented severe CHD case, with additional savings from reduced family burden and societal costs.

Indirect financial benefits encompass improved operational efficiency, enhanced clinical reputation, and potential revenue opportunities from expanded service capabilities. Healthcare systems implementing advanced monitoring technologies may attract additional patients, improve clinical outcomes metrics, and qualify for value-based care bonus payments. These indirect benefits can substantially improve overall ROI calculations, particularly for healthcare systems serving competitive markets or pursuing quality improvement initiatives.

Risk-adjusted ROI analysis accounts for uncertainties in system performance, adoption rates, and clinical outcomes to provide realistic projections for decision-making purposes. Monte Carlo simulations incorporating distributions for key parameters generate probability ranges for ROI outcomes and identify critical success factors. Scenario analyses evaluate ROI under optimistic, base case, and conservative assumptions to inform risk management strategies and implementation planning.

The temporal distribution of costs and benefits significantly influences ROI calculations, with substantial upfront investments preceding gradual accumulation of cost savings over multiple years. Net present value analysis utilizing appropriate discount rates provides accurate assessment of investment attractiveness compared to alternative healthcare technology investments. Payback period analysis identifies the timeframe required to recover initial investments, informing financing and cash flow planning decisions.

### 7.6.4 Value-Based Care Integration

The alignment of AI-driven CHD monitoring systems with value-based care models creates opportunities for sustainable financing and improved clinical outcomes. Value-based contracts that reward prevention of adverse outcomes rather than volume of services provided may better support the goals of continuous monitoring and early intervention strategies. These payment models can create financial incentives for healthcare providers to invest in advanced monitoring technologies while sharing risks and rewards with payers.

Accountable care organizations (ACOs) and bundled payment arrangements may find particular value in CHD monitoring systems due to their potential for reducing total cost of care across the patient journey. By preventing CHD cases or enabling early intervention, these systems can reduce expensive downstream treatments while improving patient satisfaction and clinical outcomes. The predictable nature of monitoring costs combined with variable savings from prevented complications aligns well with risk-sharing payment models.

Quality metrics and performance indicators for value-based contracts must be carefully designed to capture the benefits of AI-driven monitoring while ensuring clinical appropriateness and patient safety. Relevant metrics may include CHD detection rates, time to intervention, patient satisfaction scores, and long-term health outcomes. These metrics should be risk-adjusted for population characteristics and environmental factors to ensure fair comparison across different healthcare settings and patient populations.

The development of evidence-based clinical pathways and decision support tools facilitates integration with value-based care requirements while maintaining clinical quality and efficiency. Standardized protocols for interpreting AI-generated risk assessments and implementing interventions ensure consistent care delivery and optimal resource utilization. Quality improvement initiatives can continuously refine these pathways based on real-world outcomes data and emerging clinical evidence.

### 7.6.5 Insurance Coverage and Reimbursement Strategies

Achieving appropriate insurance coverage and reimbursement for AI-driven CHD monitoring requires compelling evidence of clinical effectiveness, cost-effectiveness, and improved patient outcomes. Payers increasingly demand rigorous health economic evidence demonstrating value before approving coverage for innovative medical technologies. The development of comprehensive reimbursement dossiers incorporating clinical trial data, economic analyses, and real-world evidence is essential for successful coverage decisions.

Current procedural terminology (CPT) codes and diagnosis-related group (DRG) classifications may require updates to appropriately capture and reimburse AI-driven monitoring services. New technology assessment processes by the Centers for Medicare & Medicaid Services (CMS) and private payers typically require substantial clinical and economic evidence before establishing coverage policies. Early engagement with payers during technology development can inform evidence requirements and facilitate smoother coverage approval processes.

Coverage with evidence development (CED) programs may provide pathways for conditional coverage while additional real-world evidence is collected to support broader coverage decisions. These programs allow patient access to innovative technologies while generating evidence on clinical effectiveness and cost-effectiveness in routine clinical practice. CED programs can bridge the gap between initial clinical trials and comprehensive coverage approval while ensuring appropriate utilization and patient safety.

International variations in healthcare systems and reimbursement mechanisms require tailored coverage strategies for global deployment of CHD monitoring technologies. Single-payer systems may evaluate technologies through health technology assessment (HTA) processes that emphasize cost-effectiveness and budget impact. Multi-payer systems may require separate coverage negotiations with multiple insurance companies and government programs. Understanding local coverage requirements and evidence standards is essential for successful market access in different countries.

### 7.6.6 Financing Models and Implementation Strategies

Diverse financing models can support the deployment of AI-driven CHD monitoring systems while addressing capital constraints and risk management concerns of healthcare organizations. Traditional capital purchase models may be appropriate for large healthcare systems with adequate financial resources and technical capabilities. However, alternative financing approaches may better serve smaller organizations, resource-limited settings, or risk-averse healthcare systems.

Leasing arrangements and technology-as-a-service models can reduce upfront capital requirements while providing access to the latest monitoring technologies and ongoing technical support. These models may include maintenance, updates, and clinical support services as part of monthly or annual fees, simplifying budget planning and reducing operational complexity. Risk-sharing arrangements with technology vendors can align incentives for successful implementation and clinical outcomes achievement.

Public-private partnerships may facilitate deployment in underserved areas and resource-limited settings where traditional financing approaches are insufficient. Government funding, international development agencies, and philanthropic organizations may provide initial capital investment while private sector partners contribute technical expertise and ongoing support. These partnerships can ensure sustainable operations while addressing health equity concerns and expanding access to advanced monitoring capabilities.

## 7.7 Conclusions

The development of AI-driven biosensor networks for real-time prenatal monitoring represents a significant advancement in CHD risk assessment and prevention capabilities. Through the integration of advanced sensor technologies, sophisticated artificial intelligence algorithms, and comprehensive clinical validation, these systems offer unprecedented opportunities for early detection and intervention.

The clinical validation studies demonstrate clear improvements in CHD risk prediction accuracy compared to traditional approaches, with the potential for significant reductions in adverse outcomes through early intervention. The system's ability to continuously monitor multiple risk factors simultaneously provides a comprehensive approach to understanding the complex etiology of congenital heart disease.

Implementation challenges including regulatory approval, healthcare integration, and cost-effectiveness must be carefully addressed to ensure successful clinical adoption. However, the potential benefits for improving maternal-fetal health outcomes, reducing healthcare costs, and advancing our understanding of CHD etiology justify continued investment in these innovative technologies.

Future research priorities should focus on expanding the evidence base for intervention strategies, improving algorithm performance across diverse populations, and developing sustainable deployment models for global health applications. The convergence of artificial intelligence, sensor technology, and precision medicine creates unprecedented opportunities for revolutionizing prenatal care and preventing congenital heart disease.

As we continue to refine and deploy these advanced monitoring systems, we move closer to a future where CHD prevention is based on comprehensive, real-time risk assessment rather than limited retrospective analysis. This transformation has the potential to significantly reduce the global burden of congenital heart disease and improve health outcomes for children and families worldwide.

The successful implementation of AI-driven biosensor networks for CHD prevention will require sustained collaboration between engineers, clinicians, researchers, and policymakers. Through these collaborative efforts, we can translate technological innovations into meaningful improvements in maternal-fetal health and continue advancing our understanding of one of the most challenging congenital anomalies affecting newborns worldwide.

## REFERENCES


Ahmed, S., Islam, M. J., Islam, K. M. K., Uddin, J., Khandoker, F., Fariha, T., & Hezbullah, M. (2025). Awareness, knowledge, and attitude towards basic life support among healthcare professional students in Bangladesh. *PLOS Global Public Health*, *5*(9), e0005126. DOI: 10.1371/journal.pgph.0005126 PMID: 40892842

. Alam, M. M., & Latifi, S. (2025). A Systematic Review of Techniques for Early-Stage Alzheimer's Disease Diagnosis Using Machine Learning and Deep Learning. Journal of Data Science and Intelligent Systems. DOI: 10.47852/bonviewJDSIS52025037

Alam, M. M., & Latifi, S. (2025). Early Detection of Alzheimer's Disease Using Generative Models: A Review of GANs and Diffusion Models in Medical Imaging. *Algorithms*, *18*(7), 434. DOI: 10.3390/a18070434

Baesmat, K. H. (2024, April). Impedance Analysis of Adaptive Distance Relays Using Machine Learning. In International Conference on Information Technology-New Generations (pp. 457-461). Cham: Springer Nature Switzerland. DOI: 10.1007/978-3-031-56599-1_57

Baesmat, K. H. (2026). IoT-Enabled Smart Grid Analytics for Sustainable Energy ESG Reporting and Performance Optimization: A Business Intelligence Framework. In Data-Driven ESG Strategy Implementation Through Business Intelligence (pp. 319-354). IGI Global Scientific Publishing.DOI: 10.4018/979-8-3373-5142-1.ch012

Baesmat, K. H., & Latifi, S. (2023, August). A new hybrid method for electrical load forecasting based on deviation correction and MRMRMS. In International Conference On Systems Engineering (pp. 293-303). Cham: Springer Nature Switzerland. DOI: 10.1007/978-3-031-40579-2_29

Bagohser, M., Mustafa, T., Alsmirat, M., Al-Ali, A., & Al Jawarneh, I. M. (2025). A cost-effective framework for predicting parking availability using geospatial data and machine learning. In *2025 16th International Conference on Information and Communication Systems (ICICS)* (pp. 1–6). IEEE. DOI: 10.1109/ICICS65354.2025.11073109

Chowdhury, D., Johnson, J. N., Baker-Smith, C. M., Jaquiss, R. D., Mahendran, A. K., Curren, V., & Shaffer, K. (2021). Health care policy and congenital heart disease: 2020 focus on our 2030 future. *Journal of the American Heart Association*, *10*(20), e020605. DOI: 10.1161/JAHA.120.020605 PMID: 34622676

Farrokhi, Z. (2026). AI-Powered Grid Analytics for Sustainable Energy Management in ESG Frameworks. In Data-Driven ESG Strategy Implementation Through Business Intelligence (pp. 279-318). IGI Global Scientific Publishing. DOI: 10.4018/979-8-3373-5142-1.ch011

Farrokhi, Z., Baesmat, K. H., & Regentova, E. E. (2024). Enhancing urban intelligence energy management: Innovative load forecasting techniques for electrical networks. *Journal of Power and Energy Engineering*, *12*, 72–88. DOI: 10.4236/jpee.2024.1211005

Farrokhi, Z., Kalhor, A., & Masouleh, M. T. (2018). Implementation and Evaluation of Object Identification Techniques on Nao Robot Platform. https://aeuso.org/includes/files/articles/Vol8_Iss29_3947-3958_Implementation_and_Evaluation_of_Ob.pdf

Gilboa, S. M., Salemi, J. L., Nembhard, W. N., Fixler, D. E., & Correa, A. (2010). Mortality resulting from congenital heart disease among children and adults in the United States, 1999 to 2006. *Circulation*, *122*(22), 2254–2263. DOI: 10.1161/CIRCULATIONAHA.110.947002 PMID: 21098447

Guo, L., Zhao, Y., Huang, Q., Huang, J., Tao, Y., Chen, J., & Liu, H. (2024). Electrochemical protein biosensors for disease marker detection: Progress and opportunities. *Microsystems & Nanoengineering*, *10*(1), 65. DOI: 10.1038/s41378-024-00700-w PMID: 38784375

Habib, A. R. R., Alam, M. M., & Islam, M. R. (2021, December). Design of a Mobile Aeration System for Aquaculture and Proof of Concept. In 2021 International Conference on Computer, Communication, Chemical, Materials and Electronic Engineering (IC4ME2) (pp. 1-4). IEEE. DOI: 10.1109/IC4ME253898.2021.9768594

Hassanpouri Baesmat, K., Farrokhi, Z., Chmaj, G., & Regentova, E. E. (2025). Parallel Multi-Model Energy Demand Forecasting with Cloud Redundancy: Leveraging Trend Correction, Feature Selection, and Machine Learning. *Forecasting*, *7*(2), 25. DOI: 10.3390/forecast7020025

Hassanpouri Baesmat, K., & Shiri, A. (2019). A new combined method for future energy forecasting in electrical networks. *International Transactions on Electrical Energy Systems*, *29*(3), e2749. DOI: 10.1002/etep.2749

Hudaib, A., & Yousef, M. (2025). Hybrid GWO-SA feature selection for Type II diabetes prediction using machine and deep learning models. In *2025 16th International Conference on Information and Communication Systems (ICICS)* (pp. 1–6). IEEE. DOI: 10.1109/ICICS65354.2025.11073115

Islam, M. S., Alam, M. M., Ahamed, A., & Meerza, S. I. A. (2023, April). Prediction of diabetes at early stage using interpretable machine learning. In *SoutheastCon 2023* (pp. 261–265). IEEE., DOI: 10.1109/SoutheastCon51012.2023.10115152

Jamali, H., Dascalu, S. M., & Harris, F. C. (2024, May). AI-Driven Analysis and Prediction of Energy Consumption in NYC's Municipal Buildings. In 2024 IEEE/ACIS 22nd International Conference on Software Engineering Research, Management and Applications (SERA) (pp. 277-283). IEEE. DOI: 10.1109/SERA61261.2024.10685594

Jamali, H., Dascalu, S. M., & Harris, F. C., Jr. (2024, March). Fostering joint innovation: a global online platform for ideas sharing and collaboration. In International Conference on Information Technology-New Generations (pp. 305-312). Cham: Springer Nature Switzerland. DOI: 10.1007/978-3-031-56599-1_40

Jamali, H., Dascalu, S. M., Harris, F. C., & Feil-Seifer, D. (2025, May). Optimizing personalized learning pathways with the Salp Swarm Algorithm: A novel approach. In 2025 6th International Conference on Artificial Intelligence, Robotics and Control (AIRC) (pp. 291-297). IEEE. DOI: 10.1109/AIRC64931.2025.11077498

Jamali, H., DeBolt, A. L., Dalton, H., Layosa, J. K., Macy, I. R., Shill, P. C., & Wu, R. (2025, June). FORE: A student-centered framework for accessible robotics education through simulation and interactive learning. In *2025 ASEE Annual Conference & Exposition.* DOI: 10.18260/1-2--56585

Jamali, H., Karimi, A., & Haghighizadeh, M. (2018, February). A new method of cloud-based computation model for mobile devices: energy consumption optimization in mobile-to-mobile computation offloading. In *Proceedings of the 6th International Conference on Communications and Broadband Networking* (pp. 32-37). DOI: 10.1145/3193092.3193103

Jamali, H., Shill, P. C., Feil-Seifer, D., Harris, F. C., Jr., & Dascalu, S. M. (2023, October). A schedule of duties in the cloud space using a modified salp swarm algorithm. In IFIP International Internet of Things Conference (pp. 62-75). Cham: Springer Nature Switzerland. DOI: 10.1007/978-3-031-45878-1_5

Kermani, A., Jamshidi, A. M., Mahdavi, Z., Dashtaki, A. A., Zand, M., Nasab, M. A., & Khan, B. (2023). Energy management system for smart grid in the presence of energy storage and photovoltaic systems. *International Journal of Photoenergy, 2023*(1), 5749756. DOI: 10.1155/2023/5749756

Khandoker, F., & Grigsby, T. J. (2025). Methodological Approaches in Studying Type-2 Diabetes-Related Health Behaviors—A Systematic Review. *Applied Sciences (Basel, Switzerland), 15*(19), 10567. DOI: 10.3390/app151910567

. Khandoker, F., Uddin, J., Fariha, T., & Shumi, S. S. (2024). Importance of Psychological Well-being after disasters in Bangladesh: A Narrative Review. Int. J. Sci. Res. in Multidisciplinary Studies Vol, 10(10). Google Scholar

Kwapil, T. R., Chapman, J. P., Chapman, L. J., & Miller, M. B. (1996). Deviant olfactory experiences as indicators of risk for psychosis. *Schizophrenia Bulletin*, *22*(2), 371–380. DOI: 10.1093/schbul/22.2.371 PMID: 8782292

Liu, Y., Chen, S., Zühlke, L., Black, G. C., Choy, M. K., Li, N., & Keavney, B. D. (2019). Global birth prevalence of congenital heart defects 1970–2017: Updated systematic review and meta-analysis of 260 studies. *International Journal of Epidemiology*, *48*(2), 455–463. DOI: 10.1093/ije/dyz009 PMID: 30783674

Liu, Z., Li, X., Li, N., Li, S., Deng, K., Lin, Y., & Zhu, J. (2013). Association between maternal exposure to housing renovation and offspring with congenital heart disease: A multi-hospital case–control study. *Environmental Health : A Global Access Science Source*, *12*(1), 25. DOI: 10.1186/1476-069X-12-25 PMID: 23522351

Mahdavi, Z., Samavat, T., Javanmardi, A. S. J., Dashtaki, M. A., Zand, M., Nasab, M. A., & Khan, B. (2024). Providing a control system for charging electric vehicles using ANFIS. *International Transactions on Electrical Energy Systems*, *2024*(1), 9921062. DOI: 10.1155/2024/9921062

Padmanaban, S., Nasab, M. A., Samavat, T., Nasab, M. A., & Zand, M. (2023). Securing smart power grids against cyber-attacks. In *IoT and Analytics in Renewable Energy Systems* (Vol. 1, pp. 17–36). CRC Press., DOI: 10.1201/9781003331117

Padmanaban, S., Nasab, M. A., Samavat, T., Zand, M., & Nasab, M. A. (2023). Artificial intelligence techniques for smart power systems. In *IoT and Analytics in Renewable Energy Systems* (Vol. 1, pp. 107–123). CRC Press., DOI: 10.1201/9781003331117

Padmanaban, S., Nasab, M. A., Samavat, T., Zand, M., Nasab, M. A., & Hashemi, E. (2023). Cyber security in smart energy networks. In *IoT and Analytics in Renewable Energy Systems* (Vol. 2, pp. 309–325). CRC Press., DOI: 10.1201/9781003374121

Prakash, K. B., Padmanaban, S., & Mitolo, M. (2023). *Smart and Power Grid Systems–Design Challenges and Paradigms*. River Publishers., DOI: 10.1201/9781003339557

Samavat, T., Nazari, M., Fuhong, L., & Yang, L. (2025). Optimizing stand-alone PV systems: A metaheuristic-enhanced fuzzy approach for adaptive MPPT. *China Communications*, *22*(1), 61–74. DOI: 10.23919/JCC.fa.2024-0224.202501

Uddin, J., Fariha, T., Shumi, S. S., & Khandoker, F. (2024). Factors contributing to Alzheimer's disease in older adult populations: A narrative review. DOI: 10.20944/preprints202406.1892.v1

Chapter 11

# 3D Reconstruction of Cardiovascular Anatomy for Investigating the Etiology of Congenital Heart Disease

**Irina Andra Tache**
https://orcid.org/0000-0002-6260-2264
*Politehnica University of Bucharest, Romania*

**Severus Constantin Olteanu**
https://orcid.org/0000-0003-4562-2682
*Politehnica University of Bucharest, Romania*

## ABSTRACT

*Congenital heart diseases (CHD) are a major cause of morbidity and mortality in children and involve abnormal development of heart chambers and valves, along with the origin, course, or structure of the vessels (aorta, pulmonary and coronary artery anomalies, anomalous pulmonary veins, vascular rings, etc.). This chapter presents an algorithm for 3D reconstruction from two uncalibrated fluoroscopic angiography views, addressing the resulting inaccuracies by using an optimization algorithm to minimize the reconstruction error. The study provides the vessels geometry (length, curvature, diameter) along with the generated quantitative coronary angiography (QCA). The 3D reconstruction errors were compensated by an optimization algorithm, and the results were validated by comparison with the vessels' absolute length acquired using dedicated angiographic software. The key*

DOI: 10.4018/979-8-3373-3735-7.ch011

*contributions of the manuscript are a detailed phenotyping that can help the linking of structure to development of the disease, proving insights into genetic studies and hemodynamic analysis.*

## 1. INTRODUCTION

The heart is the engine of life, due to its central function in blood pumping into the circulatory system. Besides this, it is the organ of sensation and sensitivity, with which human beings feel, love, suffer or hate. The psychical state is strongly connected to the physical state influencing the performances of the circulation system as it was revealed in the last decades by different studies.

The circulation system is responsible for transporting the oxygenated blood and supplying cells with nutrients and taking back the deoxygenated blood as long as the metabolic wastes. The cardiovascular or cerebral diseases are reduced to abnormalities in structure and blood transportation at the vascular level. Therefore, the clinical physician seeks to determine the geometry and functioning of the components of the circulation system.

Coronaries are the first blood vessels emerging from the ascending aorta and they have the key role of irrigating the heart muscle. Due to the high pressures resulting from the heart contraction, the blood circulates into the coronaries during diastole, and it is collected back by the coronary sinus. From the aorta, two main coronary arteries are detached: the right coronary artery that splits into right marginal and posterior interventricular artery. The left coronary artery bifurcates into the anterior descending and the circumflex artery. The left marginal artery is a branch of the circumflex artery.

From the aortic arch, the blood enters the brachiocephalic artery which bifurcates into the right common carotid artery. The left common carotid artery starts directly from the aorta, and it is responsible for the brain and eye irrigation.

The venous drainage can be separated into: superficial system (composed of dural venous sinuses located on the surface of the cerebrum) and deep system (composed of the sigmoid sinuses that travel laterally and inferiorly in an S-shaped curve which go on to form the two jugular veins).

Vessel diseases occur due to incorrect connection between vessels (fistula, overlapping of large artery), vessel's tunica narrowing (stenosis of the major arteries) and enlargement of the tunica (aneurism, varices).

Vascular diseases are the leading cause of death in industrialized countries generating enormous clinical and socioeconomic costs. Contemporary diagnostic and therapeutic management of vascular diseases is based on medical imaging technology. Along with the development of this domain, the medical profile must change in order to harmonize with the current technologies.

Cardiovascular diseases represent any disease which leads to physiological and/or morphological changes that alter the functioning of the heart and its transporting vessels. They are divided into cardiac diseases, vascular diseases of the brain and kidney, and peripheral arterial diseases (Bridget et al, 2010). The most common ones are atherosclerosis and/or hypertension which affect the vessels which feed the heart, also called coronaries. During that time, atherosclerosis can cause myocardial infarction. Plaque depositions are accumulated along the interior walls of the coronary arteries, which narrow the vessels and progressively reduce the blood flow which feeds the heart with nutrients and oxygenated blood.

Congenital Heart Disease (CHD) is the most common severe birth anomality (almost 1% of infants diagnosed) and has a genetic etiology (Narayan et al, 2024). It affects the entire cardiovascular system including the heart anatomy and the biggest arteries or veins (anomalous origin of a coronary artery from the pulmonary artery, aortic sinus, single coronary artery, coronary artery fistulas, etc.). The structural defects are a manifestation of a disrupted developmental process. The blood flow patterns that contribute to these imbalances play an essential organic and functional role.

The complexity of CHD etiology includes genetic, environmental and developmental factors. Genetic studies aim to find the root causes of the disease and often rely on precisely characterizing the phenotype (the observable traits or structure) in patients.

Medicine must be capable of tackling all these problems and give solutions. Therefore, it tends to be a new way of looking at this domain. The past and present medicine is reactive, so the results are expected to appear and then the physician prescribes the treatment. In cardiology, he gives various drugs in well-established amounts meanwhile the patient is strictly monitored using the electrocardiogram, ultrasound or essential biomarkers, in order to find the best treatment combination for the patient.

In the future, proactive medicine will provide predictions about the disease evolution of the patient based on his historical medical data and determine the best method for treatment. Therefore, it aims to develop medical imaging for accurate diagnosis and real-time simulations of surgical procedures based on large and complex sets of measurements and examinations of the patient. This will involve the construction of personal anatomical and physiological computational models of the human body, able to explain the observations, to detect the abnormalities, to predict the development of the disease and to make post-treatment analysis.

The mathematical descriptions of the blood flow are useful for having a unitary representation of the complex and diverse mechanisms of human physiology. Therefore, the need for relevant parameters' estimations has arisen.

The 3D reconstruction of the blood vessels from 2D images corrects foreshortening and overlapping for an efficient assessment of stenosis length, vessel diameter, and curvature. Moreover, precise 3D measurements offer important insight into cardiac function and can be used for effective diagnosis, therapy planning, personalized interventions and quantitative phenotypes in genetic association studies. Identifying specific genetic variants linked to 3D structural abnormalities strengthens the understanding of how those genes influence the developmental processes leading to that specific congenital defect.

The importance of the reconstruction resides in eliminating the overlapping and foreshortening of 2D vessel radiographic projection and the extraction of the real diameters and lengths of the vessels. Furthermore, for the hemodynamic parameters' identification, spatial and temporal analyses of the image series are needed.

3D reconstruction of the heart or pulmonary vessels can be applied to interventional cardiac angiography along with other imaging modalities (rotational angiography, computer tomography - CT, cardiac magnetic resonance imaging - CMR).

Interventional cardiac angiography is a fluoroscopic monoplane minimally invasive medical procedure that involves the insertion of a catheter into the femoral or radial artery, which is guided to the heart vessels. To render the vessels radiopaque, an iodine-based contrast agent was injected into the blood stream in the main arteries, such as the femoral or brachial artery.

The main densitometric assumption for the X-ray angiography quantification is the proportionality between the pixel's values and the density of the contrast agent injected into the vessels. This will enable the extraction of the following information from the angiograms: mean velocity, mean and instantaneous volumetric flow, the fractional flow reserve for the stenosis severity appreciation.

The scientific study of (Wagner et al, 2024) presents an acquisition modality and a method for real-time 3D reconstruction of catheters and guidewire devices from coronary X-ray angiography. The validation is performed on a 3D printed blood vessel phantom based on patient imaging.

Another approach (van Walsum et al, 2003) is a combination of fluoroscopic and rotational X-ray angiography based on tracking a guide wire from monoplane acquisitions for visualizing the guide wire positions in the 3D vasculature before the rotational acquisitions.

In the scientific paper of Horz et al in 2013 it is proposed a visual identification of the blood vessels hemodynamic patterns using only a difference of timing parameters from a clean noise time intensity curve. This is a simple and fast clinical standardized method for cerebral angiogram, but it is limited to the physician subjective interpretation of the degree of separation between arteries and veins.

Artificial intelligence (AI) algorithms have many applications in medical imaging, for example, in automated segmentation, predictive modelling, abnormal structure detection, etc. Their main limitations are the explainability issue, for which the human must understand how the algorithm generated the result and the bias of the method originated from the training dataset (for example the medical images were acquired mainly for white race or from a certain clinic, etc.).

A machine learning algorithm (Bayesian maximum a posteriori estimation) is applied to a Poisson distributed projection to reconstruct the 3-dimensional lumen of coronary arteries at a given moment of the cardiac cycle from rotational coronary angiography in (Hu et al, 2010).

A modern technique for cardiac modeling and segmentation from cardiac magnetic resonance imaging and cardiac computer tomography is proposed in the scientific community (Pandey et al.,2025) for 3D heart reconstruction based on a hybrid model of deep learning algorithms and computational techniques.

Multimodal machine learning provides algorithms that can link imaging modalities with genetics, functional data (for example, fractional flow reserve that assesses the severity of a coronary lesion) and clinical parameters extracted from electronic health records. This enables a holistic evaluation of the patient profile.

Yang et al in 2025 explains the integration in the clinical workflow of different approaches and algorithms of data preparation and fusion for advancing the cardiovascular disease management. It is revealed different contributions in image fusion such as, echocardiography with Computer Tomography / Coronary Computed Tomography Angiography - CCTA (Zeb et at, 2023), echocardiography with single photon emission computed tomography – SPECT or with positron emission tomography - PET (Dahl et al, 2021), (Thackeray et al, 2015), echoardiography with CMR (Nagueh et al, 2016), (Wagner et al, 2003), CT with SPETCT/PET (Gould et al, 2017), CCTA with CMR (Karim et al, 2018), SPETCT/PET with CMR (Rischpler et al, 2015)

In the current study, it is emplied a classical image processing techniques to perform a 3D reconstruction algorithm from two views of fluoroscopic angiography as a diagnosis tool for coronary artery disease and could be extended to congenital heart impairments. Even if the method does not employ AI capacity, it offers fast rendering due to the low computation power consumption that makes it suitable for real-time applications in modern or old versions of medical equipment. Also, it doesn't need a physician to annotate the dataset and a large quantity of images to train the model. Usually, the annotated datasets suffer from interobserver variability, which introduces another source of bias in the model prediction.

Two different case studies were presented for a patient with normal coronary arteries and another one with stenosis lesions on a major vessel. The user must manually select the regions of interest in both angiographic projections. If there are visual inaccuracies in the reconstruction, especially for the coronary arteries because they have large motion artifacts, as the systole and diastole phase changes, they were solved using a non-linear optimization algorithm, in which new parameters of the mathematical model of 3D reconstruction were identified.

Nevertheless, the proposed solution offers a more detailed visualization tool for improving the diagnosis of the vessel lesions (stenosis, aneurysm, etc.) and for identification of eventual impairments at the level of vascular structure. Also, the results can be further used for hemodynamic analysis of blood vessels such as blood velocity and flow assessments. Studying the abnormal flow patterns using computational fluid dynamics (CFD) can help researchers understand how altered mechanical forces during the cardiac cycle might contribute to the progression of the disease or to a specific morphology of a congenital defect. Also, While the initial cause could be genetic, the subsequent abnormal flow could exacerbate or shape the final anatomical outcome, thus being part of the disease process influenced by the primary etiology.

The medical imaging for children includes a series of challenges such as radiation exposure that damage the structure of the cell, external motion artefacts that may need sedation, very small vessel sizes it can be difficult to be diagnosed. The importance of providing an accurate 3D reconstruction method of cardiovascular arteries in congenital heart disease is revealed by medical scientific literature and insights about investigating its etiology.

## 2. 3D RECONSTRUCTION TECHNIQUE FOR INTERVENTIONAL CARDIAC ANGIOGRAPHY: PRINCIPLES AND APPLICATION TO CARDIOVASCULAR SYSTEM

### 2.1. Medical Context

To diagnose and plan surgeries for vascular conditions defects, it is essential to obtain both hemodynamic and geometric data. Angiograms can provide crucial information such as vessel radius, cross-sectional area, length, velocity, volumetric flow rate, fractional flow reserve along with the possibility of the 3D reconstruction.

The history of angiography starts with the radiography discovered by Rontgen in 1885 when he makes his first trails using a cathodic tube to brighten a fluorescent screen. This phenomenon was produced because the tube also emitted x-ray radiation. They are electromagnetic waves with lengths of Angstrom orders and with photons energies of some kilo-electron volts (eVs), where $1\text{eV} = 1{,}602 \cdot 10^{-19} J$.

Because the blood vessels are not naturally radiographic, in the clinical radiographic standard, the vessel opacification is obtained by introducing a catheter into a main artery, such as the femoral or branchial artery and navigate throughout the vascular network until the vessel of interest is reached. Then a quantity of 4 to 10 ml of iodine contrast solution is injected for studying the blood flow filling and emptying of the target vessels. Both the toxicity of the contrast agent and the irradiation of both patient and medical staff, limit the duration of this clinical procedure.

Interventional cardiac angiography comprises a C-arm system comprising a detector and X-ray source rotating around the patient was used to acquire fluoroscopic images in Figure 1. The isocenter is the center of the reference coordinates system of the equipment (OXYZ) and it is usually located on the region of interest of the patient. The X-ray source direction is parallel to one of the primary axes (OX or OY).

The imaging apparatus provides temporal images series for about several seconds. In the daily clinic, the physician manipulates the angiograph in order to obtain the best views of the vessels. He rotates the C-arm system around the patient, increases or decreases the magnification of vessels in the images, moves the table for better positioning the patient.

For the small coronaries, the X-ray source can be located near the patient chest to obtain vessels' magnification. Therefore, the distances between source and detector (SID) and source to object (SOD) can vary during the clinical examinations. Moreover, the C-arm system rotates around the isocenter into two directions:

- one around OX from the patient's right arm (RAO) to the left arm (LAO) entiled primary angulation axes defined by the alpha angle;
- another one around the OZ, from the patient's cranium (CRAN) to the feet (CAUD), named the secondary angulation axis, quantified by the beta angle.

*Figure 1. The X-ray angiograph along with its principal distances (adapted from Wächter, 2009)*

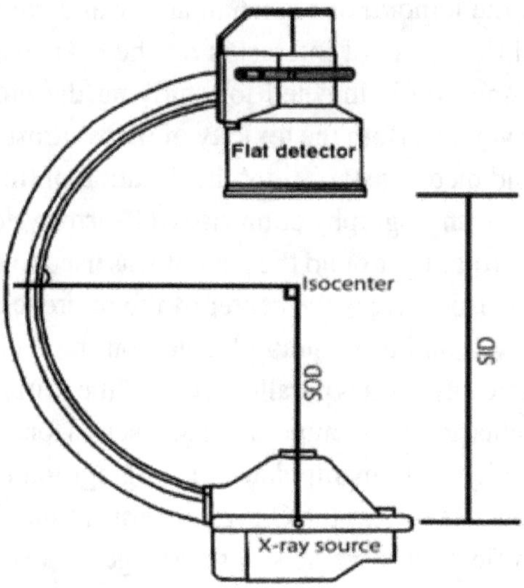


The actual developments in angiography are tackling its major limitations through the years, such as scatter spreading of radiation due to polychromatic beams, geometric distortions due to image intensifier detectors and the motion artifacts. In the first case, the construction of the mono-chromatic source could limit the noise introduced by X-ray scattering, in the second case, the replacement of the old detector with the flat panel detector which directly offers a digital image without geometrical distortions and in the third case, the most difficult one, the electrocardiogram gating during the image acquisition can help the experts to select only images where the motion is less significant, such as in the late diastole phase of the cardiac cycle for the coronarography case.

Still, the motion artifacts represent the major drawback of the cardiac angiography, because it can come from different ways: the movement of the medical equipment, especially the table during the acquisitions, the complex and unpredictable motions of the patient, the respiration and the heart blood pumping.

## 2.2. Blood vessel detection approaches

The vessel detection methods from interventional cardiac angiography include three different approaches: densitometric, model, and edge-based methods. The advantages and disadvantages of these approaches are presented in Table 1.

*Table 1. Vessels detection methods*

| METHOD | ADVANTAGES | DISAVANTAGES |
|---|---|---|
| **Densitometric approach** | The detection is not affected by the equipment noise.<br>Can be applied for small vessels and for cross-sectional area measurements from a single view. | It is applicable to digitally subtraction angiography (DSA).<br>The constant resolution must be calibrated.<br>Difficult for images affected by motion artifacts and vessel foreshortening. |
| **Model based approach** | Suitable for DSA as long as for non-subtracted images which imply background modeling with a low order polynomial.<br>It is applied for small vessels. | It needs many image series for a statistical generation of a reliable geometrical model.<br>It is a time-consuming procedure. |
| **Edge based approach** | It is less dependent on the variations of contrast agent concentration.<br>The image intensities calibration is not mandatory.<br>It is a fast and relatively simple method. | Can inherit blurring effects due to artifacts of the X-ray acquisition system.<br>It needs a constant filling of the vessel for better results (Wächter, 2009). |

Human beings can differentiate a few dozen gray levels and some thousands of colors, so this aspect leads to the need of an angiogram enhancement using colors for a better diagnostic interpretation. Some attempts are made in the development of pseudo-coloring which is treated in scientific literature as a mapping operation of each gray level to a color using a predetermined table or function. Khan et al. in 2008 has used the width of the vessels to provide false colors. Firstly, they have computed the Hessian matrix of the image for getting the geometrical structures and based on the eigenvalues they construct the rule for coloring. Because the hue saturation intensity model failed to reveal the overlapping vessels, the transparent colors were used. Another application is the pixels' classification which can also be used for advanced vessel labeling and building a vascular atlas.

## 2.3. 3D reconstruction modeling from X-ray angiography

Human beings have a stereoscopic vision, capturing the 3D sequence from slightly different angles with both eyes and fusion the data into the brain for recomposing the scene. This principle is exploited by scientists in computer vision.

Three-dimensional (3D) reconstruction has been extensively investigated in recent years owing to the development of digital medical imaging. In the scientific literature for the monoplane system can be mentioned (Movassaghi et al, 2004, Shechter, 2004, Sprague et al, 2006, Brost et al, 2009a, Brost et al, 2009b, Yang, 2009), the biplane system (Dumay et al, 1994, Esthappan et al, 1998, Radeva et al, 1998, Cheriet et al, 1999, Hoffmann et al, 2000, Law et al, 2003, Shechter et al,

2003, Bourantas et al, 2005), or the rotational system (Graß et al, 2001, Blondel et al, 2002, Blondel et al, 2006, Movassaghi et al, 2006, Garcia, 2007, Wächter, 2009).

In medical scientific papers, the rotational acquisition is used to generate an accurate 3D reconstruction of the vessels and the 2D fluoroscopic projections for extracting the wash-in and wash-out phase of the contrast agent. From the 3D reconstruction, the real lengths and diameters of the vessels are computed and from the time image series, the bolus transport time is determined. By fusion the two data types, the velocity can be computed and used as boundary conditions into the computational fluid dynamics models (Hentschke et al, 2011). Another approach appertains to Wächter-Stehle et al in 2012 who extract the velocity from the parametric image. This functional image has on its rows the time density curves and on its columns the distance density curves. The velocity is used in the physical model of blood flow and contrast agent transport. These methods have the disadvantage of requiring the irradiation of the patients two times, one for generating the rotational images and another one for the monoplane fluoroscopic projections. Also, they are time consuming.

Because rotational angiography is not so popular in daily clinics and it is limited to certain vascular diseases' diagnosis, the monoplane angiography is used in this study. The images are uncalibrated and need further processing in order to overcome their two main limitations: 2D projection and the non-physiological information about the blood vessels. Therefore, a mathematical modeling of the 3D vessels' reconstruction which permits an in-depth inspection of the complex vascular network is proposed as long as the two representations of the functional information which reflect the hemodynamic patterns.

The 3D reconstruction error from two projection views of the vessel centerline had important magnitudes owing to the mismatching of the correspondence points in both views and less accurate location parameters of the C-arm angiograph because of the possible movement of the patient's table during acquisitions. In addition, some errors can be associated with a mismatch between the endpoint selections. In addition, the implementation of epipolar geometry for computing each corresponding point of the vessel centerline in both views could minimize the 3D reconstruction errors.

Precise 3D anatomical understanding of the great vessels (aorta, pulmonary artery, systemic/pulmonary veins) along with specific vascular anomaly such as anomalous origins/courses of arteries, complex vascular rings or collaterals can provide crucial insights into which developmental steps went wrong and when during child gestation.

Different evolution pathways give rise to specific 3D structural outcomes. Analyzing the detailed 3D structure can help pinpoint the likely point of divergence from normal development, informing hypotheses about the underlying genetic or environmental factors (etiology).

Other potential imaging modalities for 3D reconstruction of the heart and coronary vessels are cardiac CT, with the advantages of fast acquisition and motion correction methods and cardiac MRI with dynamic sequences that reveal soft tissues for evaluating perfusion function, and congenital anomalies.

## 2.4. A 3D reconstruction model from two interventional cardiac angiography projections

### 2.4.1. Homogenous Coordinates

There are two main types of coordinates encountered in computer vision: Cartesian and homogenous. Homogeneous coordinates are introduced for the camera projection matrix description. Given an image point $p_{2D} = [p_x, p_y]$, it can be represented in the homogeneous coordinates $\widetilde{p_{2D}} \in \mathbb{R}^3$ as follows:

$$\widetilde{p_{2D}} = \varepsilon \cdot \left[p_x p_y \ 1\right] \tag{1}$$

Where ε is a scaling factor with the property $\varepsilon \in \mathbb{R}\backslash\{0\}$.

The Euclidean transform is $g{:}\mathbb{R}^m \rightarrow \mathbb{R}^m$, where $g(x) \rightarrow R_M \cdot x + t$, $R_M \in \mathbb{R}^{mxm}$ is the rotation matrix with the following properties: $R_M^{-1} = R_M^T$ and its determinant is equal to 1 and $t \in \mathbb{R}^m$ is the translation vector. For the homogeneous coordinates, the Euclidean transform can be described as follows:

$$p_{3D} = R_M \cdot \widetilde{p_{2D}} + t \tag{2}$$

Where $p_{3D}$ is the spatial point in Euclidean coordinates. Equation (2) can be translated into homogeneous coordinates as follows:

$$\widetilde{p_{3D}} = \begin{bmatrix} R_M & t \\ 0 & 1 \end{bmatrix} \cdot \widetilde{p_{2D}} \tag{3}$$

### 2.4.2. The algorithm workflow

The projection matrix (M) is defined as the 3D point mapping of image points:

$$M = K_{im}\left[R_M | t\right] \tag{4}$$

Where $M \in \mathbb{R}^{3\times4}$, $K_{im} \in \mathbb{R}^{3\times3}$ is the camera intrinsic parameter matrix and comprises the perspective projection matrix. $R_M \in \mathbb{R}^{3\times3}$ is the rotational matrix and $t \in \mathbb{R}^3$ is the translation vector, which forms both the matrix of the camera's extrinsic parameters and the orientation of the imaging apparatus relative to the world coordinate system.

Reconstruction requires a specific geometric setup of the imaging system. Digital Imaging and Communications in Medicine (DICOM) files contain essential parameters for each image series. The metadata included the distance between source and detector, distance between source to object, source-to-patient distance, pixel spacing measured in millimeters, and primary and secondary angles (alpha and beta).

Typically, the imaging equipment has a fixed distance between the source and isocenter (distance between source to object). Nevertheless, the precision of these measurements is questionable, particularly when considering the movement of the patient's table during the imaging process.

The 3D reconstruction algorithm based on [Brost et al. in 2009 a,b] assumes a 3D projection of the spatial point $\widetilde{p_{3D}} = [p_{3D}{}^T, 1]^T$ onto the 2D point $\widetilde{p_{2D}}$, all expressed in homogeneous coordinates as:

$$\widetilde{p_{2D}} = M \bullet \widetilde{p_{3D}} \tag{5}$$

Where M is the projection matrix.

Knowing that the last element in vector $\widetilde{p_{3D}}$ is 1, equation (2) can be rewritten as:

$$\widetilde{p_{2D}} = K_{im}\left(R_M \bullet p_{3D} + t\right) \tag{6}$$

The spatial point in Cartesian coordinates is defined by equation (7):

$$p_{3D} = R_M{}^{-1} \bullet \left(K_{im}{}^{-1} \bullet \widetilde{p_{2D}} - t\right) \tag{7}$$

Where $p_{2D} = [x_2, y_2]$ represents the coordinates of the image point.

The disparity between the actual 2D point coordinates marked in both images and those derived from the back-projection of the spatial point is known as the reconstruction error. This discrepancy can be significant, particularly for uncalibrated angiograms, as the extrinsic and intrinsic parameters of the DICOM file may be inaccurate owing to the potential movement of the patient's table during image capture. Other factors contributing to this error include deliberate or unintentional patient movements, such as breathing or heartbeat. Furthermore, as noted by (Yang, 2009) the isocenters of the two angiographic views were not aligned, and their imaging axes were not perpendicular to each other. In 2009, Wächter pointed out that gravitational and inertial forces affect the spherical rotation of the C-arm system around its isocenter.

To address these issues, it is necessary to re-estimate the reconstruction parameters by minimizing the objective function. This function is formulated as the Euclidean distance error between the skeleton image coordinates and the corresponding back-projection coordinates of the 3D reconstruction process.

The Levenberg-Marquardt nonlinear algorithm was employed by (Tache, 2017) to solve the optimization problem, chosen for its efficient computational times in solving the sum of squared residual functions (Lourakis, 2005). Eleven parameters were proposed for optimization: distance between source and detector along with distance between source to object (occasionally substituted with the source-to-patient distance), rotation angles for both projections, image plan center coordinates (Ox, Oy), and table motion translation vector, t.

### 2.4.3. Epipolar Geometry

The principle of correspondence of two points located in two different images acquired with two cameras located at a known distance, which tags the same 3D point, is employed by epipolar geometry. For angiograms, the analyzed object is the vessels' middle line, which corresponds to a skeleton. Subsequently, two different projection views ($I_1$ and $I_2$ from Figure 2) from which the vessels' skeleton was extracted are considered in the following.

*Figure 2. Exemplification of the epipolar geometry*

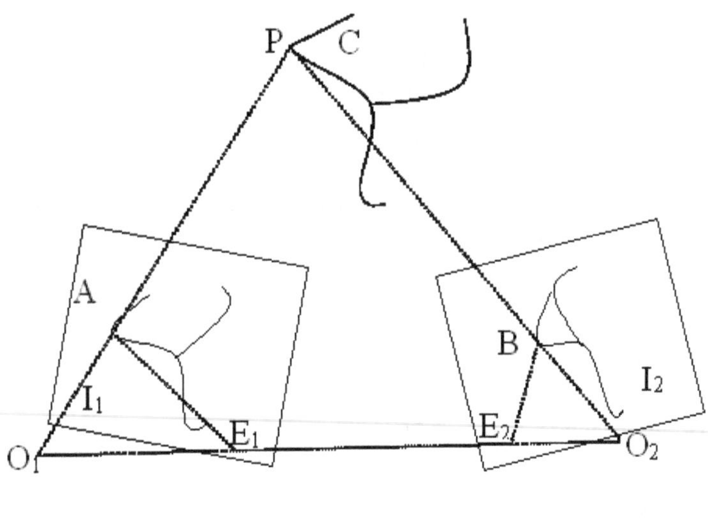


Point A from image $I_1$ and the centers of the two X-ray sources $O_1$ and $O_2$ form the epipolar plane. The intersection of the epipolar plane with the image plane $I_2$ forms the epipolar line. Point B from image $I_2$ must lie on the epipolar line as in Figure 2 in order to assure the pixels' correspondences between the two views. The

2D coordinates from the two projections are manually selected by an expert and will enable the computation of the spatial point. Errors can occur due to incorrect matching of the correspondence points due to human error.

## 2. HEMODYNAMIC ANALYSIS FROM X-RAY CORONARY ANGIOGRAPHY

The term hemodynamics is composed of the particle 'hemo' which means blood and dynamics which means motion. This term is very important for understanding the physiology of the circulation system and the appearance of vascular diseases. In fact, any vascular problem is related to a perturbation of the blood flow in specific regions of the vessel network. The factors that can influence the blood flow into the vessels are physical and emotional stress, gravitational champs, etc.

Many brilliant mathematicians and physicists were implicated in the understanding of the blood flow problem. Newton discovered the fluid viscosity, which is related to the velocity gradient, Euler formulated the fluid flow equations, Poiseuille mathematically described the flow into the capillary tubes, Bernoulli found the velocity equation when the pressure is known and finally, Navier – Stokes established the general equations of fluid flowing. Even with all these efforts, the real physics of blood flow is much more complex, especially when the blood properties are taken into consideration.

The direction of the flow is given by the higher pressure, hence, the blood flows from higher to lower pressures. Another important observation is that the pressure drops long distances because of the friction between the wall and fluid along with the friction of the fluid layers.

It's important to notice that the volumetric flow is proportionally dependent on the fourth power of the radius (Silverthorn, 2012). Some limitations are imposed since the arteries are not straight tubes because they can bifurcate and the blood flow into the large arteries is not always laminar (the case of aorta). Also, after a stenosis, the flow is turbulent.

There are two main methods for measuring blood volume: geometrical and densitometric approaches. Geometrical measurements are based on 3D vessel reconstruction from monoplane, biplane, or rotational angiography. The last technique involves the risk of small vessel exclusion. Considering the length of the vessel segment as L and the cross-sectional area as S, the volume is equal to:

$$V = S \bullet L \tag{8}$$

## 3.1. Densitometric measurements

Densitometric measurements assume that the volume is approximated by the peak value of the time-density curve -TDC ($t_{max}$). This limitation appears to be due to the lower injection rates, which cannot instantly and completely replace the blood in the region of interest (ROI). The volume of the undiluted contrast agent from a region of interest (ROI) is:

$$V = \frac{Q_{ROI}}{c_{iod}} = \frac{TDC(t_{max})}{c_{iod}} = \frac{D_{max}}{c_{iod}} \tag{9}$$

Where $Q_{ROI}$ is the densitometric blood flow for the region of interest, $c_{iod}$ is the iodine concentration of the undiluted contrast agent, $t_{max}$ is the time at which the contrast agent completely replaces the blood, and $D_{max}$ is the corresponding density. According to Rutishauser et al. (1967), the average blood flow exhibits a direct relationship with volume and an inverse relationship with time, as follows:

$$Q = \frac{V}{\bar{t}} \approx \frac{V}{\Delta t} \tag{10}$$

Where $\Delta t$ is an alternative timing difference parameter that approximates the mean transit time $\bar{t}$.

The Stewart–Hamilton dye dilution method for bolus injection applies a global mass conservation law for computing the constant volume flow rate $Q_v$ as:

$$Q_v = \frac{V}{\int_0^T c_v(t)dt} \tag{11}$$

Where V is the total volume of the indicator or contrast material injected into the circulation system, and $c_v(t)$ is the instantaneous volume concentration along the axial locations of the outlet vessel.

For prolonged and constant injection of the contrast agent (Zierler, 1962), the flow rate was determined using the following equation:

$$Q_v = \frac{Q_i}{c_{max}} \tag{12}$$

Where $Q_i$ is the injection flow rate, and $c_{max}$ is the maximum value of the curve $c_v(t)$.

The first-pass distribution theory begins with Fick's principle, which states that the contrast agent mass absorbed by an organ $m(\tau)$ is equal to the difference between the injected mass into the circulation and the remaining mass, as follows:

$$m(\tau) = m_a(\tau) - m_v(\tau) \tag{13}$$

where $m_v$ is the venous mass and $m_a$ is the arterial mass, expressed as follows:

$$m_a(\tau) = \int_0^{\tau} Q_a(t) \bullet c_a(t)dt$$

(dt) (14)

Where $Q_a(t)$ is the arterial blood flow rate, and $c_a(t)$ is the arterial concentration of the contrast agent. Analogously, the venous mass is computed, and the final mass of the contrast material is determined as follows:

$$m(\tau) = \int_0^{\tau} Q_a(t) \bullet c_a(t)dt - \int_0^{\tau} Q_v(t) \bullet c_v(t)dt \tag{15}$$

Where $Q_v(t)$ is the venous flow rate, and $c_v(t)$ is the venous concentration.

For pulsatile flow, the venous concentration can be neglected for a small amount of time because the contrast agent still resides in the organ, the arterial flow rate is replaced by $\overline{Q}$ which is the average volumetric mean flow, and the arterial concentration is replaced by $\overline{C}$ which is the average concentration. Therefore, equation (12) becomes:

$$\overline{Q} = \frac{m(\tau)}{\overline{C} \bullet \tau} \tag{16}$$

In 1990, Marinus et al. applied this method to angiographic data. The assumption of linear proportionality between the pixel values and iodine mass from the X-ray path implies image calibration. The average concentration was then determined at the location of non-overlapping vessels with a perfusion bed that was close to the injection site. A variation in concentration over time was observed. In 1996, Molloi et al. used this algorithm to quantify the coronary blood flow from DSA.

Acute coronary diseases can be hidden in the resting state and can be revealed in the hyperemic state, which is characterized by physical effort and can be induced by injecting papaverine or similar drugs into the blood circulation of the patient.

Myocardial ischemia represents an imbalance between the coronary flow and myocardial metabolic demands. It can be diagnosed by evaluating the coronary flow reserve (CFR) as the ratio of blood flow in the hyperemic ($Q_1$) and normal (Q2) states of the same artery. This helps physicians quantify severe artery stenosis and is a medical protocol for deciding on stent implementation. Considering a constant circulation volume for both states, Vogel et al. (1984) proposed the following equation for computing CFR:

$$CFR = \frac{Q_1}{Q_2} = \frac{Q_1/V}{Q_2/V} \approx \frac{\overline{t_2}}{\overline{t_1}} \qquad (8)$$

The blood flow ratio was inversely proportional to the corresponding transit time ($\overline{t_1}, \overline{t_2}$) computed from the time density curves generated for the proximal and distal ROI.

In 2002, Schrijver et al. determined the relative coronary flow reserve (RCFR) as the ratio of CFRs computed for the hyperemic state (h) and the normal state (0). By considering the constant volume assumption under both conditions, the RCFR becomes:

$$\mathrm{RCFR}_{1,2} = \frac{\overline{t_2^{(h)}}}{\overline{t_1^{(h)}}} \bullet \frac{\overline{t_1^{(0)}}}{\overline{t_2^{(0)}}} \qquad (9)$$

The equation is approximate for normal patients, except for those with severe coronary diseases, due to the changes produced at the myocardial level, especially in the hyperemic state. The consequences include volume enlargement distal to the stenosis and vessel vasodilatation.

## 3.2. Quantitative coronary angiography

Geometric measurements were performed using interventional cardiac angiography through QCA analysis (Figure 3). This is an objective evaluation of the vessel dimensions (profile of the diameters along the vessel length), from which some relevant parameters can be determined. In modern angiography, this value is determined after 3D reconstruction of the vessel segment (Gurav et al, 2024).

*Figure 3. Quantitative coronary angiography of a vessel segment*

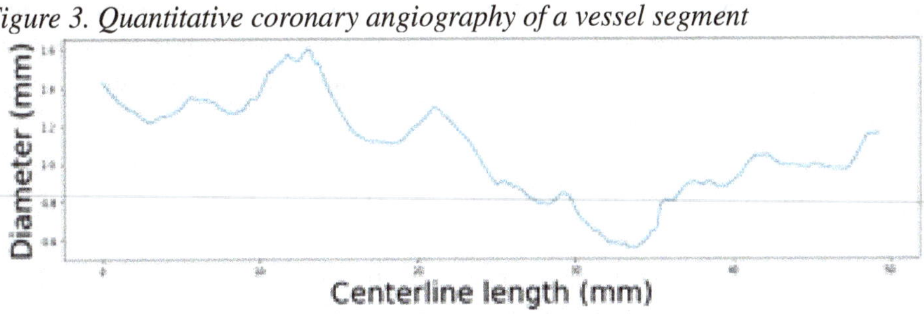

## 3. AN 3D RECONSTRUCTION TOOL FOR CONGENITAL HEART DISEASE PHENOTYPE CHARACTERIZATION

The congenital heart disease diagnosis benefits from the advances in medical images such as echocardiography, X-ray coronary angiography, cardiac magnetic resonance, cardiac computed tomography along with the innovative technical methods such as 3-dimensional modeling, virtual surgery simulation, patient specific digital twin and artificial intelligence for risk stratification (Sachdeva et al, 2024).

### 3.1. Imaging Setup

X-ray coronary angiography was collected from six patients at a hospital in Bucharest. The image data characteristics were as follows: spatial resolution is 512x512, temporal resolution, 15 images/s; contrast resolution 256, and number of images per series, 70.

The coronary vessels are very small, with diameters of 1.9 – 4.5 mm making them difficult to visualize on monoplane angiography. 3D reconstruction and hemodynamic analysis can facilitate medical investigations and diagnoses of cardiovascular diseases.

To diagnose and plan surgeries for vascular conditions defects, it is essential to obtain both hemodynamic and geometric data. Angiograms can provide crucial information such as vessel radius, cross-sectional area, length, velocity, volumetric flow rate, and fractional flow reserve.

### 3.2. The proposed solution

A MATLAB® graphical user interface (GUI) was developed to enable users to generate centerlines for vessels in both views along with 2D length measurements. Furthermore, the GUI offers segment border delineation using either densitometric techniques or the Canny edge-detection algorithm. A geometric approach was implemented to calculate the radius and cross-sectional area.

A key feature of this software is its ability to create a 3D reconstruction of the vessel segment to ascertain its actual trajectory. This reconstruction process allows the uploading of two views of cardiac angiography. The complex motion of the coronaries during the cardiac cycle complicates the problem.

To exemplify the algorithm, a 3D reconstruction of the left main coronary artery is presented. The vessel was tagged into different projections because it had the catheter tip as a reference, where the contrast agent was injected. This vessel has fewer motions during the cardiac cycle, and the selected images for reconstruction were acquired from the late diastole phase.

The imagistic specialist identified the intermediate points along the vessel centerline, and their coordinates were derived from a cubic spline divided into 100 parts. To assess the quality of the 3D reconstruction, a distance error was calculated. Subsequently, an optimization algorithm was tested, and the adjusted parameters were disclosed.

Specific parameters for each projection, such as distance between source and detector and distance between source to object, were initialized based on the distance from the source to the patient, which could modify the image magnification factor as long as the alpha and beta angles. The global parameters include the coordinates of the center of the image plane (ox, oy) and the translation vector for the table movement with coordinates [mx, my, mz].

The 3D reconstruction of the circumflex coronary centerline tagged into two projections pertaining to different cardiac phases is presented in the following. This example was provided to test the efficiency of the reconstruction algorithm when the correspondences between the points were made with fewer errors because both images contained the same cardiac cycle phase, and a reference was provided. Optimization was also performed by varying all three components of the motion vector.

Table 2 presents all the parameters of the optimization algorithm. Various iterations were evaluated by altering the coordinates of the table motion vector. The initial version of the algorithm corresponded to the default 3D reconstruction without any optimization.

Version 1 involves variations in all three coordinates of the translation vector. Version 2 modifies only the 0X and 0Z coordinates (mx, mz). Version 3 also involves variations in the 0X and 0Y components, respectively. In version 4, only the 0X component was considered, in contrast to version 5, where only the 0Z component was considered.

*Table 2. Optimization parameters for the 3D reconstruction algorithm*

| Versions | Pr. | distance between source and detector [mm] | distance between source to object [mm] | Alpha [°] | Beta [°] | ox | oy | mx | my | mz |
|---|---|---|---|---|---|---|---|---|---|---|
| Initial | 1 | 1112 | 785 | 1.6 | -39 | 256 | 256 | - | - | - |
| | 2 | 1045 | 783 | -27 | -15 | | | | | |
| v1 – [mx,my,mz] | 1 | 1112 | 784 | 5.9 | -13 | 256 | 258 | 2 | -10 | -5 |
| | 2 | 1044 | 785 | -30 | -40 | | | | | |
| v2 – [mx,mz] | 1 | 1112 | 784 | 32 | -13 | 255 | 245 | -1 | - | -4 |
| | 2 | 1037 | 794 | -43 | -64 | | | | | |

continued on following page

*Table 2. Continued*

| Versions | Pr. | distance between source and detector [mm] | distance between source to object [mm] | Alpha [°] | Beta [°] | ox | oy | mx | my | mz |
|---|---|---|---|---|---|---|---|---|---|---|
| v3 – [mx,my] | 1 | 1112 | 785 | 39 | 1.5 | 255 | 266 | -3 | -3 | - |
| | 2 | 1036 | 794 | -43 | -56 | | | | | |
| v4 – [mx] | 1 | 1112 | 785 | 60 | 8.3 | 259 | 255 | -4 | - | - |
| | 2 | 1024 | 810 | -24 | -62 | | | | | |
| v5 – [mz] | 1 | 1112 | 785 | 34 | -19 | 241 | 238 | - | - | -5 |
| | 2 | 1032 | 800 | -42 | -67 | | | | | |

Table 2 reveals significant alterations in the isocenter coordinates and rotation angles during optimization. Specifically, angle α exhibited mean changes of -32.6° and 7.8 °for the first and second projections, respectively, while angle β showed mean changes of -32° and 35.7 °for the first and second projections, respectively.

The isocenter serves as the center of the reference coordinate system, and its variation underscores the complexity of the acquisition process. Notably, the C-arm system does not rotate strictly around the isocenter; the table may be adjusted by the physician during acquisitions to obtain optimal views of the patient's heart. Additionally, vessel motion during the cardiac cycle may contribute to the modification of the translation vector.

Furthermore, minimal adjustments were made to the distance between source and detector and distance between source to object values. However, for the second projection, the distance between source to object was corrected more substantially, with a mean adjustment of 13.6 mm. The center of the image plane shifted from its initial coordinates by an average of 2 pixels along the 0X axis and 3 pixels along the 0Y axis.

In Table 3, the distance errors computed as the sums of Euclidean distances between consecutive points of the centerlines are given in millimeters.

*Table 3. Quantification of the optimization process*

| Version | Projection 1 | Projection 2 |
|---|---|---|
| | Error [mm] | Error [mm] |
| Initial | 24.42 | 28.63 |
| v1 – [mx,my,mz] | 0.50 | 0.60 |
| v2 – [mx,mz] | 0.79 | 0.99 |

continued on following page

*Table 3. Continued*

| Version | Projection 1 | Projection 2 |
|---|---|---|
| | Error [mm] | Error [mm] |
| v3 – [mx,my] | 0.51 | 0.62 |
| v4 – [mx] | 1.63 | 2.24 |
| v5 – [mz] | 1.88 | 2.46 |

The reconstruction error for the case without optimization was augmented, with the first projection at approximately 24.4 mm and the second projection at approximately 28.6 mm. Given the small dimensions of the coronary arteries, these errors are clinically significant.

For the optimization versions, the minimum errors were encountered for the variations of the motion table vector in all three axes with a mean of 0.55 mm for both projections, followed by version 3 (with the OX and OY coordinates) with a mean of 0.57 mm for both projections. This is probably due to the fact that the displacement of the isocenter on the 0Y axes is more important. The maximum error appeared for version 5, where only the motion on the 0Z axis was considered. There, the isocenter does not move significantly in this direction.

In Table 4, the vessel centerline is selected in two projections as follows: the back projections for the initial reconstruction of the 3D centerline are marked in white lines, the back projections after the optimization are marked in magenta, and the vessel segment selection in the 2D projection is marked in green. Finally, at the bottom, the 3D centerlines are plotted for both projections. The best match between the centerlines can be observed for the optimized version of the algorithm, where the back projections are almost superimposed on the initial 2D centerline.

*Table 4. Visualisation of the initial and optimized version of 3d reconstruction*

| | |
|---|---|
| 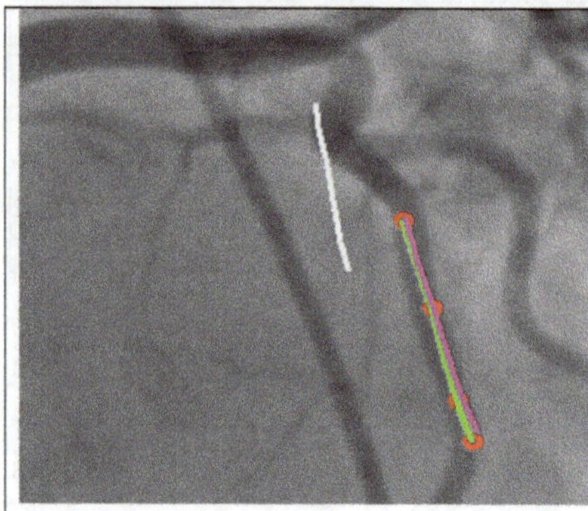 | 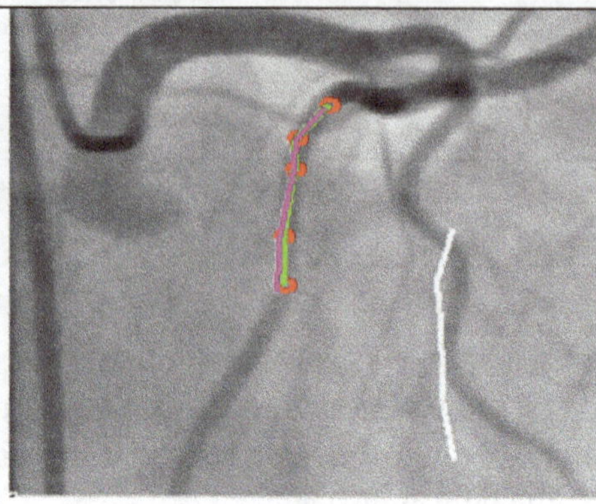 |
| Projection 1 of the vessel segment on a circumflex artery | Projection 2 of the vessel segment on a circumflex artery |
| 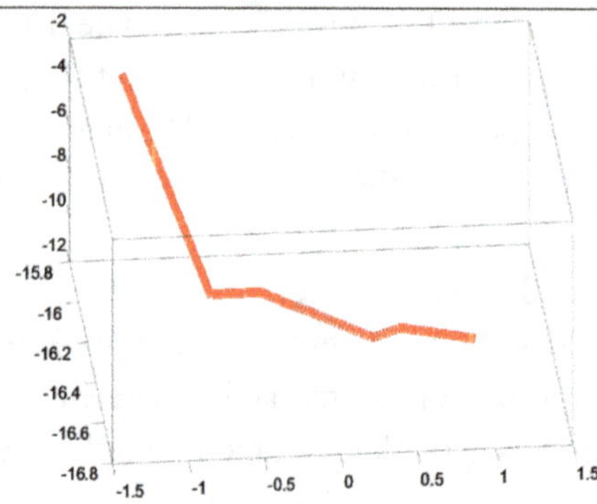 | 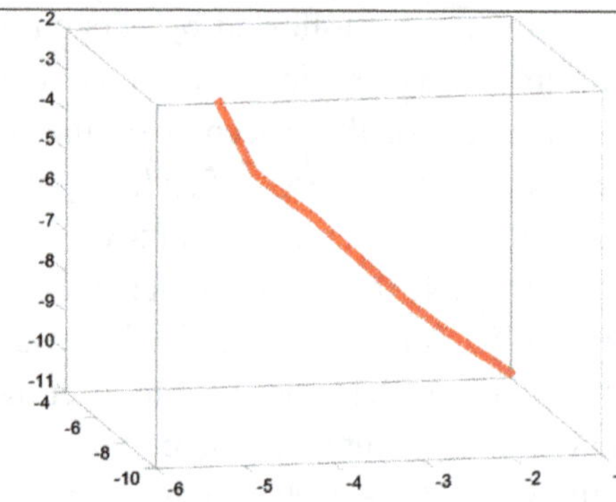 |
| Initial 3D reconstruction | 3D reconstruction after optimization step |

Table 5 presents a graphical comparison of the optimization results. In this table, the back projections for version 2 are indicated by yellow lines, whereas those for version 3 are marked in red, demonstrating good alignment with the initial centerlines. The back projections for version 4 are represented by the blue lines. Version 5 was excluded from the study because of its high error rates.

*Table 5. Comparison of the optimization versions*

| | |
|---|---|
| 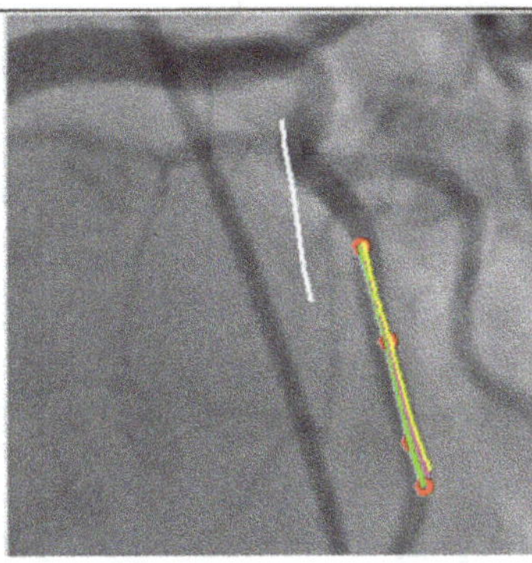 | 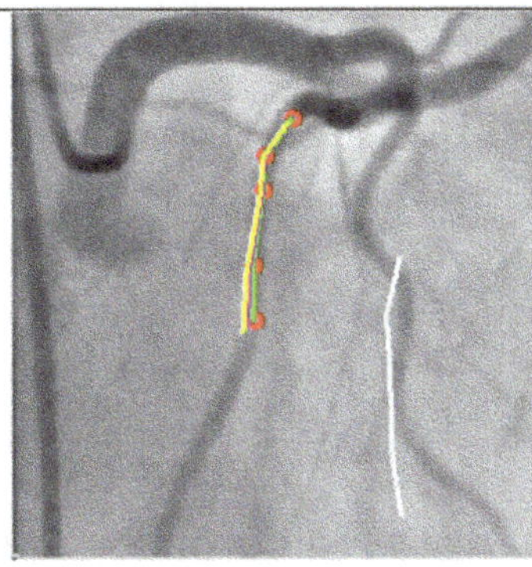 |
| **Projection 1 – v2** | **Projection 1 – v2** |
| 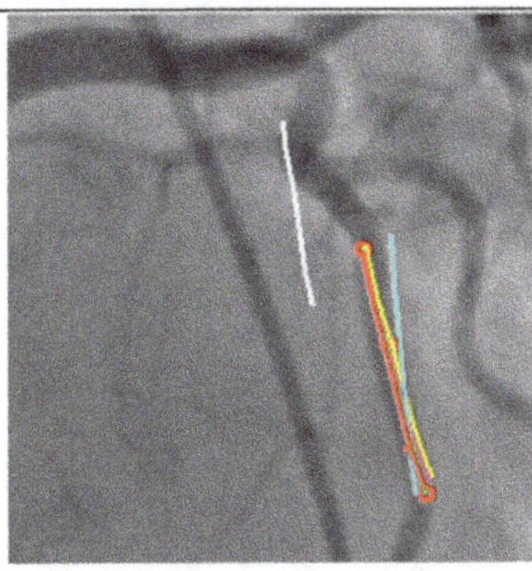 | 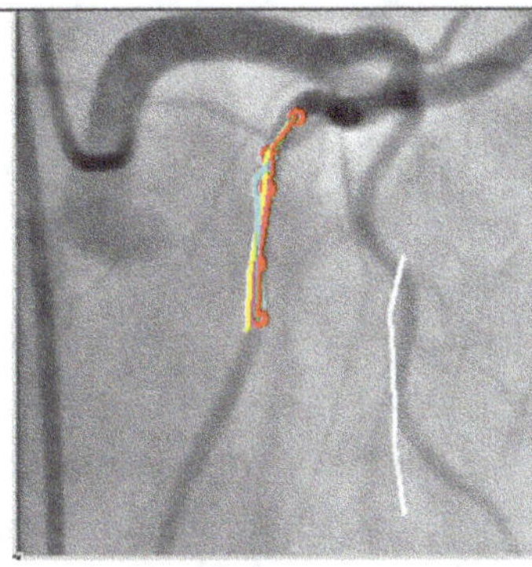 |
| **Projection 1 – v3** | **Projection 1 – v3** |
| 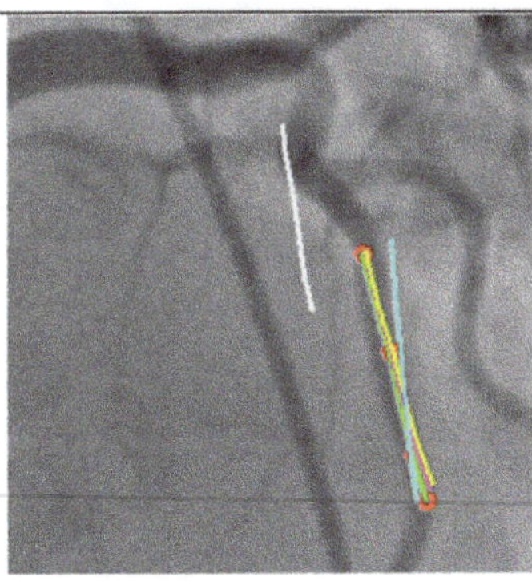 | 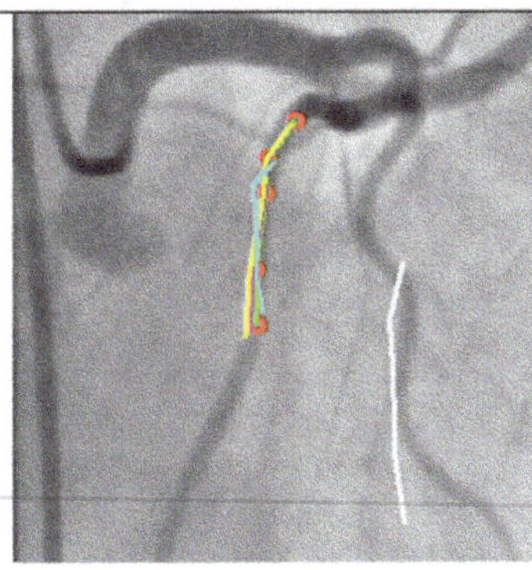 |
| **Projection 1 – v4** | **Projection 1 – v4** |

Given that the metric dimensions of each pixel are known, two-dimensional distances in millimeters and three-dimensional lengths can be computed for further analysis.

The graphical application succeeded in reproducing the results obtained using dedicated software installed on the angiographic equipment. The physician tagged the endpoints of the vessel in an image series and the second projection view. The software implements epipolar geometry to automatically detect the corresponding vessel points in the second view. The resulting lengths of the vessel segments were considered the ground truth.

## 3.3. Quantitative coronary angiography for normal and stenosis arteries

To illustrate the QCA analysis, two cases were examined: the first was a normal artery, as shown in Table 4, whereas the second focused on a stenotic vessel, where the validation was performed against the results generated by the angiograph software application.

### 4.3.1. Normal artery case

A segment of the circumflex coronary artery without stenosis was tagged in two projections. To determine the absolute path of the vessel segment, a 3D reconstruction was performed, and the results are listed in Table 6.

*Table 6. 3D dimensional reconstruction of a normal vessel's edges*

| 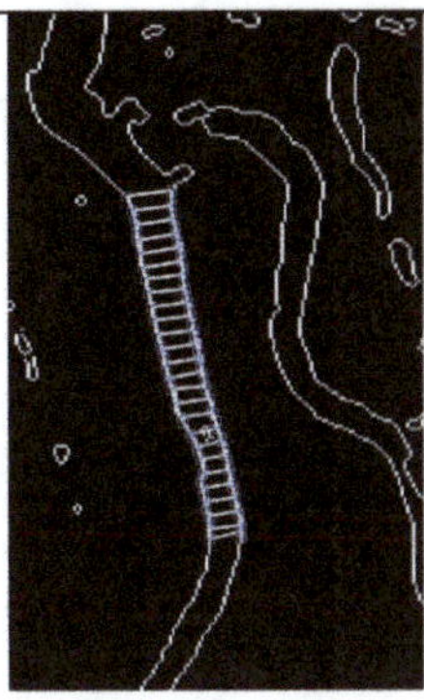 | 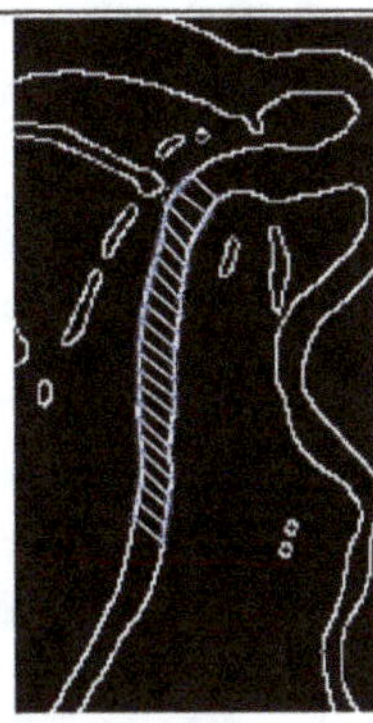 | 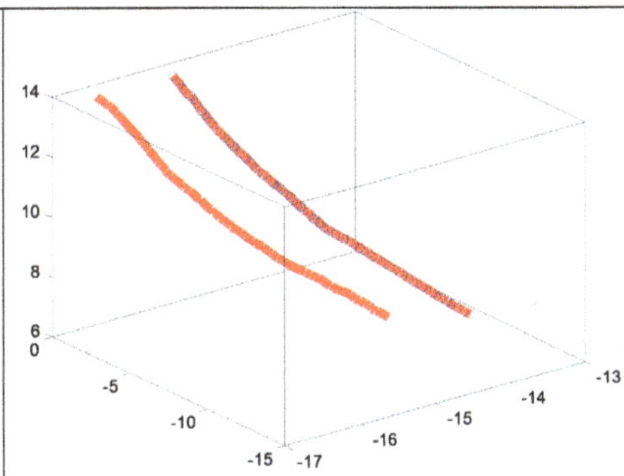 |
|---|---|---|
| First projection of the circumflex coronary | Second projection of the circumflex coronary | 3D reconstruction from the two views |

The normalized QCA graphic has on abscise the normalized vessel's segment length and on its ordinate the variation of the normalized cross-sectional areas along the vessel as presented in Figure 4. As was expected, the cross-sectional areas don't differ significantly due to the absence of stenosis on the vessel. With the geometric approach, the vessel's length is computed for both projections as 3.43 cm for the first view and 3.52 cm for the second view and after the 3D reconstruction as 3.68 cm.

The entire process of finding the vessel segment geometry and generating the quantification coronary angiography lasted approximately 9.5 seconds.

*Figure 4. QCA of the 3D reconstruction vessel's segment*

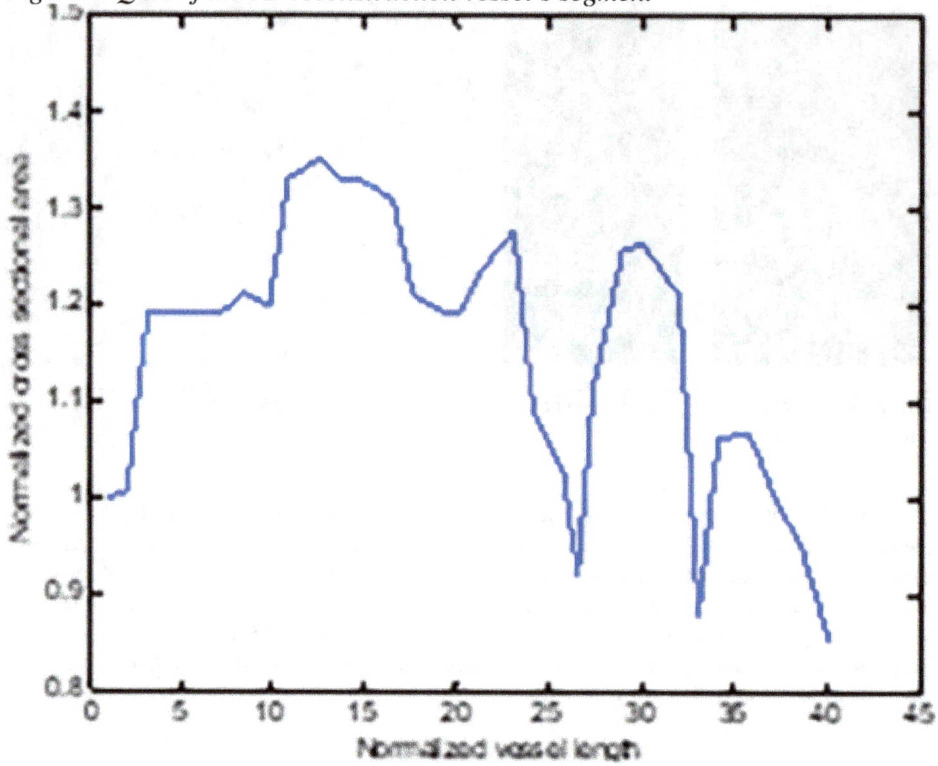


computational fluid dynamics analysis using the velocity or flow estimation as boundary conditions.

### 4.3.2. Stenosis artery case

An artery with pronounced stenosis was chosen as the reference for testing the algorithm in the disease cases. Medical acquisition data included a medical report on the severity of stenosis provided by the equipment software and the visual diagnosis of the physician.

A segment comprising the stenosis was tagged into two projections. To determine the radius evolution along the segment, a 3D reconstruction was performed, and the results are presented in Table 7.

*Table 7. 3D dimensional reconstruction of a stenosis vessel's edges*

| 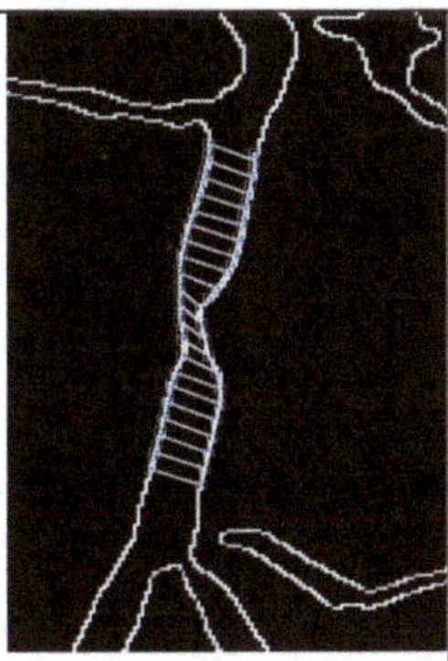 | 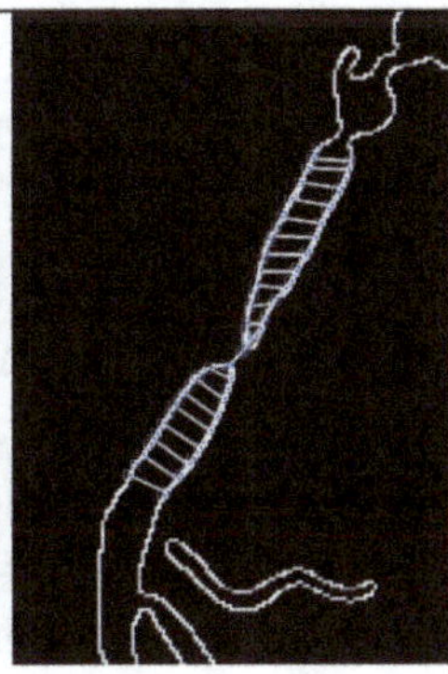 | 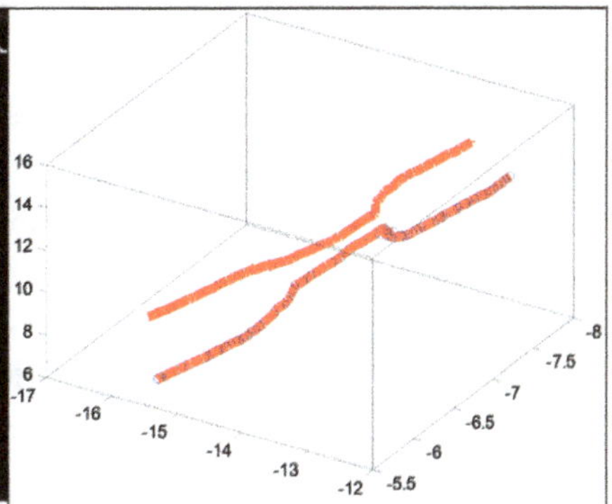 |
|---|---|---|
| Cross sectional axes along the vessel in the first projection | Cross sectional axes along the vessel in the second projection | 3D reconstruction of radius evolution from two views |

The QCA graphic was generated and compared with that extracted from the medical report and Siemens Axiom Artis Zee angiograph software, and the results are shown in Figure 5. The maximum and minimum cross-sectional areas are shown in both graphics to help the physician better quantify the stenosis.

*Figure 5. The comparison between the QCA determination from the 3D reconstruction algorithm (a) and the corresponding one performed on the angiograph (b)*

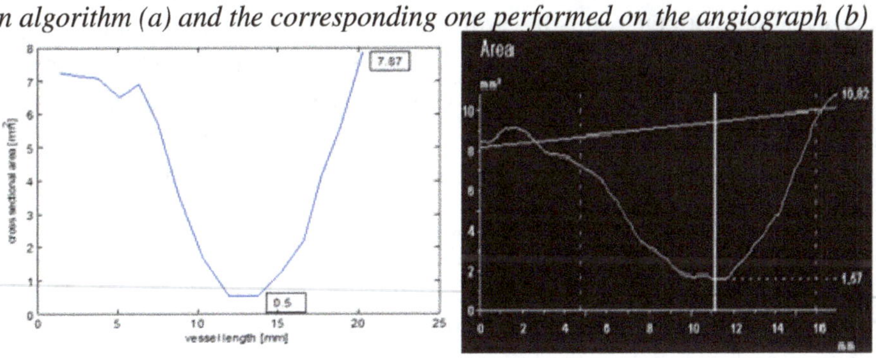


The percentage area of stenosis was approximately 80-90% based on the physician's visual inspection. For a more objective perspective, the QCA graphic was generated, and the parameter of stenosis severity (SS) was determined using the following equation:

$$SS\left(\%\right) = \frac{S_{max} - S}{S_{max}} \bullet 100 \tag{19}$$

Where $S_{max}$ is the maximum cross-sectional area, and $S_{min}$ is the minimum cross-sectional area.

As shown in Figure 5(a), $S_{max}$ is 7.87 $mm^2$ and $S_{min}$ is 0.5 $mm^2$, which means that the parameter SS is 93%. In Figure 5 (b), $S_{max}$ is 10.82 $mm^2$ and $S_{min}$ is 1.57 $mm^2$, indicating a stenosis of 92%. The results are consistent with these three reports. This analysis also validates the centerline and border detection algorithms and their 3D reconstruction.

The data were acquired in the normal state of the patient, and the relative coronary flow reserve estimation from angiography could not be determined because of the lack of data from the hyperemic state. Still, 3D models can reveal communication of intricate congenital malformations, particularly for lesions involving twists, loops, or abnormal connections.

## 4.4. Challenges and Future Directions

The challenges of the presented techniques are patient movement artifacts especially for children, difficulties in capturing small vessels, potentially faster heart rates due to medical investigations, radiation dose considerations both for patients and physicians, the need for high-quality spatial and temporal resolution. The validation is based on visual inspection which makes it dependent on clinician's expertise and high-resolution imaging.

The presented workflow includes the vessel diameters and lengths detection in 3D space along with QCA profile. Still, the method has limitations in fully capturing the complexity of the 3D anatomy from 2D projections. The blood flow and velocity, the angles between branching vessels, relative positions of great arteries, relation of a vascular ring to the trachea/esophagus, tortuosity indices, surface areas and volumes of structures are not explicitly computed in this study, and they could be beneficial in pediatric cardiology.

The characterizing of the vessel shape, tortuosity, and potential stenoses can be applied to congenital vessel issues (e.g., coarctation of the aorta, pulmonary artery stenosis, vascular rings, anomalous coronary origins).

Future work can include the following:

- developing standardized pipelines for automated 3D reconstruction and analysis across large multicenter cohorts.

- integration of the presented results with other data modalities such as clinical and genetic data, cellular imaging, fetal imaging, functional data onto the 3D models, can be done using multimodal artificial intelligence models.
- create collaborative studies with clinicians or pilot deployments to underline real-world feasibility and medical outcomes.

## 4. DISCUSSION AND CONCLUSIONS

The vascular system is a complex structure that is regulated by several factors: chemical, biological and mechanical. It is necessary to understand the interaction of these factors in order to shape the physiological and anatomic properties of the blood flow through the vessels.

In this chapter, the focus is on the blood vessels' pathologies due to their worrisome spreading in both developing and industrialized countries. The abnormal functioning of the circulatory systems is revealed geometrically in the structure of the vessels and hemodynamically in the perturbations of the blood flow. There is a need for a good spatial resolution image for detecting even the small vessels and for a functional image which can give information about hemodynamic patterns. The idea is to create or adapt some post-processing methods for actual medical imaging for tackling both needs.

The goal of this study is not to replace the physicians, therefore the human intelligence, but to help them to investigate the medical images in order to establish the diagnosis of some important vascular diseases, such as atherosclerosis and congenital heart disease.

Human intelligence has enabled the construction of extraordinary things which raise the human condition and the life expectancy, but sometimes it finds its helplessness in the solving of some problems which strictly relate to its organism, such as the physiology and pathophysiology of blood circulation.

Human vision has consistently captivated researchers, leading to the emergence of computer vision. A significant advancement in this discipline is the restoration of stereoscopic vision. This process is characterized by the analogy of two eyes to two closely positioned cameras. The images captured by these cameras are then synthesized by a computer, as the brain does, using a specialized algorithm to reproduce a three-dimensional image.

Vascular diseases are reflected by problems in transporting the blood into the vessels, also called hemodynamic disorders. Medical imaging is an indispensable procedure in the diagnosis and treatment evaluation of these diseases. In the last years, digital medical imaging has opened a new multidisciplinary field of research where medical staff as long as engineers are struggling to solve the problems of accurate detection and healing of different kinds of diseases.

The possibility to detect blood flow, which is an important physiological parameter will enhance medical images. The temporal and spatial analyses will generate a huge amount of one-dimensional signals and images to be processed and stored. Computational fluid dynamics models will capture these parameters as boundary conditions for analyzing the physiological systems of the human body and will generate predictions of the vascular diseases evolutions.

The important improvements made in medical imaging and the development of high-power computational algorithms and machines, favor these approaches. The ultrasound imaging of the heart can quantify some hemodynamic parameters, but their image quality is poor, especially in investigating the small vessels such as the coronary vessels. A more accurate alternative is the cardiac catheterization which is a more invasive technique which gives only velocity or pressure measurements.

A minimally invasive method which gives geometry, and the flow parameters of the blood vessels can be the X-ray angiography. It has a good spatial and temporal resolution, and it has a signal to noise ratio superior to other imagistic methods, such as the ultrasound images. Still, from the point of view of image processing, the x-ray emission and detection give a series of noises hard to quantify and eliminate.

For atherosclerosis, the physician visually identifies the problematic vessel into the angiograms, and the vascular analysis can be performed locally, for shortening the computing time. Therefore, a manual selection of the vessels' centerline can be performed by the specialist into a dedicated graphical user interface. Moreover, there is also implemented a semi-automatic radius estimation, using the densitometric information of the lines perpendicular to the centerline and a more automatic method based on Canny edge detection.

3D reconstruction from two angiographic projection views of congenital heart disease patients can contribute to unraveling the underlying etiological factors. Also, 3D reconstruction is very important in catheterization laboratories for measuring the absolute vessel length and radius to quantify stenosis severity. Subsequently, the geometric parameters, absolute velocity, and blood flow can be determined from the acquired data.

The location parameters of the C-arm system and the mismatch between the corresponding points in both views were corrected using an optimization algorithm. Finally, the results were validated by comparing the lengths of the vessels computed using dedicated software installed on the angiograph.

The QCA graphic was determined using an automatic method for radius detection compared to the one generated by the Siemens Axiom Artis Zee software implemented on the angiograph, which assumes a manual selection of the centerline and a semi-automatic method to find the vessel edges.

Nevertheless, challenges remain, including vessel tortuosity and pulsating multi-directional flow. Furthermore, complications arise from the need for geometric and densitometric data calibration along with issues related to the uneven distribution of contrast agents within the vessels.

The methods described herein do not require invasive procedures or supplementary data beyond monoplane series angiography. These non-invasive methods provide valuable information for children or adults with congenital heart defects to create detailed 3D models of anomalous vessels, for mapping complex congenital defects for surgical planning, for understanding coronary patterns, and for performing Comparing the 3D morphology of acquired versus congenital lesions using similar analysis techniques might highlight fundamental differences in their structural characteristics, reflecting their different etiologies (developmental error vs. degenerative/inflammatory process). Conversely, finding unexpected similarities might prompt investigation into shared underlying pathways or later remodeling processes.

Accurate 3D reconstructions are vital for planning complex surgeries for congenital heart defects and associated vascular anomalies. Studying the post-surgical 3D anatomy and blood flow can help assess the effectiveness of the intervention.

Understanding how a specific congenital impairment in 3D structure impacts surgical outcomes can indirectly inform the severity and clinical consequences associated with the manifestation of etiology. This can be valuable for prognosis and patient counseling related to the specific type of defect caused by certain etiologies.

Advanced imaging analysis techniques such as 3D reconstruction are useful to gain a deeper, more accurate understanding of the complex 3D anatomy of congenital vascular abnormalities and their functional consequences, which in turn can provide crucial data and insights that inform the study of why these defects occur. The integration of advanced imaging analysis with genetic and developmental data can unlock the secrets of how congenital heart disease originates.

## ACKNOWLEDGMENTS

The research was supported by the grant from The Executive Agency for Higher Education, Research, Development and Innovation Funding (UEFISCDI) contract no. PN-IV-P7-7.1-PED-2024-1882 entitled HEARTS - Holistic evaluation of coronary collaterals patency in correlation with myocardial viability using artificial intelligence-based system.

## REFERENCES

Bourantas, C. V., Kourtis, I. C., Plissiti, M. E., Fotiadis, D. I., Katsouras, C. S., Papafaklis, M. I., & Michalis, L. K. (2005). A method for 3D reconstruction of coronary arteries using biplane angiography and intravascular ultrasound images. *Computerized Medical Imaging and Graphics*, *29*(8), 597–606. DOI: 10.1016/j.compmedimag.2005.07.001 PMID: 16278063

Blondel, C., Malandain, G., Vaillant, R., & Ayache, N. (2006). Reconstruction of coronary arteries from a single rotational X-ray projection sequence. *IEEE Transactions on Medical Imaging*, *25*(5), 653–663. DOI: 10.1109/tmi.2006.873224 PMID: 16689269

Blondel, C., Vaillant, R., Devernay, F., Malandain, G., & Ayache, N. (2002). Automatic trinocular 3D reconstruction of coronary artery centerlines from rotational X-ray angiography. In *Proc* (pp. 1073–1078). Computer Assisted Radiology and Surgery., DOI: 10.1007/978-3-642-56168-9_139

Bridget, K., & Fuster, V. (2010). *Promoting Cardiovascular Health in the Developing World: A Critical Challenge to Achieve Global Health*. National Academies Press., DOI: 10.1093/ww/9780199540884.013.u251090

Brost, A., Strobel, N., Yatziv, L., Gilson, W., Meyer, B., Hornegger, J., Lewin, J., & Wacker, F. (2009b), Geometric Accuracy of 3-D X-Ray Image-Based Localization from Two C-Arm Views, Workshop on Geometric Accuracy In Image Guided Interventions-Medical Image Computing and Computer Assisted Interventions, MICCAI, pp. 12-19

Brost, A., Strobel, N., Yatziv, L., Gilson, W., Meyer, B., Hornegger, J., Lewin, J., & Wacker, F. (2009a). *Accuracy of x-ray image-based 3D localization from two C-arm views: a comparison between an ideal system and a real device, Medical Imaging 2009: Visualization, Image-Guided Procedures, and Modeling* (Vol. 726). SPIE., DOI: 10.1117/12.811147

Cheriet, F., & Meunier, J. (1999). Self-calibration of a biplane X-ray imaging system for an optimal three dimensional reconstruction. *Computerized Medical Imaging and Graphics*, *23*, 133–141. DOI: 10.1016/s0895-6111(99)00006-3 PMID: 10397356

Dahl, A., Hernandez-Meneses, M., & Perissinotti, A.. (2021). Echocardiography and FDG-PET/CT scan in gram-negative bacteremia and cardiovascular infections. *Current Opinion in Infectious Diseases*, *34*, 728–736. DOI: 10.1097/qco.0000000000000781 PMID: 34751186

Dumay, A. C. M., & Reiber, J. H. C., Gerbrands, Jan J. (1994). Determination of Optimal Angiographic Viewing Angles: Basic Principles and Evaluation Study. *IEEE Transactions on Medical Imaging*, *13*(1). Advance online publication. DOI: 10.1109/42.276141 PMID: 18218480

Esthappan, J., Harauchi, H., & Hoffmann, K. R. (1998). Evaluation of imaging geometries calculated from biplane images. *Medical Physics*, *25*(6), 965–975. DOI: 10.1118/1.598275 PMID: 9650187

Garcia, J. A., Chen, J., Hansgen, A., Wink, O., Movassaghi, B., & Messenger, J. C. (2007). Rotational angiography (RA) and three-dimensional imaging (3-DRA): An available clinical tool. *The International Journal of Cardiovascular Imaging*, *23*, 9–13. DOI: 10.1007/s10554-006-9088-5 PMID: 16779617

Gould, K. L., & Johnson, N. P. (2017). Coronary CT angiography with PET perfusion imaging: Hybrid or hype? *JACC: Cardiovascular Imaging*, *10*, 1371–1373. DOI: 10.1016/j.jcmg.2016.09.033 PMID: 28528157

Graß, M., Schmitt, H., Rasche, V., Haehnel, S., Schramm, O., Hartmann, M., & Sartor, K. (2001), A method for 3D flow determination based on X-ray rotational angiography, International Congress Series 1230, pp. 408–414, https://doi.org/DOI: 10.1016/s0531-5131(01)00091-7

Gurav, A., Revaiah, P. C., Tsai, T. Y., Miyashita, K., Tobe, A., Oshima, A., Sevestre, E., Garg, S., Aben, J. P., Reiber, J. H. C., Morel, M. A., Lee, C. W., Koo, B. K., Biscaglia, S., Collet, C., Bourantas, C., Escaned, J., Onuma, Y., & Serruys, P. W. (2024, November 25). Coronary angiography: A review of the state of the art and the evolution of angiography in cardio therapeutics. *Frontiers in Cardiovascular Medicine*, *11*, 1468888. DOI: 10.3389/fcvm.2024.1468888 PMID: 39654943

Hentschke, C. M., Serowy, S., Janiga, G., Rose, G., & Tönnies, K. D. (2011), Estimating blood flow velocity in angiographic image data, Proc. SPIE Volume 7964, Medical Imaging 2011: Visualization, Image-Guided Procedures, and Modelling, 79640Y, https://doi.org/DOI: 10.1117/12.878019

Hoffmann, K. R., Sen, A., Lan, L., Chua, K. G., Esthappan, J., & Mazzucco, M. (2000). A system for determination of 3D vessel tree centerlines from biplane images. *International Journal of Cardiac Imaging, 16*, 315–330. DOI: 10.1023/a:1026528209003 PMID: 11215917

Horz, T., & Kowarschik, M. (2013), Temporal Difference encoding for angiographic image sequences, United States Patent no US2013/0077839 A1

Hu, Y., Xie, L., Nunes, J. C., Bellanger, J. J., Bedossa, M., & Toumoulin, C. (2010). ECG gated tomographic reconstruction for 3-D rotational coronary angiography. *Annual International Conference of the IEEE Engineering in Medicine and Biology Society, 2010*, 3614–3617. DOI: 10.1109/iembs.2010.5627449 PMID: 21096844

Karim, R., Blake, L.-E., & Inoue, J.. (2018). Algorithms for left atrial wall segmentation and thickness—Evaluation on an open-source CT and MRI image database. *Medical Image Analysis*. PMID: 30208355

Khan, M.A.U., Khan, R.B., Bilal, S., Jamil A., ShahA. M., (2008), Enhancement of Angiogram Images using Pseudo Color Processing, Information Technology Journa,l Volume(1), pp. 210 - 214

Law, A. K. W., Zhu, H., & Chan, F. H. Y. (2003), 3D Reconstruction of Coronary Artery using Biplane Angiography, Proceedings of the 25, Annual Intemational Conference of the IELE 1MUS Cancun, Mexico

Lourakis, M. I. A. (2005). *A Brief Description of the Levenberg-Marquardt Algorithm Implemened by levmar, free paper, Institute of Computer Science Foundation for Research and Technology - Hellas (FORTH)*. GREECE.

Movassaghi, B., Garcia, J. A., Grass, M., Schaefer, D., Rasche, V., Wink, O., Chen, J. Y., Groves, B. M., Messenger, J. C., & Carroll, J. D. (2006). Three-dimensional gated reconstructed images of the coronary arteries based on rotational coronary angiography: First in human results. *Circulation, 114*, 507–507.

Movassaghi, B., Rasche, V., Grass, M., Viergever, M. A., & Niessen, W. J. (2004). A quantitative analysis of 3-D coronary modeling from two or more projection images. *IEEE Transactions on Medical Imaging, 23*(12), 1517–1531. PMID: 15575409

Nagueh, S. F., Smiseth, O. A., & Appleton, C. P.. (2016). Recommendations for the evaluation of left ventricular diastolic function by Echocardiography: An update from the American Society of Echocardiography and the European Association of Cardiovascular Imaging. *European Heart Journal Cardiovascular Imaging, 17*, 1321–1360. PMID: 27422899

Narayan, P., Richter, F., & Morton, S. (2024). Genetics and etiology of congenital heart disease. *Current Topics in Developmental Biology, 156*, 297–331. DOI: 10.1016/bs.ctdb.2024.01.009 PMID: 38556426

Pandey, R. K., & Rathore, Y. K. (2025, May). Deep learning in 3D cardiac reconstruction: A systematic review of methodologies and dataset. *Medical & Biological Engineering & Computing, 63*(5), 1271–1287. DOI: 10.1007/s11517-024-03273-y PMID: 39753994

Radeva, P., Toledo, R., Von Land, C., & Villanueva, J. (1998). *3D vessel reconstruction from biplane angiograms using snakes, Comput.* Cardiol., DOI: 10.1109/cic.1998.731988

Rischpler, C., Nekolla, S. G., & Kunze, K. P.. (2015). PET/MRI of the heart. *Seminars in Nuclear Medicine, 45*, 234–247. DOI: 10.1053/j.semnuclmed.2014.12.004 PMID: 25841278

Sachdeva R, Armstrong AK, Arnaout R, Grosse-Wortmann L, Han BK, Mertens L, Moore RA, Olivieri LJ, Parthiban A, Powell AJ. (2024) Novel Techniques in Imaging Congenital Heart Disease: JACC Scientific Statement. J Am Coll Cardiol. Jan 2;83(1):63-81, https://doi.org/ DOI: 10.1016/j.jacc.2023.10.025

Shechter, G. (2004). *Respiratory Motion of the Heart: Implications for Magnetic Resonance Coronary Angiography, PhDThesis*. Johns Hopkins University.

Shechter, G., & Devernay, F., Coste-Manière, Quyyumi, E.A., McVeigh, E.R. (2003). Three-Dimensional Motion Tracking of Coronary Arteries in Biplane Cineangiograms. *IEEE Transactions on Medical Imaging, 22*(4), 493. DOI: 10.1109/tmi.2003.809090 PMID: 12774895

Silverthorn, D. U. (2012), Human Physiology: An Integrated Approach, 6th Edition, Chapter 14

Sprague, K., Drangova, M., Lehmann, G., Slomka, P., Levin, D., Chow, B., & deKemp, R. (2006). Coronary X-ray angiographic reconstruction and image orientation. *Medical Physics, 33*, 707–718. DOI: 10.1118/1.2143352 PMID: 16878574

Tache, I. A. (2017). *Three-Dimensional Reconstruction and Hemodynamic Information Extraction from Monoplane Angiography, Patient-specific Hemodynamic Computations: Application to Personalized Diagnosis of Cardiovascular Pathologies*. Springer International Publishing., DOI: 10.1007/978-3-319-56853-9_6

Thackeray, J. T., Derlin, T., & Haghikia, A.. (2015). Molecular imaging of the Chemokine receptor CXCR4 after acute myocardial infarction. *JACC: Cardiovascular Imaging, 8*, 1417–1426. DOI: 10.1016/j.jcmg.2015.09.008 PMID: 26577262 van Walsum, T., Schaap, M., Neefjes, L. A., de Graaf, M. A., Dijkstra, J., van der Giessen, A. G., Niessen, W. J. (2003). Three-dimensional guide wire visualization from 3DRA using monoplane fluoroscopic imaging, Proceedings Volume 5029, Medical Imaging 2003: Visualization, Image-Guided Procedures, and Display

Wächter, I. (2009), 3D Reconstruction of Cerebral Blood Flow and Vessel Morphology from X-Ray Rotational Angiography, Phd thesis, Department of Medical Physics and Bioengineering, University College London

Wagner, A., Mahrholdt, H., & Holly, T. A.. (2003). Contrast-enhanced MRI and routine single photon emission computed tomography (SPECT) perfusion imaging for detection of subendocardial myocardial infarcts: An imaging study. *Lancet, 361*, 374–379. DOI: 10.1016/s0140-6736(03)12389-6 PMID: 12573373

Wagner, M. G., Kutlu, A. Z., Davis, B., Raval, A. N., Laeseke, P. F., & Speidel, M. A. (2024). Topology observing 3D device reconstruction from continuous-sweep limited angle fluoroscopy. *Medical Physics, 51*(4), 2882–2892. DOI: 10.1002/mp.16954 PMID: 38308822

Yang, J., Wang, Y., Liu, Y., Tang, S., & Chen, W. (2009). Novel Approach for 3-D Reconstruction of Coronary Arteries from Two Uncalibrated Angiographic Images. *IEEE Transactions on Image Processing, 18*(7). Advance online publication. DOI: 10.1109/tip.2009.2017363 PMID: 19414289

Yang, X. Y., Li, Y. M., Wang, J. Y., Jia, Y. H., Yi, Z., & Chen, M. (2025, July 17). Utilizing multimodal artificial intelligence to advance cardiovascular diseases. *Precision Clinical Medicine, 8*(3), pbaf016. Advance online publication. DOI: 10.1093/pcmedi/pbaf016 PMID: 40799363

Zeb, I., Uqaily, R., & Gonuguntla, K.. (2023). Multimodality assessment of high- vs. low-gradient aortic stenosis using echocardiography and cardiac CT. *Journal of Cardiovascular Computed Tomography, 17*, 421–428. PMID: 37806845

Zhang, Z. (1996). *Epipolar Geometry in Stereo, Motion and Object Recognition: A Unified Approach*. Springer.

Chapter 12

# Integrating AI and Edge Computing in Congenital Heart Disease Management

**Sachin Jain**
https://orcid.org/0000-0002-2948-7858
*Ajay Kumar Garg Engineering College, Ghaziabad, India*

**Vishal Jain**
https://orcid.org/0000-0003-1126-7424
*Kuala Lumpur University of Science and Technology, Malaysia & Vivekananda Institute of Professional Studies, New Delhi, India*

**Danish Ather**
https://orcid.org/0000-0003-1596-5553
*Amity University, Tashkent, Uzbekistan*

**Golnoosh Manteghi**
*Faculty of Architecture and Built Environment, Kuala Lumpur University of Science and Technology, Malaysia*

**Abu Bakar Abdul Hamid**
https://orcid.org/0009-0007-5177-8145
*Kuala Lumpur University of Science and Technology, Malaysia*

## ABSTRACT

*Heart disease at birth is still one of the most common birth defects, affecting 8–10 out of every 1,000 live births around the world. Even though paediatric cardiology*

DOI: 10.4018/979-8-3373-3735-7.ch012

*and surgery have gotten better, it is still hard to find heart problems early, make a correct diagnosis, and treat them effectively, especially in places with few resources. CHD has a complicated cause that includes genetic, environmental, and exposomic factors. This chapter gives an in-depth look at how Artificial Intelligence (AI) and edge computing are changing the way CHD management is done. First, we look at what causes syndromic and non-syndromic congenital heart disease. Then, we talk about progress in preconception and prenatal screening, such as foetal echocardiography. Integration of AI and edge computing in CHD management holds transformative potential, with practical implications including earlier detection, enhanced accessibility to specialist-level care, reduced healthcare costs, and improved outcomes through standardized protocols.*

## 1. INTRODUCTION TO CONGENITAL HEART DISEASE (CHD)

Congenital heart disease (CHD) refers to a broad spectrum of structural abnormalities of the heart and great vessels that are present at birth. These defects arise from errors during the embryonic development of the cardiovascular system. CHD is the most common type of birth defect, with a global prevalence of approximately 8 to 12 cases per 1,000 live births, and this figure can be higher in prenatal assessments due to pregnancies that do not reach term(Niyogi et al., 2025). The anatomical and physiological complexity of CHD is vast, ranging from simple lesions, such as an atrial septal defect (a hole between the upper chambers of the heart), which may require minimal or no intervention, to highly complex malformations, such as hypoplastic left heart syndrome (underdevelopment of the left side of the heart), which are life-threatening and necessitate a series of complex surgical interventions for survival.

The classification of CHD is typically based on the underlying pathophysiology, which includes defects that cause: (1) increased pulmonary blood flow (e.g., ventricular septal defect, patent ductus arteriosus), (2) decreased pulmonary blood flow, often leading to cyanosis (e.g., Tetralogy of Fallot, pulmonary atresia), (3) obstruction of blood flow out of the heart (e.g., coarctation of the aorta, aortic stenosis), and (4) complex mixing of oxygenated and deoxygenated blood (e.g., transposition of the great arteries, single ventricle defects).

Over the past several decades, monumental advancements in pediatric cardiology, cardiac surgery, and intensive care have dramatically improved survival rates for individuals with CHD. What was once a universally fatal condition in its severe forms has been transformed into a chronic, manageable disease.

## 1.1. Current Challenges in CHD Management

Even though there has been progress, managing congenital heart disease is still a long, hard, and frustrating process for patients, their families, and healthcare systems.

- **Diagnostic Challenges:** Even though prenatal ultrasound and postnatal screening have made early detection better, it can be hard to figure out what's wrong. It's important to get a correct diagnosis as soon as possible for the best outcomes, but this is often hard to do because the early signs aren't always easy to spot, non-specialized centres don't have a lot of them, and there aren't enough paediatric cardiovascular specialists, especially in places with limited resources (Niyogi et al., 2025). Complex imaging methods like echocardiography and cardiac magnetic resonance imaging (CMR) can be hard to interpret because they require a lot of knowledge and can vary from observer to observer (Karatzia et al., 2022).
- **Lifelong Monitoring and Unpredictable Trajectories:** People who have congenital heart defects (CHDs), especially those with moderate to severe defects, need to be watched over their whole lives. They always have a chance of long-term problems, like arrhythmias, heart failure, pulmonary hypertension, thromboembolic events, and having to have more surgery (Niyogi et al., 2025)(Bozyel et al., 2024). The clinical course is often hard to predict, with stable periods broken up by sudden worsening. Current monitoring methods, which rely on regular clinic visits and imaging studies, don't always pick up on the small, slow changes in the body that happen before something big happens. This means that care is reactive instead of proactive (Vu et al., 2025).
- **Resource and Expertise Limitations:** A small group of highly specialised tertiary care centres handle most of the care for people with complex CHD. This concentration of knowledge makes it hard for many families to get the care they need because of where they live or how to get there (Elvas et al., 2025). Also, the huge amount of data that comes from imaging studies, hemodynamic assessments, and long-term follow-up is very hard for clinicians to handle, which can cause diagnostic delays and mistakes (Gearhart et al., 2025).
- **The Interstage Vulnerability:** Infants with single ventricle physiology, like hypoplastic left heart syndrome, may be the clearest example of how limited current monitoring is. These babies go home for a while called the "interstage" after their first surgery as newborns, which is called the Norwood procedure. This is before their second surgery. There are more deaths than ever before. This is a very dangerous time. These weak babies are in a dangerous physiological state, and small changes in their health can cause it to quickly

and severely worsen. The current standard of care, which includes checking the patient's weight and oxygen levels at home every so often, isn't always enough to spot impending crises in time (Elvas et al., 2025).

## 1.2. The Promise of Emerging Technologies: AI and Edge Computing

To deal with these big problems, we need to change the way we manage congenital heart disease from one that is reactive and focused on the hospital to one that is proactive, personalised, and focused on the patient. So this is where the coming together of two game-changing technologies, AI and Edge Computing, holds unimaginable promise.

The fields of artificial intelligence (AI), especially machine learning (ML) and deep learning (DL), are all about making computers that can learn complicated patterns and make smart choices from huge amounts of data (Ren et al., 2025). When it comes to congenital heart disease, AI can look at large amounts of medical data, like pictures, physiological signals, and electronic health records, to make diagnoses more accurate, guess how patients will do, and make personalised treatment plans that go beyond what humans can do (Hizem et al., 2025).

It is a type of decentralised computing that moves processing and storage closer to where the data comes from, in this case, the patient (Ren et al., 2025). Edge computing does analysis on or near the device itself instead of sending raw data from sensors and wearable tech to a central cloud to be processed. This method cuts down on latency (delay) by a large amount, protects data better, and makes monitoring systems more reliable, especially in places where internet access is slow (Vu et al., 2025).

The integration of these two technologies creates a powerful synergy known as **Edge-AI** or the Artificial Intelligence of Things (AIoT)(Hizem et al., 2025). By using advanced AI models on small, low-power edge devices, we can create smart, always-on monitoring systems that monitor patients' health in real time at the point of care. This combination could improve CHD treatment by detecting complications early, allowing doctors to treat them, and informing patients and their families. This chapter will discuss AI and edge computing's roles, but more importantly, how they can work together to change congenital heart disease treatment from prenatal diagnosis to lifelong management.

## 2. THE ROLE OF ARTIFICIAL INTELLIGENCE IN REVOLUTIONIZING CHD CARE

Using advanced AI models on small, low-power edge devices, we can create smart, continuous monitoring systems that check patients' health at the point of care. This combination could revolutionise CHD treatment by detecting complications early, allowing doctors to prevent them, and informing patients and their families. In this chapter, we will discuss AI and edge computing and how they can work together to change congenital heart disease treatment from prenatal diagnosis to lifelong management (Gearhart et al., 2025). AI can see patterns that humans can't, which is helpful when treating congenital heart disease (CHD), which has many small differences in anatomy and blood flow and requires lifelong management (Vu et al., 2025). AI is used in CHD from diagnosis to prognostic modelling.

### 2.1. AI-Powered Diagnostics in CHD

A correct and timely diagnosis is the most important part of managing a congenital heart defect (CHD). AI algorithms, especially deep learning models, have done a great job of making diagnostic processes faster, more accurate, and more consistent.

#### 2.1.1. Enhancing Prenatal and Neonatal Screening

Prenatal ultrasounds are the earliest time that CHD can be found. But foetal echocardiography is a very specialised skill, and the rates at which congenital heart defects are found vary a lot. Sonographers and obstetricians can use AI to help them do their jobs better. Deep learning models can automatically identify normal anatomical views, flag abnormalities, and group certain CHD types after being trained on thousands of foetal heart images (Niyogi et al., 2025). This can improve screening consistency, reduce missed diagnoses, and ensure high-risk pregnancies are referred to paediatric cardiology specialists for counselling and delivery planning (Williams et al., 2025).

AI goes beyond imaging. Also used for genetic screening. AI algorithms can find congenital heart disease-risky genetic variants and complex gene interactions in large genomic datasets. This helps determine a family's prenatal risk and provide better advice (Bozyel et al., 2024). AI-enhanced ECG analysis is promising for post-natal screening. ECGs are easy and painless, but newborn heart disease screening ECGs can be confusing. Deep learning models can detect significant congenital heart disease in neonatal ECGs as well as paediatric cardiologists. This allows for low-cost, large-scale baby screening (Vu et al., 2025).

### 2.1.2. Automated Image Analysis and Interpretation

Postnatal screening with AI-enhanced electrocardiogram (ECG) analysis is promising. ECGs for newborn heart disease screening are simple and painless, but they can be confusing. Deep learning models have been shown to detect significant congenital heart disease in neonatal ECGs as well as paediatric cardiologists. This allows for mass, low-cost baby screening.

- **Echocardiography:** Deep learning models, especially CNNs, excel at image analysis. They can automate critical tasks like segmenting cardiac chambers, calculating functional parameters like ejection fraction, and identifying anatomical abnormalities (Niyogi et al., 2025). This automation not only saves significant time but also improves the reproducibility and standardization of measurements. Explainable AI models are now demonstrating clinical utility in real-time image classification, even in the challenging neonatal and infant populations(Bozyel et al., 2024).
- **Cardiac MRI and CT:** CMR provides detailed anatomical and functional information crucial for managing complex CHD. However, post-processing CMR scans to extract quantitative data can take longer than the scan itself(Gearhart et al., 2025). AI can dramatically accelerate this workflow. Deep learning pipelines have been developed for automated contouring of ventricles in complex single-ventricle patients, a task that is particularly laborious when done manually(Nemani et al., 2024). Similarly, in cardiac CT, AI algorithms can perform automated coronary calcium scoring and characterize atherosclerotic plaques, which is becoming increasingly relevant for the aging ACHD population(Nemani et al., 2024). By using AI for image reconstruction, it is also possible to generate high-quality images from undersampled data, potentially reducing scan times and the need for sedation in young children(Niyogi et al., 2025).

### 2.1.3. Advanced ECG and Hemodynamic Analysis

Beyond basic screening, AI can extract far more information from physiological signals than is possible with conventional methods. AI programmes can look at ECG waveforms and find small patterns that could mean arrhythmias, which are a common long-term problem for people with congenital heart disease. Deep learning can also do more than just human interpretation. For example, an AI model trained on ECGs can figure out a patient's risk of future bad events, even if a human expert sees the ECG as normal. AI is also being used for more advanced signal processing for hemodynamic assessment. This makes it easier and more accurate to look at data from cardiac catheterizations and other invasive monitoring procedures.

## 2.2. AI in Treatment Planning and Intervention

After a diagnosis is made, the next most important thing is to come up with the best way to treat the problem. For complicated CHD, this usually means complicated surgeries or catheter-based procedures. AI can help doctors make these important decisions by giving them powerful tools.

### 2.2.1. Personalized Surgical and Interventional Planning

CHD anatomy is so diverse that a "one-size-fits-all" surgery is rarely enough. AI personalises pre-procedure planning. Advanced segmentation algorithms on CT or MRI scans allow AI to create 3D models of each patient's heart and great vessels. These virtual models can help surgeons and interventional cardiologists visualise complex anatomy, test different surgical approaches, and anticipate issues before making an incision. This can improve surgery accuracy, safety, and results. AI can simulate the effects of surgery on blood flow or determine where and how big a stent or valve should be.

### 2.2.2. Clinical Decision Support Systems (CDSS)

AI-powered Clinical Decision Support Systems (CDSS) use patient data like medical history, imaging results, lab tests, and genomics to make evidence-based treatment recommendations. They can help the clinical team smartly with these systems. A CDSS could analyse a patient's profile and suggest a treatment or warn doctors about a drug interaction based on thousands of previous cases. These systems are meant to supplement clinicians' knowledge and ensure decisions are based on the most current evidence (Bozyel et al., 2024).

*Equation 1: Example of a Simplified Risk Prediction Formula*

CDSS risk prediction models are crucial. . While real-world models are highly complex, a simplified logistic regression equation can illustrate the concept:

$$P(Event) = 1 / (1 + e(\beta \ + \beta X \ + \beta X \ + ... + \beta X \ ))$$

Where:
P(Event) is the probability of a specific outcome (e.g., 1-year mortality).
\`e\` is the base of the natural logarithm.
\`$\beta_0$\` is the intercept.
\`$\beta_1$\`, \`$\beta_2$\`, ..., \`β \` are the coefficients for each predictor variable, determined by the machine learning model during training.
\`$X_1$\`, \`$X_2$\`, ..., \`X \` are the patient-specific predictor variables (e.g., \`$X_1$\`=age at surgery, \`$X_2$\`=ventricular ejection fraction, \`$X_3$\`=presence of a genetic syndrome).
This equation takes multiple patient factors, weights them according to their learned importance (\`β\` coefficients), and outputs a personalized risk score, which can then be used to guide clinical decisions.

## 2.3. AI for Prognosis and Long-Term Management

The journey for a patient with CHD does not end after surgery. Lifelong monitoring and management of chronic complications are paramount. AI is uniquely capable of analyzing longitudinal data to predict future events and personalize follow-up care.

### 2.3.1. Risk Stratification and Outcome Prediction

One of the most powerful applications of AI is in predicting the future. By training machine learning models on large, multicenter clinical datasets, researchers can develop highly accurate models for risk stratification. These models can predict a wide range of outcomes, such as the likelihood of developing heart failure, the risk of sudden cardiac death, or the 5-year transplant-free survival rate for infants with specific conditions like hypoplastic left heart syndrome (Niyogi et al., 2025).

### 2.3.2. Predictive Analytics for Postoperative Care

After surgery, AI can help in the intensive care unit (ICU). Bedside monitor data like heart rate, blood pressure, and oxygen saturation can be constantly monitored by algorithms to detect small signs of worsening hours before a person notices them. The ICU team can act quickly with these early warning systems for sepsis and cardiac arrest. AI can predict patient reactions to drugs and ventilator settings to improve care. This can lead to more personalised and effective critical care.

*Figure 1. Flow Chart of an AI-based Clinical Decision Support System for CHD*

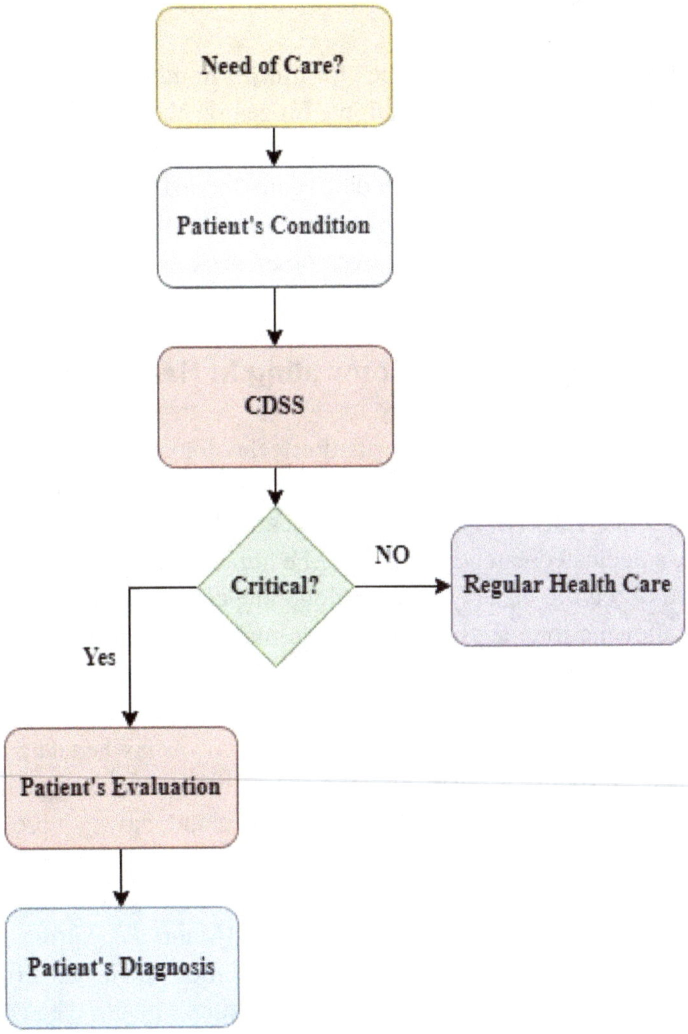

Flow chart in Figure 1 outlines the workflow of an integrated AI-driven CDSS for CHD management. It begins with the aggregation of diverse patient data. This data is fed into an AI core consisting of several machine learning models for diagnosis, risk prediction, and treatment simulation. The outputs from the AI core are synthesized with a knowledge base of clinical guidelines to generate actionable recommendations. These recommendations are presented to the clinician through an intuitive interface, who then makes the final, informed decision, leading to a personalized care plan for the patient.

## 3. EDGE COMPUTING: BRINGING COMPUTATION CLOSER TO THE PATIENT

While AI provides the "intelligence" for transforming CHD care, its effectiveness, especially for real-time applications, hinges on the ability to process data quickly, reliably, and securely. The traditional cloud computing model, where data is transmitted from a device to a distant data center for analysis, presents significant limitations in the context of continuous health monitoring. Edge computing emerges as a critical enabling technology that overcomes these barriers by fundamentally changing where data processing occurs(Niyogi et al., 2025).

### 3.1. Fundamentals of Edge Computing in Healthcare

Edge computing is a distributed information technology (IT) architecture in which client data is processed at the periphery of the network, as close to the originating source as possible.(Yeh et al., 2025) In healthcare, the "edge" can be the patient's smartphone, a dedicated gateway device in the home, or even the wearable sensor itself. Instead of relying on a centralized cloud, the computational workload is decentralized, allowing for analysis and decision-making to happen locally.

The key benefits of this paradigm shift are profound:

- **Reduced Latency:** Latency is the time delay between when data is collected and when a response is received. For a critically ill infant with CHD at home, every second counts. Transmitting data to the cloud, having it processed, and waiting for an alert to be sent back can introduce critical delays. Edge computing enables near-instantaneous analysis of vital signs, allowing for real-time anomaly detection and immediate alerts.(Maurya & Verma, 2025) This can be the difference between a timely intervention and a catastrophic event.
- **Enhanced Data Privacy and Security:** Children's health data is exceptionally sensitive.(Williams et al., 2025) The cloud-centric model requires trans-

mitting large volumes of raw, identifiable physiological data over the internet, increasing the attack surface for potential data breaches. With edge computing, most of the raw data is processed and analyzed locally on a device the patient or family controls.(Karimov & Zaim Gökbay, 2025) Only essential information, such as summarized insights or critical alerts, needs to be transmitted to the hospital, significantly minimizing privacy risks.

- **Improved Reliability and Continuity of Care:** Cloud-based monitoring systems are dependent on a stable, high-bandwidth internet connection. In rural areas or for families with unreliable internet access, this can lead to intermittent monitoring and gaps in data. Edge devices can continue to monitor, process data, and even trigger local alarms (e.g., on a parent's smartphone) without an active internet connection, ensuring a continuous safety net for the patient. The device can store data locally and upload it to the hospital's servers whenever a connection becomes available (Ren et al., 2025).
- **Bandwidth and Cost Efficiency:** Continuously streaming high-frequency physiological data from multiple sensors to the cloud can consume a significant amount of internet bandwidth and incur substantial data transmission costs. By processing data at the edge, the volume of data that needs to be transmitted can be reduced by up to 76%, making long-term monitoring more scalable and affordable (Yeh et al., 2025).

## 3.2. Applications of Edge Computing in Cardiac Monitoring

The conceptual benefits of edge computing translate into tangible, life-saving applications for patients with CHD, particularly in the context of remote patient monitoring (RPM).

### 3.2.1. Real-time Analysis of Wearable Sensor Data

The proliferation of non-invasive wearable biosensors has opened the door to continuous physiological monitoring outside the hospital.(Ren et al., 2025) These sensors, which can be integrated into patches, garments, or smartwatches, can measure a variety of vital signs:

- **Electrocardiogram (ECG):** For heart rate and rhythm analysis.
- **Photoplethysmography (PPG):** An optical technique used in most smartwatches and pulse oximeters to measure heart rate, heart rate variability, and blood oxygen saturation (SpO2).
- **Accelerometers/Gyroscopes:** To monitor activity levels, sleep patterns, and detect falls.

- **Temperature Sensors:** To track core body temperature.

An edge computing device (e.g., a home hub or smartphone) can collect data streams from these wearables and perform real-time analysis directly within the patient's home. Lightweight machine learning models running on the edge device can continuously screen for predefined anomalies, such as tachyarrhythmias, bradycardia, or significant oxygen desaturation (Karatzia et al., 2022).

### 3.2.2. Edge-Powered Implantable Devices

For patients with a high risk of life-threatening arrhythmias, implantable devices like pacemakers and implantable cardioverter-defibrillators (ICDs) are common. The next generation of these devices is incorporating more powerful onboard processors, turning them into sophisticated edge computing nodes. These devices can analyze intracardiac electrograms in real-time to not only deliver immediate therapy when needed but also to detect subtle, pro-arrhythmic patterns that could predict future events. By performing this analysis on the device, battery life is conserved (as data transmission is minimized), and patient privacy is inherently protected.

### 3.2.3. Enabling Remote Patient Monitoring (RPM) at Scale

Edge computing is the key to making large-scale, effective RPM programs for CHD a practical reality. Studies have shown that edge-enabled RPM solutions can significantly reduce hospital readmission rates for cardiovascular patients.(Pozza et al., 2024) For the fragile interstage single ventricle population, a home monitoring system powered by edge computing can provide a level of surveillance that approaches that of an ICU. A home gateway device can collect data from multiple sensors, analyze it in real-time, and use a traffic-light system (red-yellow-green) on a parent's app to indicate the infant's status, providing peace of mind and clear guidance on when to seek medical help. (Niyogi et al., 2025)This immediate feedback loop empowers parents to become active participants in their child's care Table 1 shows the comparison of cloud vs. edge computing for CHD monitoring.

*Table 1. Comparison of Cloud vs. Edge Computing for CHD Monitoring*

| Feature | Cloud Computing Model | Edge Computing Model | Implication for CHD Management |
|---|---|---|---|
| **Data Processing Location** | Centralized, remote data centers | Decentralized, on or near the patient's device | **Edge:** Enables processing independent of internet connectivity. |
| **Latency** | High (seconds to minutes) | Very Low (milliseconds) | **Edge:** Critical for immediate alerts in life-threatening situations. |
| **Data Privacy** | Raw data transmitted over the internet; higher risk | Raw data remains local; only insights are transmitted; lower risk | **Edge:** Safer for sensitive pediatric data. |
| **Internet Dependency** | High; continuous connection required for real-time analysis | Low; can operate offline and sync later | **Edge:** More reliable for patients in areas with poor connectivity. |
| **Bandwidth Requirement** | High; requires streaming of all raw sensor data | Low; transmits only processed results or alerts | **Edge:** More scalable and cost-effective for long-term, multi-sensor monitoring. |
| **Autonomy** | Device is a simple data collector; "dumb" terminal | Device has local intelligence and can make decisions | **Edge:** Creates a more robust and resilient monitoring ecosystem. |

## 4. THE SYNERGY: INTEGRATING AI AND EDGE COMPUTING FOR COMPREHENSIVE CHD MANAGEMENT

While AI and edge computing are powerful technologies in their own right, their true transformative potential is unleashed when they are integrated. This fusion, often termed Edge-AI, creates intelligent systems that can perceive, reason, and act in real-time within the patient's own environment. This synergy allows for the deployment of sophisticated AI-driven insights directly at the point of care, shifting the paradigm from intermittent, reactive check-ups to continuous, proactive, and personalized surveillance.

### 4.1. The Edge-AI (or AIoT) Architecture for CHD

A robust Edge-AI system for CHD management can be conceptualized as a multi-layered architecture, ensuring that data is processed efficiently and securely at the most appropriate location.

*Figure 2. Integrated Edge-AI Architecture for Remote CHD Monitoring*

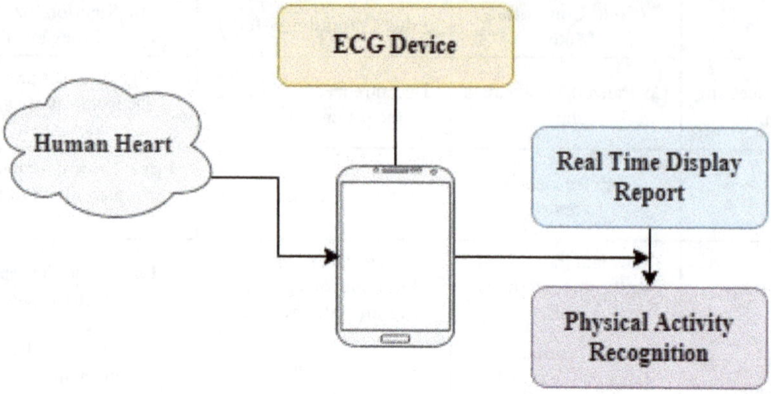


Diagram in Figure 2 illustrates a typical Edge-AI architecture. At the edge (the patient's home), data from various wearable sensors are collected by a central edge device. A lightweight but powerful AI model runs directly on this device, performing real-time analysis to detect anomalies. It provides immediate feedback and alerts to the caregiver's app. Only processed data, summaries, and critical alerts are sent to the cloud/hospital layer. There, the data is securely stored, integrated with the Electronic Health Record (EHR), and visualized on a clinical dashboard for the cardiology team to review. This layered approach maximizes responsiveness and privacy at the edge while enabling long-term and population-level analysis in the cloud.

This architecture consists of three primary layers:

1. **Data Acquisition Layer:** This layer comprises the body-worn sensors and other devices that capture raw physiological and behavioral data. Wearable patches for ECG and breathing, pulse oximeters for SpO2, smart scales for daily weight, and even video cameras for watching how people eat or move are all examples of this (Niyogi et al., 2025).
2. **Edge-AI Processing Layer:** For real-time monitoring, this is what it all works on. A dedicated hub, a tablet, or a powerful smartphone can be used as an edge device. This is where the pre-trained AI models are stored. A lot of the time, these models are tweaked to work best on hardware with limited resources. This is called TinyML. The edge device collects data, processes signals, and finds strange behaviour using AI, all without needing to connect to the cloud (Hizem et al., 2025).
3. **Centralized Analytics and EHR Integration Layer:** This layer, which can be in the hospital's secure cloud or on premise servers, does a number of important things. It receives and archives the summarized insights and alerts from the edge

devices, providing a longitudinal record of the patient's health. This aggregated data can be integrated into the hospital's EHR system, visualized on a clinical dashboard for review, and used to train and refine even more powerful AI models that can identify population-level trends (Williams et al., 2025).

## 4.2. Use Case: A Closed-Loop Monitoring System for Interstage Single Ventricle Patients

The high-risk interstage period for infants with single ventricle physiology is a perfect use case for an Edge-AI system.

1. **Continuous Data Collection:** A patch that measures ECG, heart rate, and breathing rate is sent home with the baby, along with a sock-based pulse oximeter that measures SpO2. A smart scale automatically records their weight daily.
2. **On-Device AI Analysis:** A dedicated gateway in the home collects these data streams via Bluetooth. A multi-modal AI model running on the gateway continuously analyzes these signals in real-time. It has been trained to recognize not just simple threshold breaches (e.g., SpO2 $< 75\%$) but also more complex, subtle patterns that may precede decompensation, such as a gradual increase in resting heart rate combined with decreasing heart rate variability and a plateau in weight gain (Gearhart et al., 2025).
3. **Immediate Alerts and Feedback:** If the edge AI model detects a high-risk pattern, it triggers an immediate, escalating alert. First, an alarm sounds on the parent's smartphone app with clear instructions (e.g., "Check on your baby now. If they are sleeping peacefully, re-check saturations in 5 minutes. If they appear distressed, call the cardiology nurse line immediately."). If the pattern is critical, the system can automatically send a high-priority alert directly to the on-call cardiology team's dashboard.

This closed-loop system provides a constant layer of intelligent surveillance, empowering parents and enabling clinical teams to intervene at the earliest sign of trouble, potentially preventing hospital readmissions and mortality.

### Algorithm 1: Edge-based Anomaly Detection in Vital Signs

#### *Step 1: Initialize Buffers and Parameters*

Create circular buffers to store recent heart rate (HR) and oxygen saturation ($SpO_2$) values.

Example: hr_buffer size = 300 → stores 5 minutes of HR data if sampling every 1 second.

spo2_buffer size = 300 → stores 5 minutes of $SpO_2$ data.

*Step 2: Load Pre-trained AI Models*

Load lightweight AI models suitable for edge devices:
anomaly_detection_model → detects multi-modal anomalies from HR & $SpO_2$ trends.
arrhythmia_model → classifies ECG rhythms (e.g., SVT, VT).

*Step 3: Main Loop for Continuous Monitoring*

Continuously process incoming patient data packets from a streaming source (patientDataStream).

*Step 4: Ingest and Preprocess Data*

Extract timestamp, ECG signal, HR value, and $SpO_2$ value from each data packet.
Apply preprocessing if needed (e.g., normalization, filtering).

*Step 5: Update Data Buffers*

Add latest HR and $SpO_2$ readings to the respective circular buffers.
This ensures a rolling window of recent data for trend analysis.

*Step 6: Run AI Inference at Edge*

Arrhythmia Check (every 2 seconds):
Feed the latest ECG signal to arrhythmia_model.
If prediction indicates critical rhythm (SVT or VT), generate a CRITICAL alert.
Multi-modal Anomaly Check (every 30 seconds):
Extract features from recent HR & $SpO_2$ trends.
Feed features into anomaly_detection_model.
Generate alerts based on anomaly score:
Score > 0.9 → HIGH alert
Score > 0.7 → MEDIUM alert

### 4.3. Federated Learning: Collaborative AI without Compromising Privacy

One of the greatest challenges in applying AI to CHD is data scarcity. While CHD is the most common birth defect, specific subtypes can be quite rare. Training a robust AI model requires a large and diverse dataset, which a single hospital may not possess. Historically, this would necessitate pooling patient data into a central repository, a process fraught with ethical, legal, and logistical hurdles related to patient privacy (Gearhart et al., 2025).

**Federated Learning (FL)** provides an elegant solution to this problem. It is a decentralized machine learning approach that enables model training across multiple locations without ever moving the raw data (Alasmari et al., 2025). The traditional centralized approach, where sensitive patient data from multiple hospitals must be sent to a central server to train a model. The bottom panel illustrates federated learning. Each hospital gets an initial AI model from a central server. Each hospital uses its own private data to train the model in its own area. They don't send back data; instead, they send back the updated model parameters (the "learnings"). These changes are sent to the central server, which then improves the global model and sends it back to the hospitals. This process is repeated, which lets people train models together without ever sharing patient information (Williams et al., 2025).

An initial AI model is sent to each hospital by a central server. Each hospital trains the model with data that is only available to that hospital. They only send the updated model parameters back instead of the data (the "learnings"). The updates are sent to the central server, which then makes a better global model and sends it back to the hospitals. This process happens again and again, which lets people train models together without ever sharing patient information (Maurya & Verma, 2025).

## 5. CHALLENGES, ETHICAL CONSIDERATIONS, AND FUTURE DIRECTIONS

AI and edge computing cannot solve all CHD management issues. To implement it responsibly and successfully, you must overcome technical, practical, and moral issues. We must be cautious, deliberate, and patient when approaching this new technology's promise.

### 5.1. Technical and Practical Challenges

- **Data Quality, Heterogeneity, and Standardization:** Learning makes AI models good. Medical data is inconsistent, comes from different devices and

EHR systems, and is often mislabeled. It is difficult to create large, well-organized CHD datasets for AI model training. This requires a lot of money for data infrastructure and institution cooperation (Gearhart et al., 2025).

- **Model Generalizability and Robustness:** An AI model trained on data from one hospital's patients may not work well with patients at another hospital with different demographics or clinical practises. Making sure models work well with a wide range of people is difficult and requires outside experts to check them with new data before they are used in clinical settings. Federated learning can help, but it must be planned to avoid bias (Williams et al., 2025).
- **Integration into Clinical Workflows:** A complex AI algorithm is useless if it doesn't fit clinicians' daily work. New systems must be simple, provide useful information, and prevent clinicians from developing "alert fatigue," which results from hearing many unnecessary alarms. User-centered interfaces and clear value propositions are crucial for clinician adoption (Niyogi et al., 2025).
- **Hardware and Power Constraints:** Deploying complex AI models on low-power, resource-constrained edge devices is a significant technical challenge. This requires specialized expertise in model optimization and compression (e.g., quantization, pruning) to ensure that the device can perform real-time inference without rapidly draining its battery. The hardware itself must also be robust, comfortable, and suitable for long-term use by pediatric patients, from fragile neonates to active adolescents (Ren et al., 2025).

## 5.2. Ethical and Regulatory Imperatives

The application of powerful predictive technologies to a vulnerable pediatric population raises a host of ethical, legal, and social implications (ELSI) that must be proactively addressed (Jamil Abusamra et al., 2025).

### 5.2.1. Data Privacy and Security

As discussed, pediatric health data is highly sensitive. While edge computing mitigates some risks, security must be a foundational design principle at every level of the system—from the sensor to the edge device to the cloud. Robust encryption, secure authentication protocols, and clear data governance policies are non-negotiable. Crucially, obtaining meaningful informed consent from parents for the collection and use of their child's continuous physiological data is a complex ethical requirement that needs careful consideration (Williams et al., 2025).

### 5.2.2. Algorithmic Bias and Fairness

AI systems learn from historical data, and if that data reflects existing societal or healthcare biases, the AI will learn and potentially amplify those biases. For example, if a risk prediction model is trained predominantly on data from one ethnic group, it may be less accurate for patients from other groups, thus exacerbating health disparities. It is imperative to train and validate AI models on diverse and representative datasets and to continuously audit them for fairness and equity (Karatzia et al., 2022).

### 5.2.3. Transparency and Explainability (XAI)

Many advanced deep learning models operate as "black boxes," meaning it is difficult to understand precisely how they arrive at a particular prediction. In a high-stakes clinical environment, this is problematic. If an AI system recommends a course of action, the clinician needs to understand the underlying rationale to trust the recommendation and take responsibility for the final decision. The field of Explainable AI (XAI) is focused on developing techniques to make AI models more interpretable, providing insights into which features in the data most influenced a model's output.

### 5.2.4. Accountability and Regulatory Pathways

Who is responsible when an AI system makes an error that leads to patient harm? Is it the clinician who followed the recommendation, the hospital that implemented the system, or the developer who created the algorithm? Establishing clear lines of accountability is a complex legal and ethical challenge. Furthermore, AI algorithms and the wearable devices they rely on are increasingly being regulated as medical devices. Navigating the regulatory pathways, such as clearance from the U.S. Food and Drug Administration (FDA), is a rigorous process that requires extensive validation to prove the safety and efficacy of these technologies, especially for pediatric use (Karatzia et al., 2022). Table 2 shows the ethical, legal, and social implications (ELSI) of AI/Edge in pediatric cardiology

*Table 2. Ethical, Legal, and Social Implications (ELSI) of AI/Edge in Pediatric Cardiology*

| Domain | Key Consideration | Mitigation Strategies and Best Practices |
|---|---|---|
| Consent & Autonomy | Obtaining meaningful consent from parents for continuous data collection and predictive modeling. The evolving autonomy of the child. | Dynamic consent models; clear, multi-layered explanations of data use; processes for data withdrawal. Establish age-appropriate assent procedures. |
| Privacy & Security | Protection of highly sensitive, lifelong pediatric health data from breaches and misuse. | End-to-end encryption; federated learning to avoid data pooling; robust access controls; regular security audits. |
| Bias & Fairness | Algorithms may perpetuate or amplify existing health disparities if trained on biased data. | Use of diverse, representative training datasets; algorithmic auditing for bias; transparency in model performance across demographic subgroups. |
| Transparency (XAI) | The "black box" nature of some AI models hindering clinical trust and understanding. | Development and use of explainable AI methods; providing clinicians with confidence scores and the key factors influencing a prediction. |
| Accountability | Determining liability in the event of an AI-related error causing patient harm. | Clear regulatory frameworks; defining the roles and responsibilities of developers, institutions, and clinicians; robust post-market surveillance. |
| Psychosocial Impact | Potential for increased parental anxiety due to constant monitoring and alerts; risk of data-driven stigma or discrimination. | User-centered design to avoid alert fatigue; providing psychosocial support for families; strong legal protections against genetic/health data discrimination. |

## 5.3. Future Vision: The Dawn of the "Digital Twin" in CHD

Looking ahead, the ultimate culmination of integrating AI, edge computing, and multi-modal data may be the creation of a "digital twin" for each patient with CHD. A digital twin is a dynamic, virtual replica of a patient's cardiovascular system, continuously updated with real-world data.

- **Concept:** This virtual model would integrate the patient's specific anatomy from imaging, their genetic and proteomic data, and, crucially, real-time physiological data streamed from their wearable and implantable edge devices(Hizem et al., 2025).
- **Functionality:** The digital twin would serve as a personalized simulation platform. Clinicians could test the potential hemodynamic effects of a new medication or simulate different surgical approaches *in silico* before performing them on the actual patient. The model could forecast the patient's disease trajectory over years or decades, identifying the optimal timing for interven-

tions to preserve cardiac function and prevent complications(Hizem et al., 2025).

- **The Role of Edge-AI:** The Edge-AI ecosystem would be the "nervous system" for the digital twin, constantly feeding it with the high-fidelity, real-world data it needs to stay synchronized with the patient's current physiological state. This continuous flow of data from the edge is what would make the digital twin a living, evolving model rather than a static snapshot in time.

While the concept of a comprehensive digital twin is still on the horizon, it represents the ultimate goal of personalized, predictive, and preventative medicine in CHD. It is a future where treatment is no longer based on population averages but is exquisitely tailored to the unique, evolving biology of each individual patient.

## 6. CONCLUSION

The management of congenital heart disease, a journey that spans from prenatal life through adulthood, stands at the cusp of a profound transformation. It has been hard in the past to deal with complicated diagnoses, unpredictable long-term outcomes, and the limitations of a hospital-centered, episodic care model. But now, the huge benefits of combining AI and edge computing are starting to shine through. This convergence is not just a small step forward; it's a big change that will lead to a future of healthcare that is more proactive, predictive, personalised, and participatory (Niyogi et al., 2025).

AI's ability to find complex patterns in very large datasets is improving our ability to diagnose diseases. This means that coronary heart disease can be found earlier and more accurately than ever before. It is giving doctors more power by giving them advanced tools for planning surgeries, figuring out who is at risk, and making clinical decisions based on data. This should make interventions safer and more effective. By predicting future problems, AI gives us a chance to stop treating problems after they happen and start using preventative strategies that are tailored to each patient's specific risk profile (Niyogi et al., 2025).

Edge computing is what makes it possible to bring this intelligence right to the patient, breaking down the hospital walls. Edge computing makes a constant, smart safety net that is especially important for the most vulnerable patients by letting real-time, on-device analysis of continuous physiological data from wearable sensors. This decentralised method makes things more reliable, cuts down on important wait times for help, and most importantly, protects the privacy of private paediatric health information (Nemani et al., 2024).

The real power, though, comes from how Edge-AI works together. This integration creates a closed-loop ecosystem where a patient's health can be constantly tracked, intelligent algorithms can pick up on small changes from their baseline, and caregivers and clinical teams can get useful information quickly. With privacy-protecting methods like federated learning, this ecosystem can help people from all over the world work together to solve the problems that come with not having enough data about rare diseases. This will speed up the development of strong and fair AI solutions (Gearhart et al., 2025).

Bringing this transformative vision to life will take a coordinated, cross-disciplinary effort. It needs paediatric cardiologists, computer scientists, bioengineers, ethicists, and regulatory bodies to work together (Nemani et al., 2024). We need to solve big technical problems in the areas of standardising data and designing hardware. More importantly, we need to take action to address the very important ethical issues of algorithmic fairness, transparency, and accountability to make sure that these powerful technologies help to reduce health disparities instead of making them worse (Bozyel et al., 2024). To move forward, we need to make sure that everything is thoroughly tested, that user-centered design is followed, and that we always put the health and trust of patients and their families first (Maurya & Verma, 2025).

We need to make sure that everything we do is thoroughly tested, that we always put the needs and trust of patients and their families first, and that we never stop focusing on these things. It will empower clinicians with deeper insights, equip families with more effective tools for care, and, most importantly, offer individuals born with heart defects the promise of a longer, healthier, and more secure life.

## REFERENCES


Alasmari, S., AlGhamdi, R., Tejani, G. G., Kumar Sharma, S., & Mousavirad, S. J. (2025). Federated learning-based multimodal approach for early detection and personalized care in cardiac disease. *Frontiers in Physiology, 16,* 1563185. DOI: 10.3389/fphys.2025.1563185 PMID: 40337245

Bozyel, S., Şimşek, E., Koçyiğit, D., Güler, A., Korkmaz, Y., Şeker, M., Ertürk, M., & Keser, N. (2024). Artificial Intelligence-Based Clinical Decision Support Systems in Cardiovascular Diseases. *The Anatolian Journal of Cardiology, 28*(2), 74–86. DOI: 10.14744/AnatolJCardiol.2023.3685 PMID: 38168009

Elvas, L. B., Almeida, A., & Ferreira, J. C. (2025). The Role of AI in Cardiovascular Event Monitoring and Early Detection: Scoping Literature Review. *JMIR Medical Informatics, 13*(1), e64349. DOI: 10.2196/64349 PMID: 40048151

Gearhart, A., Anjewierden, S., Buddhe, S., & Tandon, A. (2025). Review of the Current State of Artificial Intelligence in Pediatric Cardiovascular Magnetic Resonance Imaging. *Children (Basel, Switzerland), 12*(4), 416. DOI: 10.3390/children12040416 PMID: 40310065

Hizem, M., Bousbia, L., Ben Dhiab, Y., Aoueileyine, M. O. E., & Bouallegue, R. (2025). Reliable ECG Anomaly Detection on Edge Devices for Internet of Medical Things Applications. *Sensors (Basel), 25*(8), 2496. DOI: 10.3390/s25082496 PMID: 40285186

Jamil Abusamra, H. N., Ali, S. H. M., Khidir Elhussien, W. A., Ahmed Mirghani, A. M., Alameen Ahmed, A. A., & Abdelrahman Ibrahim, M. E. (2025). Ethical and Practical Considerations of Artificial Intelligence in Pediatric Medicine: A Systematic Review. *Cureus, 17*(2). Advance online publication. DOI: 10.7759/cureus.79024 PMID: 40104456

Karatzia, L., Aung, N., & Aksentijevic, D. (2022). Artificial intelligence in cardiology: Hope for the future and power for the present. *Frontiers in Cardiovascular Medicine, 9,* 945726. DOI: 10.3389/fcvm.2022.945726 PMID: 36312266

Karimov, E., & Zaim Gökbay, İ. (2025). Enhancing Pediatric Congenital Heart Disease Outcomes: The Role of Machine Learning Models and AI-Driven Methodologies. *Cam and Sakura Medical Journal,* 1–8. https://doi.org/DOI: 10.4274/csmedj.galenos.2025.2025-7-1

Maurya, A., & Verma, K. (2025). FedSec+: An Advanced Privacy-Enhanced Cardiovascular Disease Prediction Model using Federated Learning. *AIP Conference Proceedings, 3253*(1), 30033. DOI: 10.1063/5.0248335

Nemani, S., Goyal, S., Sharma, A., & Kothari, N. (2024). Artificial intelligence in pediatric airway - A scoping review. *Saudi Journal of Anaesthesia, 18*(3), 410–416. DOI: 10.4103/sja.sja_110_24 PMID: 39149736

Niyogi, S. G., Nag, D. S., Shah, M. M., Swain, A., Naskar, C., Srivastava, P., & Kant, R. (2025). Role of artificial intelligence in congenital heart disease. *World Journal of Clinical Pediatrics, 14*(3). Advance online publication. DOI: 10.5409/wjcp.v14.i3.105926 PMID: 40881074

Pozza, A., Zanella, L., Castaldi, B., & Di Salvo, G. (2024). How Will Artificial Intelligence Shape the Future of Decision-Making in Congenital Heart Disease? *Journal of Clinical Medicine, 13*(10), 2996. DOI: 10.3390/jcm13102996 PMID: 38792537

Ren, H., Jing, F., Ma, Y., Wang, R., He, C., Wang, Y., Zhou, J., & Sun, Y. (2025). Harnessing artificial intelligence of things for cardiac sensing: Current advances and network-based perspectives. *Frontiers in Public Health, 13*, 1569887. DOI: 10.3389/fpubh.2025.1569887 PMID: 40740375

Vu, T., Kokubo, Y., Inoue, M., Yamamoto, M., Mohsen, A., Martin-Morales, A., Dawadi, R., Inoue, T., Tay, J. T., Yoshizaki, M., Watanabe, N., Kuriya, Y., Matsumoto, C., Arafa, A., Nakao, Y. M., Kato, Y., Teramoto, M., & Araki, M. (2025). Machine Learning Model for Predicting Coronary Heart Disease Risk: Development and Validation Using Insights From a Japanese Population–Based Study. *JMIR Cardio, 9*(1), e68066. DOI: 10.2196/68066 PMID: 40354648

Williams, M. C., MacArthur, J. A. L., Forsyth, R., & Petersen, S. E. (2025). New ways to use imaging data in cardiovascular research: Survey of opinions on federated learning and synthetic data. *European Heart Journal. Imaging Methods and Practice, 3*(1), qyaf012. Advance online publication. DOI: 10.1093/ehjimp/qyaf012 PMID: 40066149

Yeh, Y.-T., Ock, J., & Farimani, A. B. (2025). Text to Band Gap: Pre-trained Language Models as Encoders for Semiconductor Band Gap Prediction. *ArXiv Preprint ArXiv:2501.03456*. https://arxiv.org/abs/2501.03456

# Compilation of References


Abdelfattah, A. M., Park, C., & Choi, M. Y. (2014). Update on non-canonical microRNAs. *Biomolecular Concepts*, *5*(4), 275–287. DOI: 10.1515/bmc-2014-0012

Abu-Halima, M., Meese, E., Abdul-Khaliq, H., & Raedle-Hurst, T. (2021). MicroRNA-183-3p Is a Predictor of Worsening Heart Failure in Adult Patients With Transposition of the Great Arteries and a Systemic Right Ventricle. *Frontiers in Cardiovascular Medicine*, *8*, 730364. DOI: 10.3389/fcvm.2021.730364

Abu-Halima, M., Meese, E., Keller, A., Abdul-Khaliq, H., & Rädle-Hurst, T. (2017). Analysis of circulating microRNAs in patients with repaired Tetralogy of Fallot with and without heart failure. *Journal of Translational Medicine*, *15*, 156. DOI: 10.1186/s12967-017-1255-z

Abu-Halima, M., Wagner, V., Rishik, S., Raedle-Hurst, T., Meese, E., & Abdul-Khaliq, H. (2022). Expression profiling analysis reveals key microRNA-mRNA interactions in patients with transposition of the great arteries and systemic left and right ventricles. *Frontiers in Cardiovascular Medicine*, *9*, 1056427. DOI: 10.3389/fcvm.2022.1056427

Ahamad, S., & Kukshal, P. (2025). Summary of initiatives for treating congenital heart disease: Enhancing quality of life and bridging the knowledge gap. *Annals of the National Academy of Medical Sciences (India)*, *61*(1), 40–44. DOI: 10.25259/ANAMS_242_2024

Aherne, N. J., Rangaswamy, G., & Thirion, P. (2013). Prostate cancer in a male with Holt-Oram syndrome: First clinical association of the TBX5 mutation. *Case Reports in Urology*, *405343*. Advance online publication. DOI: 10.1155/2013/405343 PMID: 23984174

Ahmad, S., Zafar, I., Shafiq, S., Sehar, L., Khalil, H., Matloob, N., Hina, M., Muntaha, S. T., Khan, H., Khan, N. U., Rana, S., Unar, A., Azmat, M., Shafiq, M., Jardan, Y. A. B., Dauelbait, M., & Bourhia, M. (2025). Deep learning-based computational approach for predicting ncRNAs-disease associations in metaplastic breast cancer diagnosis. *BMC Cancer*, *25*(1), 830. DOI: 10.1186/s12885-025-14113-z PMID: 40329245

Ahmed, F. (2019). Congenital Heart Defects in ART-conceived Infants: A Study from Bangladesh. *Journal of Obstetrics and Gynaecology Bangladesh*, *34*(1), 45–49. DOI: 10.3329/jogb.v34i1.41985

Ahmed, S., Islam, M. J., Islam, K. M. K., Uddin, J., Khandoker, F., Fariha, T., & Hezbullah, M. (2025). Awareness, knowledge, and attitude towards basic life support among healthcare professional students in Bangladesh. *PLOS Global Public Health*, *5*(9), e0005126. DOI: 10.1371/journal.pgph.0005126 PMID: 40892842

Akanda, M. R., Sabuj, M. S. S., Salam, S. A., & Jahan, E. (2025). Molecular interplay of gene network dynamics, epigenetic regulation, and therapeutic mapping in cardiovascular disease. *Cardiovascular Drugs and Therapy*, •••, 1–14. DOI: 10.1007/s10557-025-07739-5 PMID: 40540082

Akat, K. M., Moore-McGriff, D., Morozov, P., Brown, M., Gogakos, T., Correa Da Rosa, J., Mihailovic, A., Sauer, M., Ji, R., Ramarathnam, A., Totary-Jain, H., Williams, Z., Tuschl, T., & Schulze, P. C. (2014). Comparative RNA-sequencing analysis of myocardial and circulating small RNAs in human heart failure and their utility as biomarkers. *Proceedings of the National Academy of Sciences of the United States of America*, *111*(30), 11151–11156. DOI: 10.1073/pnas.1401724111 PMID: 25012294

Alam, M. M., & Latifi, S. (2025). Early Detection of Alzheimer's Disease Using Generative Models: A Review of GANs and Diffusion Models in Medical Imaging. *Algorithms*, *18*(7), 434. DOI: 10.3390/a18070434

Alasmari, S., AlGhamdi, R., Tejani, G. G., Kumar Sharma, S., & Mousavirad, S. J. (2025). Federated learning-based multimodal approach for early detection and personalized care in cardiac disease. *Frontiers in Physiology*, *16*, 1563185. DOI: 10.3389/fphys.2025.1563185 PMID: 40337245

Alemu, R., Sharew, N. T., Arsano, Y. Y., Ahmed, M., Tekola-Ayele, F., Mersha, T. B., & Amare, A. T. (2025). Multi-omics approaches for understanding gene-environment interactions in noncommunicable diseases: Techniques, translation, and equity issues. *Human Genomics*, *19*(1), 8. DOI: 10.1186/s40246-025-00718-9 PMID: 39891174

Ali, Z. (2020). Congenital Heart Disease in ART Babies: A Single-center Study from Pakistan. *Pakistan Journal of Medical Sciences*, *36*(5), 890–894. DOI: 10.12669/pjms.36.5.2559 PMID: 32704258

Alkahtani, H. K., Haq, I. U., Ghadi, Y. Y., Innab, N., Alajmi, M., & Nurbapa, M. (2024). Precision diagnosis: An automated method for detecting congenital heart diseases in children from phonocardiogram signals employing deep neural network. *IEEE Access : Practical Innovations, Open Solutions*, *12*, 76053–76064.

Ameen, M., Sundaram, L., Shen, M., Banerjee, A., Kundu, S., Nair, S., Shcherbina, A., Gu, M., Wilson, K. D., Varadarajan, A., Vadgama, N., Balsubramani, A., Wu, J. C., Engreitz, J. M., Farh, K., Karakikes, I., Wang, K. C., Quertermous, T., Greenleaf, W. J., & Kundaje, A. (2022). Integrative single-cell analysis of cardiogenesis identifies developmental trajectories and non-coding mutations in congenital heart disease. *Cell*, *185*(26), 4937–4953.e23. DOI: 10.1016/j.cell.2022.11.028 PMID: 36563664

Ananthakumar, B., Nagaraja, B. G., Umesh, S. M., & Raghavan, R. (2025). Predictive Medicine. *Predictive Algorithms for Rehabilitation and Assistive Systems*, 291–314. https://doi.org/DOI: 10.4018/979-8-3373-0194-5.ch011

Ananthakumar, B., Nanjundeshwara, N., Lakshmaiah, A., & Raghavan, R. (2024). Synthetic Gene Circuits as a Promising Approach in Cancer Immunotherapy. *Critical Developments in Cancer Immunotherapy*, 391–418. https://doi.org/DOI: 10.4018/979-8-3693-3976-3.ch011

Ananthakumar, B., Nanjundeshwara, N., Lakshmaiah, A., & Raghavan, R. (2025). Nanocarriers for Delivering Nucleic Acids in Plants. *Nanocarriers in Plant Science and Agriculture*, 207–234. https://doi.org/DOI: 10.4018/979-8-3693-9869-2.ch008

Appiah, D., Sang, J., Olayemi, O. E., Broni, E. K., Baykoca-Arslan, B., Ebong, I. A., & Kim, C. (2024). Infertility treatments and cyanotic congenital heart defects among livebirths in the USA: Findings from a contemporary cohort. *Human Reproduction (Oxford, England)*, *39*(9), 2115–2123. DOI: 10.1093/humrep/deae161 PMID: 39008825

Armendariz, D. A., Goetsch, S. C., Sundarrajan, A., Sivakumar, S., Wang, Y., Xie, S., Munshi, N. V., & Hon, G. C. (2023). CHD-associated enhancers shape human cardiomyocyte lineage commitment. *eLife*, *12*, e86206. DOI: 10.7554/eLife.86206 PMID: 37096669

Ashiq, S., Hyder, S. N., Ashiq, K., & Sabar, M. F. (2023). Role of Vascular Endothelial Growth Factor as a Potential Biomarker in Congenital Heart Defects: A Systematic Review. *The journal of Tehran Heart Center*, *18*(4), 237–243. https://doi.org/DOI: 10.18502/jthc.v18i4.14822

Athar, M. (2024). Potentials of artificial intelligence in familial hypercholesterolemia: Advances in screening, diagnosis, and risk stratification for early intervention and treatment. *International Journal of Cardiology*, *412*, 132315. PMID: 38972488

Azhdari, M., & zur Hausen, A. (2025). Wnt/β-catenin and notch signaling pathways in cardiovascular disease: Mechanisms and therapeutics approaches. *Pharmacological Research, 211*, 107565. DOI: 10.1016/j.phrs.2024.107565 PMID: 39725339

Baesmat, K. H. (2024, April). Impedance Analysis of Adaptive Distance Relays Using Machine Learning. In International Conference on Information Technology-New Generations (pp. 457-461). Cham: Springer Nature Switzerland. https://doi.org/DOI: 10.1007/978-3-031-56599-1_57

Baesmat, K. H. (2026). IoT-Enabled Smart Grid Analytics for Sustainable Energy ESG Reporting and Performance Optimization: A Business Intelligence Framework. In Data-Driven ESG Strategy Implementation Through Business Intelligence (pp. 319-354). IGI Global Scientific Publishing.https://doi.org/DOI: 10.4018/979-8-3373-5142-1.ch012

Baesmat, K. H., & Latifi, S. (2023, August). A new hybrid method for electrical load forecasting based on deviation correction and MRMRMS. In International Conference On Systems Engineering (pp. 293-303). Cham: Springer Nature Switzerland. DOI: 10.1007/978-3-031-40579-2_29

Bagohser, M., Mustafa, T., Alsmirat, M., Al-Ali, A., & Al Jawarneh, I. M. (2025). A cost-effective framework for predicting parking availability using geospatial data and machine learning. In *2025 16th International Conference on Information and Communication Systems (ICICS)* (pp. 1–6). IEEE. DOI: 10.1109/ICICS65354.2025.11073109

Bahado-Singh, R., Ashrafi, N., Ibrahim, A., Aydas, B., Yilmaz, A., Friedman, P., & Turkoglu, O. (2025). Precision fetal cardiology detects cyanotic congenital heart disease using maternal saliva metabolome and artificial intelligence. *Scientific Reports*, *15*(1), 2060. PMID: 39814838

Bajan, S., & Hutvagner, G. (2020). RNA-Based Therapeutics: From Antisense Oligonucleotides to miRNAs. *Cells*, *9*(1), 137. DOI: 10.3390/cells9010137

Baker, B. H., Zhang, S., Simon, J. M., McLarnan, S. M., Chung, W. K., & Pearson, B. L. (2023). Environmental carcinogens disproportionally mutate genes implicated in neurodevelopmental disorders. *Frontiers in Neuroscience*, *17*. Advance online publication. DOI: 10.3389/fnins.2023.1106573 PMID: 37599994

Baker, V. L., Dyer, S., Chambers, G. M., Keller, E., Banker, M., de Mouzon, J., Elgindy, E., Bai, F. M., Ishihara, O., Jwa, S. C., Kupka, M. S., Zegers-Hochschild, F., & Adamson, G. D. (2025). International Committee for Monitoring Assisted Reproductive Technologies (ICMART): World report for cycles conducted in 2017-2018. *Human Reproduction (Oxford, England)*, *40*(6), 1110–1126. DOI: 10.1093/humrep/deaf049 PMID: 40239109

Banerjee, S., Prabhu Basrur, N., & Rai, P. S. (2021). Omics technologies in personalized combination therapy for cardiovascular diseases: Challenges and opportunities. *Personalized Medicine*, *18*(6), 595–611. DOI: 10.2217/pme-2021-0087 PMID: 34689602

Banker, M., Arora, P., Banker, J., Benani, H., Shah, S., & Lalitkumar, P. G. L. (2019). Prevalence of structural birth defects in IVF-ICSI pregnancies resulting from autologous and donor oocytes in Indian sub-continent: Results from 2444 births. *Acta Obstetricia et Gynecologica Scandinavica*, *98*(6), 715–721. DOI: 10.1111/aogs.13541 PMID: 30663773

Bastos, J. M., Colaço, B., Baptista, R., Gavina, C., & Vitorino, R. (2025). Innovations in heart failure management: The role of cutting-edge biomarkers and multi-omics integration. *Journal of Molecular and Cellular Cardiology Plus*, *11*, 100290. DOI: 10.1016/j.jmccpl.2025.100290 PMID: 40129519

Bayne, J., Garry, J., & Albert, M. A. (2023). Brief review: Racial and ethnic disparities in cardiovascular care with a focus on congenital heart disease and precision medicine. *Current Atherosclerosis Reports*, *25*(5), 189–195. PMID: 36964821

Belhadjer, Z., Pontailler, M., Hily, M., Gaudin, R., Raisky, O., Bonnet, D., & Houyel, L. (2025). The particular anatomy of atrioventricular septal defect with a common valvar orifice in patients with Down syndrome: An echocardiographic study. *International Journal of Cardiology*, *423*. Advance online publication. DOI: 10.1016/j.ijcard.2025.133003 PMID: 39892564

Berliner, J. L., & Fay, A. M. (2007). Risk assessment and genetic counselling for hereditary breast and ovarian cancer: Recommendations of the National Society of Genetic Counsellors. *Journal of Genetic Counseling*, *16*(3), 241–260. PMID: 17508274

Bhat, P., Dhyani, V. S., Lakshmi, V., Uppangala, S., Adiga, S. K., Adiga, P., Kumar, P., & Gupta, A. (2025). Congenital anomalies observed in children conceived through assisted reproductive technology—A systematic review and meta-analysis. *Journal of Assisted Reproduction and Genetics*, *42*(5), 1547–1565. DOI: 10.1007/s10815-025-03454-0 PMID: 40163274

Bhuvana, G. N., Umesh, S. M., & Raghavan, R. (2025). Expanding the frontiers of Schistosomiasis Treatment: The promise of Nanoparticle-Based Therapies. *Journal of Vector Borne Diseases, 10*(4103/jvbd.jvbd_180_23). https://doi.org/DOI: 10.4103/jvbd.jvbd_180_23

Bi, F., Gao, C., & Guo, H. (2024). Epigenetic regulation of cardiovascular diseases induced by behavioural and environmental risk factors: Mechanistic, diagnostic, and therapeutic insights. *FASEB bioAdvances*, *6*(11), 477–502. PMID: 39512842

Billi, M., De Marinis, E., Gentile, M., Nervi, C., & Grignani, F. (2024). Nuclear miRNAs: Gene Regulation Activities. *International Journal of Molecular Sciences*, *25*(11), 6066. DOI: 10.3390/ijms25116066

Biradar, S., Suresh, C., Nanjundeshwara, N., & Raghavan, R. (2025). Spatially Variable Genes. *Spatially Variable Genes in Cancer*, 1–28. https://doi.org/DOI: 10.4018/979-8-3693-7728-4.ch001

Bi, W., Xiao, Y., Wang, X., Cui, L., Song, G., Yang, Z., Zhang, Y., & Ren, W. (2022). The association between assisted reproductive technology and cardiac remodeling in fetuses and early infants: A prospective cohort study. *BMC Medicine*, *20*(1), 104. DOI: 10.1186/s12916-022-02303-6 PMID: 35361200

Blondel, C., Malandain, G., Vaillant, R., & Ayache, N. (2006). Reconstruction of coronary arteries from a single rotational X-ray projection sequence. *IEEE Transactions on Medical Imaging*, *25*(5), 653–663. DOI: 10.1109/tmi.2006.873224 PMID: 16689269

Blondel, C., Vaillant, R., Devernay, F., Malandain, G., & Ayache, N. (2002). Automatic trinocular 3D reconstruction of coronary artery centerlines from rotational X-ray angiography. In *Proc* (pp. 1073–1078). Computer Assisted Radiology and Surgery., DOI: 10.1007/978-3-642-56168-9_139

Blue, G. M., Kirk, E. P., Giannoulatou, E., Sholler, G. F., Dunwoodie, S. L., Harvey, R. P., & Winlaw, D. S. (2017). Advances in the genetics of congenital heart disease: A clinician's guide. *Journal of the American College of Cardiology*, *69*(7), 859–870. PMID: 28209227

Bolkier, Y., Nevo-Caspi, Y., Salem, Y., Vardi, A., Mishali, D., & Paret, G. (2016). Micro-RNA-208a, -208b, and -499 as Biomarkers for Myocardial Damage After Cardiac Surgery in Children. Pediatric Critical Care Medicine: A Journal of the Society of Critical Care Medicine and the World Federation of Pediatric Intensive and Critical Care Societies, 17(4), e193-197. https://doi.org/DOI: 10.1097/PCC.0000000000000644

Bourantas, C. V., Kourtis, I. C., Plissiti, M. E., Fotiadis, D. I., Katsouras, C. S., Papafaklis, M. I., & Michalis, L. K. (2005). A method for 3D reconstruction of coronary arteries using biplane angiography and intravascular ultrasound images. *Computerized Medical Imaging and Graphics*, *29*(8), 597–606. DOI: 10.1016/j.compmedimag.2005.07.001 PMID: 16278063

Bourdon, G., Lenne, X., Godart, F., Storme, L., Theis, D., Subtil, D., Bruandet, A., & Rakza, T. (2024). Epidemiology of congenital heart defects in France from 2013 to 2022 using the PMSI-MCO (French Medical Information System Program in Medicine, Surgery, and Obstetrics) database. *PLoS One*, *19*(4), e0298234. DOI: 10.1371/journal.pone.0298234 PMID: 38626139

Bozyel, S., Şimşek, E., Koçyiğit, D., Güler, A., Korkmaz, Y., Şeker, M., Ertürk, M., & Keser, N. (2024). Artificial Intelligence-Based Clinical Decision Support Systems in Cardiovascular Diseases. *The Anatolian Journal of Cardiology*, *28*(2), 74–86. DOI: 10.14744/AnatolJCardiol.2023.3685 PMID: 38168009

Bradley, E. A., Khan, A., McNeal, D. M., Bravo-Jaimes, K., Khanna, A., Cook, S., Opotowsky, A. R., John, A., Lee, M., Pasquali, S., Daniels, C. J., Pernick, M., Kirkpatrick, J. N., & Gurvitz, M. (2022). Operational and Ethical Considerations for a National Adult Congenital Heart Disease Database. *Journal of the American Heart Association*, *11*(7), e022338. DOI: 10.1161/JAHA.121.022338 PMID: 35301853

Brameier, M., Herwig, A., Reinhardt, R., Walter, L., & Gruber, J. (2011). Human box C/D snoRNAs with miRNA like functions: Expanding the range of regulatory RNAs. *Nucleic Acids Research*, *39*(2), 675–686. DOI: 10.1093/nar/gkq776

Breton, C. V., Landon, R., Kahn, L. G., Enlow, M. B., Peterson, A. K., Bastain, T., Braun, J., Comstock, S. S., Duarte, C. S., Hipwell, A., Ji, H., LaSalle, J. M., Miller, R. L., Musci, R., Posner, J., Schmidt, R., Suglia, S. F., Tung, I., Weisenberger, D., & Fry, R. (2021). Exploring the evidence for epigenetic regulation of environmental influences on child health across generations. *Communications Biology*, *4*(1), 1–15. DOI: 10.1038/s42003-021-02316-6 PMID: 34158610

Bridget, K., & Fuster, V. (2010). *Promoting Cardiovascular Health in the Developing World: A Critical Challenge to Achieve Global Health*. National Academies Press., DOI: 10.1093/ww/9780199540884.013.u251090

Brost, A., Strobel, N., Yatziv, L., Gilson, W., Meyer, B., Hornegger, J., Lewin, J., & Wacker, F. (2009b), Geometric Accuracy of 3-D X-Ray Image-Based Localization from Two C-Arm Views, Workshop on Geometric Accuracy In Image Guided Interventions-Medical Image Computing and Computer Assisted Interventions, MICCAI, pp. 12-19

Brost, A., Strobel, N., Yatziv, L., Gilson, W., Meyer, B., Hornegger, J., Lewin, J., & Wacker, F. (2009a). *Accuracy of x-ray image-based 3D localization from two C-arm views: a comparison between an ideal system and a real device, Medical Imaging 2009: Visualization, Image-Guided Procedures, and Modeling* (Vol. 726). SPIE., DOI: 10.1117/12.811147

Buikema, J. W., Zwetsloot, P.-P. M., Doevendans, P. A., Domian, I. J., & Sluijter, J. P. G. (2014). Wnt/β-Catenin Signaling during Cardiac Development and Repair. *Journal of Cardiovascular Development and Disease, 1*(1), 98–110. DOI: 10.3390/jcdd1010098

Burnicka-Turek, O., Steimle, J. D., Huang, W., Felker, L., Kamp, A., Kweon, J., Peterson, M., Reeves, R. H., Maslen, C. L., Gruber, P. J., Yang, X. H., Shendure, J., & Moskowitz, I. P. (2016). Cilia gene mutations cause atrioventricular septal defects by multiple mechanisms. *Human Molecular Genetics, 25*(14), 3011–3028. DOI: 10.1093/hmg/ddw155 PMID: 27340223

Burridge, P. W., Sharma, A., & Wu, S. M. (2021). Epigenetic regulation of cardiac development and congenital heart disease. *Developmental Cell, 56*(2), 146–161. DOI: 10.1016/j.devcel.2020.11.016

Byalahunasishetter, B. I., N., V., P., S., C., M., S., S., & Raghavan, R. (2025). Spatial Omics and Bioprinting. *Innovations in Precision Medicine and Genomics*, 85–110. https://doi.org/DOI: 10.4018/979-8-3693-5787-3.ch003

Byun, G., Choi, Y., Lee, J.-T., & Bell, M. L. (2025). Effects of Prenatal Exposure to PM2.5 Chemical Components on Adverse Birth Outcomes and Under-5 Mortality in South Korea. *Epidemiology (Cambridge, Mass.), 36*(4), 531. DOI: 10.1097/EDE.0000000000001868 PMID: 40257114

Cajachagua-Torres, K. N., Blaauwendraad, S. M., El Marroun, H., Demmelmair, H., Koletzko, B., Gaillard, R., & Jaddoe, V. W. V. (2022). Fetal Exposure to Maternal Smoking and Neonatal Metabolite Profiles. *Metabolites, 12*(11), 1101. DOI: 10.3390/metabo12111101 PMID: 36422240

Cao, Y., Wen, J., Li, Y., Chen, W., Wu, Y., Li, J., & Huang, G. (2019). Uric acid and sphingomyelin enhance autophagy in iPS cell-originated cardiomyocytes through lncRNA MEG3/miR-7-5p/EGFR axis. *Artificial Cells, Nanomedicine, and Biotechnology, 47*(1), 3774–3785. DOI: 10.1080/21691401.2019.1667817

Carvalho, J. S., Axt-Fliedner, R., Chaoui, R., Copel, J. A., Cuneo, B. F., Goff, D., Gordin Kopylov, L., Hecher, K., Lee, W., Moon-Grady, A. J., Mousa, H. A., Munoz, H., Paladini, D., Prefumo, F., Quarello, E., Rychik, J., Tutschek, B., Wiechec, M., & Yagel, S. (2023). ISUOG Practice Guidelines (updated): Fetal cardiac screening. *Ultrasound in Obstetrics & Gynecology*, *61*(6), 788–803. DOI: 10.1002/uog.26224 PMID: 37267096

Casciaro, C., Hamada, H., Bloise, E., & Matthews, S. G. (2024). The paternal contribution to shaping the health of future generations. *Trends in Endocrinology and Metabolism*, *0*(0). Advance online publication. DOI: 10.1016/j.tem.2024.10.007 PMID: 39562264

Cau, R., Pisu, F., Suri, J. S., & Saba, L. (2025). Addressing hidden risks: Systematic review of artificial intelligence biases across racial and ethnic groups in cardiovascular diseases. *European Journal of Radiology*, *183*, 111867. PMID: 39637580

Cavaillé, J., Buiting, K., Kiefmann, M., Lalande, M., Brannan, C. I., Horsthemke, B., Bachellerie, J.-P., Brosius, J., & Hüttenhofer, A. (2000). Identification of brain-specific and imprinted small nucleolar RNA genes exhibiting an unusual genomic organization. *Proceedings of the National Academy of Sciences of the United States of America*, *97*(26), 14311–14316. DOI: 10.1073/pnas.250426397

CDC. (2024, October 22). Data and Statistics. Congenital Heart Defects (CHDs). https://www.cdc.gov/heart-defects/data/index.html

Chaix, M. A., Andelfinger, G., & Khairy, P. (2016). Genetic testing in congenital heart disease: A clinical approach. *World Journal of Cardiology*, *8*(2), 180. PMID: 26981213

Cheloufi, S., Dos Santos, C. O., Chong, M. M. W., & Hannon, G. J. (2010). A dicer-independent miRNA biogenesis pathway that requires Ago catalysis. *Nature*, *465*(7298), 584–589. DOI: 10.1038/nature09092

Cheng, M., Wang, J., Liu, X., Wang, Y., Wu, Q., Wang, F., Li, P., Wang, B., Zhang, X., & Xie, W. (2024). Development and Validation of a Deep-Learning Network for Detecting Congenital Heart Disease from Multi-View Multi-Modal Transthoracic Echocardiograms. *Research (Washington, D.C.)*, *7*, 0319. https://doi.org/DOI: 10.34133/research.0319

Chen, H. H., & Stewart, A. F. R. (2025). Identifying Structural Variants and Their Contribution to Cardiovascular Disease Risk: The Long and the Short of It. *Journal of the American Heart Association*, *14*(4), e039948. DOI: 10.1161/JAHA.124.039948 PMID: 39950435

Chen, W., & Li, S. (2017). Circulating microRNA as a Novel Biomarker for Pulmonary Arterial Hypertension Due to Congenital Heart Disease. *Pediatric Cardiology, 38*(1), 86–94. DOI: 10.1007/s00246-016-1487-3

Chen, Y.-L., Pascuzzi, N., Ruiz, A., & Chen, K.-H. E. (2025). Mirtrons in Human Cancers. *Onco*, *5*(1), 7. DOI: 10.3390/onco5010007

Chen, Y., Xiao, D., Zhang, L., Cai, C. L., Li, B. Y., & Liu, Y. (2021). The Role of Tbx20 in Cardiovascular Development and Function. *Frontiers in Cell and Developmental Biology*, *9*, 638542. DOI: 10.3389/fcell.2021.638542 PMID: 33585493

Cheriet, F., & Meunier, J. (1999). Self-calibration of a biplane X-ray imaging system for an optimal three dimensional reconstruction. *Computerized Medical Imaging and Graphics*, *23*, 133–141. DOI: 10.1016/s0895-6111(99)00006-3 PMID: 10397356

Chinni, B. K., & Manlhiot, C. (2024). Emerging analytical approaches for personalized medicine using machine learning in pediatric and congenital heart disease. *The Canadian Journal of Cardiology*, *40*(10), 1880–1896. PMID: 39097187

Choudhury, T. Z., Gilbert, B. L., & Garg, V. (2025). Genetic and Environmental Contributors To Congenital Heart Disease. *Current Treatment Options in Cardiovascular Medicine*, *27*(1), 36. DOI: 10.1007/s11936-025-01091-5 PMID: 40438121

Chowdhury, D., Johnson, J. N., Baker-Smith, C. M., Jaquiss, R. D., Mahendran, A. K., Curren, V., & Shaffer, K. (2021). Health care policy and congenital heart disease: 2020 focus on our 2030 future. *Journal of the American Heart Association*, *10*(20), e020605. DOI: 10.1161/JAHA.120.020605 PMID: 34622676

Chu, R., Chen, W., Song, G., Yao, S., Xie, L., Song, L., Zhang, Y., Chen, L., Zhang, X., Ma, Y., Luo, X., Liu, Y., Sun, P., Zhang, S., Fang, Y., Dong, T., Zhang, Q., Peng, J., Zhang, L., & Kong, B. (2020). Predicting the Risk of Adverse Events in Pregnant Women With Congenital Heart Disease. *Journal of the American Heart Association*, *9*(14). Advance online publication. DOI: 10.1161/jaha.120.016371 PMID: 32662348

Cifuentes, D., Xue, H., Taylor, D. W., Patnode, H., Mishima, Y., Cheloufi, S., Ma, E., Mane, S., Hannon, G. J., Lawson, N. D., Wolfe, S. A., & Giraldez, A. J. (2010). A novel miRNA processing pathway independent of Dicer requires Argonaute2 catalytic activity. *Science*, *328*(5986), 1694–1698. DOI: 10.1126/science.1190809

Coley, A. B., DeMeis, J. D., Chaudhary, N. Y., & Borchert, G. M. (2022). Small Nucleolar Derived RNAs as Regulators of Human Cancer. *Biomedicines*, *10*(8), 1819. DOI: 10.3390/biomedicines10081819

Condrat, C. E., Thompson, D. C., Barbu, M. G., Bugnar, O. L., Boboc, A., Cretoiu, D., Suciu, N., Cretoiu, S. M., & Voinea, S. C. (2020). miRNAs as Biomarkers in Disease: Latest Findings Regarding Their Role in Diagnosis and Prognosis. *Cells, 9*(2), 276. DOI: 10.3390/cells9020276

Cooke, M. S., Hu, C.-W., Chang, Y.-J., & Chao, M.-R. (2018). Urinary DNA adductomics – A novel approach for exposomics. *Environment International, 121*, 1033–1038. DOI: 10.1016/j.envint.2018.10.041 PMID: 30392940

Crook, S., Dragan, K., Woo, J. L., Neidell, M., Nash, K. A., Jiang, P., Zhang, Y., Sanchez, C. M., Cook, S., Hannan, E. L., Newburger, J. W., Jacobs, M. L., Petit, C. J., Goldstone, A., Vincent, R., Walsh-Spoonhower, K., Mosca, R., Kumar, T. K. S., & Devejian, N., … The New York State Congenital Heart Surgery Collaborative for Longitudinal Outcomes & Utilization of Resources (CHS-COLOUR). (2024). Impact of Social Determinants of Health on Predictive Models for Outcomes After Congenital Heart Surgery. *Journal of the American College of Cardiology, 83*(24), 2440–2454. DOI: 10.1016/j.jacc.2024.03.430 PMID: 38866447

Crouch, D. J., & Bodmer, W. F. (2020). Polygenic inheritance, GWAS, polygenic risk scores, and the search for functional variants. *Proceedings of the National Academy of Sciences of the United States of America, 117*(32), 18924–18933. PMID: 32753378

Dahl, A., Hernandez-Meneses, M., & Perissinotti, A.. (2021). Echocardiography and FDG-PET/CT scan in gram-negative bacteremia and cardiovascular infections. *Current Opinion in Infectious Diseases, 34*, 728–736. DOI: 10.1097/qco.0000000000000781 PMID: 34751186

de Rooij, L. A., Mastebroek, D. J., ten Voorde, N., van der Wall, E., van Diest, P. J., & Moelans, C. B. (2022). The microRNA Lifecycle in Health and Cancer. *Cancers (Basel), 14*(23), 5748. DOI: 10.3390/cancers14235748

de Ruiter, S. C., Tschiderer, L., Grobbee, D. E., Willeit, P., den Ruijter, H. M., Schmidt, A. F., & Peters, S. A. E. (2025). Mendelian Randomisation: Concepts, Opportunities, Challenges, and Future Directions. *Global Heart, 20*(1). Advance online publication. DOI: 10.5334/gh.1438 PMID: 40547872

Dehghanbanadaki, H., Jimbo, M., Fendereski, K., Kunisaki, J., Horns, J. J., Ramsay, J. M., & Hotaling, J. M. (2025). Transgenerational effects of paternal exposures: The role of germline de novo mutations. *Andrology, 13*(1), 101–118.

Di Mauro, V., Crasto, S., Colombo, F. S., Di Pasquale, E., & Catalucci, D. (2019). Wnt signalling mediates miR-133a nuclear re-localization for the transcriptional control of Dnmt3b in cardiac cells. *Scientific Reports, 9*(1), 9320. DOI: 10.1038/s41598-019-45818-4

Diener, C., Keller, A., & Meese, E. (2022). Emerging concepts of miRNA therapeutics: From cells to clinic. *Trends in Genetics*, *38*(6), 613–626. DOI: 10.1016/j.tig.2022.02.006

Doe, C. M., Relkovic, D., Garfield, A. S., Dalley, J. W., Theobald, D. E. H., Humby, T., Wilkinson, L. S., & Isles, A. R. (2009). Loss of the imprinted snoRNA mbii-52 leads to increased 5htr2c pre-RNA editing and altered 5HT2CR-mediated behaviour. *Human Molecular Genetics*, *18*(12), 2140–2148. DOI: 10.1093/hmg/ddp137

Dogan, M. V., Knight, S., Dogan, T. K., Knowlton, K. U., & Philibert, R. (2021). External validation of integrated genetic-epigenetic biomarkers for predicting incident coronary heart disease. *Epigenomics*, *13*(14), 1095–1112. DOI: 10.2217/epi-2021-0123 PMID: 34148365

Doherty, B. T., Koelmel, J. P., Lin, E. Z., Romano, M. E., & Godri Pollitt, K. J. (2021). Use of Exposomic Methods Incorporating Sensors in Environmental Epidemiology. *Current Environmental Health Reports*, *8*(1), 34–41. DOI: 10.1007/s40572-021-00306-8 PMID: 33569731

Dolk, H., McCullough, N., Callaghan, S., Casey, F., Craig, B., Given, J., Loane, M., Lagan, B. M., Bunting, B., Boyle, B., & Dabir, T. (2020). Risk factors for congenital heart disease: The Baby Hearts Study, a population-based case-control study. *PLoS One*, *15*(2), e0227908. DOI: 10.1371/journal.pone.0227908 PMID: 32092068

Domingo, J., Baeza-Centurion, P., & Lehner, B. (2019). The causes and consequences of genetic interactions (epistasis). *Annual Review of Genomics and Human Genetics*, *20*(1), 433–460. PMID: 31082279

Dubey, G., Singh, M., Singh, H., Agarwal, M., Chandel, S. S., Mishra, A., Singh, R. P., & Kukreti, N. (2024). Emerging roles of SnoRNAs in the pathogenesis and treatment of autoimmune disorders. *Pathology, Research and Practice*, *253*, 154952. DOI: 10.1016/j.prp.2023.154952

Dumay, A. C. M., & Reiber, J. H. C., Gerbrands, Jan J. (1994). Determination of Optimal Angiographic Viewing Angles: Basic Principles and Evaluation Study. *IEEE Transactions on Medical Imaging*, *13*(1). Advance online publication. DOI: 10.1109/42.276141 PMID: 18218480

Ehrlich, L., & Prakash, S. K. (2022). Copy-number variation in congenital heart disease. *Current Opinion in Genetics & Development*, *77*, 101986. DOI: 10.1016/j.gde.2022.101986 PMID: 36202051

Ejaz, H., Thyyib, T., Ibrahim, A., Nishat, A., & Malay, J. (2024). Role of artificial intelligence in early detection of congenital heart diseases in neonates. *Frontiers in Digital Health, 5*, 1345814. PMID: 38274086

Elmagrpy, Z., Rayani, A., Shah, A., Habas, E., & Aburawi, E. H. (2011). Down syndrome and congenital heart disease: Why the regional difference as observed in the Libyan experience? *Cardiovascular Journal of Africa, 22*(6), 306–309. DOI: 10.5830/CVJA-2010-072 PMID: 22159317

Elvas, L. B., Almeida, A., & Ferreira, J. C. (2025). The Role of AI in Cardiovascular Event Monitoring and Early Detection: Scoping Literature Review. *JMIR Medical Informatics, 13*(1), e64349. DOI: 10.2196/64349 PMID: 40048151

Espinoza-Lewis, R. A., & Wang, D.-Z. (2012). MicroRNAs in Heart Development. *Current Topics in Developmental Biology, 100*, 279–317. DOI: 10.1016/B978-0-12-387786-4.00009-9

Esthappan, J., Harauchi, H., & Hoffmann, K. R. (1998). Evaluation of imaging geometries calculated from biplane images. *Medical Physics, 25*(6), 965–975. DOI: 10.1118/1.598275 PMID: 9650187

Estill, M., Hauser, R., Nassan, F. L., Moss, A., & Krawetz, S. A. (2019). The effects of di-butyl phthalate exposure from medications on human sperm RNA among men. *Scientific Reports, 9*(1), 12397. DOI: 10.1038/s41598-019-48441-5 PMID: 31455814

Evertz, R., Lange, T., Backhaus, S. J., Schulz, A., Beuthner, B. E., Topci, R., & Schuster, A. (2022). Artificial intelligence enabled fully automated CMR function quantification for optimized risk stratification in patients undergoing transcatheter aortic valve replacement. *Journal of Interventional Cardiology, 2022*(1), 1368878. PMID: 35539443

Fan, D., Pang, S., Chen, J., Shan, J., Cheng, Q., & Yan, B. (2021). Identification and functional study of GATA4 gene regulatory variants in atrial septal defects. *BMC Cardiovascular Disorders, 21*(1), 321. DOI: 10.1186/s12872-021-02136-w PMID: 34193080

Fang, Q., Fan, H., Li, Q., Zhang, M., Zhou, Z., Du, J., & Huang, J. (2025). Multi-Omic Insight Into the Molecular Networks in the Pathogenesis of Coronary Artery Disease. *Journal of the American Heart Association*. Advance online publication. DOI: 10.1161/jaha.124.037203 PMID: 40135555

Farhan, S. M., & Hegele, R. A. (2013). Genetics 101 for cardiologists: Rare genetic variants and monogenic cardiovascular disease. *The Canadian Journal of Cardiology, 29*(1), 18–22. PMID: 23200093

Farrokhi, Z. (2026). AI-Powered Grid Analytics for Sustainable Energy Management in ESG Frameworks. In Data-Driven ESG Strategy Implementation Through Business Intelligence (pp. 279-318). IGI Global Scientific Publishing. https://doi.org/DOI: 10.4018/979-8-3373-5142-1.ch011

Farrokhi, Z., Kalhor, A., & Masouleh, M. T. (2018). Implementation and Evaluation of Object Identification Techniques on Nao Robot Platform. https://aeuso.org/includes/files/articles/Vol8_Iss29_3947-3958_Implementation_and_Evaluation_of_Ob.pdf

Farrokhi, Z., Baesmat, K. H., & Regentova, E. E. (2024). Enhancing urban intelligence energy management: Innovative load forecasting techniques for electrical networks. *Journal of Power and Energy Engineering*, *12*, 72–88. DOI: 10.4236/jpee.2024.1211005

Fazekas-Pongor, V., Csáky-Szunyogh, M., Fekete, M., Mészáros, Á., Cseh, K., & Pénzes, M. (2020). Congenital heart diseases and parental occupational exposure in a Hungarian case-control study in 1997 to 2002. *Congenital Anomalies*, *61*(2), 55–62. DOI: 10.1111/cga.12401 PMID: 33140474

Fazekas-Pongor, V., Fekete, M., Csáky-Szunyogh, M., Cseh, K., & Pénzes, M. (2021). Parental occupational exposure and congenital heart diseases in a Hungarian case–control study. *International Archives of Occupational and Environmental Health*, *94*(3), 515–527. DOI: 10.1007/s00420-020-01589-4 PMID: 33170344

Fernández-Sanlés, A., Sayols-Baixeras, S., Subirana, I., Degano, I. R., & Elosua, R. (2017). Association between DNA methylation and coronary heart disease or other atherosclerotic events: A systematic review. *Atherosclerosis*, *263*, 325–333. DOI: 10.1016/j.atherosclerosis.2017.05.022 PMID: 28577936

Fitzsimons, L. A., Brewer, V. L., & Tucker, K. L. (2022). Hedgehog morphogens act as growth factors critical to pre- and postnatal cardiac development and maturation: How primary cilia mediate their signal transduction. *Cells*, *11*(12), 1879. PMID: 35741008

Flynt, A. S., Greimann, J. C., Chung, W.-J., Lima, C. D., & Lai, E. C. (2010). MicroRNA Biogenesis via Splicing and Exosome-Mediated Trimming in Drosophila. *Molecular Cell*, *38*(6), 900–907. DOI: 10.1016/j.molcel.2010.06.014

Fotiou, E., Williams, S., Martin-Geary, A., Robertson, D. L., Tenin, G., Hentges, K. E., & Keavney, B. (2019). Integration of large-scale genomic data sources with evolutionary history reveals novel genetic loci for congenital heart disease. *Circulation. Genomic and Precision Medicine*, *12*(10), e002694. PMID: 31613678

Fountzilas, E., Pearce, T., Baysal, M. A., Chakraborty, A., & Tsimberidou, A. M. (2025). Convergence of evolving artificial intelligence and machine learning techniques in precision oncology. *NPJ Digital Medicine*, *8*(1). Advance online publication. DOI: 10.1038/s41746-025-01471-y PMID: 39890986

Fuller, A. M., & Qian, L. (2014). MiRiad Roles for MicroRNAs in Cardiac Development and Regeneration. *Cells*, *3*(3), 724–750. DOI: 10.3390/cells3030724

Funamoto, M., Imanishi, M., Tsuchiya, K., & Ikeda, Y. (2023). Roles of histone acetylation sites in cardiac hypertrophy and heart failure. *Frontiers in Cardiovascular Medicine*, *10*, 1133611. DOI: 10.3389/fcvm.2023.1133611 PMID: 37008337

Fu, X.-D. (2014). Non-coding RNA: A new frontier in regulatory biology. *National Science Review*, *1*(2), 190–204. DOI: 10.1093/nsr/nwu008

Galdini, A., Fesslova, V. M. E., Gaeta, G., Candiani, M., Pozzoni, M., Chiarello, C., & Cavoretto, P. I. (2021). Prevalence of Congenital Heart Defects in Pregnancies Conceived by Assisted Reproductive Technology: A Cohort Study. *Journal of Clinical Medicine*, *10*(22), 5363. DOI: 10.3390/jcm10225363 PMID: 34830645

Gál, L., Schamberger, A., Wachtl, G., & Orbán, T. I. (2024). The Effect of Alternative Splicing Sites on Mirtron Formation and Arm Selection of Precursor microRNAs. *International Journal of Molecular Sciences*, *25*(14), 7643. DOI: 10.3390/ijms25147643

Garcia, J. A., Chen, J., Hansgen, A., Wink, O., Movassaghi, B., & Messenger, J. C. (2007). Rotational angiography (RA) and three-dimensional imaging (3-DRA): An available clinical tool. *The International Journal of Cardiovascular Imaging*, *23*, 9–13. DOI: 10.1007/s10554-006-9088-5 PMID: 16779617

Garcia, Y. E., Sjögren, B., & Osei-Owusu, P. (2025). G protein regulation by RGS proteins in the pathophysiology of dilated cardiomyopathy. *American Journal of Physiology. Heart and Circulatory Physiology*, *328*(2), H348–H360. DOI: 10.1152/ajpheart.00653.2024 PMID: 39772618

Garg, V., Kathiriya, I. S., Barnes, R., Schluterman, M. K., King, I. N., Butler, C. A., Rothrock, C. R., Eapen, R. S., Hirayama-Yamada, K., Joo, K., Matsuoka, R., Cohen, J. C., & Srivastava, D. (2003). GATA4 mutations cause human congenital heart defects and reveal an interaction with TBX5. *Nature*, *424*(6947), 443–447. DOI: 10.1038/nature01827 PMID: 12845333

Garg, V., Muth, A. N., Ransom, J. F., Schluterman, M. K., Barnes, R., King, I. N., Grossfeld, P. D., & Srivastava, D. (2005). Mutations in NOTCH1 cause aortic valve disease. *Nature*, *437*(7056), 270–274. DOI: 10.1038/nature03940 PMID: 16025100

Garreau, M., Weidner, J., Hamilton, R., Kolosionek, E., Toki, N., Stavenhagen, K., Paris, C., Bonetti, A., Czechtizky, W., Gnerlich, F., & Rydzik, A. (2024). Chemical modification patterns for microRNA therapeutic mimics: A structure-activity relationship (SAR) case-study on miR-200c. *Nucleic Acids Research, 52*(6), 2792–2807. DOI: 10.1093/nar/gkae141

Gautam, Y., Johansson, E., & Mersha, T. B. (2022). Multi-Omics Profiling Approach to Asthma: An Evolving Paradigm. *Journal of Personalized Medicine, 12*(1), 66. DOI: 10.3390/jpm12010066 PMID: 35055381

Gearhart, A., Anjewierden, S., Buddhe, S., & Tandon, A. (2025). Review of the Current State of Artificial Intelligence in Pediatric Cardiovascular Magnetic Resonance Imaging. *Children (Basel, Switzerland), 12*(4), 416. DOI: 10.3390/children12040416 PMID: 40310065

Gelb, B. D. (2022). Prospects for precision genetic medicine in congenital heart disease. *Current Opinion in Genetics & Development, 77*, 101983. PMID: 36115276

Giannubilo, S. R., Marzioni, D., Tossetta, G., Montironi, R., Meccariello, M. L., & Ciavattini, A. (2024). The "Bad Father": Paternal Role in Biology of Pregnancy and in Birth Outcome. *Biology (Basel), 13*(3), 165. DOI: 10.3390/biology13030165 PMID: 38534435

Gifford, C. A., Ranade, S. S., Samarakoon, R., Salunga, H. T., De Soysa, T. Y., Huang, Y. U., & Srivastava, D. (2019). Oligogenic inheritance of a human heart disease involving a genetic modifier. *Science, 364*(6443), 865–870. PMID: 31147515

Gilboa, S. M., Salemi, J. L., Nembhard, W. N., Fixler, D. E., & Correa, A. (2010). Mortality resulting from congenital heart disease among children and adults in the United States, 1999 to 2006. *Circulation, 122*(22), 2254–2263. DOI: 10.1161/CIRCULATIONAHA.110.947002 PMID: 21098447

Giorgione, V., Parazzini, F., Fesslova, V., Cipriani, S., Candiani, M., Inversetti, A., Sigismondi, C., Tiberio, F., & Cavoretto, P. (2018). Congenital heart defects in IVF/ICSI pregnancy: Systematic review and meta-analysis. *Ultrasound in Obstetrics & Gynecology, 51*(1), 33–42. DOI: 10.1002/uog.18932 PMID: 29164811

Girolami, F., Frisso, G., Benelli, M., Crotti, L., Iascone, M., Mango, R., & Olivotto, I. (2018). Contemporary genetic testing in inherited cardiac disease: Tools, ethical issues, and clinical applications. *The Journal of Cardiovascular Medicine, 19*(1), 1–11. PMID: 29176389

Giudicessi, J. R., Kullo, I. J., & Ackerman, M. J. (2021). Precision cardiovascular medicine: State of the science and future outlook. *Journal of the American Heart Association, 10*(16), e021314. DOI: 10.1161/JAHA.121.021314

González-Moyotl, N., Huesca-Gómez, C., Torres-Paz, Y. E., Fuentevilla-Álvarez, G., Romero-Maldonado, S., Sámano, R., Soto, M. E., Martínez-Rosas, M., Domínguez-López, A., & Gamboa, R. (2024). Paediatrics congenital heart disease is associated with plasma miRNAs. *Pediatric Research, 96*(5), 1220–1227. DOI: 10.1038/s41390-024-03230-3

González-Peña, S. M., Calvo-Anguiano, G., Martínez-de-Villarreal, L. E., Ancer-Rodríguez, P. R., Lugo-Trampe, J. J., Saldivar-Rodríguez, D., Hernández-Almaguer, M. D., Calzada-Dávila, M., Guerrero-Orjuela, L. S., & Campos-Acevedo, L. D. (2021). Maternal Folic Acid Intake and Methylation Status of Genes Associated with Ventricular Septal Defects in Children: Case-Control Study. *Nutrients, 13*(6), 2071. DOI: 10.3390/nu13062071 PMID: 34204335

Gorini, F., & Tonacci, A. (2025). Ambient air pollution and congenital heart disease: Updated evidence and future challenges. *Antioxidants, 14*(1), 48. PMID: 39857382

Gould, K. L., & Johnson, N. P. (2017). Coronary CT angiography with PET perfusion imaging: Hybrid or hype? *JACC: Cardiovascular Imaging, 10*, 1371–1373. DOI: 10.1016/j.jcmg.2016.09.033 PMID: 28528157

Graß, M., Schmitt, H., Rasche, V., Haehnel, S., Schramm, O., Hartmann, M., & Sartor, K. (2001), A method for 3D flow determination based on X-ray rotational angiography, International Congress Series 1230, pp. 408–414, https://doi.org/DOI: 10.1016/s0531-5131(01)00091-7

Grunert, M., Appelt, S., Dunkel, I., Berger, F., & Sperling, S. R. (2019). Altered microRNA and target gene expression related to Tetralogy of Fallot. *Scientific Reports, 9*(1), 19063. DOI: 10.1038/s41598-019-55570-4

*GSE129216*. (2019). https://www.ncbi.nlm.nih.gov/geo/query/acc.cgi?acc=GSE129216

Gullo, G., Scaglione, M., Laganà, A. S., Perino, A., Andrisani, A., Chiantera, V., Cucinella, G., Gitas, G., Barra, F., & Riemma, G. (2023). Assisted Reproductive Techniques and Risk of Congenital Heart Diseases in Children: A Systematic Review and Meta-analysis. *Reproductive Sciences (Thousand Oaks, Calif.), 30*(10), 2896–2906. DOI: 10.1007/s43032-023-01252-6 PMID: 37145300

Guo, F. (2012). Chapter Five—Drosha and DGCR8 in MicroRNA Biogenesis. In Guo, F., & Tamanoi, F. (Eds.), *The Enzymes* (Vol. 32, pp. 101–121). Academic Press., DOI: 10.1016/B978-0-12-404741-9.00005-2

Guo, L., Zhao, Y., Huang, Q., Huang, J., Tao, Y., Chen, J., & Liu, H. (2024). Electrochemical protein biosensors for disease marker detection: Progress and opportunities. *Microsystems & Nanoengineering*, *10*(1), 65. DOI: 10.1038/s41378-024-00700-w PMID: 38784375

Guo, Z., Maki, M., Ding, R., Yang, Y., Zhang, B., & Xiong, L. (2014). Genome-wide survey of tissue-specific microRNA and transcription factor regulatory networks in 12 tissues. *Scientific Reports*, *4*, 5150. DOI: 10.1038/srep05150

Gupta, R., Joshi, P., Mohan, V., Reddy, K. S., & Yusuf, S. (2008). Social determinants of cardiovascular disease outcomes in Indians: The CREATE registry. *European Heart Journal*, *29*(5), 668–675. DOI: 10.1093/eurheartj/ehm635

Gurav, A., Revaiah, P. C., Tsai, T. Y., Miyashita, K., Tobe, A., Oshima, A., Sevestre, E., Garg, S., Aben, J. P., Reiber, J. H. C., Morel, M. A., Lee, C. W., Koo, B. K., Biscaglia, S., Collet, C., Bourantas, C., Escaned, J., Onuma, Y., & Serruys, P. W. (2024, November 25). Coronary angiography: A review of the state of the art and the evolution of angiography in cardio therapeutics. *Frontiers in Cardiovascular Medicine*, *11*, 1468888. DOI: 10.3389/fcvm.2024.1468888 PMID: 39654943

Gu, S., Jin, L., Zhang, Y., Huang, Y., Zhang, F., Valdmanis, P. N., & Kay, M. A. (2012). The loop position of shRNAs and pre-miRNAs is critical for the accuracy of Dicer processing in vivo. *Cell*, *151*(4), 900–911. DOI: 10.1016/j.cell.2012.09.042

GVS, A. C., Ananthakumar, B., & Raghavan, R. (2025). Enhancing Assistive Technologies With Neuromorphic Computing. *Revolutionizing AI with Brain-Inspired Technology: Neuromorphic Computing*, 207–232. https://doi.org/DOI: 10.4018/979-8-3693-6303-4.ch009

Habib, A. R. R., Alam, M. M., & Islam, M. R. (2021, December). Design of a Mobile Aeration System for Aquaculture and Proof of Concept. In 2021 International Conference on Computer, Communication, Chemical, Materials and Electronic Engineering (IC4ME2) (pp. 1-4). IEEE. DOI: 10.1109/IC4ME253898.2021.9768594

Håkansson, K. E. J., Goossens, E. A. C., Trompet, S., van Ingen, E., de Vries, M. R., van der Kwast, R. V. C. T., Ripa, R. S., Kastrup, J., Hohensinner, P. J., Kaun, C., Wojta, J., Böhringer, S., Le Cessie, S., Jukema, J. W., Quax, P. H. A., & Nossent, A. Y. (2019). Genetic associations and regulation of expression indicate an independent role for 14q32 snoRNAs in human cardiovascular disease. *Cardiovascular Research*, *115*(10), 1519–1532. DOI: 10.1093/cvr/cvy309

Han, F. (2025). Sudden cardiac death in congenital heart disease—A narrative review and update. *Frontiers in Cardiovascular Medicine*, *12*. Advance online publication. DOI: 10.3389/fcvm.2025.1539958 PMID: 40371062

Han, P. L., Jiang, L., Cheng, J. L., Shi, K., Huang, S., Jiang, Y., & Yang, Z. G. (2024). Artificial intelligence-assisted diagnosis of congenital heart disease and associated pulmonary arterial hypertension from chest radiographs: A multi-reader multi-case study. *European Journal of Radiology*, *171*, 111277. PMID: 38160541

Han, S., & Dong, H. (2022). A temporal window attention-based window-dependent long short-term memory network for multivariate time series prediction. *Entropy (Basel, Switzerland)*, *25*(1), 10. DOI: 10.3390/e25010010 PMID: 36673150

Hansen, M., Kurinczuk, J. J., Klerk, N., Burton, P., & Bower, C. (2013). Assisted reproductive technology and major birth defects in Western Australia. *Obstetrics and Gynecology*, *121*(4), 852–863. DOI: 10.1097/AOG.0b013e31828738e5 PMID: 22996103

Hăşmăşanu, M. G., Procopciuc, L. M., Matyas, M., Zonda, G. I., & Zaharie, G. C. (2023). Genetic Polymorphisms of Vascular Endothelial Growth Factor in Neonatal Pathologies: A Systematic Search and Narrative Synthesis of the Literature. *Children (Basel, Switzerland)*, *10*(4), 744. DOI: 10.3390/children10040744 PMID: 37189993

Hassanpouri Baesmat, K., Farrokhi, Z., Chmaj, G., & Regentova, E. E. (2025). Parallel Multi-Model Energy Demand Forecasting with Cloud Redundancy: Leveraging Trend Correction, Feature Selection, and Machine Learning. *Forecasting*, *7*(2), 25. DOI: 10.3390/forecast7020025

Hassanpouri Baesmat, K., & Shiri, A. (2019). A new combined method for future energy forecasting in electrical networks. *International Transactions on Electrical Energy Systems*, *29*(3), e2749. DOI: 10.1002/etep.2749

Hata, A., & Kang, H. (2015). Functions of the bone morphogenetic protein signaling pathway through microRNAs [Review]. *International Journal of Molecular Medicine*, *35*(3), 563–568. DOI: 10.3892/ijmm.2015.2060

Havens, M. A., Reich, A. A., Duelli, D. M., & Hastings, M. L. (2012). Biogenesis of mammalian microRNAs by a non-canonical processing pathway. *Nucleic Acids Research*, *40*(10), 4626–4640. DOI: 10.1093/nar/gks026

Hayama-Terada, M., Aochi, Y., Ikehara, S., Kimura, T., Yamagishi, K., Sato, T., & Iso, H. (2023). Paternal occupational exposures and infant congenital heart defects in the Japan Environment and Children's Study. *Environmental Health and Preventive Medicine*, *28*, 12–12. DOI: 10.1265/ehpm.22-00202 PMID: 36740268

Helbig, C., Ueberham, M., Becker, A. M., Schlink, U., & Kraemer, U. (2021). Wearable sensors for human environmental exposure in urban settings. *Current Pollution Reports*, *7*(4), 417–433. DOI: 10.1007/s40726-021-00186-4

Helm, B. M., & Ware, S. M. (2024). Clinical Decision Analysis of Genetic Evaluation and Testing in 1013 Intensive Care Unit Infants with Congenital Heart Defects Supports Universal Genetic Testing. *Genes*, *15*(4), 505. DOI: 10.3390/genes15040505 PMID: 38674439

Henningsen, A.-K. A., Opdahl, S., Wennerholm, U.-B., Tiitinen, A., Rasmussen, S., Romundstad, L. B., Bergh, C., Gissler, M., Forman, J. L., & Pinborg, A. (2023). Risk of congenital malformations in live-born singletons conceived after intracytoplasmic sperm injection: A Nordic study from the CoNARTaS group. *Fertility and Sterility*, *120*(5), 1033–1041. DOI: 10.1016/j.fertnstert.2023.07.003 PMID: 37442533

Hentschke, C. M., Serowy, S., Janiga, G., Rose, G., & Tönnies, K. D. (2011), Estimating blood flow velocity in angiographic image data, Proc. SPIE Volume 7964, Medical Imaging 2011: Visualization, Image-Guided Procedures, and Modelling, 79640Y, https://doi.org/DOI: 10.1117/12.878019

Hikspoors, J. P. J. M., Kruepunga, N., Mommen, G. M. C., Köhler, S. E., Anderson, R. H., & Lamers, W. H. (2022). A pictorial account of the human embryonic heart between 3.5 and 8 weeks of development. *Communications Biology*, *5*(1), 226. DOI: 10.1038/s42003-022-03153-x PMID: 35277594

Hizem, M., Bousbia, L., Ben Dhiab, Y., Aoueileyine, M. O. E., & Bouallegue, R. (2025). Reliable ECG Anomaly Detection on Edge Devices for Internet of Medical Things Applications. *Sensors (Basel)*, *25*(8), 2496. DOI: 10.3390/s25082496 PMID: 40285186

Hoagland, A., & Kipping, S. (2024). Challenges in Promoting Health Equity and Reducing Disparities in Access Across New and Established Technologies. *The Canadian Journal of Cardiology*, *40*(6), 1154–1167. DOI: 10.1016/j.cjca.2024.02.014 PMID: 38417572

Hoffmann, K. R., Sen, A., Lan, L., Chua, K. G., Esthappan, J., & Mazzucco, M. (2000). A system for determination of 3D vessel tree centerlines from biplane images. *International Journal of Cardiac Imaging*, *16*, 315–330. DOI: 10.1023/a:1026528209003 PMID: 11215917

Holt, D. B., El-Bokl, A., Stromberg, D., & Taylor, M. D. (2025). Role of artificial intelligence in congenital heart disease and interventions. *Journal of the Society for Cardiovascular Angiography & Interventions*, *4*(3), 102567. PMID: 40230672

Homsy, J., Zaidi, S., Shen, Y., Ware, J. S., Samocha, K. E., Karczewski, K. J., DePalma, S. R., McKean, D., Wakimoto, H., Gorham, J., Jin, S. C., Deanfield, J., Giardini, A., Porter, G. A.Jr, Kim, R., Bilguvar, K., López-Giráldez, F., Tikhonova, I., Mane, S., & Chung, W. K. (2015). De novo mutations in congenital heart disease with neurodevelopmental and other congenital anomalies. *Science*, *350*(6265), 1262–1266. DOI: 10.1126/science.aac9396 PMID: 26785492

Horenstein, M. S., Diaz-Frias, J., & Guillaume, M. (2024). Tetralogy of Fallot. In *StatPearls*. StatPearls Publishing., https://www.ncbi.nlm.nih.gov/books/NBK513288/

Horz, T., & Kowarschik, M. (2013), Temporal Difference encoding for angiographic image sequences, United States Patent no US2013/0077839 A1

Hudaib, A., & Yousef, M. (2025). Hybrid GWO-SA feature selection for Type II diabetes prediction using machine and deep learning models. In *2025 16th International Conference on Information and Communication Systems (ICICS)* (pp. 1–6). IEEE. DOI: 10.1109/ICICS65354.2025.11073115

Huesca-Gomez, C., Gonzalez-Moyotl, N., Romero-Maldonado, S., Samano, R., & Gamboa, R. (2025). Role of circulating microRNAs in tetralogy of Fallot. Postepy W Kardiologii Interwencyjnej = Advances in Interventional Cardiology, 21(2), 247–254. https://doi.org/DOI: 10.5114/aic.2025.151804

Hughes, A., Shandhi, M. M. H., Master, H., Dunn, J., & Brittain, E. (2023). Wearable Devices in Cardiovascular Medicine. *Circulation Research*, *132*(5), 652–670. DOI: 10.1161/CIRCRESAHA.122.322389 PMID: 36862812

Hu, Y., Xie, L., Nunes, J. C., Bellanger, J. J., Bedossa, M., & Toumoulin, C. (2010). ECG gated tomographic reconstruction for 3-D rotational coronary angiography. *Annual International Conference of the IEEE Engineering in Medicine and Biology Society*, *2010*, 3614–3617. DOI: 10.1109/iembs.2010.5627449 PMID: 21096844

Hynes, C., & Kakumani, P. K. (2024). Regulatory role of RNA-binding proteins in microRNA biogenesis. *Frontiers in Molecular Biosciences*, *11*. Advance online publication. DOI: 10.3389/fmolb.2024.1374843

Imani, P., Grigoryan, H., Dudoit, S., Shu, X.-O., Wong, J., Zhang, L., Zhang, J., Hu, W., Cai, Q., Gao, Y., Blechter, B., Rahman, M., Zheng, W., Rothman, N., Lan, Q., & Rappaport, S. M. (2025). HSA Adductomics in the Shanghai Women's Health Study Links Lung Cancer in Never-Smokers with Air Pollution, Redox Biology, and One-Carbon Metabolism. *Antioxidants*, *14*(3), 335. DOI: 10.3390/antiox14030335 PMID: 40227422

Inouye, M., Abraham, G., Nelson, C. P., Wood, A. M., Sweeting, M. J., Dudbridge, F., & Samani, N. J. (2021). Genomic risk prediction of coronary artery disease in 480,000 adults: Implications for CHD research. *European Heart Journal*, *42*(2), 136–145. DOI: 10.1093/eurheartj/ehaa1025

Islam, M. S., Alam, M. M., Ahamed, A., & Meerza, S. I. A. (2023, April). Prediction of diabetes at early stage using interpretable machine learning. In *SoutheastCon 2023* (pp. 261–265). IEEE., DOI: 10.1109/SoutheastCon51012.2023.10115152

Islam, Z., Aslam, M., Khan, A. U., & Rehman, M. (2025). Genetic testing and its role in precision medicine: Understand disease risk and tailoring treatments. *Indus Journal of Bioscience Research*, *3*(1), 461–470.

Ivey, K. N., & Srivastava, D. (2015). microRNAs as Developmental Regulators. *Cold Spring Harbor Perspectives in Biology*, *7*(7), a008144. DOI: 10.1101/cshperspect.a008144

Izquierdo-Condoy, J. S., Arias-Rodríguez, F. D., Díaz-Chamba, W. I., Mena-Noroña, D. A., Toaquiza, L. C., Espín-Sambache, B., Valdivieso-Andrade, E. J., Cangas-Isacaz, A., García-Cañarte, S., Rubio-Niera, M., & Ortiz-Prado, E. (2025). Epidemiological characterization of congenital heart disease at different altitudes in Ecuador: A four-year retrospective study in a pediatric referral hospital. *Frontiers in Public Health*, *13*. Advance online publication. DOI: 10.3389/fpubh.2025.1497253 PMID: 39944066

Jamali, H., Dascalu, S. M., & Harris, F. C. (2024, May). AI-Driven Analysis and Prediction of Energy Consumption in NYC's Municipal Buildings. In 2024 IEEE/ACIS 22nd International Conference on Software Engineering Research, Management and Applications (SERA) (pp. 277-283). IEEE. DOI: 10.1109/SERA61261.2024.10685594

Jamali, H., Dascalu, S. M., & Harris, F. C., Jr. (2024, March). Fostering joint innovation: a global online platform for ideas sharing and collaboration. In International Conference on Information Technology-New Generations (pp. 305-312). Cham: Springer Nature Switzerland. DOI: 10.1007/978-3-031-56599-1_40

Jamali, H., Dascalu, S. M., Harris, F. C., & Feil-Seifer, D. (2025, May). Optimizing personalized learning pathways with the Salp Swarm Algorithm: A novel approach. In 2025 6th International Conference on Artificial Intelligence, Robotics and Control (AIRC) (pp. 291-297). IEEE. DOI: 10.1109/AIRC64931.2025.11077498

Jamali, H., Shill, P. C., Feil-Seifer, D., Harris, F. C., Jr., & Dascalu, S. M. (2023, October). A schedule of duties in the cloud space using a modified salp swarm algorithm. In IFIP International Internet of Things Conference (pp. 62-75). Cham: Springer Nature Switzerland. DOI: 10.1007/978-3-031-45878-1_5

Jamali, H., Watson, J., Dascalu, S. M., & Harris, F. C. (2025, April). Harmonized Data Drive: Standardizing and Unifying Smart Car Information Storage for Enhanced Forensics and Interoperability. In 2025 13th International Symposium on Digital Forensics and Security (ISDFS) (pp. 1-6). IEEE. https://doi.org/DOI: 10.1109/ISDFS65363.2025.11012079

Jamali, H., DeBolt, A. L., Dalton, H., Layosa, J. K., Macy, I. R., Shill, P. C., & Wu, R. (2025, June). FORE: A student-centered framework for accessible robotics education through simulation and interactive learning. In *2025 ASEE Annual Conference & Exposition*. https://doi.org/DOI: 10.18260/1-2--56585

Jamali, H., Karimi, A., & Haghighizadeh, M. (2018, February). A new method of cloud-based computation model for mobile devices: energy consumption optimization in mobile-to-mobile computation offloading. In *Proceedings of the 6th International Conference on Communications and Broadband Networking* (pp. 32-37). https://doi.org/DOI: 10.1145/3193092.3193103

Jamil Abusamra, H. N., Ali, S. H. M., Khidir Elhussien, W. A., Ahmed Mirghani, A. M., Alameen Ahmed, A. A., & Abdelrahman Ibrahim, M. E. (2025). Ethical and Practical Considerations of Artificial Intelligence in Pediatric Medicine: A Systematic Review. *Cureus*, *17*(2). Advance online publication. DOI: 10.7759/cureus.79024 PMID: 40104456

Jentink, J., Loane, M. A., Dolk, H., Barisic, I., Garne, E., Morris, J. K., & de Jong-van den Berg, L. T.EUROCAT Antiepileptic Study Working Group. (2010). Valproic acid monotherapy in pregnancy and major congenital malformations. *The New England Journal of Medicine*, *362*(23), 2185–2193. DOI: 10.1056/NEJMoa0907328 PMID: 20558369

Jia, L., Limeng, D., Xiaoyin, T., Junwen, W., Xintong, Z., Gang, X., Yun, B., & Hong, G. (2022). A Novel Splicing Mutation c.335–1 G>A in the Cardiac Transcription Factor NKX2-5 Leads to Familial Atrial Septal Defect Through miR-19 and PYK2. *Stem Cell Reviews and Reports*, *18*(8), 2646–2661. DOI: 10.1007/s12015-022-10400-5

Jiang, X.-Y., Feng, Y.-L., Ye, L.-T., Li, X.-H., Feng, J., Zhang, M.-Z., Shelat, H. S., Wassler, M., Li, Y., Geng, Y.-J., & Yu, X.-Y. (2017). Inhibition of Gata4 and Tbx5 by Nicotine-Mediated DNA Methylation in Myocardial Differentiation. *Stem Cell Reports*, *8*(2), 290–304. DOI: 10.1016/j.stemcr.2016.12.016 PMID: 28111280

Jiang, Y., Zhuang, J., Lin, Y., Wang, X., Chen, J., & Han, F. (2019). Long noncoding RNA SNHG6 contributes to ventricular septal defect formation via negative regulation of miR-101 and activation of Wnt/β-catenin pathway. *Die Pharmazie*, *74*(1), 23–28. DOI: 10.1691/ph.2019.8736 PMID: 30782246

Ji, L., Hou, H., Zhu, K., Liu, X., Liu, Y., Wang, Q., Li, J., Liu, H., Zhang, Q., Lv, J., Alexander, R., Wang, W., & Li, D. (2019). NOTCH1 Gene MicroRNA Target Variation and Ventricular Septal Defect Risk. *OMICS: A Journal of Integrative Biology*, *23*(1), 28–35. DOI: 10.1089/omi.2018.0171

Jin, S., Yoon, S. Z., Choi, Y. J., Kang, G., & Choi, S. U. (2024). Prenatal exposure to air pollutants and the risk of congenital heart disease: A Korean national health insurance database-based study. *Scientific Reports*, *14*(1), 16940. DOI: 10.1038/s41598-024-63150-4 PMID: 39043676

Jin, Y., Ai, L., Chai, X., Tang, P., Zhang, W., Yang, L., Hu, Y., Xu, Y., & Li, S. (2021). Maternal Circulating Exosomal miRNAs as Non-invasive Biomarkers for the Prediction of Fetal Ventricular Septal Defect. *Frontiers in Genetics*, *12*, 717208. DOI: 10.3389/fgene.2021.717208

Jonas, R. A. (2025). Twenty-five-year milestone for the ECHSA database: Time to focus on patient survival rather than procedural success. *European Journal of Cardio-Thoracic Surgery*, *67*(4), ezaf136. Advance online publication. DOI: 10.1093/ejcts/ezaf136 PMID: 40220325

Joshi, R. O., Chellappan, S., & Kukshal, P. (2020). Exploring the Role of Maternal Nutritional Epigenetics in Congenital Heart Disease. *Current Developments in Nutrition*, *4*(11), nzaa166. Advance online publication. DOI: 10.1093/cdn/nzaa166 PMID: 33294766

Joubert, B. R., Felix, J. F., Yousefi, P., Bakulski, K. M., Just, A. C., Breton, C., Reese, S. E., Markunas, C. A., Richmond, R. C., Xu, C. J., Küpers, L. K., Oh, S. S., Hoyo, C., Gruzieva, O., Söderhäll, C., Salas, L. A., Baïz, N., Zhang, H., Lepeule, J., & London, S. J. (2016). DNA Methylation in Newborns and Maternal Smoking in Pregnancy: Genome-wide Consortium Meta-analysis. *American Journal of Human Genetics*, *98*(4), 680–696. DOI: 10.1016/j.ajhg.2016.02.019 PMID: 27040690

Juarez, P. D., Hood, D. B., Song, M.-A., & Ramesh, A. (2020). Use of an Exposome Approach to Understand the Effects of Exposures From the Natural, Built, and Social Environments on Cardio-Vascular Disease Onset, Progression, and Outcomes. *Frontiers in Public Health, 8*, 379. DOI: 10.3389/fpubh.2020.00379 PMID: 32903514

Kabesch, M., & Tost, J. (2020). Recent findings in the genetics and epigenetics of asthma and allergy. *Seminars in Immunopathology, 42*(1), 43–60. DOI: 10.1007/s00281-019-00777-w PMID: 32060620

Kalisch-Smith, J. I., Ved, N., & Sparrow, D. B. (2020). Environmental Risk Factors for Congenital Heart Disease. *Cold Spring Harbor Perspectives in Biology, 12*(3), a037234. DOI: 10.1101/cshperspect.a037234 PMID: 31548181

Kalisch-Smith, J. I., Ved, N., & Sparrow, D. B. (2020). Environmental risk factors for congenital heart disease. *Cold Spring Harbor Perspectives in Biology, 12*(3), a037234. PMID: 31548181

Kaltsas, A., Markou, E., Kyrgiafini, M.-A., Zikopoulos, A., Symeonidis, E. N., Dimitriadis, F., Zachariou, A., Sofikitis, N., & Chrisofos, M. (2025). Oxidative-Stress-Mediated Epigenetic Dysregulation in Spermatogenesis: Implications for Male Infertility and Offspring Health. *Genes, 16*(1), 1. Advance online publication. DOI: 10.3390/genes16010093 PMID: 39858640

Kamath, B. M., Baker, A., Houwen, R., Todorova, L., & Kerkar, N. (2018). Systematic review: The epidemiology, natural history, and burden of Alagille syndrome. *Journal of Pediatric Gastroenterology and Nutrition, 67*(2), 148–156. DOI: 10.1097/MPG.0000000000001958 PMID: 29543694

Kan, Z., Yan, W., Wang, N., Fang, Y., Gao, H., & Song, Y. (2022). Identification of circRNA-miRNA-mRNA Regulatory Network and Crucial Signaling Pathway Axis Involved in Tetralogy of Fallot. *Frontiers in Genetics, 13*, 917454. DOI: 10.3389/fgene.2022.917454

Karabayir, I., & Akbilgic, O. (2025). Generalizability of electrocardiographic artificial intelligence. *npj Cardiovascular Health, 2*(1), 38.

Karas Kuželički, N., & Doljak, B. (2024). Congenital Heart Disease and Genetic Changes in Folate/Methionine Cycles. *Genes, 15*(7), 872. DOI: 10.3390/genes15070872 PMID: 39062651

Karatzia, L., Aung, N., & Aksentijevic, D. (2022). Artificial intelligence in cardiology: Hope for the future and power for the present. *Frontiers in Cardiovascular Medicine, 9*, 945726. DOI: 10.3389/fcvm.2022.945726 PMID: 36312266

Karimov, E., & Zaim Gökbay, İ. (2025). Enhancing Pediatric Congenital Heart Disease Outcomes: The Role of Machine Learning Models and AI-Driven Methodologies. *Cam and Sakura Medical Journal*, 1–8. https://doi.org/DOI: 10.4274/csmedj.galenos.2025.2025-7-1

Karim, R., Blake, L.-E., & Inoue, J.. (2018). Algorithms for left atrial wall segmentation and thickness—Evaluation on an open-source CT and MRI image database. *Medical Image Analysis*. PMID: 30208355

Kars, M. E., Stein, D., Stenson, P. D., Cooper, D. N., Chung, W. K., Gruber, P. J., Seidman, C. E., Shen, Y., Tristani-Firouzi, M., Gelb, B. D., & Itan, Y. (2025). Deciphering the digenic architecture of congenital heart disease using trio exome sequencing data. *American Journal of Human Genetics, 112*(3), 583–598. DOI: 10.1016/j.ajhg.2025.01.024 PMID: 39983722

Kashyap, S., & Tripathi, P. (2023). Assisted Reproductive Technology (Regulation) Act 2021: Critique and Contestations. *Asian Bioethics Review*, *16*(2), 149–164. DOI: 10.1007/s41649-023-00253-6 PMID: 38586570

Kawamura, J., Yamakuchi, M., Ueno, K., Hashiguchi, T., & Okamoto, Y. (2025). MiR-25-3p regulates pulmonary arteriovenous malformation after Glenn procedure in patients with univentricular heart via the PHLPP2-HIF-1α axis. *Scientific Reports*, *15*(1), 4138. DOI: 10.1038/s41598-025-88840-5

Kelly, R. G. (2023). The heart field transcriptional landscape at single-cell resolution. *Developmental Cell, 58*(4), 257–266. DOI: 10.1016/j.devcel.2023.01.010 PMID: 36809764

Kemp-Casey, A., Hart, R., Milne, E., Bower, C., Walls, M. L., Yovich, J. L., Burton, P., Liu, Y., Barblett, H., & Hansen, M. (2025). Are assisted reproductive technology pregnancies more likely to be exposed to teratogenic medication? A whole-population study. *Australian and New Zealand Journal of Obstetrics and Gynaecology*, *65*(3), 390–397. DOI: 10.1111/ajo.13911 PMID: 39651600

Kermani, A., Jamshidi, A. M., Mahdavi, Z., Dashtaki, A. A., Zand, M., Nasab, M. A., & Khan, B. (2023). Energy management system for smart grid in the presence of energy storage and photovoltaic systems. *International Journal of Photoenergy*, *2023*(1), 5749756. DOI: 10.1155/2023/5749756

Khan, M.A.U., Khan, R.B., Bilal, S., Jamil A., ShahA. M., (2008), Enhancement of Angiogram Images using Pseudo Color Processing, Information Technology Journa,l Volume(1), pp. 210 - 214

Khandoker, F., & Grigsby, T. J. (2025). Methodological Approaches in Studying Type-2 Diabetes-Related Health Behaviors—A Systematic Review. *Applied Sciences (Basel, Switzerland), 15*(19), 10567. DOI: 10.3390/app151910567

Khurana, E., Fu, Y., Chakravarty, D., Demichelis, F., Rubin, M. A., & Gerstein, M. (2016). Role of non-coding sequence variants in cancer. *Nature Reviews. Genetics, 17*(2), 93–108. PMID: 26781813

Kido, T., Sikora-Wohlfeld, W., Kawashima, M., Kikuchi, S., Kamatani, N., Patwardhan, A., & Butte, A. J. (2018). Are minor alleles more likely to be risk alleles? *BMC Medical Genomics, 11*(1), 3. PMID: 29351777

Kim, Y. Y., Min, H., Kim, H., Choi, Y. M., Liu, H. C., & Ku, S.-Y. (2017). Differential MicroRNA Expression Profile of Human Embryonic Stem Cell-Derived Cardiac Lineage Cells. *Tissue Engineering and Regenerative Medicine, 14*(2), 163–169. DOI: 10.1007/s13770-017-0051-4

Kirk, E. P., Sunde, M., Costa, M. W., Rankin, S. A., Wolstein, O., Castro, M. L., Butler, T. L., Hyun, C., Guo, G., Otway, R., Mackay, J. P., Waddell, L. B., Cole, A. D., Hayward, C., Keogh, A., Macdonald, P., Griffiths, L., Fatkin, D., Sholler, G. F., & Harvey, R. P. (2007). Mutations in cardiac T-box factor gene TBX20 are associated with diverse cardiac pathologies, including defects of septation and valvulogenesis and cardiomyopathy. *American Journal of Human Genetics, 81*(2), 280–291. DOI: 10.1086/519530 PMID: 17668378

Kirschner, M. B., Edelman, J. J. B., Kao, S. C.-H., Vallely, M. P., Van Zandwijk, N., & Reid, G. (2013). The Impact of Hemolysis on Cell-Free microRNA Biomarkers. *Frontiers in Genetics, 4*. Advance online publication. DOI: 10.3389/fgene.2013.00094

Kocher, K., Ngwa, J., Bhattacharya, S., Donofrio, M., Limperopoulos, C., & Andescavage, N. (2025). Epigenomic signatures of accelerated epigenetic aging are associated with congenital heart disease in newborns. *BMC Medical Genomics, 18*(1), 121. PMID: 40722095

Komatsu, M., Sakai, A., Komatsu, R., Matsuoka, R., Yasutomi, S., Shozu, K., Dozen, A., Machino, H., Hidaka, H., Arakaki, T., Asada, K., Kaneko, S., Sekizawa, A., & Hamamoto, R. (2021). Detection of Cardiac Structural Abnormalities in Fetal Ultrasound Videos Using Deep Learning. *Applied Sciences (Basel, Switzerland), 11*(1), 371. DOI: 10.3390/app11010371

Kotowska-Zimmer, A., Pewinska, M., & Olejniczak, M. (2021). Artificial miRNAs as therapeutic tools: Challenges and opportunities. *Wiley Interdisciplinary Reviews. RNA, 12*(4), e1640. DOI: 10.1002/wrna.1640

Krishnan, U., Dhurandhar, V., & Joshi, S. (2025). Clinical profile and outcome of pediatric heart surgeries at a tertiary care center. *Frontiers in Pediatrics*, *13*, 1543755. DOI: 10.3389/fped.2025.1543755 PMID: 40464041

Krismanuel, H. (2025). Air pollution and cardiovascular diseases: Mechanisms, evidence, and mitigation strategies. *Journal of Medicine and Life*, *18*(5), 411–427. DOI: 10.25122/jml-2025-0018 PMID: 40599138

Kukshal, P., Joshi, R. O., Kumar, A., Ahamad, S., Murthy, P. R., Sathe, Y., Manohar, K., Guhathakurta, S., & Chellappan, S. (2023). Case–control association study of congenital heart disease from a tertiary paediatric cardiac centre from North India. *BMC Pediatrics*, *23*(1), 290. DOI: 10.1186/s12887-023-04095-x PMID: 37322441

Kumar, S. (2020). Prevalence of Congenital Heart Disease in ART-conceived Infants: A North India Cohort Study. *Indian Journal of Pediatrics*, *87*(3), 207–212. DOI: 10.1007/s12098-019-03125-2 PMID: 31900850

Kuppusamy, K. T., Jones, D. C., Sperber, H., Madan, A., Fischer, K. A., Rodriguez, M. L., Pabon, L., Zhu, W.-Z., Tulloch, N. L., Yang, X., Sniadecki, N. J., Laflamme, M. A., Ruzzo, W. L., Murry, C. E., & Ruohola-Baker, H. (2015). Let-7 family of microRNA is required for maturation and adult-like metabolism in stem cell-derived cardiomyocytes. *Proceedings of the National Academy of Sciences of the United States of America*, *112*(21), E2785–E2794. DOI: 10.1073/pnas.1424042112

Kwapil, T. R., Chapman, J. P., Chapman, L. J., & Miller, M. B. (1996). Deviant olfactory experiences as indicators of risk for psychosis. *Schizophrenia Bulletin*, *22*(2), 371–380. DOI: 10.1093/schbul/22.2.371 PMID: 8782292

Kwon, C., Arnold, J., Hsiao, E. C., Taketo, M. M., Conklin, B. R., & Srivastava, D. (2007). Canonical Wnt signaling is a positive regulator of mammalian cardiac progenitors. *Proceedings of the National Academy of Sciences of the United States of America*, *104*(26), 10894–10899. DOI: 10.1073/pnas.0704044104

Kwon, C., Han, Z., Olson, E. N., & Srivastava, D. (2005). MicroRNA1 influences cardiac differentiation in Drosophila and regulates Notch signaling. *Proceedings of the National Academy of Sciences of the United States of America*, *102*(52), 18986–18991. DOI: 10.1073/pnas.0509535102

Ladewig, E., Okamura, K., Flynt, A. S., Westholm, J. O., & Lai, E. C. (2012). Discovery of hundreds of mirtrons in mouse and human small RNA data. *Genome Research*, *22*(9), 1634–1645. DOI: 10.1101/gr.133553.111

Lage, K., Greenway, S. C., Rosenfeld, J. A., Wakimoto, H., Gorham, J. M., Segrè, A. V., & Larsen, L. A. (2012). Genetic and environmental risk factors in congenital heart disease functionally converge in protein networks driving heart development. *Proceedings of the National Academy of Sciences of the United States of America, 109*(35), 14035–14040. PMID: 22904188

Lahm, H., Jia, M., Dreßen, M., Wirth, F., Puluca, N., Gilsbach, R., Keavney, B. D., Cleuziou, J., Beck, N., Bondareva, O., Dzilic, E., Burri, M., König, K. C., Ziegelmüller, J. A., Abou-Ajram, C., Neb, I., Zhang, Z., Doppler, S. A., Mastantuono, E., & Krane, M. (2021). Congenital heart disease risk loci identified by genome-wide association study in European patients. *The Journal of Clinical Investigation, 131*(2), e141837. DOI: 10.1172/JCI141837 PMID: 33201861

Lai, C. T. M., Ng, E. K. O., Chow, P., Kwong, A., & Cheung, Y. (2013). Circulating microRNA expression profile and systemic right ventricular function in adults after atrial switch operation for complete transposition of the great arteries. *BMC Cardiovascular Disorders, 13*, 73. DOI: 10.1186/1471-2261-13-73

Lai, C. T. M., Ng, E. K. O., Chow, P., Kwong, A., & Cheung, Y. (2017). Circulating MicroRNA in patients with repaired tetralogy of Fallot. *European Journal of Clinical Investigation, 47*(8), 574–582. DOI: 10.1111/eci.12778

Lakshmaiah, A., Korrapati, C., Suresh, C., & Raghavan, R. (2025). Synthetic Biology and AI. *Spatially Variable Genes in Cancer*, 265–290. https://doi.org/DOI: 10.4018/979-8-3693-7728-4.ch010

Lakshmanan, S., & Gimelli, A. (2023). Cancer risk in adult congenital heart disease. *International Journal of Cardiology: Congenital Heart Disease, 12*, 100441. 10.1016/j.ijcchd.2023.100441

Law, A. K. W., Zhu, H., & Chan, F. H. Y. (2003), 3D Reconstruction of Coronary Artery using Biplane Angiography, Proceedings of the 25, Annual Intemational Conference of the IELE 1MUS Cancun, Mexico

Leirgul, E., Fomina, T., Greve, G., Tell, G. S., Sandberg, M., & Øyen, N. (2025). Trends in Birth Prevalence of Congenital Heart Defects in Norway—A Population Study 1994–2014. *Acta Paediatrica, n/a*(n/a). https://doi.org/DOI: 10.1111/apa.70235

Lemieux, A., Khalilipalandi, S., Lauzon-Schnittka, J., Taillefer, V., Tousignant, A., Perreault, L., Rego, K., Dubois, M., Watelle, L., Roy, L.-O., & Dallaire, F. (2024). Meta-Analysis of Risk Factors for Congenital Heart Disease: Part 2, Maternal Medication, Reproductive Technologies, and Familial and Fetal Factors. *The Canadian Journal of Cardiology, 40*(12), 2496–2511. DOI: 10.1016/j.cjca.2024.09.011 PMID: 39288833

Leonard, R., Zhao, Y., Eliason, S., Zimmerman, K., Batz, A., Hatcher, C. J., Weiss, R. M., Sweat, M., Li, X., & Amendt, B. A. (2025). Single-nuclei multiomics analysis identifies abnormal cardiomyocytes in a murine model of cardiac development. *Nature Communications*, *16*, 6947. DOI: 10.1038/s41467-025-62208-9

Liang, Y., Pan, Z., Zhu, M., Gao, R., Wang, Y., Cheng, Y., & Zhang, N. (2023). Exposure to essential and non-essential trace elements and risks of congenital heart defects: A narrative review. *Frontiers in Nutrition*, *10*, 1121826. PMID: 36998909

Lian, X., Hsiao, C., Wilson, G., Zhu, K., Hazeltine, L. B., Azarin, S. M., Raval, K. K., Zhang, J., Kamp, T. J., & Palecek, S. P. (2012). Robust cardiomyocyte differentiation from human pluripotent stem cells via temporal modulation of canonical Wnt signaling. *Proceedings of the National Academy of Sciences of the United States of America*, *109*(27), E1848–E1857. DOI: 10.1073/pnas.1200250109

Li, D., Ji, L., Liu, L., Liu, Y., Hou, H., Yu, K., Sun, Q., & Zhao, Z. (2014). Characterization of circulating microRNA expression in patients with a ventricular septal defect. *PLoS One*, *9*(8), e106318. DOI: 10.1371/journal.pone.0106318

Li, D., Li, T., Wang, Y., Pan, F., Chen, J., Ruan, J., & Xu, W. (2025). Greenness exposure mitigate PM2.5-associated congenital heart defects in China: A mediation analysis of chemical composition and seasonal-spatial vulnerability. *International Journal of Hygiene and Environmental Health*, *269*, 114624. DOI: 10.1016/j.ijheh.2025.114624 PMID: 40684539

Li, H., Zhou, M., Sun, Y., Yang, J., Zeng, X., Qiu, Y., Xia, Y., Zheng, Z., Yu, J., Feng, Y., Shi, Z., Huang, T., Tan, L., Lin, R., Li, J., Fan, X., Ye, J., Duan, H., Shi, S., & Shu, Q. (2024). A Patient Similarity Network (CHDmap) to Predict Outcomes After Congenital Heart Surgery: Development and Validation Study. *JMIR Medical Informatics*, *12*, e49138. DOI: 10.2196/49138 PMID: 38297829

Li, J., Cao, Y., Ma, X., Wang, H., Zhang, J., Luo, X., Chen, W., Wu, Y., Meng, Y., Zhang, J., Yuan, Y., Ma, D., & Huang, G. (2013). Roles of miR-1-1 and miR-181c in ventricular septal defects. *International Journal of Cardiology*, *168*(2), 1441–1446. DOI: 10.1016/j.ijcard.2012.12.048

Li, J., Liu, Y., Huang, H., & Jin, L. (2024). Cardiovascular health of offspring conceived by assisted reproduction technology: A comprehensive review. *Frontiers in Cardiovascular Medicine*, *11*. Advance online publication. DOI: 10.3389/fcvm.2024.1287060 PMID: 38292241

Li, J.-Y., Li, X.-C., & Tang, Y.-L. (2021). Upregulation of miR-128 Mediates Heart Injury by Activating Wnt/β-catenin Signaling Pathway in Heart Failure Mice. *Organogenesis*, *17*(3–4), 27–39. DOI: 10.1080/15476278.2021.2020018

Li, K.-X., Li, J.-R., Zuo, S.-J., Li, X., Chen, X.-T., Xiao, P.-Y., Li, H.-T., Sun, L., Qian, T., Zhang, H.-M., Zhu, D., Yu, X.-Y., Chen, G., & Jiang, X.-Y. (2024). Identification of miR-20b-5p as an inhibitory regulator in cardiac differentiation via TET2 and DNA hydroxymethylation. *Clinical Epigenetics, 16*(1), 42. DOI: 10.1186/s13148-024-01653-7

Lim, T. B., Foo, S. Y. R., & Chen, C. K. (2021). The role of epigenetics in congenital heart disease. *Genes, 12*(3), 390. PMID: 33803261

Linabery, A. M., Blair, C. K., Gamis, A. S., Olshan, A. F., Heerema, N. A., & Ross, J. A. (2008). Congenital abnormalities and acute leukemia among children with Down syndrome: A Children's Oncology Group study. *Cancer Epidemiology, Biomarkers & Prevention, 17*(10), 2572–2577. DOI: 10.1158/1055-9965.EPI-08-0284 PMID: 18829445

Linares, D., Luna, B., Loayza, E., del Callejo, A., Garcia-Sejas, M., Erostegui, C., & Taboada, G. (2025). High altitude exposure and the birth prevalence of congenital anomalies in newborns with Down syndrome. *Early Human Development, 205*, 106270. DOI: 10.1016/j.earlhumdev.2025.106270 PMID: 40280041

Lindley, K. J. (2025). Introduction to the Compendium on Lifelong Care in Women: Applying a Sex- and Gender-Lens to Practice. *Circulation Research, 136*(6), 551–552. DOI: 10.1161/CIRCRESAHA.125.326335 PMID: 40080537

Linglart, L., & Bonnet, D. (2022). Epigenetics and Congenital Heart Diseases. *Journal of Cardiovascular Development and Disease, 9*(6), 185. DOI: 10.3390/jcdd9060185 PMID: 35735814

Linglart, L., & Bonnet, D. (2022). Epigenetics and congenital heart diseases. *Journal of Cardiovascular Development and Disease, 9*(6), 185. PMID: 35735814

Lin, J., Zhao, D., Liang, Y., Liang, Z., Wang, M., Tang, X., Zhuang, H., Wang, H., Yin, X., Huang, Y., Yin, L., & Shen, L. (2024). Proteomic analysis of plasma total exosomes and placenta-derived exosomes in patients with gestational diabetes mellitus in the first and second trimesters. *BMC Pregnancy and Childbirth, 24*(1). Advance online publication. DOI: 10.1186/s12884-024-06919-9 PMID: 39478498

Lin, M., Guo, J., Gu, Z., Tang, W., Tao, H., You, S., Jia, D., Sun, Y., & Jia, P. (2025). Machine learning and multi-omics integration: Advancing cardiovascular translational research and clinical practice. *Journal of Translational Medicine, 23*(1), 388. DOI: 10.1186/s12967-025-06425-2 PMID: 40176068

Lismer, A., Siklenka, K., Lafleur, C., Dumeaux, V., & Kimmins, S. (2020). Sperm histone H3 lysine 4 trimethylation is altered in a genetic mouse model of transgenerational epigenetic inheritance. *Nucleic Acids Research*, *48*(20), 11380–11393. DOI: 10.1093/nar/gkaa712 PMID: 33068438

Liu, B., Lu, Y., Wang, Q., Dai, Y., & Liu, L. (2024). Cancer in 22q11.2 deletion syndrome: A case report and literature review. *European Journal of Medical Genetics*, *70*, 104959. DOI: 10.1016/j.ejmg.2024.104959 PMID: 38969060

Liu, J., Litt, L., Segal, M. R., Kelly, M. J., Pelton, J. G., & Kim, M. (2011). Metabolomics of oxidative stress in recent studies of endogenous and exogenously administered intermediate metabolites. *International Journal of Molecular Sciences*, *12*(10), 6469–6501. DOI: 10.3390/ijms12106469 PMID: 22072900

Liu, L., Pu, Y., Fan, J., Yan, Y., Liu, W., Luo, K., Wang, Y., Zhao, G., Chen, T., Puiu, P. D., & Huang, H. (2024). Wearable Sensors, Data Processing, and Artificial Intelligence in Pregnancy Monitoring: A Review. *Sensors (Basel)*, *24*(19), 6426. DOI: 10.3390/s24196426 PMID: 39409471

Liu, X., Li, M., Peng, Y., Hu, X., Xu, J., Zhu, S., Yu, Z., & Han, S. (2016). miR-30c regulates proliferation, apoptosis and differentiation via the Shh signaling pathway in P19 cells. *Experimental & Molecular Medicine*, *48*(7), e248. DOI: 10.1038/emm.2016.57

Liu, Y., Chen, S., Zühlke, L., Black, G. C., Choy, M. K., Li, N., & Keavney, B. D. (2019). Global birth prevalence of congenital heart defects 1970–2017: Updated systematic review and meta-analysis of 260 studies. *International Journal of Epidemiology*, *48*(2), 455–463. PMID: 30783674

Liu, Z., Li, X., Li, N., Li, S., Deng, K., Lin, Y., & Zhu, J. (2013). Association between maternal exposure to housing renovation and offspring with congenital heart disease: A multi-hospital case–control study. *Environmental Health : A Global Access Science Source*, *12*(1), 25. DOI: 10.1186/1476-069X-12-25 PMID: 23522351

Li, Y., Du, J., Deng, S., Liu, B., Jing, X., Yan, Y., & She, Q. (2024). The molecular mechanisms of cardiac development and related diseases. *Signal Transduction and Targeted Therapy*, *9*(1), 368. PMID: 39715759

Li, Z., Wang, D., Jin, L., Zhang, J., Xue, T., & Jin, L. (2025). Maternal exposure to fine particulate matter in the air and risk for fetal congenital heart defects: A case-control study. *Reproductive Toxicology (Elmsford, N.Y.)*, *132*, 108816. DOI: 10.1016/j.reprotox.2024.108816 PMID: 39638263

Lockridge, O. (2023). Overview of Adductomics in Toxicology. *Current Protocols, 3*(2), e672. DOI: 10.1002/cpz1.672 PMID: 36799690

Long, L., Xiao, Y., Yin, X., Gao, S., Zhou, L., & Liu, H. (2020). Expression of serum miR-27b and miR-451 in patients with congenital heart disease associated pulmonary artery hypertension and risk factor analysis. *Experimental and Therapeutic Medicine, 20*(4), 3196–3202. DOI: 10.3892/etm.2020.9042

Lourakis, M. I. A. (2005). *A Brief Description of the Levenberg-Marquardt Algorithm Implemened by levmar, free paper, Institute of Computer Science Foundation for Research and Technology - Hellas (FORTH)*. GREECE.

Lozano-Velasco, E., Inácio, J. M., Sousa, I., Guimarães, A. R., Franco, D., Moura, G., & Belo, J. A. (2024). miRNAs in Heart Development and Disease. *International Journal of Molecular Sciences, 25*(3), 1673. DOI: 10.3390/ijms25031673

MacGrogan, D., Münch, J., & de la Pompa, J. L. (2018). Notch and interacting signalling pathways in cardiac development, disease, and regeneration. *Nature Reviews. Cardiology, 15*(11), 685–704. PMID: 30287945

MacKenzie, E. (2024). *The role of rare genetic variants in aortic valve stenosis* (Master's thesis). McGill University.

Mahdavi, Z., Samavat, T., Javanmardi, A. S. J., Dashtaki, M. A., Zand, M., Nasab, M. A., & Khan, B. (2024). Providing a control system for charging electric vehicles using ANFIS. *International Transactions on Electrical Energy Systems, 2024*(1), 9921062. DOI: 10.1155/2024/9921062

Maiorino, E., & Loscalzo, J. (2023). Phenomics and Robust Multiomics Data for Cardiovascular Disease Subtyping. *Arteriosclerosis, Thrombosis, and Vascular Biology, 43*(7), 1111–1123. DOI: 10.1161/ATVBAHA.122.318892 PMID: 37226730

Malkawi, A., Almarzooq, Z., Al-Mallah, M. H., & Al'Aref, S. J. (2022). Artificial Intelligence-Based Cardiovascular Risk Stratification. In *Artificial Intelligence in Cardiothoracic Imaging* (pp. 403–419). Springer International Publishing.

Malta, M., AlMutiri, R., Martin, C. S., & Srour, M. (2023). Holoprosencephaly: Review of embryology, clinical phenotypes, etiology and management. *Children (Basel, Switzerland), 10*(4), 647. PMID: 37189898

Manivannan, S., Mansfield, C., & Zhang, X.. (2022). Single-cell transcriptomic profiling unveils dysregulation of cardiac progenitor cells and cardiomyocytes in a mouse model of maternal hyperglycemia. *Communications Biology, 5*, 820. DOI: 10.1038/s42003-022-03779-x PMID: 35970860

Mannarino, S., Calcaterra, V., Puricelli, F., Cecconi, G., Chillemi, C., Raso, I., Cordaro, E., & Zuccotti, G. (2025). The Role of miRNA Expression in Congenital Heart Disease: Insights into the Mechanisms and Biomarker Potential. *Children (Basel, Switzerland)*, *12*(5), 611. DOI: 10.3390/children12050611 PMID: 40426790

Mariana, M., & Cairrao, E. (2020). Phthalates Implications in the Cardiovascular System. *Journal of Cardiovascular Development and Disease*, *7*(3), 26. DOI: 10.3390/jcdd7030026 PMID: 32707888

Marino, N., Putignano, G., Cappilli, S., Chersoni, E., Santuccione, A., Calabrese, G., & Santus, E. (2023). Towards AI-driven longevity research: An overview. *Frontiers in Aging*, *4*, 1057204. PMID: 36936271

Maris, M. T., Koçar, A., Willems, D. L., Pols, J., Tan, H. L., Lindinger, G. L., & Bak, M. A. (2024). Ethical use of artificial intelligence to prevent sudden cardiac death: An interview study of patient perspectives. *BMC Medical Ethics*, *25*(1), 42. PMID: 38575931

Marracino, L., Fortini, F., Bouhamida, E., Camponogara, F., Severi, P., Mazzoni, E., Patergnani, S., D'Aniello, E., Campana, R., Pinton, P., Martini, F., Tognon, M., Campo, G., Ferrari, R., Vieceli Dalla Sega, F., & Rizzo, P. (2021). Adding a "Notch" to Cardiovascular Disease Therapeutics: A MicroRNA-Based Approach. *Frontiers in Cell and Developmental Biology*, *9*. Advance online publication. DOI: 10.3389/fcell.2021.695114

Ma, S., Zeng, A. G. X., Haibe-Kains, B., Goldenberg, A., Dick, J. E., & Wang, B. (2025). Moving towards genome-wide data integration for patient stratification with Integrate Any Omics. *Nature Machine Intelligence*, *7*(1), 29–42. DOI: 10.1038/s42256-024-00942-3

Mattapally, S., Nizamuddin, S., & Murthy, K. S.. (2015). c.620C>T mutation in GATA4 is associated with congenital heart disease in South India. *BMC Medical Genetics*, *16*, 7. DOI: 10.1186/s12881-015-0152-7 PMID: 25928801

Maurya, A., & Verma, K. (2025). FedSec+: An Advanced Privacy-Enhanced Cardiovascular Disease Prediction Model using Federated Learning. *AIP Conference Proceedings*, *3253*(1), 30033. DOI: 10.1063/5.0248335

Maute, R. L., Schneider, C., Sumazin, P., Holmes, A., Califano, A., Basso, K., & Dalla-Favera, R. (2013). tRNA-derived microRNA modulates proliferation and the DNA damage response and is down-regulated in B cell lymphoma. *Proceedings of the National Academy of Sciences of the United States of America*, *110*(4), 1404–1409. DOI: 10.1073/pnas.1206761110

McAllan, A. L., Pillman, K. A., Gearing, L. J., & Gantier, M. P. (2025). IsomiR stoichiometry changes as disease biomarkers. *Molecular Therapy. Nucleic Acids, 36*(3), 102578. DOI: 10.1016/j.omtn.2025.102578

Meng, X., Du, W., & Sun, Z. (2024). Fine particulate matter-induced cardiac developmental toxicity [Review]. *Experimental and Therapeutic Medicine, 29*(1), 6. DOI: 10.3892/etm.2024.12756 PMID: 39534282

Meng, X., Song, M., Zhang, K., Lu, W., Li, Y., Zhang, C., & Zhang, Y. (2024). Congenital heart disease: Types, pathophysiology, diagnosis, and treatment options. *MedComm, 5*(7), e631. DOI: 10.1002/mco2.631

Mick, E., Shah, R., Tanriverdi, K., Murthy, V., Gerstein, M., Rozowsky, J., Kitchen, R., Larson, M. G., Levy, D., & Freedman, J. E. (2017). Stroke and Circulating Extracellular RNAs. *Stroke, 48*(4), 828–834. DOI: 10.1161/STROKEAHA.116.015140

Miranda, J., Paules, C., Noell, G., Youssef, L., Paternina-Caicedo, A., Crovetto, F., Cañellas, N., Garcia-Martín, M. L., Amigó, N., Eixarch, E., Faner, R., Figueras, F., Simões, R. V., Crispi, F., & Gratacós, E. (2023). Similarity network fusion to identify phenotypes of small-for-gestational-age fetuses. *iScience, 26*(9), 107620. DOI: 10.1016/j.isci.2023.107620 PMID: 37694157

Mishra, R., Verma, A., Sharma, B., & Sharma, P. (2025). An Overview of Transdermal Patches: Opportunities and Obstacles in Modern Drug Delivery. *Asian Journal of Research in Medical and Pharmaceutical Sciences, 14*(3), 18–29. DOI: 10.9734/ajrimps/2025/v14i3314

Misra, C., Sachan, N., McNally, C. R., Koenig, S. N., Nichols, H. A., Guggilam, A., Lucchesi, P. A., Pu, W. T., Srivastava, D., & Garg, V. (2012). Congenital heart disease–causing Gata4 mutation displays functional deficits in vivo. *PLOS Genetics, 8*(5), e1002690. DOI: 10.1371/journal.pgen.1002690 PMID: 22589735

Mitchell, L. E. (2022). Maternal genetic factors in the development of congenital heart defects. *Current Opinion in Genetics & Development, 76*, 101961. PMID: 35882070

Mo, J., Liu, X., Huang, Y., He, R., Zhang, Y., & Huang, H. (2022). Developmental origins of adult diseases. *Medical Review (Berlin, Germany), 2*(5), 450–470. DOI: 10.1515/mr-2022-0027 PMID: 37724166

Moreau, J. L. M., Kesteven, S., Martin, E. M. M. A., Lau, K. S., Yam, M. X., O'Reilly, V. C., del Monte-Nieto, G., Baldini, A., Feneley, M. P., Moon, A. M., Harvey, R. P., Sparrow, D. B., Chapman, G., & Dunwoodie, S. L. (2019). Gene-environment interaction impacts on heart development and embryo survival. *Development, 146*(4), dev172957. Advance online publication. DOI: 10.1242/dev.172957 PMID: 30787001

Morrell, N. W., Bloch, D. B., Ten Dijke, P., Goumans, M. J. T., Hata, A., Smith, J., & Bloch, K. D. (2016). Targeting BMP signalling in cardiovascular disease and anaemia. *Nature Reviews. Cardiology, 13*(2), 106–120. PMID: 26461965

Morton, S. U., Quiat, D., Seidman, J. G., & Seidman, C. E. (2022). Genomic frontiers in congenital heart disease. *Nature Reviews. Cardiology, 19*(1), 26–42. PMID: 34272501

Motairek, I., Makhlouf, M. H. E., Rajagopalan, S., & Al-Kindi, S. (2023). The Exposome and Cardiovascular Health. *The Canadian Journal of Cardiology, 39*(9), 1191–1203. DOI: 10.1016/j.cjca.2023.05.020 PMID: 37290538

Mouat, J. S., Li, S., Myint, S. S., Laufer, B. I., Lupo, P. J., Schraw, J. M., & LaSalle, J. M. (2023). Epigenomic signature of major congenital heart defects in newborns with Down syndrome. *Human Genomics, 17*(1), 92. PMID: 37803336

Movassaghi, B., Garcia, J. A., Grass, M., Schaefer, D., Rasche, V., Wink, O., Chen, J. Y., Groves, B. M., Messenger, J. C., & Carroll, J. D. (2006). Three-dimensional gated reconstructed images of the coronary arteries based on rotational coronary angiography: First in human results. *Circulation, 114*, 507–507.

Movassaghi, B., Rasche, V., Grass, M., Viergever, M. A., & Niessen, W. J. (2004). A quantitative analysis of 3-D coronary modeling from two or more projection images. *IEEE Transactions on Medical Imaging, 23*(12), 1517–1531. PMID: 15575409

Munshi, N. V. (2012). Gene regulatory networks in cardiac conduction system development. *Circulation Research, 110*(11), 1525–1537. PMID: 22628576

Münsterberg, A., & Hoppler, S. (2016). WNT and BMP regulate roadblocks toward cardiomyocyte differentiation: Lessons learned from embryos inform human stem cell differentiation. *Stem Cell Investigation, 3*, 33. DOI: 10.21037/sci.2016.07.03

Musunuru, K., Kathiresan, S., & Khera, A. V. (2021). Genetics and cardiovascular disease: The next decade. *Journal of the American College of Cardiology, 77*(3), 406–420. DOI: 10.1016/j.jacc.2020.11.034

Nagashri, N., Archana, L., & Raghavan, R. (2024). Microbial Volatile Compounds (MVOCs) in Food Industries and Food Safety Applications. *Innovations, Securities, and Case Studies Across Healthcare, Business, and Technology*, 75–96. https://doi .org/DOI: 10.4018/979-8-3693-1906-2.ch005

Nagueh, S. F., Smiseth, O. A., & Appleton, C. P.. (2016). Recommendations for the evaluation of left ventricular diastolic function by Echocardiography: An update from the American Society of Echocardiography and the European Association of Cardiovascular Imaging. *European Heart Journal Cardiovascular Imaging, 17*, 1321–1360. PMID: 27422899

Nail, H. M., Chiu, C.-C., Leung, C.-H., Ahmed, M. M. M., & Wang, H.-M. D. (2023). Exosomal miRNA-mediated intercellular communications and immunomodulatory effects in tumor microenvironments. *Journal of Biomedical Science, 30*(1), 69. DOI: 10.1186/s12929-023-00964-w

Naito, A. T., Shiojima, I., Akazawa, H., Hidaka, K., Morisaki, T., Kikuchi, A., & Komuro, I. (2006). Developmental stage-specific biphasic roles of Wnt/β-catenin signaling in cardiomyogenesis and hematopoiesis. *Proceedings of the National Academy of Sciences of the United States of America, 103*(52), 19812–19817. DOI: 10.1073/pnas.0605768103

Najjar, R. (2023). Redefining radiology: A review of artificial intelligence integration in medical imaging. *Diagnostics (Basel), 13*(17), 2760. PMID: 37685300

Nakayama, K. H., Hou, L., & Huang, N. F. (2014). Role of extracellular matrix signaling cues in modulating cell fate commitment for cardiovascular tissue engineering. *Advanced Healthcare Materials, 3*(5), 628–641. PMID: 24443420

Nanjundeshwara, N., Lakshmaiah, A., & Raghavan, R. (2025). Aflatoxigenic Fungi. *Aflatoxigenic Fungi*, 225–239. https://doi.org/DOI: 10.1201/9781003487043-29

Narayan, P., Richter, F., & Morton, S. (2024). Genetics and etiology of congenital heart disease. *Current Topics in Developmental Biology, 156*, 297–331. DOI: 10.1016/bs.ctdb.2024.01.009 PMID: 38556426

Natarelli, L., & Weber, C. (2022). A Non-Canonical Link between Non-Coding RNAs and Cardiovascular Diseases. *Biomedicines, 10*(2), 445. DOI: 10.3390/ biomedicines10020445

National Organization for Rare Disorders. (2020). Holt-Oram syndrome. In *NORD Rare Disease Database*. https://rarediseases.org/rare-diseases/holt-oram-syndrome/

Nemani, S., Goyal, S., Sharma, A., & Kothari, N. (2024). Artificial intelligence in pediatric airway - A scoping review. *Saudi Journal of Anaesthesia, 18*(3), 410–416. DOI: 10.4103/sja.sja_110_24 PMID: 39149736

Ney, G., Gross, A., Livinski, A., Kratz, C. P., & Stewart, D. R. (2022). Cancer incidence and surveillance strategies in individuals with RASopathies. *American Journal of Medical Genetics. Part C, Seminars in Medical Genetics, 190*(4), 530–540. DOI: 10.1002/ajmg.c.32018 PMID: 36533693

Nicoll, R. (2018). Environmental Contaminants and Congenital Heart Defects: A Re-Evaluation of the Evidence. *International Journal of Environmental Research and Public Health, 15*(10), 2096. DOI: 10.3390/ijerph15102096 PMID: 30257432

Nikolova, E., Laleva, L., Milev, M., Spiriev, T., Stoyanov, S., Ferdinandov, D., Mitev, V., & Todorova, A. (2024). miRNAs and related genetic biomarkers according to the WHO glioma classification: From diagnosis to future therapeutic targets. *Non-Coding RNA Research, 9*(1), 141–152. DOI: 10.1016/j.ncrna.2023.10.003

Niyogi, S. G., Nag, D. S., Shah, M. M., Swain, A., Naskar, C., Srivastava, P., & Kant, R. (2025). Role of artificial intelligence in congenital heart disease. *World Journal of Clinical Pediatrics, 14*(3). Advance online publication. DOI: 10.5409/wjcp.v14.i3.105926 PMID: 40881074

Nogel, M. (2025). Sustainable and equal integration of genomics into healthcare. *Journal of Infrastructure. Policy and Development, 9*(1), 10090.

Nordestgaard, L. T., Wolford, B. N., de Gonzalo-Calvo, D., Sopić, M., Devaux, Y., Matic, L., Wettinger, S. B., Schmid, J. A., Amigó, N., Masana, L., Catapano, A. L., Kardassis, D., & Magni, P. (2025). Multiomics in atherosclerotic cardiovascular disease. *Atherosclerosis, 408*, 120414. DOI: 10.1016/j.atherosclerosis.2025.120414 PMID: 40663987

Nossent, A. Y., Ektefaie, N., Wojta, J., Eichelberger, B., Kopp, C., Panzer, S., & Gremmel, T. (2019). Plasma Levels of snoRNAs are Associated with Platelet Activation in Patients with Peripheral Artery Disease. *International Journal of Molecular Sciences, 20*(23), 5975. DOI: 10.3390/ijms20235975

Nowak, K., Oluwayiose, O. A., Houle, E., Maxwell, D. L., Sawant, S., Paskavitz, A., Ford, J. B., Minguez-Alarcon, L., Calafat, A. M., Hauser, R., & Pilsner, J. R. (2024). Urinary concentrations of phthalate and phthalate alternative metabolites and sperm DNA methylation: A multi-cohort and *meta*-analysis of men in preconception studies. *Environment International, 192*, 109049. DOI: 10.1016/j.envint.2024.109049 PMID: 39393261

Nusrat, A., & Wu, M. (2025). Epicardium-myocardium crosstalk orchestrates heart development. *Frontiers in Cell and Developmental Biology, 13.* Advance online publication. DOI: 10.3389/fcell.2025.1655878 PMID: 41070347

Nussbaumer, G., & Benesch, M. (2022). Hepatoblastoma in molecularly defined, congenital diseases. *American Journal of Medical Genetics. Part A, 188*(9), 2527–2535. DOI: 10.1002/ajmg.a.62767 PMID: 35478319

O'Brien, J. E., Kibiryeva, N., Zhou, X.-G., Marshall, J. A., Lofland, G. K., Artman, M., Chen, J., & Bittel, D. C. (2012). Noncoding RNA expression in myocardium from infants with tetralogy of Fallot. *Circulation: Cardiovascular Genetics, 5*(3), 279–286. DOI: 10.1161/CIRCGENETICS.111.961474

O'Brien, J., Hayder, H., Zayed, Y., & Peng, C. (2018). Overview of MicroRNA Biogenesis, Mechanisms of Actions, and Circulation. *Frontiers in Endocrinology, 9*, 402. DOI: 10.3389/fendo.2018.00402

O'Sullivan, J. W., Raghavan, S., Marquez-Luna, C., Luzum, J. A., Damrauer, S. M., Ashley, E. A., O'Donnell, C. J., Willer, C. J., & Natarajan, P., & American Heart Association Council on Genomic and Precision Medicine; Council on Clinical Cardiology; Council on Arteriosclerosis, Thrombosis and Vascular Biology; Council on Cardiovascular Radiology and Intervention; Council on Lifestyle and Cardiometabolic Health; and Council on Peripheral Vascular Disease. (2022). Polygenic Risk Scores for Cardiovascular Disease: A Scientific Statement From the American Heart Association. *Circulation, 146*(8), e93–e118. DOI: 10.1161/CIR.0000000000001077 PMID: 35862132

Odogwu, N. M., Hagen, C., & Nelson, T. J. (2023). Transcriptome studies of congenital heart diseases: Identifying current gaps and therapeutic frontiers. *Frontiers in Genetics, 14*, 1278747. DOI: 10.3389/fgene.2023.1278747 PMID: 38152655

Okamura, K., Hagen, J. W., Duan, H., Tyler, D. M., & Lai, E. C. (2007). The Mirtron Pathway Generates microRNA-Class Regulatory RNAs in Drosophila. *Cell, 130*(1), 89–100. DOI: 10.1016/j.cell.2007.06.028

Olson, E. N. (2006). Gene regulatory networks in the evolution and development of the heart. *Science, 313*(5795), 1922–1927. PMID: 17008524

Oluwayiose, O. A., Marcho, C., Wu, H., Houle, E., Krawetz, S. A., Suvorov, A., Mager, J., & Richard Pilsner, J. (2021). Paternal preconception phthalate exposure alters sperm methylome and embryonic programming. *Environment International, 155*, 106693. DOI: 10.1016/j.envint.2021.106693 PMID: 34120004

Ouyang, Z., & Wei, K. (2021). miRNA in cardiac development and regeneration. *Cell Regeneration (London, England)*, *10*, 14. DOI: 10.1186/s13619-021-00077-5

Øyen, N., Diaz, L. J., Leirgul, E., Boyd, H. A., Priest, J., Mathiesen, E. R., Quertermous, T., Wohlfahrt, J., & Melbye, M. (2016). Prepregnancy Diabetes and Offspring Risk of Congenital Heart Disease: A Nationwide Cohort Study. *Circulation*, *133*(23), 2243–2253. DOI: 10.1161/CIRCULATIONAHA.115.017465 PMID: 27166384

Ozhan, G., & Weidinger, G. (2015). Wnt/β-catenin signaling in heart regeneration. *Cell Regeneration (London, England)*, *4*(1), 4–3. PMID: 26157574

P., A., D., K. M., M., J., P., S., & Raghavan, R. (2025). The Cancer Exposome. *Cancer Exposomics and Environmental Influences on Carcinogenesis*, 161–192. https://doi.org/DOI: 10.4018/979-8-3373-2165-3.ch004

Paddison, P. J., Caudy, A. A., Bernstein, E., Hannon, G. J., & Conklin, D. S. (2002). Short hairpin RNAs (shRNAs) induce sequence-specific silencing in mammalian cells. *Genes & Development*, *16*(8), 948–958. DOI: 10.1101/gad.981002

Padmanaban, S., Nasab, M. A., Samavat, T., Zand, M., & Nasab, M. A. (2023). Artificial intelligence techniques for smart power systems. In *IoT and Analytics in Renewable Energy Systems* (Vol. 1, pp. 107–123). CRC Press., DOI: 10.1201/9781003331117

Page, D. J., Miossec, M. J., Williams, S. G., Monaghan, R. M., Fotiou, E., Cordell, H. J., Sutcliffe, L., Topf, A., Bourgey, M., Bourque, G., Eveleigh, R., Dunwoodie, S. L., Winlaw, D. S., Bhattacharya, S., Breckpot, J., Devriendt, K., Gewillig, M., Brook, J. D., & Setchfield, K. J., Bu'Lock, F. A., … Keavney, B. D. (2019). Whole Exome Sequencing Reveals the Major Genetic Contributors to Nonsyndromic Tetralogy of Fallot. *Circulation Research*, *124*(4), 553–563. DOI: 10.1161/CIRCRESAHA.118.313250 PMID: 30582441

Pal, M., & Parija, S. (2021). Prediction of Heart Diseases using Random Forest. *Journal of Physics: Conference Series*, *1817*(1), 012009. DOI: 10.1088/1742-6596/1817/1/012009

Palma, A., Morais, S., Silva, P. V., & Pires, A. (2023). Congenital heart defects and preterm birth: Outcomes from a referral center. *Revista Portuguesa de Cardiologia*, *42*(5), 403–410. DOI: 10.1016/j.repc.2022.05.009 PMID: 36828187

Pandey, R. K., & Rathore, Y. K. (2025, May). Deep learning in 3D cardiac reconstruction: A systematic review of methodologies and dataset. *Medical & Biological Engineering & Computing*, *63*(5), 1271–1287. DOI: 10.1007/s11517-024-03273-y PMID: 39753994

Pandolfini, L., Barbieri, I., Bannister, A. J., Hendrick, A., Andrews, B., Webster, N., Murat, P., Mach, P., Brandi, R., Robson, S. C., Migliori, V., Alendar, A., d'Onofrio, M., Balasubramanian, S., & Kouzarides, T. (2019). METTL1 Promotes let-7 MicroRNA Processing via m7G Methylation. *Molecular Cell, 74*(6), 1278–1290. e9. DOI: 10.1016/j.molcel.2019.03.040

Patel, A. P., & Natarajan, P. (2019). Completing the genetic spectrum influencing coronary artery disease: From germline to somatic variation. *Cardiovascular Research, 115*(5), 830–843. PMID: 30789660

Patel, A., Sharma, R., & Kumar, S. (2025). Risk factor profiling in congenital heart disease: Maternal and environmental determinants. *Medical Science Journal, 15*(5), 234–241.

Paternostro, C., Springer, S., Kasprian, G., Yerlikaya-Schatten, G., & Reischer, T. (2023). Clinical Course and Outcome of Prenatally Detected 22q11.2 Deletion Syndrome—A Retrospective Analysis. *Diagnostics (Basel), 13*(13), 2244. DOI: 10.3390/diagnostics13132244 PMID: 37443638

Penaloza, J. S., Moreland, B., Gaither, J. B., Landis, B. J., Ware, S. M., McBride, K. L., & White, P.CCVM Consortium. (2025). Identification of Long Noncoding RNA Candidate Disease Genes Associated With Clinically Reported Copy Number Variants in Congenital Heart Disease. *Journal of the American Heart Association, 14*(6), e039177. DOI: 10.1161/JAHA.124.039177 PMID: 40079339

Peng, W., Yi, X., Peng, Y., Lu, H., & Liu, H. (2024). Developmental toxicity and mechanism of dibutyl phthalate on the development of subintestinal vessels in zebrafish. *Scientific Reports, 14*(1), 28464. DOI: 10.1038/s41598-024-80088-9 PMID: 39558027

Peng, Y., Song, L., Zhao, M., Harmelink, C., Debenedittis, P., Cui, X., Wang, Q., & Jiao, K. (2014). Critical roles of miRNA-mediated regulation of TGFβ signalling during mouse cardiogenesis. *Cardiovascular Research, 103*(2), 258–267. DOI: 10.1093/cvr/cvu126

Pereira, S. A., & Antunes, A. M. M. (2019). Special Issue "Adductomics: Elucidating the Environmental Causes of Disease.". *High-Throughput, 8*(3), 17. DOI: 10.3390/ht8030017 PMID: 31370290

Pierpont, M. E., Brueckner, M., Chung, W. K., Garg, V., Lacro, R. V., McGuire, A. L., Mital, S., Priest, J. R., Pu, W. T., Roberts, A., Ware, S. M., Gelb, B. D., & Russell, M. W., American Heart Association Council on Cardiovascular Disease in the Young, Council on Cardiovascular and Stroke Nursing, & Council on Genomic and Precision Medicine. (2018). Genetic basis for congenital heart disease: Revisited: A scientific statement from the American Heart Association. *Circulation*, *138*(21), e653–e711. DOI: 10.1161/CIR.0000000000000606 PMID: 30571578

Pietruszyńska-Reszetarska, A., Pietruszyński, R., Majsterek, I., Popławski, T., Skrzypek, M., Kolesińska, B., Waśko, J., Kapusta, J., Watała, C., & Irzmański, R. (2024). Coronary Artery Disease Is Related to Methylation Disorders Caused by the c.1286A>C *MTHFR* Polymorphism and to Low Serum 5-MTHF and Folic Acid Concentrations—Preliminary Results. *Reports*, *7*(1), 6. DOI: 10.3390/reports7010006 PMID: 40729255

Pinborg, A., Wennerholm, U. B., & Bergh, C. (2023). Long-term outcomes for children conceived by assisted reproductive technology. *Fertility and Sterility*, *120*(3 Pt 1), 449–456. DOI: 10.1016/j.fertnstert.2023.04.022 PMID: 37086833

Pi, X., Wang, J., Chu, L., Zhang, G., & Zhang, W. (2025). Prediction of high-risk pregnancy based on machine learning algorithms. *Scientific Reports*, *15*(1), 15561. DOI: 10.1038/s41598-025-00450-3 PMID: 40319080

Plotnikova, O., Baranova, A., & Skoblov, M. (2019). Comprehensive Analysis of Human microRNA–mRNA Interactome. *Frontiers in Genetics*, *10*, 933. DOI: 10.3389/fgene.2019.00933

Plusquin, M., Chadeau-Hyam, M., Ghantous, A., Alfano, R., Bustamante, M., Chatzi, L., Cuenin, C., Gulliver, J., Herceg, Z., Kogevinas, M., Nawrot, T. S., Pizzi, C., Porta, D., Relton, C. L., Richiardi, L., Robinson, O., Sunyer, J., Vermeulen, R., Vriens, A., & Vineis, P. (2018). DNA methylome marks of exposure to particulate matter at three time points in early life. *Environmental Science & Technology*, *52*(9), 5427–5437. DOI: 10.1021/acs.est.7b06447 PMID: 29597345

Poon, E. N., Hao, B., Guan, D., Jun Li, M., Lu, J., Yang, Y., Wu, B., Wu, S. C., Webb, S. E., Liang, Y., Miller, A. L., Yao, X., Wang, J., Yan, B., & Boheler, K. R. (2018). Integrated transcriptomic and regulatory network analyses identify microRNA-200c as a novel repressor of human pluripotent stem cell-derived cardiomyocyte differentiation and maturation. *Cardiovascular Research*, *114*(6), 894–906. DOI: 10.1093/cvr/cvy019

Potiris, A., Perros, P., Drakaki, E., Mavrogianni, D., Machairiotis, N., Sfakianakis, A., Karampitsakos, T., Vrachnis, D., Antonakopoulos, N., Panagopoulos, P., Drakakis, P., & Stavros, S. (2024). Investigating the Association of Assisted Reproduction Techniques and Adverse Perinatal Outcomes. *Journal of Clinical Medicine, 13*(2), 328. DOI: 10.3390/jcm13020328 PMID: 38256462

Pozza, A., Zanella, L., Castaldi, B., & Di Salvo, G. (2024). How Will Artificial Intelligence Shape the Future of Decision-Making in Congenital Heart Disease? *Journal of Clinical Medicine, 13*(10), 2996. DOI: 10.3390/jcm13102996 PMID: 38792537

Pozza, A., Zanella, L., Castaldi, B., & Di Salvo, G. (2024). How will artificial intelligence shape the future of decision-making in congenital heart disease? *Journal of Clinical Medicine, 13*(10), 2996. PMID: 38792537

Prakash, K. B., Padmanaban, S., & Mitolo, M. (2023). *Smart and Power Grid Systems–Design Challenges and Paradigms*. River Publishers., DOI: 10.1201/9781003339557

Priest, J. R., Ashley, E. A., & Giraldez, A. J. (2022). Genetics of congenital heart disease: Current knowledge and future directions. *Nature Reviews. Cardiology, 19*(5), 331–348. DOI: 10.1038/s41569-021-00668-5

Protopapas, E., Padalino, M., Tobota, Z., Ebels, T., Speggiorin, S., Horer, J., Kansy, A., Jacobs, J. P., Fragata, J., Maruszewski, B., Vida, V., & Sarris, G. (2025). The European Congenital Heart Surgeons Association congenital cardiac database: A 25-year summary of congenital heart surgery outcomes†. *European Journal of Cardio-Thoracic Surgery, 67*(4), ezaf119. Advance online publication. DOI: 10.1093/ejcts/ezaf119 PMID: 40193525

Qian, Y., Shao, H., Ying, X., Huang, W., & Hua, Y. (2020). The Endocrine Disruption of Prenatal Phthalate Exposure in Mother and Offspring. *Frontiers in Public Health, 8*. Advance online publication. DOI: 10.3389/fpubh.2020.00366 PMID: 32984231

Qin, J., Guo, N., Tong, J., & Wang, Z. (2021). Function of histone methylation and acetylation modifiers in cardiac hypertrophy. *Journal of Molecular and Cellular Cardiology, 159*, 120–129. DOI: 10.1016/j.yjmcc.2021.06.011 PMID: 34175302

Qu, Y., Deng, X., Lin, S., Han, F., Chang, H. H., Ou, Y., & Liu, X. (2022). Using innovative machine learning methods to screen and identify predictors of congenital heart diseases. *Frontiers in Cardiovascular Medicine, 8*, 797002. PMID: 35071361

Radeva, P., Toledo, R., Von Land, C., & Villanueva, J. (1998). *3D vessel reconstruction from biplane angiograms using snakes, Comput*. Cardiol., DOI: 10.1109/cic.1998.731988

Radhakrishna, U., Albayrak, S., Zafra, R., Baraa, A., Vishweswaraiah, S., Veerappa, A. M., Mahishi, D., Saiyed, N., Mishra, N. K., Guda, C., Ali-Fehmi, R., & Bahado-Singh, R. O. (2019). Placental epigenetics for evaluation of fetal congenital heart defects: Ventricular Septal Defect (VSD). *PLoS One*, *14*(3), e0200229. DOI: 10.1371/journal.pone.0200229

Raghavan, R., & Ahamad, S. (2025). Developmental Origins of Health and Disease. *Cancer Exposomics and Environmental Influences on Carcinogenesis*, 1–34. https://doi.org/DOI: 10.4018/979-8-3373-2165-3.ch001

Raghavan, R., Moger, S. S., Umesh, S., & Bhuvana, G. N. (2025). Revolutionizing Pain Management. *Unveiling Technological Advancements and Interdisciplinary Solutions for Pain Care*, 129–164. https://doi.org/DOI: 10.4018/979-8-3693-9501-1.ch005

Ramachandran, V., Bhagavatheeswaran, S., Shanmugam, S., Vasudevan, M., Ragunathan, M., Cherian, K. M., Munirajan, A. K., Ravi, S., & Balakrishnan, A. (2022). Deep sequencing unveils altered cardiac miRNome in congenital heart disease. *Molecular Genetics and Genomics*, *297*(4), 1123–1139. DOI: 10.1007/s00438-022-01908-z

Ramírez-Fuentes, T. C., Jaime-Cruz, R., Patiño-Morales, C. C., Villavicencio-Guzmán, L., Corona, J. C., Revilla-Monsalve, M. C., Jarillo-Luna, R. A., & Salazar-García, M. (2025). Morphological Alterations of Conal Ridges and Differential Expression of AP2α in the Offspring Hearts of Experimental Diabetic Rats. *International Journal of Molecular Sciences*, *26*(11), 5061. DOI: 10.3390/ijms26115061 PMID: 40507872

Rana, N., Sharma, K., & Sharma, A. (2025). Diagnostic strategies using AI and ML in cardiovascular diseases: Challenges and future perspectives. In *Deep Learning and Computer Vision: Models and Biomedical Applications* (Vol. 1, pp. 135–165). Springer Nature Singapore.

Rasouli, S., Radgoodarzi, M., Azarbad, R., Ghazvini, A., Sotoudeheian, M., Taghizadeh, M., & Dakkali, M. S. (2024). Congenital Heart Defects in Pregnancies Conceived by Assisted Reproductive Technology: Comparing Functional and Structural Defects. *Cureus*, *16*(2), e54810. DOI: 10.7759/cureus.54810 PMID: 38529454

Rathi, A. (2018). Incidence of Congenital Heart Defects in ART Pregnancies in Mumbai: A Retrospective Study. *Journal of Obstetrics and Gynaecology of India*, *68*(5), 363–367. DOI: 10.1007/s13224-018-1134-3

Reddy, C. D., Van den Eynde, J., & Kutty, S. (2022, June). Artificial intelligence in perinatal diagnosis and management of congenital heart disease. [). WB Saunders.]. *Seminars in Perinatology*, *46*(4), 151588. PMID: 35396036

Registry, S. L. A. R. T. (2021). Congenital Heart Disease and ART Pregnancy Outcomes: A National Cohort Study. *Sri Lanka Journal of Obstetrics and Gynaecology*, *43*(2), 123–128. DOI: 10.4038/sljog.v43i2.808

Ren, H., Jing, F., Ma, Y., Wang, R., He, C., Wang, Y., Zhou, J., & Sun, Y. (2025). Harnessing artificial intelligence of things for cardiac sensing: Current advances and network-based perspectives. *Frontiers in Public Health*, *13*, 1569887. DOI: 10.3389/fpubh.2025.1569887 PMID: 40740375

Richter, F., Morton, S. U., Kim, S. W., & MacArthur, D. G. (2022). Functional impact of noncoding variants in congenital disorders. *Nature Reviews. Genetics*, *23*(1), 59–71. DOI: 10.1038/s41576-021-00415-4

Rischpler, C., Nekolla, S. G., & Kunze, K. P.. (2015). PET/MRI of the heart. *Seminars in Nuclear Medicine*, *45*, 234–247. DOI: 10.1053/j.semnuclmed.2014.12.004 PMID: 25841278

Rivera-Madera, A., Peña-Martínez, E. G., Messon-Bird, J. L., Pomales-Matos, D. A., Echevarría-Bonilla, O. L., Sanabria-Alberto, L., Peterson-Peguero, E. A., & Rodríguez-Martínez, J. A. (2025). Congenital heart disease missense mutations in the TBX5 DNA-binding domain alter thermal stability and DNA-binding affinity. https://doi.org/DOI: 10.1101/2025.05.16.654568

Rodríguez-Pérez, J. M., Ortega-Zhindón, D. B., Villamil-Castañeda, C., Lara-Ortiz, J. S., Borgonio-Cuadra, V. M., Cervantes-Salazar, J. L., Calderón-Colmenero, J., Escalante-Ruiz, Z. N., Retama-Méndez, E., Hernández-García, Y. C., & Pérez-Hernández, N. (2025). Congenital Heart Diseases: Recent Insights into Epigenetic Mechanisms. *Cells*, *14*(11), 820. DOI: 10.3390/cells14110820 PMID: 40497996

Romanò, A., Pagiatakis, C., Gornati, R., Bernardini, G., & Papait, R. (2025). Epigenetics: A link between toxicants and diseases. *iScience*, *28*(6), 112613. DOI: 10.1016/j.isci.2025.112613 PMID: 40487436

Ruan, Y., Liu, X., Zhu, H., Lu, Y., Liu, X., Han, J., Sun, L., Zhang, Y., Gu, X., Zhao, Y., Li, L., Ran, S., Chen, J., Yu, Q., Xu, Y., Xia, H., & He, Y. (2021). Noninherited Factors in Fetal Congenital Heart Diseases Based on Bayesian Network: A Large Multicenter Study. *Congenital Heart Disease*, *16*(6), 529–549. DOI: 10.32604/chd.2021.015862

Russell, M. W., Chung, W. K., Kaltman, J. R., & Miller, T. A. (2018). Advances in the understanding of the genetic determinants of congenital heart disease and their impact on clinical outcomes. *Journal of the American Heart Association*, *7*(6), e006906. PMID: 29523523

S., G. V., C., A., Biradar, S., & Raghavan, R. (2025). Neuroscience-Driven Solutions for Speech Impairment. *Advancing Medical Research Through Neuroscience*, 119–146. https://doi.org/DOI: 10.4018/979-8-3693-5464-3.ch006

S.Običan, L. Maggio, Holt-oram Syndrome. Obstetric Imaging: Fetal Diagnosis and Care, 2018, pp. 557–559, https://doi.org/DOI: 10.1016/B978-0-323-44548-1.00132-7

Sachdeva R, Armstrong AK, Arnaout R, Grosse-Wortmann L, Han BK, Mertens L, Moore RA, Olivieri LJ, Parthiban A, Powell AJ. (2024) Novel Techniques in Imaging Congenital Heart Disease: JACC Scientific Statement. J Am Coll Cardiol. Jan 2;83(1):63-81, https://doi.org/ DOI: 10.1016/j.jacc.2023.10.025

Safdar, M., Ullah, M., Wahab, A., Hamayun, S., Rehman, M. U., Khan, M. A., & Naeem, M. (2024). Genomic insights into heart health: Exploring the genetic basis of cardiovascular disease. *Current Problems in Cardiology*, *49*(1), 102182. PMID: 37913933

Safi-Stibler, S., & Gabory, A. (2020). Epigenetics and the Developmental Origins of Health and Disease: Parental environment signalling to the epigenome, critical time windows and sculpting the adult phenotype. *Seminars in Cell & Developmental Biology*, *97*, 172–180. DOI: 10.1016/j.semcdb.2019.09.008 PMID: 31587964

Sahoo, K., & Sundararajan, V. (2024). Methods in DNA methylation array dataset analysis: A review. *Computational and Structural Biotechnology Journal*, *23*, 2304–2325. DOI: 10.1016/j.csbj.2024.05.015 PMID: 38845821

Salim, U., Kumar, A., Kulshreshtha, R., & Vivekanandan, P. (2022a). Biogenesis, characterization, and functions of mirtrons. *Wiley Interdisciplinary Reviews. RNA*, *13*(1), e1680. DOI: 10.1002/wrna.1680

Samavat, T., Nazari, M., Fuhong, L., & Yang, L. (2025). Optimizing stand-alone PV systems: A metaheuristic-enhanced fuzzy approach for adaptive MPPT. *China Communications*, *22*(1), 61–74. DOI: 10.23919/JCC.fa.2024-0224.202501

Sargisian, N., Petzold, M., Furenäs, E., Gissler, M., Spangmose, A. L., Malchau Lauesgaard, S., Opdahl, S., Pinborg, A., Henningsen, A.-K. A., Westvik-Johari, K., Rönö, K., Bergh, C., & Wennerholm, U.-B. (2024). Congenital heart defects in children born after assisted reproductive technology: A CoNARTaS study. *European Heart Journal*, *45*(45), 4840–4858. DOI: 10.1093/eurheartj/ehae572 PMID: 39326528

Sarwar, S., Aslam, S., Khalid, H., Hameed, M. A., & Khan, J., & Shabana. (2025). Polygenic risk score (PRS) analysis of genetic variants in a pediatric Pakistani population with ventricular septal defects (VSDs). *The Egyptian Journal of Medical Human Genetics*, *26*(1). Advance online publication. DOI: 10.1186/s43042-025-00661-3

Saxena, A., Relan, J., Agarwal, R., Awasthy, N., Azad, S., Chakrabarty, M., Dagar, K. S., Devagourou, V., Dharan, B. S., Gupta, S. K., Iyer, K. S., Jayranganath, M., Joshi, R., Kannan, B., Katewa, A., Kohli, V., Kothari, S. S., Krishnamoorthy, K. M., Kulkarni, S., & Vijaykumar, R. (2019). Indian guidelines for indications and timing of intervention for common congenital heart diseases: Revised and updated consensus statement of the Working group on management of congenital heart diseases. *Annals of Pediatric Cardiology*, *12*(3), 254–286. DOI: 10.4103/apc.APC_32_19 PMID: 31516283

Scher, M. S. (2024). Interdisciplinary fetal-neonatal neurology training applies neural exposome perspectives to neurology principles and practice. *Frontiers in Neurology*, *14*, 1321674. PMID: 38288328

Schuette, J., Zaccagni, H., Donohue, J., Bushnell, J., Veneziale, K., Gaies, M., & Tabbutt, S. (2022). Assessing data accuracy in a large multi-institutional quality improvement registry: An update from the Pediatric Cardiac Critical Care Consortium (PC4). *Cardiology in the Young*, *32*(11), 1742–1747. PMID: 34961570

Scott, M. S., & Ono, M. (2011). From snoRNA to miRNA: Dual function regulatory non-coding RNAs. *Biochimie*, *93*(11), 1987–1992. DOI: 10.1016/j.biochi.2011.05.026

Sethi, Y., Patel, N., Kaka, N., Desai, A., Kaiwan, O., Sheth, M., & Emran, T. B. (2022). Artificial intelligence in pediatric cardiology: A scoping review. *Journal of Clinical Medicine*, *11*(23), 7072. PMID: 36498651

Sethi, Y., Patel, N., Kaka, N., Kaiwan, O., Kar, J., Moinuddin, A., & Cavalu, S. (2023). Precision medicine and the future of cardiovascular diseases: A clinically oriented comprehensive review. *Journal of Clinical Medicine*, *12*(5), 1799. PMID: 36902588

Sevim Bayrak, C., Zhang, P., Tristani-Firouzi, M., Gelb, B. D., & Itan, Y. (2020). De novo variants in exomes of congenital heart disease patients identify risk genes and pathways. *Genome Medicine*, *12*(1). Advance online publication. DOI: 10.1186/s13073-019-0709-8 PMID: 31941532

Seyhan, A. A. (2024). Trials and Tribulations of MicroRNA Therapeutics. *International Journal of Molecular Sciences*, *25*(3), 1469. DOI: 10.3390/ijms25031469

Shabana, N. A., Shahid, S. U., & Irfan, U. (2020). Genetic contribution to congenital heart disease (CHD). *Pediatric Cardiology*, *41*(1), 12–23. PMID: 31872283

Shang, R., Lee, S., Senavirathne, G., & Lai, E. C. (2023). microRNAs in action: Biogenesis, function and regulation. *Nature Reviews. Genetics*, *24*(12), 816–833. DOI: 10.1038/s41576-023-00611-y

Sharma, P. (2019). Congenital Heart Disease in IVF Pregnancies: An Institutional Experience from Delhi. *Indian Heart Journal*, *71*(2), 119–124. DOI: 10.1016/j.ihj.2019.02.019

Sharma, P., Mishra, R., Sharma, B., Kumari, A., & Modgil, S. (2025). Health Sciences: Advancing Healthcare through Interdisciplinary Approaches and Innovation. *International Journal of Multidisciplinary: Applied Business and Education Research*, *6*(5), 2309–2316. DOI: 10.11594/ijmaber.06.05.17

Shechter, G. (2004). *Respiratory Motion of the Heart: Implications for Magnetic Resonance Coronary Angiography, PhDThesis*. Johns Hopkins University.

Shechter, G., & Devernay, F., Coste-Manière, Quyyumi, E.A., McVeigh, E.R. (2003). Three-Dimensional Motion Tracking of Coronary Arteries in Biplane Cineangiograms. *IEEE Transactions on Medical Imaging*, *22*(4), 493. DOI: 10.1109/tmi.2003.809090 PMID: 12774895

Shi, H., Book, W., Raskind-Hood, C., Downing, K. F., Farr, S. L., Bell, M. N., Sameni, R., Rodriguez, F. H.III, & Kamaleswaran, R. (2023). A machine learning model for predicting congenital heart defects from administrative data. *Birth Defects Research*, *115*(18), 1693–1707. DOI: 10.1002/bdr2.2245 PMID: 37681293

Shih, S. Y., Sun, F. K., & Lee, H. Y. (2019). Temporal pattern attention for multivariate time series forecasting. *Machine Learning*, *108*(8), 1421–1441. DOI: 10.1007/s10994-019-05815-0

Shruti, K., Shrey, K., & Vibha, R. (2011). Micro RNAs: Tiny sequences with enormous potential. *Biochemical and Biophysical Research Communications*, *407*(3), 445–449. DOI: 10.1016/j.bbrc.2011.03.058

Sierant, M. C., Jin, S. C., Bilguvar, K., Morton, S. U., Dong, W., Jiang, W., Lu, Z., Li, B., López-Giráldez, F., Tikhonova, I., Zeng, X., Lu, Q., Choi, J., Zhang, J., Nelson-Williams, C., Knight, J. R., Zhao, H., Cao, J., Mane, S., & Lifton, R. P. (2025). Genomic analysis of 11,555 probands identifies 60 dominant congenital heart disease genes. *Proceedings of the National Academy of Sciences of the United States of America*, *122*(13), e2420343122. Advance online publication. DOI: 10.1073/pnas.2420343122 PMID: 40127276

Silverthorn, D. U. (2012), Human Physiology: An Integrated Approach, 6th Edition, Chapter 14

Singh, R. (2022). Congenital Heart Disease in ART Babies: A Study from Pune. *Heart Asia, 14*(1), 23. DOI: 10.1136/heartasia-2021-010524

Sinibaldi, L., Garone, G., Mandarino, A., Iarossi, G., Chioma, L., Dentici, M. L., Merla, G., Agolini, E., Micalizzi, A., Mancini, C., Niceta, M., Macchiaiolo, M., Diodato, D., Onesimo, R., Blandino, R., Delogu, A. B., De Rosa, G., Trevisan, V., Iademarco, M., & Calcagni, G. (2023). Congenital heart defects in CTNNB1 syndrome: Raising clinical awareness. *Clinical Genetics, 104*(5), 528–541. DOI: 10.1111/cge.14404 PMID: 37455656

Snijder, C. A., Vlot, I. J., Burdorf, A., Obermann-Borst, S. A., Helbing, W. A., Wildhagen, M. F., Steegers, E. A. P., & Steegers-Theunissen, R. P. M. (2012). Congenital heart defects and parental occupational exposure to chemicals. *Human Reproduction (Oxford, England), 27*(5), 1510–1517. DOI: 10.1093/humrep/des043 PMID: 22357765

Soliman, O., Acharya, Y., Gilard, M., Duffy, G., Wijns, W., Kannan, V., & Sultan, S. (2024). Systematic review of cardiovascular neurocristopathy—Contemporary insights and future perspectives. *Frontiers in Cardiovascular Medicine, 11*. Advance online publication. DOI: 10.3389/fcvm.2024.1333265 PMID: 38660479

Solovieva, T., & Bronner, M. E. (2025). Congenital heart defects differ following left versus right avian cardiac neural crest ablation. *Developmental Biology, 519*, 30–37. DOI: 10.1016/j.ydbio.2024.12.003 PMID: 39667652

Song, M., Wang, H., Liu, C., Jin, S., Liu, B., & Sun, W. (2024). Non-coding RNAs as regulators of the Hippo pathway in cardiac development and cardiovascular disease. *Frontiers in Pharmacology, 15*. Advance online publication. DOI: 10.3389/fphar.2024.1348280

Song, Y., Higgins, H., Guo, J., Harrison, K., Schultz, E. N., Hales, B. J., Moses, E. K., Goldblatt, J., Pachter, N., & Zhang, G. (2018). Clinical significance of circulating microRNAs as markers in detecting and predicting congenital heart defects in children. *Journal of Translational Medicine, 16*, 42. DOI: 10.1186/s12967-018-1411-0

Spendlove, S. J., Bondhus, L., Lluri, G., Sul, J. H., & Arboleda, V. A. (2022). Polygenic risk scores of endo-phenotypes identify the effect of genetic background in congenital heart disease. *HGG Advances, 3*(3), 100112. DOI: 10.1016/j.xhgg.2022.100112 PMID: 35599848

Sperling, S. R. (2011). Systems biology approaches to heart development and congenital heart disease. *Cardiovascular Research, 91*(2), 269–278. PMID: 21527437

Spinner, N. B., Loomes, K. M., Krantz, I. D., Adam, M. P., Feldman, J., & Mirzaa, G. M. (2000). Alagille syndrome. In M. P. Adam, J. Feldman, G. M. Mirzaa, et al. (Eds.), *GeneReviews®* [Internet]. University of Washington, Seattle. (Updated 2024, January 4). https://www.ncbi.nlm.nih.gov/books/NBK1273/

Sprague, K., Drangova, M., Lehmann, G., Slomka, P., Levin, D., Chow, B., & deKemp, R. (2006). Coronary X-ray angiographic reconstruction and image orientation. *Medical Physics, 33*, 707–718. DOI: 10.1118/1.2143352 PMID: 16878574

Spurrell, C. H., Barozzi, I., Kosicki, M., Mannion, B. J., Blow, M. J., Fukuda-Yuzawa, Y., Slaven, N., Afzal, S. Y., Akiyama, J. A., Afzal, V., Tran, S., Plajzer-Frick, I., Novak, C. S., Kato, M., Lee, E. A., Garvin, T. H., Pham, Q. T., Kronshage, A. N., Lisgo, S., & Visel, A. (2022). Genome-wide fetalization of enhancer architecture in heart disease. *Cell Reports, 40*(12), 111400. DOI: 10.1016/j.celrep.2022.111400 PMID: 36130500

Sridhar, P., Gan, H. H., & Schlick, T. (2008). A computational screen for C/D box snoRNAs in the human genomic region associated with Prader-Willi and Angelman syndromes. *Journal of Biomedical Science, 15*(6), 697–705. DOI: 10.1007/s11373-008-9271-x

Stingone, J. A., Luben, T. J., Carmichael, S. L., Aylsworth, A. S., Botto, L. D., Correa, A., Gilboa, S. M., Langlois, P. H., Nembhard, W. N., Richmond-Bryant, J., Shaw, G. M., & Olshan, A. F., & National Birth Defects Prevention Study. (2017). Maternal Exposure to Nitrogen Dioxide, Intake of Methyl Nutrients, and Congenital Heart Defects in Offspring. *American Journal of Epidemiology, 186*(6), 719–729. DOI: 10.1093/aje/kwx139 PMID: 28520847

Sucharov, C. C., Sucharov, J., Karimpour-Fard, A., Nunley, K., Stauffer, B. L., & Miyamoto, S. D. (2015). miRNA Expression in Hypoplastic Left Heart Syndrome. *Journal of Cardiac Failure, 21*(1), 83–88. DOI: 10.1016/j.cardfail.2014.09.013

Sumwiza, K., Twizere, C., Rushingabigwi, G., Bakunzibake, P., & Bamurigire, P. (2023). Enhanced cardiovascular disease prediction model using random forest algorithm. *Informatics in Medicine Unlocked, 41*, 101316. DOI: 10.1016/j.imu.2023.101316

Sun, C., & Kontaridis, M. I. (2018). Physiology of Cardiac Development: From Genetics to Signaling to Therapeutic Strategies. *Current Opinion in Physiology, 1*, 123–139. DOI: 10.1016/j.cophys.2017.09.002

Sun, G., & Li, Y. (2019). Exposure to DBP induces the toxicity in early development and adverse effects on cardiac development in zebrafish (*Danio rerio*). *Chemosphere, 218*, 76–82. DOI: 10.1016/j.chemosphere.2018.11.095 PMID: 30469006

Sun, L., Ke, M., Yin, M., Zeng, Y., Ji, Y., Hu, Y., Fu, S., & Zhang, C. (2023). Extracellular vesicle-encapsulated microRNA-296-3p from cancer-associated fibroblasts promotes ovarian cancer development through regulation of the PTEN/AKT and SOCS6/STAT3 pathways. *Cancer Science, 115*(1), 155–169. DOI: 10.1111/cas.16014

Sun, Q., Ren, X., Sun, Z., & Duan, J. (2021). The critical role of epigenetic mechanism in $PM_{2.5}$-induced cardiovascular diseases. *Genes and Environment : the Official Journal of the Japanese Environmental Mutagen Society*, *43*(1), 47. DOI: 10.1186/s41021-021-00219-w PMID: 34654488

Suri, J. S., Paul, S., Maindarkar, M. A., Puvvula, A., Saxena, S., Saba, L., & Paraskevas, K. I. (2022). Cardiovascular/stroke risk stratification in Parkinson's disease patients using atherosclerosis pathway and artificial intelligence paradigm: A systematic review. *Metabolites, 12*(4), 312. PMID: 35448500

Synnergren, J., Améen, C., Lindahl, A., Olsson, B., & Sartipy, P. (2011). Expression of microRNAs and their target mRNAs in human stem cell-derived cardiomyocyte clusters and in heart tissue. *Physiological Genomics, 43*(10), 581–594. DOI: 10.1152/physiolgenomics.00074.2010

Szot, J. O., Campione, M., & Sparrow, D. B. (2020). Oligogenic inheritance in human congenital heart disease. *Human Molecular Genetics, 29*(R2), R145–R151. DOI: 10.1093/hmg/ddaa179

Tache, I. A. (2017). *Three-Dimensional Reconstruction and Hemodynamic Information Extraction from Monoplane Angiography, Patient-specific Hemodynamic Computations: Application to Personalized Diagnosis of Cardiovascular Pathologies*. Springer International Publishing., DOI: 10.1007/978-3-319-56853-9_6

Talmud, P. J. (2007). Gene–environment interaction and its impact on coronary heart disease risk. *Nutrition, Metabolism, and Cardiovascular Diseases, 17*(2), 148–152. PMID: 17306734

Tang, Q., Liao, D., & Zheng, B. (2025). DBR1 orchestrates the fate of lariat RNA: Debranching-dependent turnover and function. *Nucleic Acids Research, 53*(13), gkaf639. Advance online publication. DOI: 10.1093/nar/gkaf639

Tararbit, K., Houyel, L., Bonnet, D., Vigan, C., Lelong, N., Goffinet, F., & Khoshnood, B. (2013). The risk for four specific congenital heart defects associated with assisted reproductive techniques: A population-based evaluation. *Human Reproduction (Oxford, England)*, *28*(2), 367–374. DOI: 10.1093/humrep/des400 PMID: 23178272

Tararbit, K., Lelong, N., Thieulin, A. C., Houyel, L., Bonnet, D., Goffinet, F., & Khoshnood, B. (2014). Assessing the role of multiple pregnancies in the association between tetralogy of Fallot and assisted reproductive techniques: A path-analysis approach. *Orphanet Journal of Rare Diseases*, *9*, 27. DOI: 10.1186/1750-1172-9-27 PMID: 24555734

Tarazon, E., Perez Carrillo, L., Alvarez, I., Gimenez Escamilla, I., Delgado Arija, M., Gonzalez, I., Portoles, M., & Rosello-Lleti, E. (2023). Analysis of the snoRNA profile in ischemic and dilated cardiomyopathy. European Heart Journal, 44(Supplement_2), ehad655.729. https://doi.org/DOI: 10.1093/eurheartj/ehad655.729

Tartaglia, M., Zampino, G., & Gelb, B. D. (2010). Noonan syndrome: Clinical aspects and molecular pathogenesis. *Molecular Syndromology*, *1*(1), 2–26. DOI: 10.1159/000276766 PMID: 20648242

Tcheandjieu, C.. (2022). Large-scale multi-ancestry genome-wide association study of coronary artery disease. *Nature Genetics*, *54*(9), 1372–1383. DOI: 10.1038/s41588-022-01118-1

Thackeray, J. T., Derlin, T., & Haghikia, A.. (2015). Molecular imaging of the Chemokine receptor CXCR4 after acute myocardial infarction. *JACC: Cardiovascular Imaging*, *8*, 1417–1426. DOI: 10.1016/j.jcmg.2015.09.008 PMID: 26577262

Thompson, J.-L. M., Tarr, I. S., Rath, E. M., Troup, M., Ip, E. K. K., Dunwoodie, S. L., Winlaw, D., Giannoulatoudslo, E., Nassar, N., Kirk, E., Chapman, G., Blue, G., Sholler, G., Lain, S., Blue, G. M., Winlaw, D. S., Dunwoodie, S. L., & Giannoulatou, E. (2025). Polygenic Inheritance for Common Comorbidities Associated With Congenital Heart Disease. *JACC Advances*, *4*(4), 101673. DOI: 10.1016/j.jacadv.2025.101673 PMID: 40120216

Thornton, J. M., Shah, N. M., Lillycrop, K. A., Cui, W., Johnson, M. R., & Singh, N. (2024). Multigenerational diabetes mellitus. *Frontiers in Endocrinology*, *14*. Advance online publication. DOI: 10.3389/fendo.2023.1245899 PMID: 38288471

Tian, Y., Cohen, E. D., & Morrisey, E. E. (2010). The Importance of Wnt Signaling in Cardiovascular Development. *Pediatric Cardiology*, *31*(3), 342–348. DOI: 10.1007/s00246-009-9606-z

Tian, Y., Liu, Y., Wang, T., Zhou, N., Kong, J., Chen, L., Snitow, M., Morley, M., Li, D., Petrenko, N., Zhou, S., Lu, M., Gao, E., Koch, W. J., Stewart, K. M., & Morrisey, E. E. (2015). A microRNA-Hippo pathway that promotes cardiomyocyte proliferation and cardiac regeneration in mice. *Science Translational Medicine*, *7*(279), 279ra38. Advance online publication. DOI: 10.1126/scitranslmed.3010841

Tingting, T., Wenjing, F., Qian, Z., Hengquan, W., Simin, Z., Zhisheng, J., & Shunlin, Q. (2020). The TGF-β pathway plays a key role in aortic aneurysms. *Clinica Chimica Acta*, *501*, 222–228. DOI: 10.1016/j.cca.2019.10.042 PMID: 31707165

Tito, C., De Falco, E., Rosa, P., Iaiza, A., Fazi, F., Petrozza, V., & Calogero, A. (2021). Circulating microRNAs from the Molecular Mechanisms to Clinical Biomarkers: A Focus on the Clear Cell Renal Cell Carcinoma. *Genes*, *12*(8), 1154. DOI: 10.3390/genes12081154

Titov, I. I., & Vorozheykin, P. S. (2018). Comparing miRNA structure of mirtrons and non-mirtrons. *BMC Genomics*, *19*(3), 114. DOI: 10.1186/s12864-018-4473-8

Tocantins, C., Diniz, M. S., Grilo, L. F., & Pereira, S. P. (2022). The birth of cardiac disease: Mechanisms linking gestational diabetes mellitus and early onset of cardiovascular disease in offspring. *WIREs Mechanisms of Disease*, *14*(4), e1555. DOI: 10.1002/wsbm.1555 PMID: 35304833

Tomasello, L., Distefano, R., Nigita, G., & Croce, C. M. (2021). The MicroRNA Family Gets Wider: The IsomiRs Classification and Role. *Frontiers in Cell and Developmental Biology*, *9*, 668648. DOI: 10.3389/fcell.2021.668648

Torrorey-Sawe, R. (2025). *Global bioethics: Addressing current challenges, innovations, and the needs of underserved populations.*

Toscano, A., & Moras, P. (2024). Artificial intelligence in congenital heart disease. *Intelligence-Based Cardiology and Cardiac Surgery*, 279–284. https://doi.org/DOI: 10.1016/b978-0-323-90534-3.00042-1

Tran, R., Forman, R., Mossialos, E., Nasir, K., & Kulkarni, A. (2022). Social Determinants of Disparities in Mortality Outcomes in Congenital Heart Disease: A Systematic Review and Meta-Analysis. *Frontiers in Cardiovascular Medicine*, *9*, 829902. DOI: 10.3389/fcvm.2022.829902 PMID: 35369346

Trasande, L., Nelson, M. E., Alshawabkeh, A., Barrett, E. S., Buckley, J. P., Dabelea, D., Dunlop, A. L., Herbstman, J. B., Meeker, J. D., Naidu, M., Newschaffer, C., Padula, A. M., Romano, M. E., Ruden, D. M., Sathyanarayana, S., Schantz, S. L., Starling, A. P., Hamra, G. B., Smith, P. B., & Karr, C. (2024). Prenatal phthalate exposure and adverse birth outcomes in the USA: A prospective analysis of births and estimates of attributable burden and costs. *The Lancet. Planetary Health*, *8*(2), e74–e85. DOI: 10.1016/S2542-5196(23)00270-X PMID: 38331533

Tutarel, O., Dangwal, S., Bretthauer, J., Westhoff-Bleck, M., Roentgen, P., Anker, S. D., Bauersachs, J., & Thum, T. (2013). Circulating miR-423_5p fails as a biomarker for systemic ventricular function in adults after atrial repair for transposition of the great arteries. *International Journal of Cardiology*, *167*(1), 63–66. DOI: 10.1016/j.ijcard.2011.11.082

Tyagi, R., Verma, S., Dash, N., Attri, S. V., Sankhyan, N., & Rohit, M. K. (2022). Folate deficiency: A possible association with congenital heart defects. *Indian Journal of Pediatrics*, *89*, 1013–1015. DOI: 10.1007/s12098-022-04125-z PMID: 35175552

Uddin, J., Fariha, T., Shumi, S. S., & Khandoker, F. (2024). Factors contributing to Alzheimer's disease in older adult populations: A narrative review. https://doi.org/ DOI: 10.20944/preprints202406.1892.v1

Ueno, S., Weidinger, G., Osugi, T., Kohn, A. D., Golob, J. L., Pabon, L., Reinecke, H., Moon, R. T., & Murry, C. E. (2007). Biphasic role for Wnt/β-catenin signaling in cardiac specification in zebrafish and embryonic stem cells. *Proceedings of the National Academy of Sciences of the United States of America*, *104*(23), 9685–9690. DOI: 10.1073/pnas.0702859104

van Assen, M., Beecy, A., Gershon, G., Newsome, J., Trivedi, H., & Gichoya, J. (2024). Implications of bias in artificial intelligence: Considerations for cardiovascular imaging. *Current Atherosclerosis Reports*, *26*(4), 91–102. PMID: 38363525

van der Linde, D., Konings, E. E., Slager, M. A., Witsenburg, M., Helbing, W. A., Takkenberg, J. J., & Roos-Hesselink, J. W. (2011). Birth prevalence of congenital heart disease worldwide: A systematic review and meta-analysis. *Journal of the American College of Cardiology*, *58*(21), 2241–2247. DOI: 10.1016/j.jacc.2011.08.025 PMID: 22078432

van Walsum, T., Schaap, M., Neefjes, L. A., de Graaf, M. A., Dijkstra, J., van der Giessen, A. G., Niessen, W. J. (2003). Three-dimensional guide wire visualization from 3DRA using monoplane fluoroscopic imaging, Proceedings Volume 5029, Medical Imaging 2003: Visualization, Image-Guided Procedures, and Display

Vecoli, C., Pulignani, S., Foffa, I., & Grazia Andreassi, M. (2014). Congenital heart disease: The crossroads of genetics, epigenetics and environment. *Current Genomics, 15*(5), 390–399. PMID: 25435801

Veeramani, M., Balachandren, N., Hong, Y. H., Lee, J., Corno, A. F., Mavrelos, D., & Kastora, S. L. (2024). Assisted reproduction and congenital malformations: A systematic review and meta-analysis. *Congenital Anomalies, 64*(3), 107–115. DOI: 10.1111/cga.12561 PMID: 38577728

Ventura, A., Young, A. G., Winslow, M. M., Lintault, L., Meissner, A., Erkeland, S. J., Newman, J., Bronson, R. T., Crowley, D., Stone, J. R., Jaenisch, R., Sharp, P. A., & Jacks, T. (2008). Targeted deletion reveals essential and overlapping functions of the miR-17~92 family of miRNA clusters. *Cell, 132*(5), 875–886. DOI: 10.1016/j.cell.2008.02.019

Verma, S. (2021). Congenital Heart Defects in ART Pregnancies: A South Indian Perspective. *The Indian Journal of Medical Research, 153*(3), 354–359. DOI: 10.4103/ijmr.IJMR_652_20

Vervoort, D., Jin, H., Edwin, F., Kumar, R. K., Malik, M., Tapaua, N., & Hasan, B. S. (2023). Global access to comprehensive care for paediatric and congenital heart disease. *CJC Pediatric and Congenital Heart Disease, 2*(6), 453–463. PMID: 38205434

Vey, C., Melnik, N., Dombrowsky, G., & Hitz, M.-P. (2025). Current and future diagnostics of congenital heart disease (CHD). *Medizinische Genetik : Mitteilungsblatt des Berufsverbandes Medizinische Genetik e.V, 37*(2), 95–102. DOI: 10.1515/medgen-2025-2008 PMID: 40207043

Vitorino, R. (2024). Transforming Clinical Research: The Power of High-Throughput Omics Integration. *Proteomes, 12*(3), 25. DOI: 10.3390/proteomes12030025 PMID: 39311198

Voros, C., Papadimas, G., Theodora, M., Mavrogianni, D., Athanasiou, D., Sapantzoglou, I., Bananis, K., Athanasiou, A., Athanasiou, A., Tsimpoukelis, C., Papapanagiotou, I., Vaitsis, D., Koulakmanidis, A.-M., Daskalaki, M. A., Topalis, V., Thomakos, N., Antsaklis, P., Chatzinikolaou, F., Loutradis, D., & Daskalakis, G. (2025). From Petri Dish to Primitive Heart: How IVF Alters Early Cardiac Gene Networks and Epigenetic Landscapes. *Biomedicines, 13*(8), 2044. DOI: 10.3390/biomedicines13082044 PMID: 40868294

Voß, H., Schlumbohm, S., Barwikowski, P., Wurlitzer, M., Dottermusch, M., Neumann, P., Schlüter, H., Neumann, J. E., & Krisp, C. (2022). HarmonizR enables data harmonization across independent proteomic datasets with appropriate handling of missing values. *Nature Communications*, *13*(1). Advance online publication. DOI: 10.1038/s41467-022-31007-x PMID: 35725563

Vrijheid, M., Martinez, D., Manzanares, S., Dadvand, P., Schembari, A., Rankin, J., & Nieuwenhuijsen, M. (2021). Association between parents' socioeconomic conditions and risk of congenital heart defects in offspring: A systematic review and meta-analysis. *Journal of Epidemiology and Community Health*, *75*(11), 1091–1099. DOI: 10.1136/jech-2020-216034 PMID: 33980719

Vrijheid, M., Slama, R., Robinson, O., Chatzi, L., Coen, M., van den Hazel, P., & Vineis, P. (2020). The human exposome and health: Where are we now and where do we go from here? *Environmental Health Perspectives*, *128*(6), 065001. DOI: 10.1289/EHP4755 PMID: 32579081

Vu, T., Kokubo, Y., Inoue, M., Yamamoto, M., Mohsen, A., Martin-Morales, A., Dawadi, R., Inoue, T., Tay, J. T., Yoshizaki, M., Watanabe, N., Kuriya, Y., Matsumoto, C., Arafa, A., Nakao, Y. M., Kato, Y., Teramoto, M., & Araki, M. (2025). Machine Learning Model for Predicting Coronary Heart Disease Risk: Development and Validation Using Insights From a Japanese Population–Based Study. *JMIR Cardio*, *9*(1), e68066. DOI: 10.2196/68066 PMID: 40354648

Wächter, I. (2009), 3D Reconstruction of Cerebral Blood Flow and Vessel Morphology from X-Ray Rotational Angiography, Phd thesis, Department of Medical Physics and Bioengineering, University College London

Wagh, V., Pomorski, A., Wilschut, K. J., Piombo, S., & Bernstein, H. S. (2014). MicroRNA-363 negatively regulates the left ventricular determining transcription factor HAND1 in human embryonic stem cell-derived cardiomyocytes. *Stem Cell Research & Therapy*, *5*(3), 75. DOI: 10.1186/scrt464

Wagner, A., Mahrholdt, H., & Holly, T. A.. (2003). Contrast-enhanced MRI and routine single photon emission computed tomography (SPECT) perfusion imaging for detection of subendocardial myocardial infarcts: An imaging study. *Lancet*, *361*, 374–379. DOI: 10.1016/s0140-6736(03)12389-6 PMID: 12573373

Wagner, M. G., Kutlu, A. Z., Davis, B., Raval, A. N., Laeseke, P. F., & Speidel, M. A. (2024). Topology observing 3D device reconstruction from continuous-sweep limited angle fluoroscopy. *Medical Physics*, *51*(4), 2882–2892. DOI: 10.1002/mp.16954 PMID: 38308822

Wajahat, M., Bracken, C. P., & Orang, A. (2021). Emerging Functions for snoRNAs and snoRNA-Derived Fragments. *International Journal of Molecular Sciences, 22*(19), 10193. DOI: 10.3390/ijms221910193

Wang, B., Shi, G., Zhu, Z., Chen, H., & Fu, Q. (2018). Sexual difference of small RNA expression in Tetralogy of Fallot. *Scientific Reports, 8*, 12847. DOI: 10.1038/s41598-018-31243-6

Wang, C., Hou, X., Guan, Q., Zhou, H., Zhou, L., Liu, L., Liu, J., Li, F., Li, W., & Liu, H. (2023). RNA modification in cardiovascular disease: Implications for therapeutic interventions. *Signal Transduction and Targeted Therapy, 8*(1), 412. DOI: 10.1038/s41392-023-01638-7

Wang, G., Wang, B., & Yang, P. (2022). Epigenetics in Congenital Heart Disease. *Journal of the American Heart Association, 11*(7), e025163. DOI: 10.1161/JAHA.121.025163 PMID: 35348004

Wang, H., Chen, X., Li, Y., Xiao, S., Teng, T., Yang, S., Wang, K., & Zhang, M. (2026). Non-coding RNAs in congenital heart disease and placental development: Bridging molecular mechanisms to clinical biomarkers and therapies. *Non-Coding RNA Research, 16*, 1–20. DOI: 10.1016/j.ncrna.2025.08.006 PMID: 41080762

Wang, J., Greene, S. B., Bonilla-Claudio, M., Tao, Y., Zhang, J., Bai, Y., Huang, Z., Black, B. L., Wang, F., & Martin, J. F. (2010). Bmp Signaling Regulates Myocardial Differentiation from Cardiac Progenitors Through a MicroRNA-Mediated Mechanism. *Developmental Cell, 19*(6), 903–912. DOI: 10.1016/j.devcel.2010.10.022

Wang, J., Greene, S. B., & Martin, J. F. (2011). Bmp Signaling in Congenital Heart Disease: New Developments and Future Directions. *Birth Defects Research. Part A, Clinical and Molecular Teratology, 91*(6), 441–448. DOI: 10.1002/bdra.20785

Wang, J., Zhang, R., Cai, K., Yang, Q., Duan, W., Zhao, J., Gui, Y., & Wang, F. (2019). Susceptibility to congenital heart defects associated with a polymorphism in TBX2 3′ untranslated region in the Han Chinese population. *Pediatric Research, 85*(3), 378–383. DOI: 10.1038/s41390-018-0181-y

Wang, J., Zhang, X., Li, Y., Liu, Y., & Tao, L. (2021). Exposure to Dibutyl Phthalate and Reproductive-Related Outcomes in Animal Models: Evidence From Rodents Study. *Frontiers in Physiology, 12*. Advance online publication. DOI: 10.3389/fphys.2021.684532 PMID: 34955869

Wang, K., Tian, J., Zheng, C., Yang, H., Ren, J., Liu, Y., & Zhang, Y. (2021). Interpretable prediction of 3-year all-cause mortality in patients with heart failure caused by coronary heart disease based on machine learning and SHAP. *Computers in Biology and Medicine*, *137*, 104813. PMID: 34481185

Wang, Y. R., Yang, K., Wen, Y., Wang, P., Hu, Y., Lai, Y., & Zhao, S. (2024). Screening and diagnosis of cardiovascular disease using artificial intelligence-enabled cardiac magnetic resonance imaging. *Nature Medicine*, *30*(5), 1471–1480. PMID: 38740996

Wang, Y., Du, X., Zhou, Z., Jiang, J., Zhang, Z., Ye, L., & Hong, H. (2016). A gain-of-function ACTC1 3′UTR mutation that introduces a miR-139-5p target site may be associated with a dominant familial atrial septal defect. *Scientific Reports*, *6*, 25404. DOI: 10.1038/srep25404

Wang, Y., Fang, Y., Lu, P., Wu, B., & Zhou, B. (2021). NOTCH Signaling in Aortic Valve Development and Calcific Aortic Valve Disease. *Frontiers in Cardiovascular Medicine*, *8*, 682298. DOI: 10.3389/fcvm.2021.682298 PMID: 34239905

Wang, Y., Fu, M., Zheng, Z., Feng, J., & Zhang, C. (2025). Small Nucleolar RNAs: Biological Functions and Diseases. *MedComm*, *6*(7), e70257. DOI: 10.1002/mco2.70257

Wang, Y., Liu, J., Cui, J., Sun, M., Du, W., Chen, T., Ming, X., Zhang, L., Tian, J., Li, J., Yin, L., Liu, F., Pu, Z., Lv, B., Hou, J., & Yu, B. (2016). MiR218 Modulates Wnt Signaling in Mouse Cardiac Stem Cells by Promoting Proliferation and Inhibiting Differentiation through a Positive Feedback Loop. *Scientific Reports*, *6*(1), 20968. DOI: 10.1038/srep20968

Wang, Z., Wang, H., Zhou, S., Mao, J., Zhan, Z., & Duan, S. (2024). miRNA interplay: Mechanisms and therapeutic interventions in cancer. *MedComm. Oncology*, *3*(4), e93. DOI: 10.1002/mog2.93

Watelle, L., Roy, L.-O., Lauzon-Schnitka, J., Newell, G., Dumas, A., Nadeau, A., Xiong, W. T., Rego, K., Beaulieu, C., Groulx-Boivin, E., Roy-Lacroix, M.-È., Vaujois, L., Drolet, C., Dancea, A., Dahdah, N., Bigras, J.-L., & Dallaire, F. (2024). The Quebec Congenital Heart Disease Registry: A Model of Prospective Databank to Facilitate Research in Congenital Cardiology. *CJC Pediatric and Congenital Heart Disease*, *3*(2), 57–66. DOI: 10.1016/j.cjcpc.2023.12.001 PMID: 38774679

Wells, B. K., Garramone, G. K., Mahomed, A., & Ezin, M. (2025). Teratogenic Effects of Serotonin Receptor 2B Disruption on the Migration and Cardiac Derivatives of the Cardiac Neural Crest. *Birth Defects Research*, *117*(7), e2506. DOI: 10.1002/bdr2.2506 PMID: 40667631

Wen, H., Chandrasekaran, P., Jin, A., Pankin, J., Lu, M., Liberti, D. C., Zepp, J. A., Jain, R., Morrisey, E. E., Michki, S. N., & Frank, D. B. (2025). A spatiotemporal cell atlas of cardiopulmonary progenitor cell allocation during development. *Cell Reports*, *44*(4). Advance online publication. DOI: 10.1016/j.celrep.2025.115513 PMID: 40178979

Wennerholm, U. B., Henningsen, A. K., Romundstad, L. B., Bergh, C., Pinborg, A., Skjaerven, R., & Gissler, M. (2013). Perinatal outcomes of children born after frozen-thawed embryo transfer: A Nordic cohort study from the CoNARTaS group. *Human Reproduction (Oxford, England)*, *28*(9), 2545–2553. DOI: 10.1093/humrep/det272 PMID: 23832793

Wesołowski, S., Lemmon, G., Hernandez, E. J., Henrie, A., Miller, T. A., Weyhrauch, D., & Yandell, M. (2022). An explainable artificial intelligence approach for predicting cardiovascular outcomes using electronic health records. *PLOS Digital Health*, *1*(1), e0000004. PMID: 35373216

Westholm, J. O., & Lai, E. C. (2011). Mirtrons: microRNA biogenesis via splicing. *Biochimie*, *93*(11), 1897–1904. DOI: 10.1016/j.biochi.2011.06.017

Wijnands, K. P. J., Zeilmaker, G. A., Meijer, W. M., Helbing, W. A., & Steegers-Theunissen, R. P. M. (2014). Periconceptional parental conditions and perimembranous ventricular septal defects in the offspring. *Birth Defects Research. Part A, Clinical and Molecular Teratology*, *100*(12), 944–950. DOI: 10.1002/bdra.23265 PMID: 25196200

Wild, C. P. (2012). The exposome: From concept to utility. *International Journal of Epidemiology*, *41*(1), 24–32. DOI: 10.1093/ije/dyr236 PMID: 22296988

Willhite, C. C., Hill, R. M., & Irving, D. W. (1986). Isotretinoin-induced craniofacial malformations in humans and hamsters. *Journal of Craniofacial Genetics and Developmental Biology. Supplement*, *2*, 193–20. PMID: 3491113

Williams, M. C., MacArthur, J. A. L., Forsyth, R., & Petersen, S. E. (2025). New ways to use imaging data in cardiovascular research: Survey of opinions on federated learning and synthetic data. *European Heart Journal. Imaging Methods and Practice*, *3*(1), qyaf012. Advance online publication. DOI: 10.1093/ehjimp/qyaf012 PMID: 40066149

Winkler, I., Posod, A., Staudt, A., Huber, E., Urbanek, M., Kiechl-Kohlendorfer, U., & Griesmaier, E. (2025). MicroRNA Expression Profiles in Very Preterm Infants with Patent Ductus Arteriosus: A Pilot Study. *Neonatology*. Advance online publication. DOI: 10.1159/000546934

Wolfe, K., & Peyvandi, S. (2025). Neurodevelopmental outcomes in congenital heart disease: Modifiable and nonmodifiable substrates. *Current Opinion in Cardiology*, *40*(4), 259. DOI: 10.1097/HCO.0000000000001218 PMID: 40401446

Wolton, M., Davey, M. G., & Dietrich, S. (2025). At early stages of heart development, the first and second heart fields are a continuum of lateral head mesoderm-derived, cardiogenic cells. *Developmental Biology*, *520*, 200–223. DOI: 10.1016/j.ydbio.2025.01.009 PMID: 39848483

Wong, A. C. H., & Rasko, J. E. J. (2021). Splice and Dice: Intronic microRNAs, Splicing and Cancer. *Biomedicines*, *9*(9), 1268. DOI: 10.3390/biomedicines9091268

Wu, K.-H., Xiao, Q.-R., Yang, Y., Xu, J.-L., Zhang, F., Liu, C.-M., Zhang, Z.-M., Lu, Y.-Q., & Huang, N.-P. (2018). MicroRNA-34a modulates the Notch signaling pathway in mice with congenital heart disease and its role in heart development. *Journal of Molecular and Cellular Cardiology*, *114*, 300–308. DOI: 10.1016/j.yjmcc.2017.11.015

Wu, Q., Fu, X., Liu, G., He, X., Li, Y., & Ou, C. (2025). N7-methylguanosine modification in cancers: From mechanisms to therapeutic potential. *Journal of Hematology & Oncology*, *18*(1), 12. DOI: 10.1186/s13045-025-01665-7

Wu, Y., Jin, X., Zhang, Y., Zheng, J., & Yang, R. (2021). Genetic and epigenetic mechanisms in the development of congenital heart diseases. *World Journal of Pediatric Surgery*, *4*(2), e000196. PMID: 36474778

Wu, Y., Ma, X.-J., Wang, H.-J., Li, W.-C., Chen, L., Ma, D., & Huang, G.-Y. (2014). Expression of Cx43-related microRNAs in patients with tetralogy of Fallot. *World Journal of Pediatrics: WJP*, *10*(2), 138–144. DOI: 10.1007/s12519-013-0434-0

Wystub, K., Besser, J., Bachmann, A., Boettger, T., & Braun, T. (2013). miR-1/133a Clusters Cooperatively Specify the Cardiomyogenic Lineage by Adjustment of Myocardin Levels during Embryonic Heart Development. *PLOS Genetics*, *9*(9), e1003793. DOI: 10.1371/journal.pgen.1003793

Xiang, H., Zhuang, J., Bao, L., & Shi, Y. (2025). Variants and molecular mechanism of NOTCH1 in congenital heart disease. *Congenital Heart Disease*, *20*(2), 245–263. DOI: 10.32604/chd.2025.064366

Xie, F., Chen, X., Weng, S., Xia, T., Sun, X., Luo, T., & Li, P. (2019). Effects of two environmental endocrine disruptors di-*n*-butyl phthalate (DBP) and mono-*n*-butyl phthalate (MBP) on human sperm functions in vitro. *Reproductive Toxicology (Elmsford, N.Y.)*, *83*, 1–7. DOI: 10.1016/j.reprotox.2018.10.011 PMID: 30391722

Xie, M., Li, M., Vilborg, A., Lee, N., Shu, M.-D., Yartseva, V., Šestan, N., & Steitz, J. A. (2013). Mammalian 5′-capped microRNA precursors that generate a single microRNA. *Cell, 155*(7), 1568–1580. DOI: 10.1016/j.cell.2013.11.027

Xie, X., Huang, M., Ma, S., Xin, Q., Wang, Y., Hu, L., Zhao, H., Li, P., Liu, M., Yuan, R., Miao, Y., Zhu, Y., & Cong, W. (2025). The role of long non-coding RNAs in cardiovascular diseases: A comprehensive review. *Non-Coding RNA Research, 11*, 158–187. DOI: 10.1016/j.ncrna.2024.12.009 PMID: 39896344

Xi, Y., Lu, E., Ruan, X., Wu, R., Wu, L., Zhou, T., Gu, H., & Wu, Y. (2024). Potential candidate maternal serum miRNAs for the diagnosis of fetal congenital heart disease. *Cellular and Molecular Biology, 70*(8), 121–128. DOI: 10.14715/cmb/2024.70.8.16

Xu, F., Yang, J., Shang, J., Lan, F., Li, M., Shi, L., Shen, L., Wang, Y., & Ge, J. (2019). MicroRNA-302d promotes the proliferation of human pluripotent stem cell-derived cardiomyocytes by inhibiting LATS2 in the Hippo pathway. *Clinical Science, 133*(13), 1387–1399. DOI: 10.1042/CS20190099

Xu, J., Li, Q., Deng, L., Xiong, J., Cheng, Z., & Ye, C. (2025). Global, regional, and national epidemiology of congenital heart disease in children from 1990 to 2021. *Frontiers in Cardiovascular Medicine, 12*. Advance online publication. DOI: 10.3389/fcvm.2025.1522644 PMID: 40454242

Xu, X., Hong, P., Wang, Z., Tang, Z., & Li, K. (2021). MicroRNAs in Transforming Growth Factor-Beta Signaling Pathway Associated With Fibrosis Involving Different Systems of the Human Body. *Frontiers in Molecular Biosciences, 8*, 707461. DOI: 10.3389/fmolb.2021.707461

Yang, H., Li, Y., Chen, Q., Li, S., Yang, Y., & Lyu, G. (2025). Analyzing exosomal miRNA profiles in tetralogy of fallot fetuses' amniotic fluid. *Scientific Reports, 15*, 96. DOI: 10.1038/s41598-024-83576-0

Yang, J.-S., Maurin, T., Robine, N., Rasmussen, K. D., Jeffrey, K. L., Chandwani, R., Papapetrou, E. P., Sadelain, M., O'Carroll, D., & Lai, E. C. (2010). Conserved vertebrate mir-451 provides a platform for Dicer-independent, Ago2-mediated microRNA biogenesis. *Proceedings of the National Academy of Sciences of the United States of America, 107*(34), 15163–15168. DOI: 10.1073/pnas.1006432107

Yang, J., Wang, Y., Liu, Y., Tang, S., & Chen, W. (2009). Novel Approach for 3-D Reconstruction of Coronary Arteries from Two Uncalibrated Angiographic Images. *IEEE Transactions on Image Processing, 18*(7). Advance online publication. DOI: 10.1109/tip.2009.2017363 PMID: 19414289

Yang, S., Qin, G., He, G., Liang, M., Liang, Y., Luo, S., Yang, Z., Pang, Y., Long, F., & Tang, Y. (2025). Evaluation of first-trimester ultrasound screening strategy for fetal congenital heart disease. *Ultrasound in Obstetrics & Gynecology, 65*(4), 478–486. DOI: 10.1002/uog.29186 PMID: 40019943

Yang, X. Y., Li, Y. M., Wang, J. Y., Jia, Y. H., Yi, Z., & Chen, M. (2025, July 17). Utilizing multimodal artificial intelligence to advance cardiovascular diseases. *Precision Clinical Medicine, 8*(3), pbaf016. Advance online publication. DOI: 10.1093/pcmedi/pbaf016 PMID: 40799363

Yang, Y., Yang, H., Lian, X., Yang, S., Shen, H., Wu, S., Wang, X., & Lyu, G. (2022). Circulating microRNA: Myocardium-derived prenatal biomarker of ventricular septal defects. *Frontiers in Genetics, 13*. Advance online publication. DOI: 10.3389/fgene.2022.899034

Yan, S., Thienthanasit, R., Chen, D., Engelen, E., Brühl, J., Crossman, D. K., Kesterson, R., Wang, Q., Bouazoune, K., & Jiao, K. (2020). CHD7 regulates cardiovascular development through ATP-dependent and -independent activities. *Proceedings of the National Academy of Sciences of the United States of America, 117*(46), 28847–28858. DOI: 10.1073/pnas.2005222117 PMID: 33127760

Yasuhara, J., Bigelow, A. M., & Garg, V. (2025). Genetics of Congenital Heart Disease. *Clinics in Perinatology, 52*(3), 589–608. DOI: 10.1016/j.clp.2025.06.010 PMID: 40850718

Yasuhara, J., & Garg, V. (2021). Genetics of congenital heart disease: A narrative review of recent advances and clinical implications. *Translational Pediatrics, 10*(9), 2366–2386. DOI: 10.21037/tp-21-297 PMID: 34733677

Yeh, Y.-T., Ock, J., & Farimani, A. B. (2025). Text to Band Gap: Pre-trained Language Models as Encoders for Semiconductor Band Gap Prediction. *ArXiv Preprint ArXiv:2501.03456*. https://arxiv.org/abs/2501.03456

Ye, X., Li, M., Meng, Y., Duan, S., Zhang, S., & Zhong, K. (2025). D-tetramethrin induces cardiac looping failure in zebrafish during embryonic development. *Comparative Biochemistry and Physiology. Toxicology & Pharmacology : CBP, 294*, 110193. DOI: 10.1016/j.cbpc.2025.110193 PMID: 40086682

Yi, K., He, S. E., Guo, T., Wang, Z. Q., Zhang, X., Xu, J. G., Zhang, H. Y., Liu, W. G., & You, T. (2025). Association of MTHFD1 G1958A (rs2236225) gene polymorphism with the risk of congenital heart disease: A systematic review and meta-analysis. *BMC Medical Genomics, 18*(1), 20. DOI: 10.1186/s12920-024-02052-w PMID: 39871280

Yousefi, F., Shabaninejad, Z., Vakili, S., Derakhshan, M., Movahedpour, A., Dabiri, H., Ghasemi, Y., Mahjoubin-Tehran, M., Nikoozadeh, A., Savardashtaki, A., Mirzaei, H., & Hamblin, M. R. (2020). TGF-β and WNT signaling pathways in cardiac fibrosis: Non-coding RNAs come into focus. *Cell Communication and Signaling : CCS, 18*(1), 87. DOI: 10.1186/s12964-020-00555-4

Yu, K., Ji, Y., Wang, H., Xuan, Q. K., Li, B. B., Xiao, J. J., Sun, W., & Kong, X. Q. (2016). Association of miR-196a2, miR-27a, and miR-499 polymorphisms with isolated congenital heart disease in a Chinese population. *Genetics and Molecular Research: GMR, 15*(4). Advance online publication. DOI: 10.4238/gmr15048929

Yu, Y., Ge, X., Wang, L.-S., Wang, X.-X., & Xu, L.-C. (2023). Abnormalities of hsa-mir-16 and hsa-mir-124 Affect Mitochondrial Function and Fatty Acid Metabolism in Tetralogy of Fallot. *Combinatorial Chemistry & High Throughput Screening, 26*(2), 373–382. DOI: 10.2174/1386207325666220421104617

Zachariah, J. P., Jone, P. N., Agbaje, A. O., Ryan, H. H., Trasande, L., Perng, W., & Farzan, S. F. (2024). Environmental exposures and pediatric cardiology: A scientific statement from the American heart association. *Circulation, 149*(20), e1165–e1175.

Zachariah, J. P., Jone, P.-N., Agbaje, A. O., Ryan, H. H., Trasande, L., Perng, W., & Farzan, S. F.American Heart Association Council on Lifelong Congenital Heart Disease and Heart Health in the Young; Council on Cardiovascular and Stroke Nursing; Council on Epidemiology and Prevention; Council on Lifestyle and Cardiometabolic Health; and Council on Clinical Cardiology. (2024). Environmental Exposures and Pediatric Cardiology: A Scientific Statement From the American Heart Association. *Circulation, 149*(20), e1165–e1175. DOI: 10.1161/CIR.0000000000001234 PMID: 38618723

Zaidi, A. H., Alberts, A., Chowdhury, D., Beaty, C., Brewer, B., Chen, M. H., & de Ferranti, S. D. (2024). Trends in Gaps of Care for Patients With Congenital Heart Disease: Implications for Social Determinants of Health and Child Opportunity Index. *Journal of the American Heart Association, 13*(20), e034796. DOI: 10.1161/JAHA.124.034796 PMID: 39377195

Zaidi, S., & Brueckner, M. (2017). Genetics and genomics of congenital heart disease. *Circulation Research, 120*(6), 923–940. DOI: 10.1161/CIRCRESAHA.116.309140 PMID: 28302740

Zaqout, M., Aslem, E., Abuqamar, M., Wolf, D., & Backer, J. (2021). The impact of oral folic acid supplementation on the prevention of congenital heart defects: A systematic review and meta-analysis. *Nutrients, 13*(11), 4003. DOI: 10.3390/nu13114003 PMID: 34836257

Zdanowicz, J. A., Yildrim, G., Fonseca, A., Hecher, K., & de Sousa, M. T. (2024). Is There a Cumulative Effect for Congenital Heart Defects in Monochorionic Twins after Assisted Reproduction? – A Retrospective Analysis at a Tertiary Referral Center. *Geburtshilfe und Frauenheilkunde*, *84*(03), 274–281. DOI: 10.1055/a-2238-3181 PMID: 38455999

Zeb, I., Uqaily, R., & Gonuguntla, K.. (2023). Multimodality assessment of high- vs. low-gradient aortic stenosis using echocardiography and cardiac CT. *Journal of Cardiovascular Computed Tomography*, *17*, 421–428. PMID: 37806845

Zelli, V., Compagnoni, C., Capelli, R., Corrente, A., Cornice, J., Vecchiotti, D., Di Padova, M., Zazzeroni, F., Alesse, E., & Tessitore, A. (2021). Emerging Role of isomiRs in Cancer: State of the Art and Recent Advances. *Genes*, *12*(9), 1447. DOI: 10.3390/genes12091447

Zeng, W., Guo, H., Liu, Q., & Wong, W. H. (2025). Improving polygenic prediction from whole-genome sequencing data by leveraging predicted epigenomic features. *Proceedings of the National Academy of Sciences of the United States of America*, *122*(24), e2419202122. DOI: 10.1073/pnas.2419202122 PMID: 40504151

Zhang, B., & Schmidlin, T. (2024). Recent advances in cardiovascular disease research driven by metabolomics technologies in the context of systems biology. *NPJ Metabolic Health and Disease*, *2*(1). Advance online publication. DOI: 10.1038/s44324-024-00028-z PMID: 40603608

Zhang, J., Chang, J.-J., Xu, F., Ma, X.-J., Wu, Y., Li, W.-C., Wang, H.-J., Huang, G.-Y., & Ma, D. (2013). MicroRNA deregulation in right ventricular outflow tract myocardium in nonsyndromic tetralogy of fallot. *The Canadian Journal of Cardiology*, *29*(12), 1695–1703. DOI: 10.1016/j.cjca.2013.07.002

Zhang, M., Sun, Y., Zhao, X., Liu, R., Yang, B.-Y., Chen, G., Zhang, W., Dong, G.-H., Yin, C., & Yue, W. (2022). How Parental Predictors Jointly Affect the Risk of Offspring Congenital Heart Disease: A Nationwide Multicenter Study Based on the China Birth Cohort. *Frontiers in Cardiovascular Medicine*, *9*. Advance online publication. DOI: 10.3389/fcvm.2022.860600 PMID: 35722125

Zhang, Y., Yuan, B., Xu, Y., Zhou, N., Zhang, R., Lu, L., & Feng, Z. (2022). MiR-208b/miR-21 Promotes the Progression of Cardiac Fibrosis Through the Activation of the TGF-β1/Smad-3 Signaling Pathway: An in vitro and in vivo Study. *Frontiers in Cardiovascular Medicine*, *9*. Advance online publication. DOI: 10.3389/fcvm.2022.924629

Zhang, Z. (1996). *Epipolar Geometry in Stereo, Motion and Object Recognition: A Unified Approach*. Springer.

Zhao, M., Tang, Y., Zhou, Y., & Zhang, J. (2019). Deciphering Role of Wnt Signalling in Cardiac Mesoderm and Cardiomyocyte Differentiation from Human iPSCs: Four-dimensional control of Wnt pathway for hiPSC-CMs differentiation. *Scientific Reports*, *9*(1), 19389. DOI: 10.1038/s41598-019-55620-x

Zhao, Y., Ransom, J. F., Li, A., Vedantham, V., von Drehle, M., Muth, A. N., Tsuchihashi, T., McManus, M. T., Schwartz, R. J., & Srivastava, D. (2007). Dysregulation of cardiogenesis, cardiac conduction, and cell cycle in mice lacking miRNA-1-2. *Cell*, *129*(2), 303–317. DOI: 10.1016/j.cell.2007.03.030

Zhou, J., Liu, H., Gu, H., Cui, Y., Zhao, N., Chen, J., Gao, L., Zhang, Y., & Liu, J. (2014). Association of Cardiac Development with Assisted Reproductive Technology in Childhood: A Prospective Single-Blind Pilot Study. *Cellular Physiology and Biochemistry*, *34*(3), 988–1000. DOI: 10.1159/000366315 PMID: 25201231

Zhou, W., Yi, Y., Cao, W., Zhong, X., & Chen, L. (2025). Functions of METTL1/WDR4 and QKI as m7G modification—Related enzymes in digestive diseases. *Frontiers in Pharmacology*, *15*, 1491763. DOI: 10.3389/fphar.2024.1491763

Zia, M. F., Peter, J., Hoover, J., Chen, K. E., & Flynt, A. (2021). Human 5′-tailed Mirtrons are Processed by RNaseP (p. 2021.10.15.464553). *bioRxiv*. https://doi.org/DOI: 10.1101/2021.10.15.464553

Zong, D., Liu, X., Li, J., Ouyang, R., & Chen, P. (2019). The role of cigarette smoke-induced epigenetic alterations in inflammation. *Epigenetics & amp. Chromatin*, *12*(1). Advance online publication. DOI: 10.1186/s13072-019-0311-8 PMID: 31711545

Zu, B., Zheng, Z., & Fu, Q. (2020). Molecular diagnostics for congenital heart disease: A narrative review of the current technologies and applications. *Journal of Bio-X Research*, *3*, 92–96. DOI: 10.1097/JBR.0000000000000068

# About the Contributors

**Ramya Raghavan** is an Assistant Professor at Sri Sathya Sai University for Human Excellence, India, and an accomplished editor and researcher specializing in medical and scientific publications. As the editor for this book on Congenital Heart Disease (CHD), her work is dedicated to advancing the mission of the Sri Sathya Sai Sanjeevani Research Centre in India. Dr. Raghavan's research interests are broad and interdisciplinary, including Genetics, Biostatistics, Biophotons, and Assistive Technologies. Her current work aligns with the Developmental Origins of Health and Disease (DOHaD) paradigm, focusing on early developmental programming projects to address health disparities and promote equitable approaches to disease prevention. A key focus of her expertise is the critical intersection of the exposome and Social Determinants of Health (SDOH). Dr. Raghavan's work underscores how a holistic understanding of environmental exposures, from the molecular level to population-wide influences, is essential for addressing major global health issues like CHD. Her research specifically highlights the challenges in low- and middle-income countries (LMICs). Dr. Raghavan possesses a unique ability to bridge complex scientific concepts with broader societal impact, making her a vital voice in translating research into meaningful advancements in CHD care.

***

**Danish Ather** is an accomplished book editor with a robust academic and professional background. Currently as Professor at Amity University in Tashkent, Uzbekistan, Dr. Ather brings over 18 years of experience in teaching, research, and administration. He holds dual Ph.D. degrees in Computer Science and Computer Science & Engineering. His editorial expertise is highlighted through his role as Editor of the proceedings submitted yearly to IEEE USA for the SMART Series conferences. Dr. Ather has authored a book titled "Level up Your Programming with Core Dragon" and published 54 research papers in international journals and conferences, with 15 indexed in Scopus. He is a Senior Member of the IEEE Society and has received numerous awards, including a Certificate of Appreciation from the Ministry of Digital Technologies, Republic of Uzbekistan. His technical proficiency and dedication to advancing knowledge in fields such as IoT, AI, and programming make him a valuable asset in the realm of academic publishing.

**Sinem Durmus** is currently serving as a Research Assistant (PhD) in the Department of Medical Biochemistry, Faculty of Medicine, İzmir Katip Çelebi University, İzmir, Türkiye. She earned her PhD degree in Medical Biochemistry from the Department of Medical Biochemistry, Cerrahpaşa Faculty of Medicine, Istanbul University-Cerrahpaşa. Dr. Durmus's research primarily focuses on the role of microRNAs in the pathogenesis and diagnosis of various diseases, with a particular emphasis on cancer, cardiological disorders and rheumatological diseases. Her work aims to elucidate molecular mechanisms underlying disease development and to identify novel biomarkers with potential clinical applications. Her broader academic interests include molecular diagnostics, translational biochemistry, and the integration of molecular biomarkers into personalized medicine.

**S. Ida Evangeline**, presently working as an Assistant Professor in the Department of Electrical and Electronics Engineering at the Government College of Engineering, Tirunelveli, Tamilnadu, India. She obtained her Bachelor's in Electrical and Electronics Engineering from Manonmaniam Sundaranar University in 2003, and Master's in Power Systems Engineering from Anna University, Chennai, Tamilnadu, India in 2005. She completed her PhD degree in 2023 at Anna University, Chennai, Tamilnadu, India. She has published six research papers in international journals. Her current research interests include optimal power flow, renewable energy, soft computing, machine learning, and deep learning.

**Sachin Jain** is working as an Associate Professor in the Department of Computer Science and Engineering at Ajay Kumar Garg Engineering College, Ghaziabad. He completed his B.Tech in Computer Science and Engineering in 2007 from UPTU, Lucknow and M.Tech in Computer Science and Engineering in 2010 from GGSIPU, Delhi. He has completed his Ph.D in Computer Science and Engineering from Sharda University Greater Noida in 2025. He is a UGC-NET qualified teacher and has total 16 years of teaching experience. His research interests lie in Artificial Intelligence, Deep Learning and Machine Learning. He has published several research papers in Peer-Reviewed Journals and Conference proceedings. Dr. Jain has filed several patents for his work.

**Vishal Jain** is pursuing Postdoc from Kuala Lumpur University of Science & Technology (KLUST) (formerly known as Infrastructure University Kuala Lumpur (IUKL)), Malaysia. He is presently working as a Professor (CSE) at the Department of Computer Science & Engineering, School of Engineering & Technology, Vivekananda Institute of Professional Studies - Technical Campus, New Delhi. Before that, he worked as Professor at Sharda University, Greater Noida and Associate Professor at Bharati Vidyapeeth's Institute of Computer Applications and Management (BVICAM), New Delhi. He has associated as a member of the Faculty Board, Board of Planning and Management, Executive Council, Academic Council, Curriculum Development and Review Committee and Academic Audit of various higher education Institutions. His research areas include machine learning, information retrieval, semantic web, ontology engineering, data mining, ad hoc networks, sensor networks and network security.

**Archana Kumari** is currently working as an Assistant Professor, School of Pharmacy and Emerging Sciences at Baddi University of Emerging Sciences and Technology, Baddi, Himachal Pradesh. She holds M. Pharmacy degree with a specialization in Pharmacognosy and has two years of academic and research experience. Her areas of interest include herbal drug technology, natural product research, and phytochemistry. She has contributed to the scientific community through several review papers and book chapters in reputed publications.

**Golnoosh Manteghi** Experienced Head of the Postgraduate Program in the Faculty of Architecture and Built Environment at Infrastructure University Kuala Lumpur with a demonstrated history of research and teaching interests focus on environmental and building science thermal comfort and skilled in theoretical, numerical and experimental methods in the higher education industry. Focused on publishing peer-reviewed journal papers including supervising and examining postgraduate student's thesis. I have gained advanced skills in developing programmes in related to various standards such as Malaysian Qualification Agency (MQA). In addition, I am trained in Outcome Based Education (OBE) to develop curriculum, design assessments, and measuring Course Learning Outcome (CLO) and Programme Learning Outcome (PLO) attainments based on OBE.

**Ravinesh Mishra** is currently working as Dean, School of Pharmacy and Emerging Sciences at Baddi University of Emerging Sciences and Technology, Baddi, Himachal Pradesh. He holds a B. Pharm. from CCS University (2003), M. Pharm. from Rajiv Gandhi University of Health Sciences, Bengaluru (2007), and Ph.D. in Pharmaceutical Sciences from Jamia Hamdard University, New Delhi (2011). With over 18 years of professional experience, he has qualified GATE twice and was awarded the UGC and CSIR fellowships during his doctoral studies. He received the prestigious DST Young Scientist Award in 2010 and has also undergone short-term toxicological trainings. He has made significant contributions to pharmaceutical research with over 80 publications, 14 patents, 3 books, and 10 book chapters to his credit. He has guided several M. Pharm students and Ph.D. scholars. His achievements have been recognized with awards from the Society of Toxicology and Therapeutic Drug Monitoring & Clinical Toxicology.

**Bhartendu Sharma** is currently working as an Associate Professor, Head of Department, School of Pharmacy and Emerging Sciences at Baddi University of Emerging Sciences and Technology, Baddi, Himachal Pradesh. He holds M. Pharm in Pharmaceutical Chemistry and earned his Ph.D. in Pharmaceutical Sciences, bringing with him over 13 years of academic and research experience. He has been actively involved in both teaching and research, contributing to the development of future pharmaceutical professionals. His areas of interest include drug design and synthesis, medicinal chemistry, and pharmaceutical analysis. He has guided numerous undergraduate, postgraduate and PhD scholars and is committed to fostering research-oriented learning. Over the years, he has contributed to several research publications in reputed journals and has participated in various national and international conferences. He is dedicated to academic excellence, innovation in pharmaceutical education, and continuous professional development.

**Priya Sharma** is currently working as an Assistant Professor, School of Pharmacy and Emerging Sciences at Baddi University of Emerging Sciences and Technology, Baddi, Himachal Pradesh. She holds M. Pharm in Pharmaceutics and earned her Ph.D. in Pharmaceutical Sciences. With over 5 years of academic and research experience, she is actively involved in both teaching and guiding students in the field of pharmaceutical sciences. Her core areas of interest include novel drug delivery systems, formulation and development, and pharmaceutical technology. She has participated in several national/ international conferences and workshops and is committed to continuous learning and innovation in pharmaceutical education. She has also contributed to research publications and is keen on expanding her research profile through interdisciplinary collaborations.

**Versha Sharma** is currently working as an Assistant Professor at Himachal Pharmacy College, Maganpura, Nalagarh, Solan (Himachal Pradesh). She holds a Master's degree in Pharmaceutical Chemistry (M. Pharm) and is presently pursuing her Ph.D. Her academic and professional journey reflects a strong dedication to teaching and research in the pharmaceutical sciences. With 4.5 years of experience in academia, she has been actively involved in imparting knowledge to pharmacy students and guiding them in various aspects of pharmaceutical education. Her areas of interest include pharmaceutical chemistry, drug design, and development. She has also contributed to academic growth through participation in seminars, workshops, and research-oriented activities.

# Index

## Symbols



## A



## B



## C



## D

## E



## F



## G



## H



## I

## K



## M



## N



## O



## P



## R



## S

## T



## V



## W

www.ingramcontent.com/pod-product-compliance
Lightning Source LLC
LaVergne TN
LVHW062334300926
849161LV00007B/1685